A Textbook of
Veterinary General Pathology

(Also useful for Medical and Dental Students)

Second Edition

J.L. Vegad

Former Professor & Head,
Department of Pathology,
College of Veterinary Science & Animal Husbandry,
Jabalpur - 482 001

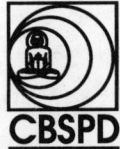

CBSPD

CBS Publishers & Distributors Pvt Ltd

New Delhi • Bengaluru • Chennai • Kochi • Kolkata • Lucknow • Mumbai
Hyderabad • Jharkhand • Nagpur • Patna • Pune • Uttarakhand

A Textbook of Veterinary General Pathology

ISBN: 978-81-239-2787-9

Copyright © Publisher

First CBS Reprint: 2015
Reprint: 2016, 2017, 2018, 2019, 2021, 2022, **2025**

Published by **Satish Kumar Jain** and produced by **Varun Jain** for

CBS Publishers & Distributors Pvt Ltd

4819/XI Prahlad Street, 24 Ansari Road, Daryaganj, New Delhi 110 002, India.
Ph: 011-23266838, 23289259   Website: www.cbspd.com
                                    e-mail: delhi@cbspd.com
Corporate Office: 204 FIE, Industrial Area, Patparganj, Delhi 110 092
Ph: 011-4934 4934   Fax: 011-4934 4935
                          e-mail: publishing@cbspd.com; publicity@cbspd.com

Branches

- **Bengaluru:** Seema House 2975, 17th Cross, KR Road, Banasankari 2nd Stage, Bengaluru 560 070, Karnataka, India
  Ph: +91-80-26771678/79   Fax: +91-80-26771680   e-mail: bangalore@cbspd.com
- **Chennai:** 18/8B, Subbarayan Street, Shenoy Nagar, Chennai 600 030, Tamil Nadu, India
  Ph: +91-44-42032115, 26681266   e-mail: chennai@cbspd.com
- **Kochi:** 42/1325, 1326, Power House Road, Opp KSEB, Power House, Ernakulum Kochi 682 018, Kerala, India
  Ph: +91-484-4059061-65,67   Fax: +91-484-4059065   e-mail: kochi@cbspd.com
- **Kolkata:** 147, Hind Ceramics Compound, 1st Floor, Nilgunj Road, Belghoria, Kolkata-700056, West Bengal, India
  Ph: +033-25633055, 033-25633056   e-mail: kolkata@cbspd.com
- **Lucknow:** Basement, Khushnuma Complex, 7 Meerabai Marg (Behind Jawahar Bhawan), Lucknow-226001, UP India
  Ph: +0522-4000032   e-mail: tiwari.lucknow@cbspd.com
- **Mumbai:** PWD Shed, Gala no 25/26, Ramchandra Bhatt Marg, Next to JJ Hospital Gate no. 2, Opp. Union Bank of India, Noorbaug, Mumbai-400009, Maharashtra, India
  Ph: 022-66661880/89   e-mail: mumbai@cbspd.com

Representatives

- Hyderabad   0-9885175004
- Patna   0-9334159340
- Jharkhand   0-9811541605
- Pune   0-9664372571
- Nagpur   0-8692091830
- Uttarakhand   0-9716462459

Printed at Mudrak, Noida, UP, India

Preface to Second Edition

The widespread popularity of the first edition, both with students and teachers, has prompted me to bring out this Second Edition. I do hope this edition proves equally useful and is received with the same fervour.

Since the first edition was published in 1995, there have been further spectacular advances in our understanding of the molecular mechanisms involved in the pathogenesis of disease processes. This accelerating pace of knowledge necessitated revision and updating of the book. The second edition has been extensively revised and most chapters are completely rewritten. As such, it contains the latest information on molecular pathology. The changes in particular include:

- An effort has been made to incorporate the most recent information on the molecular mechanisms of disease processes.
- For an easy grasp of the complicated molecular mechanisms, a large number of illustrations have been added, 79 in all, in the form of flow charts, line diagrams, and diagrammatic representations of pathological processes.
- Keeping in view the Veterinary Council of India (VCI)'s syllabus, a new chapter on *'Concretions' (Chapter 12) has been added.*
- Also, in view of the VCI syllabus, a new sub-topic **'Avian Inflammation'** has been added in the chapter on **'Inflammation'** (Chapter 4).
- The main points are given in bold type.
- In the Index, where there are more page numbers for the same topic, the number that covers the main discussion is shown in bold.

As the book deals with basic pathology, it will be very useful for medical and dental students.

I am grateful to Mr. Suneel Gomber, Manager, International Book Distributing Co., Lucknow, for the publication of this book. I extend my sincere thanks to Dr. Madhu Swamy for going through the typescript. Dr. Priti Mishra checked the index, while Mr. Anand Parmar and Mr. Vijay Parmar of Jabalpur Graphics were most generous in extending help relating to computer and other work. I am thankful to them all. I am especially grateful to my wife Nita and eldest brother Amrit Lal Vegad for the moral support and for their faith in me and my task.

J. L. Vegad

Preface to First Edition

Recent years have witnessed explosion of knowledge in molecular biology, and consequent thereupon, in the field of molecular pathology. The study of pathology is no longer confined to morphological alterations. Molecular mechanisms involved in the pathogenesis of diseases are being continuously unraveled. No area of pathology has remained untouched by the molecular strides. Since this book deals with General Pathology, that is, study of the basic pathological processes, an attempt has been made to bring out the most recent concepts of molecular mechanisms. For, it is the conceptualization of the underlying principles that is paramount in laying the foundations of systemic pathology, and in fact, medicine as a whole.

The book is intended for both undergraduate and postgraduate students. The undergraduate may, at places, find the test a little too extensive. They are advised to skip these portions. However, should they find the new information rewarding, the idea is to make it readily available at one place. I only hope I could succeed in transmitting the excitement of the remarkable insights gained into the biomolecular origins of disease processes.

The complex mechanisms have been explained in a simplified way using line diagrams, so that they are readily understood. Also, before dealing with the pathogenetic mechanisms, physiological, biochemical, and other related aspects have been briefly reviewed, for an easy comprehension of the subject. Thus, discussion of free radical mediation of cell injury is preceded by a consideration of what free radicals are; or that of mechanisms of healing by an examination of extracellular matrix, or a discussion of thrombosis by a brief consideration of haemostatic mechanisms.

Another feature of the book is that, wherever considered appropriate, aspects of human pathology have been narrated side by side. The text will therefore act as a useful exercise in comparative pathology. As such the book may serve as a good reference for medical, dentistry, and zoology students. In fact, it should prove useful to workers in all branches of science who wish to learn about the basic disease processes.

I am grateful to Dr. S. K. Ranjhan who encouraged me to write this book and to Shri C. M. Chawla of Vikas Publishing House for its publication. It is a pleasure to acknowledge the help of my colleagues

– Dr. A. K. Katiyar, Dr. H. K. B. Parekh, Dr. R. G. Dhawedkar and Dr. B.C. Sarkhel – for their many contributions. Finally, my deepest gratitude to members of my joint family for their patience and understanding. I am especially grateful to my wife Nita and my eldest brother Amritlal Vegad for the moral support, and for their faith in me and my task.

J. L. Vegad,
Department of Pathology,
College of Veterinary Science & A.H.,
Jabalpur - 482001

Abbreviations

AD	=	Anno Domini
ADCC	=	Antibody-dependent cell-mediated cytotoxicity
BC	=	Before Christ
BCR	=	B-cell receptor
BM	=	Basement membrane
CD	=	Cluster of differentiation
CTL	=	Cytotoxic T- cell
DIC	=	Disseminated intravascular coagulation
DTH	=	Delayed-type hypersensitivity
ECF	=	Eosinophil chemotactic factor
ECM	=	Extracellular matrix
EGF	=	Epidermal growth factor
F	=	French
FGF	=	Fibroblast growth factor
G	=	Greek
IFN	=	Interferon
Ig	=	Immunoglobulin
IL	=	Interleukin
IVP	=	Increased vascular permeability
L	=	Latin
LPS	=	Lipopolysaccharide
LT	=	Leukotriene
LX	=	Lipoxin
MAC	=	Membrane attack complex
MHC	=	Major histocompatibility complex
mm	=	Millimetre (thousandth part of a metre)
MPS	=	Mononuclear phagocyte system

μm	=	Micron /micrometre (one millionth of a metre)
NCF	=	Neutrophil chemotactic factor
NK cell	=	Natural killer cell
nm	=	Nanometre (one billionth of metre)
NO	=	Nitric oxide
PAF	=	Platelet activating factor
PDGF	=	Platelet-derived growth factor
PG	=	Prostaglandin
PGI_2	=	Prostacyclin
R	=	Receptor, e.g., IL-2R
TCR	=	T- cell receptor
TGF	=	Transforming growth factor
TNF	=	Tumour necrosis factor
TX	=	Thromboxane
VEGF	=	Vascular endothelial growth factor
vWF	=	von Willebrad factor

Contents

Chapter 1

Introduction

Pathology is the study of disease (G. pathos = suffering or disease + logos = study). **Disease** is that condition in which the individual suffers from discomfort (L. dis = not + ease, i.e., **not at ease**). Just as anatomy is the study of the structure and physiology its functions, **pathology is the study of structure and function of the body in disease**. Pathology therefore deals with the structural and functional changes in cells, tissues, and organs **that underlie disease**. It is a discipline that bridges basic science and clinical practice. To understand the structural and functional changes, pathologists use modern microbiological, immunological, and molecular techniques.

The **object of pathology** is to acquaint the student with the changes occurring in tissues as the result of disease. By studying pathology the student learns to apply the knowledge of basic subjects, and as one progresses to junior and senior years, one has a better understanding of the changes that take place within an animal as the result of disease. The student is then able to visualize tissue changes and appreciate why the symptoms appeared. Thus, pathology serves as a bridge between the basic subjects of anatomy, physiology, and biochemistry on the one hand, and medical, surgical, and gynaecological treatment on the other. In other words, pathology is that correlating study by which the pre-pathology courses are co-ordinated so that a better understanding of clinical subjects is possible. **Pathology is therefore central to an understanding of disease**. It explains how altered structures produce **lesions** and disordered functions **symptoms. Thus, pathology occupies a pivotal position in the study of veterinary medicine.**

Earlier, pathology was mostly confined to the study of morphological changes, both gross and microscopic. With advances in knowledge, immunological and molecular mechanisms that underlie the morphological changes became an integral part of modern pathology. Remarkable progress in molecular pathology has now clearly established that disease is produced first at a molecular level, that is, **biochemical** or **molecular lesion**. This, in turn, induces structural changes, first at an electron microscopical level

1

(**ultrastructural lesion**), then **light microscopical lesions** develop, and these when extensive, produce **gross lesions**.

Pathology is divided into "**General Pathology**" and "**Systemic or Special Pathology**". **General pathology** is concerned with the basic reactions of cells and tissues to injurious stimuli. The **systemic** or **special pathology** is the application of these basic reactions to the various body systems, or to various specific diseases. **This book deals with the basic principles of general pathology.**

Pathology covers **five aspects** of a disease process: (1) its cause (**aetiology**), (2) the mechanisms of its development (**pathogenesis**), (3) structural changes produced in cells and organs (**morphological changes**), (4) the functional consequences of the morphological changes (**clinical significance**), and (5) **result** or **termination**.

1. **Cause (Aetiology)**: There are two major classes of aetiological factors: **genetic (intrinsic)** and **acquired (extrinsic)** (infectious, nutritional, chemical, physical, etc.). However, the concept of "one cause - one disease" is no longer adequate. Genetic factors clearly affect environmentally induced diseases, and the environment may have profound influence on certain genetic diseases.

2. **Pathogenesis**: Pathogenesis is the progressive development of a disease process from the time it is initiated to its conclusion, in recovery or death. In other words, pathogenesis refers to the sequence of events in the response of the cells or tissues to the causal agent, from the initial stimulus to the ultimate expression of the disease. **The study of pathogenesis remains pivotal to the subject of pathology.**

3. **Structural and functional changes**: These are the morphological and associated functional alterations in cells or tissues. **Lesion** is the macroscopic or microscopic alteration occurring in the tissue as the result of injury, e.g., fracture in a bone is a lesion. **Pathognomonic lesion** is an alteration that indicates without doubt the cause of a particular disease. For example, button-shaped ulcers of the large intestine in swine fever; zebra markings of the large intestine in rinderpest; punched-out ulcers in the abomasum in theileriasis; and Negri body in the cells of the hippocampus and cerebellum in rabies. Disturbance in function may show itself as symptom of disease. Thus, **symptom** is a clinical sign (fever, swelling, diarrhoea, vomiting, lameness,

2

etc.) manifested by the individual as the result of tissue changes.

4. **Clinical significance**: The structural and functional changes influence normal functions and determine the clinical features (symptoms and signs), course, and prognosis of disease. **Clinical pathology** involves use of laboratory methods by clinicians to help them in arriving at a diagnosis. It includes the examination of blood, urine, faeces, exudates, skin scrapings, and biopsy material. Clinical pathology is so named because some of the work, especially the collection of material, is done at the **bed**side of patient (G. clinics, klinike = bed). **Diagnosis** is the art or act of identifying a disease from its signs and symptoms, and also through various laboratory tests. In other words, diagnosis is **to know** or recognize disease states **through** clinical signs (G. dia = **through** + gnos = **to know**). **Prognosis** is the prospect of recovery as expected from the usual cause of disease, or peculiarities of the case. That is, forecast about the likely course and outcome of a disease. In other words, prognosis is a **knowing beforehand** (L. & G. pro = **before** + gnos = **to know**), or foreknowledge of the chances of recovery.

5. **Result** or **termination**: It occurs in three ways: (1) **recovery**, (2) **death**, and (3) **invalidism**. If the damage produced by the disease is not much and is repaired, the individual recovers. If body defences are overcome and the tissue damage is great, then life cannot be maintained and individual dies. If, on the other hand, the body is not able to completely repair and the extent of injury is not so great as to kill the animal, invalidism occurs. That is, the animal continues to suffer from prolonged ill health, as in Johne's disease or tuberculosis in cattle.

Let us also consider a few other definitions, before proceeding to history of pathology in the next chapter.

Macroscopic or **gross pathology** is examination of tissue without the help of a microscope.

Microscopic pathology or **histopathology** is examination of tissue with the help of a microscope, and involves the use of stained tissue sections.

Chemical pathology is the study of chemical alterations of the body fluids and tissue that result from disease.

Postmortem examination is examination of an animal after death to establish a disease, that is, cause of its death. Postmortem

3

examination of animals and birds is called **necropsy**. The term **autopsy** is used for the postmortem examination of humans.

Morbid changes are alterations found in tissues at necropsy as a result of disease.

Biopsy is examination of tissue removed from the **living** (G. bios=**life**) animal to determine the cause of disease. Biopsy is normally performed in a suspected cancer.

Syndrome: Syndrome (G. syn = together + drome = to run) literally means 'a running together'. Thus, syndrome refers to a group of symptoms that occur together and characterize a particular abnormality, that is, they are characteristic of a certain disease.

Health and **disease**: **Health** is the condition in which the individual is in complete harmony with its environment/surroundings. **Disease** is a change in that condition, as a result the individual suffers from discomfort. In other words, disease is a condition in which an individual shows a structural, functional, or chemical deviation from the normal. However, at times it is difficult to determine if an individual is in health or disease. For example, one kidney may be absent. The remaining kidney may become twice its normal size, since it assumes the function of the missing kidney. This change is called compensatory hypertrophy, and if it comes about gradually, the individual remains clinically healthy and continues to lead a normal life. **But, pathologically, he is in disease**, because absence of a kidney is a structural deviation from the normal. **Thus, the pathologist's concept of a disease is not necessarily the same as that of a clinician.**

Cause (aetiology): Causes are of two types: **intrinsic** or **endogenous**, and **extrinsic** or **exogenous**.

The **intrinsic (endogenous) causes of disease**, also known as the **predisposing factors**, are those characteristics (genus, breed, sex, age, etc.) over which an individual has no control and which determine the type of disease present. At the basis of the first three factors, namely, genus, breed, and strain, underlie genetics and heredity.

Genus: Examples: Swine fever is a disease of the pig and no other animals are infected with it. Canine distemper is primarily a disease of the dog. It does not affect the horse, cow, sheep, or pig.

Breed: Dairy cattle are much more susceptible to diseases than beef cattle. Within the dairy cattle, certain breeds are less resistant to some diseases than others. The same is applicable with certain breeds of dogs. For example, brain tumours are common in the bulldog breeds. The boxer dog has a very high incidence of brain tumours than other breeds.

Strain: Certain strains of animals possess unusual resistance to certain diseases. For example, strains of chickens that have unusual resistance to leukosis can be produced, in contrast to other strains which have a very high mortality rate from this disease. Other examples include hernias in pigs, and calves with hydrocephalus (accumulation of fluid in the ventricles of brain). These problems are observed with greater frequency in certain family of animals than others.

Age: Certain diseases are found in a definite age group. Tumours are commonly observed in older animals. Likewise, strangles is a disease of young horses. Caecal coccidiosis in the chicken is a disease of young birds.

Sex: Reproductive diseases are more common in the female than in the male. Certain diseases (metritis, mastitis, milk fever) are confined to the female. Nephritis in the dog is 2 to 3 times more common in the male than in the female. In cattle, nephritis is more common in the female.

Colour: Cancer melanosarcomas are very common in grey and white horses, but very rare in brown or black horses. Animals with non-pigmented skin are much more susceptible to photodynamic diseases. If pigment is present in the skin, it protects the animal by preventing the sunlight from penetrating the skin, thus inhibiting the chemical reaction (see 'photosensitization', Chapter 11). **Idiosyncrasy** is an unusual reaction to some substance. Some animals exhibit an unusual reaction when a drug is administered and may even die, or show serious manifestations of unusual toxicity.

The **extrinsic (exogenous) causes of disease** are those environmental factors (physical, chemical, thermal, infectious, immunological, nutritional) that are capable of producing disease in the individual. These factors are described in Chapter 3, under "Causes of cell injury".

Chapter 2
History of Pathology

History of pathology is fascinating. Disease is as old as life itself. In fact, history of pathology (or disease) and history of medicine go hand in hand. That is, they are closely interwoven. Explorations into the past tell us how the present day knowledge was reached. What were the contributions of those dedicated souls who made supreme sacrifices so that the science flourishes, and human and animal lives are saved from the scourge of disease. They tell us how the concept of disease evolved from its most primitive form in the Stone Age to the present day. Who, in fact, were the early physicians, and how did they treat their patients? How steadily the science of anatomy, physiology and pathology progressed. How, indeed the veterinary medicine came into being? While these aspects of the history are deeply engrossing, their detailed accounts are beyond the scope of this book.

At times, it has so happened that one single event has changed the course of history and resulted in an entire revolution of medicine. These milestones of medical progress stand out quite clearly as we delve into the past. For example, circulation of blood by William Harvey was an epoch-making discovery, because it explained how nutrients and oxygen are carried to cells in the body. It also explained many other alterations observed in pathology. The work of Leeuwenhoek, Bichat and Müeller opened the field of histopathology. Virchow put forward the concept that all forms of injury start with molecular or structural alterations in cells, in his book on cellular pathology. The study of bacteria by Pasteur, Koch and Klebs demonstrated that these minute organisms were, in fact, the cause of disease. Cohnheim and Metchnikoff described the vascular and cellular changes that occurred in inflammation. Here, however, we shall consider very briefly, somewhat chronologically, only the most outstanding contributions of the glittering scientific geniuses.

Veterinary medicine, through ages, has been closely allied with human medicine, just as it is today. The diseases of animals are often the diseases of humans, and therefore their histories are closely linked.

The First Concept of Disease

Man, in stone or prehistoric age, was barbarous, brutal and cruel. He hunted animals and ate their flesh; and even indulged in cannibalism (i.e., eating of human flesh by a human). Then, he came to believe in the existence of evil spirits or demons and dreaded them. The study of demons or evil spirits is called **'demonology'**. He further believed that if man got possessed by a demon, that is, he became a demoniac, then he was taken ill and suffered disease. The cause of disease was considered to be the displeasure of evil spirits, and the treatment was directed toward appeasing them. The demons were even worshipped. Thus originated the first notion about the nature of an illness - **the demoniac concept of disease.**

He further assumed and accepted it as true that the evil spirit used to enter the head. To expel the evil spirit (exorcize), the wild medical man trephined the skull by a sharp long pointed stone. Thus, the skull surgery came into existence. The medicine and treatment were controlled by the **witch doctor,** who used secret methods, magic, spells, incantations, magical ceremonies, vegetable and animal concoctions and even noise to drive away the evil spirits, and wore hideous dress. **Thus, the first physician was a witch doctor.** In one of the caves in the Pyrenees mountains, that are between France and Spain, there is a rock painting of a witch doctor. The portrait is believed to have been made some 17 thousand years ago. And, it is from the witch doctor that the medical man of today is descended.

The Theological Concept of Disease

Then came the theory of the theological cause of disease. About 4000 B.C., in Egypt, embalming (i.e., preservation of a dead body against putrefaction) of thousands of mummies (dead bodies) was carried out. Bodies were taken into the embalming temples, and no one but the priest saw them. Though priests recognized the changes in the organs, they kept the information secret. On the other hand, they put forward the theory **that illness was the result of Divine displeasure.** That is, if man disobeyed or displeased God, he suffered God's wrath (intense anger) and became ill. By so doing, priests could maintain their theological hold on the people. Thus, the theological concept of aetiology and mysticism (spiritualism) was nourished, and **now the priest played the role of a physician.**

The Humoral Concept of Disease

With the arrival of Greek culture, a scientific study of medicine began, and rejection of demon worship occurred. **Hippocrates (460-377 B.C.)** was undoubtedly the most outstanding individual in the history of medicine. His impact on medical science was so great he is honoured as the **'Father of Medicine'**. He formulated the **'Oath of Hippocrates'**, concerning the practice and ethics of medicine. His writings formed the basis for the **'humoral theory of disease'**. He put forward that the body consists of **four humours** (four fluids): (i) **blood,** which was warm and moist like air, (ii) **phlegm,** which was cold and moist like water, (iii) **yellow bile,** which was warm and dry like fire, and (iv) **black bile,** which was cold and dry like earth. The origin of humours was interesting. The blood came from the heart, the phlegm originated in the brain, the yellow bile came from the liver, and the black bile (the most serious of all) came from the spleen. Hippocrates taught that health was due to a correct mixture, a **eucrasia** (G. eu = well + krasis = mixture) of the four fluids of body, and that **disease** was due to an incorrect mixture, **dyscrasia** (G. dys = bad).

Hippocrates explained that when phlegm that originated in the brain, begins to gravitate downward and appears at the nose, the individual has a cold. If it gravitates into the lungs, the patient has pneumonia. If it continues to gravitate into the lungs for a long period, tuberculosis is the result. When gravitation extends still lower and reaches the intestine, dysentery occurs. Finally, when the phlegm descends into the rectum, haemorrhoids occur. Diseases of the black bile were considered to be the most serious. Although the humoral theory of Hippocrates seems odd to us today, **it served as the basis for medical practice for two thousand years.** In fact, historically, it is the most important pathological theory yet propounded. It was not until the end of the nineteenth century that its hold on the medical world was finally broken, when modern physiology, pathology, and bacteriology proved it to be wrong.

Developments in Anatomy, Physiology and Pathology

Aristotle (384-322 B.C.), another Greek philosopher, was the **originator of modern anatomy and physiology.** He dissected many animals and carried out experiments in physiology. **Claudius Galen (131-206 A.D.),** a Greek physician practising in Rome, contributed greatly to human physiology and also dissected animals. He is considered as **'Father of Anatomy'.** Galen is perhaps the greatest

9

medical figure of all times. Even after his death, for thirteen centuries his teachings prevailed. Another important person of this era (period) was **Cornelius Celsus (30 B.C. - 38 A.D.)**, a Roman writer of the first century A.D. Celsus was not a physician, but had a wide variety of interests. He described **the four cardinal signs of inflammation - redness, swelling, heat, and pain.**

First Textbook on Veterinary Medicine

A Roman veterinarian, **Renatus Vegetius (450-500 A.D.)** is credited as being the first to write a textbook on veterinary medicine, known as **'Book of the Veterinary Art'**. His concepts of the diseases of animals and their control had great influence on many people, and on the animal industry of that time. Because of the book he wrote, and the impact he had on veterinary medicine, he is considered as the **'Father of Veterinary Medicine'**. However, the Roman slave Androcles, who extracted a thorn from the paw of a lion, is credited as the first veterinarian.

Century of Anatomy

Soon Divine displeasure as the cause of disease began to disappear, and people were beginning to resort to surgery, medicine, and common sense. Gradually there was elimination of superstition and fear. Medical and veterinary literature began to appear. **Antonio Benivieni (1440-1502),** an Italian, was a remarkable pioneer in reporting postmortem examinations. A gifted pathologist, he is credited as **'Father of Pathological Anatomy'**, and also as **'Founder of Pathology'** before Morgagni. **Leonardo da Vinci (1452-1519)** was the greatest artist and scientist of the Italian Renaissance (golden period of the Italian civilization). Despite being an artist, he contributed to anatomy so much that he is honoured as **'First Modern Dissector'**. He also wrote anatomy of the horse in 1499. **Andreas Vesalius (1514-1564),** a Belgian, was the most outstanding figure in European medicine after Galen and before Harvey. At the young age of 24, he became professor of anatomy at the University of Padua, in Italy. There were plenty of dissectors and dissections before Vesalius, but he alone made anatomy what it is today - a living, working science. **The 16th century is often called as the century of anatomy.**

Discovery of Blood Circulation

Sixteenth and seventeenth centuries witnessed certain monumental discoveries in medicine. **William Harvey (1578-1657),** an Englishman, described the blood vascular system and made the epoch-making **discovery of blood circulation, in 1628.** It is a gripping account of his genius. He dissected vascular system of no less than 80 different species of animals over a period of 14 years. His discovery had the greatest impact and changed the very course of medicine. It marked a new phase. Without the knowledge of blood circulation, most of the alterations in pathology could not be explained. Disturbances in circulation like hyperaemia, haemorrhage, embolism and many other alterations in pathology had remained unexplained unless circulation of the blood was understood. In fact, **no single discovery has had a more far-reaching effect on pathology than the discovery of blood circulation.**

His discovery also clarified certain myths. For example, earlier, **'artery'** was called as **'airtree'.** Etymologically, the word was coined from the belief that arteries contained air and the veins blood, and the arteries also bifurcated like the branches of a tree. (Etymology is the study of the origin and history of words and their meanings). Discovery of circulation clarified the myth; the word **'airtree'** became a misnomer (a wrong name), and was changed to **'artery'.**

Marcello Malpighi (1628-1694), an Italian, extended Harvey's work and discovered the capillaries and erythrocytes; and made masterly microscopic descriptions of the kidney, lungs, and spleen. He discovered **Malpighian layer** of the skin, and proved that the papillae of tongue are organs of taste.

Invention and Application of Microscope

An event of great significance was the **invention of the microscope by Hans and Zacharias Jannsen** in Holland (The Netherlands). Cornelius Drebbel, also of Holland, made a better microscope and the credit for the introduction of the microscope really goes to him.

The next major advance in medicine was made by **Antony van Leeuwenhoek (1632-1723),** a Dutch draper (a cloth merchant), and yet a very great microscopist. He made 200 microscopes before he was satisfied and the best magnification he could obtain was 160. However, he is not given the credit for inventing the microscope because others had demonstrated magnification of lenses long before his time. All the same, he is credited for being **the first to show that the microscope had practical importance in the study of tissues,** and other minute objects. He was the first to see protozoa under the microscope, in 1675. Without the microscope, the study of histology would be impossible. By demonstrating the practical use of the microscope, Leeuwenhoek paved the way for the minute examination of tissues. With his simple crude instrument, he observed many objects. He even demonstrated the capillary anastomosis between the arteries and veins.

First Textbook on Pathology

One of the first compilers of medical literature was a Frenchman by the name **Jean Fernel (1497-1558)**. He collected the information of his time, and was **the first to codify (organize systematically) the new knowledge of pathology.** He attempted to bring medical information into a form that could be used by others in the study of disease. He was the first to write and describe the diseases according to organs, or parts of the body. His writings formed the **'First Textbook in Pathology'**, which was the main text in teaching pathology for many years.

Jean Fernel (1497-1558) was followed by a famous Italian compiler - **Giovanni Battista Morgagni (1682-1771).** Modern pathology began with Morgagni. At the age of seventy, he published five volumes entitled **'The Seats and Causes of Disease'** - an incredible feat of achievement. In these, he systematically described 700 complete autopsies, and attempted to correlate the structural changes to the symptoms shown by the individual. This was the first time that anyone had attempted to correlate pathological alterations in the dead with the symptoms shown during life. That is, he introduced the **'anatomical concept'** into the practice of medicine. His book was an extremely important text.

Father of Histology

A young Frenchman **Marie-François Xavier Bichat (1771-1802)** opened a new field in medical science. During his brief life-span of 31 years (he died from tuberculosis), he established the foundation for the study of histology. He presented a new concept of anatomy and showed that body is composed of twenty-one tissues. The remarkable thing about Bichat's discovery was that his observations were made entirely by physical and chemical methods since he did not possess a microscope, and yet his contributions immortalized him as the **'Father of Histology'.** It is a delightful story as to how he instilled the new concept. With simple methods such as maceration, chemical disintegration using acids and bases, cooking, putrefaction and several others, he was able to divide the tissues of the body into 21 groups. The word **'tissue'** was first introduced by him. Etymologically, it is derived from the French word **'tissu'**, which means **fabric or texture**. In other words, Bichat meant that body is made up of fabrics of different textures!

Father of Immunology

Edward Jenner (1749-1823), an Englishman, discovered vaccination for smallpox, and performed his first vaccination on May 14, 1796 on a village boy, James Phipps. The immunization proved successful. The story of how he came to practise smallpox vaccination is fascinating. He observed that dairymaids (women working in a dairy), who had contracted cowpox through milking, did not suffer from smallpox. Jenner then thought of putting his observation to practice, and put forward the theory that vaccination against cowpox protects from smallpox. He thus became one of the greatest benefactors (one who does good to others) of mankind. He is honoured as the **'Father of Immunology'**. Later, Jenner also contributed on a dog disease - canine distemper.

Establishment of the First Veterinary College

Modern veterinary medicine originated in France. In 1664, man by the name **Jacques Labessie De Solleysel (1617-1680)** published the first complete book on veterinary medicine. The publication of this work, with its influence on veterinary medicine, was the outstanding event of the seventeenth century in veterinary medicine.

The second dominating veterinarian in France was **Claude Bourgelat (1712-1779).** Bourgelat was engaged in the practice of law, but was greatly interested in horses. In 1751, he wrote a book on equine medicine. He also investigated the glanders outbreak, and was successful in eradicating this disease for the French army. He was then requested to establish a veterinary college in Lyon, France, which he did. Thus, **the first modern veterinary college was established in Lyon, France, on January 1, 1762.**

First Experimental Pathologist

The next major contribution to medicine was made by a Scot - **John Hunter (1728-1793).** He is best known for his contributions on blood diseases and inflammation, gunshot wounds, and for a monograph **'venereal disease'**. He recorded 700 autopsies. He was man of great curiosity. His great zeal for experimental pathology led

13

him to infect himself with syphilis in order to study the disease more closely. He then developed typical case of the disease, which became the cause of his death. His saga of supreme sacrifice to enrich the medical science is an overpowering, spellbinding, heroic tale. He is credited as the **'First Experimental Pathologist'.**

Matthew Baillie (1761-1823), another Scot, wrote the first systematic text on pathological anatomy. In each case, the autopsy was correlated with a full case history.

Supreme Descriptive Pathologist

The Germans soon came to dominate the field of pathology. **Carl Rokitansky (1804-1878),** who lived in Vienna, is considered as **the supreme descriptive pathologist of all time.** The apogee (highest point) of gross descriptive morbid anatomy was reached by his work. He firmly established the structural basis of disease. **He had conducted 70, 000 autopsies in his life**. It was he who established postmortem techniques - the systematic examination of every organ by methods that preserved organ continuity yet revealed the lesions they contained.

Cellular Pathology

Johannes Müeller (1801-1878), a German, who lived in Berlin, was one of the first to use the microscope in the study of tissues. He impressed upon the world the necessity of examining tissues with the microscope in order to appreciate and understand the changes that were occurring

Rudolph Virchow (1821-1902) was greatest of all German scientists. His foremost contribution was the publication of his book **'Cellular Pathology', in 1858**, nearly one hundred and fifty years ago, in which he put forth the concept that all forms of injury start with molecular or structural alterations at the cellular level. All areas of pathology were clarified by his concept of cellular pathology. He gave pathology the push it needed, and from then on, its development was rapid. Thus, the rise of modern pathology and medicine is inseparably connected with his name. He is known as the **'Father of Cellular Pathology'**, or even as **'Father of Modern Pathology'.** Most of the terms used in pathology, such as thrombosis, embolism, fatty degeneration, and amyloidosis, were coined by him.

Germ Theory of Disease

The importance of infectious organisms was demonstrated by

Louis Pasteur (1822-1895) in France. He was one of the originators of the new field of bacteriology and of the theory that bacteria were the cause of some diseases - known as the **'germ theory of disease'.** His studies carried him into the field of human and animal diseases (pasteurellosis, anthrax, rabies). He showed that individuals could be successfully immunized by vaccine prepared with organisms and carried out immunization against anthrax. He established the science of bacteriology.

Robert Koch (1843-1910), a German bacteriologist, isolated many microorganisms, showed that many bacteria caused diseases, and was the first to use artificial solid media to obtain pure cultures. In 1882, he discovered the tubercle bacillus. Further, he established **'Koch's postulates',** a procedure necessary for proving a specific microorganism as the cause of a specific disease. That is, the organisms must be present in disease, must be obtained in pure culture and maintained by subculture, and on their inoculation the disease must be reproduced in healthy animals.

Although Louis Pasteur and Robert Koch did much to show that bacteria caused disease, it was **Edwin Klebs (1834-1913),** who demonstrated the importance of bacteria in pathology.

Originator of Modern Experimental Pathology

Julius Cohnheim's (1839-1884) methods of investigation were experimental, and because of this he is credited as **'Originator of Modern Experimental Pathology'.** He was a German and his contributions, particularly in the field of inflammation, are monumental. His most notable experiment concerned the vascular and cellular changes in the mesentery of the frog when acted upon by the irritant. He opened the abdomen of a frog and spread the mesentery across the stage of a microscope. He then placed a drop of dilute acetic acid on the mesentery and recorded the changes. His simple observations formed the basis for the pathology of inflammation. He was the first to provide microscopic observations of inflammation and wrote descriptions that can hardly be improved upon.

Discovery of Phagocytosis

The cellular changes in inflammation were clarified by the Russian biologist **Elie Metchnikoff (1845-1916),** in 1882. He inserted rose thorns into the larvae of a starfish. The next morning he observed a

15

grey zone around each of the rose thorns. He found this grey zone to be an accumulation of large cells, and also observed ingestion of rose thorns by these cells. Because the cells were large and possessed phagocytic properties, he named them **macrophages** (G. macro = large + phagein = to eat), in contrast to the smaller phagocytic cell, the neutrophil, which is designated as the **microphage** (G. micro = small). He thus discovered the process of phagocytosis. In 1884, he described phagocytosis of bacteria by mammalian neutrophils. He concluded that the purpose of inflammation was to bring phagocytic cells to the injured area to engulf the invading bacteria.

Discovery of Lysosomes (Suicide Bags)

Lysosomes are small vesicular bodies within a cell that contain a variety of very potent digestive enzymes. Because of the whole spectrum of acid hydrolases that they contain, lysosomes have come to dominate the events in pathology. Activation of these enzymes can lead to enzymatic digestion of every cell component (see 'Cell injury and cell death', Chapter 3). Because lysosomes, under certain circumstances, destroy the very cells that contain them, they are sometimes referred to as **'suicide bags'**.

The discovery of lysosomes is very interesting. Their existence was **first postulated** by Christian de Duve and his associates working at Louvain University, Belgium, in 1955. In fact, they were examining the enzyme content of mitochondrial fractions that could be separated from homogenates of rat liver cells by differential centrifugation. In one of the fractions, they unexpectedly found a number of digestive enzymes. After conducting many experiments, they postulated that the digestive enzymes must have been contained in some membrane-bound bodies. Realizing that the little bodies in this fraction were not mitochondria, but a new type of cytoplasmic organelle, they proposed the name lysosomes. They thought that these vesicular **bodies** contained enzymes that could **digest** cell structures (G. **lysis** = digestion, dissolution + **soma** = body), hence the name **'lysosomes'**. A few years later, existence of these postulated lysosomes, was demonstrated by electron microscope by Novikoff and his associates; and this proved that the assumption of Christian de Duve and his team was correct.

Thus, paradoxically, a structure that could be seen only with an electron microscope was discovered without its use. Likewise, Bichat, through his ingenuity earned for himself the title 'Father of Histology', without using a microscope. **It is tempting to draw a similarity between the two discoveries, and marvel at the creative genius of their discoverers.**

Discovery of Prions

'Prions' are the most recent addition to the class of agents that cause diseases in domestic animals and humans. 'Prion' is a proteinaceous infective particle. Recent work has revealed that prion is a heavily glycosylated specific protein (a polypeptide) of 30 kilodaltons (30-kD), called 'prion protein (PrP). Since it is a proteinaceous particle closely associated with infectivity, the term 'proin' was coined from 'proteinaceous infective particle'. The word 'proin' thus formed from 'pro' and 'in' was changed to 'prion' to sound rhythmic.

Although both 'prions' and 'viruses' replicate, their properties, structure, and modes of replication are fundamentally different. **Prions lack nucleic acid (RNA or DNA), and also do not produce any inflammatory or immune reaction in the host.** Thus, **prions are the most unconventional agents**. Because they lack nucleic acids, prions are remarkably resistant to many agents that normally inactivate viruses, such as ultraviolet light and standard disinfectants. In fact, **they can be classified as an entirely separate category. For his discovery of 'prions', Stanley Prusiner,** professor of Biochemistry at the University of California, San Francisco, USA, **won the 1997 Nobel Prize in Physiology and Medicine.** Both, in domestic animals and humans, prions cause a group of diseases known as **'transmissible spongiform encephalopathies (TSEs)'** (see 'Prions', Chapter 15).

To conclude, history of pathology has sequentially passed through the **'demoniac', 'theological or theistic'** and **'humoral' phases**, and is now in the **'cellular and molecular' phase**. However, the rapid strides made recently in the field of molecular biology, and consequent thereupon in the field of molecular pathology, make one wonder if pathology is not again swinging somewhat in the direction of humoral pathology. More and more diseases are being explained by effects of the released chemical mediators as well as by antigen-antibody reactions and endocrine glands. Thus, diseases are manifestations of humoral products like various interleukins, tumour necrosis factor, several other cytokines, hormones, leukotrienes, prostaglandins, thromboxane A2, nitric oxide, and a host of others carried in the blood.

17

Chapter 3

Cell Injury and Cell Death

Introduction

More than a hundred years ago, Rudolph Virchow, **'Father of Cellular Pathology'**, put forward the concept that disease begins at the cellular level. This has been abundantly established since then, by the phenomenal progress made in the field of molecular pathology. As all forms of tissue injury commence with molecular and structural changes in **cells**, we shall begin consideration of pathology with an examination of disease at the cellular and molecular levels.

The normal cell lives in a hostile environment. In other words, it exists in a state of striking disequilibrium with its external environment. For example, the **concentration of calcium ions outside the cell is 10,000 times higher than that inside**. If all this calcium were to enter the cell, it will prove toxic, and kill the cell. This can happen during cell injury. It is the plasma membrane of the cell that constitutes the structural and functional barrier, which separates the intracellular from the hostile extracellular environment. It maintains a constant internal ionic composition, against very large chemical gradients between the intracellular and extracellular components. The membrane selectively admits small molecules, while throws out others.

Definitions

The normal cell has to live within a fairly narrow range of function and structure. Even then, it is able to handle normal physiological demands, so-called **normal homeostasis** (L. staying same). Somewhat more excessive physiological stresses, or some pathological stimuli, bring about **adaptation**. That is, the cell modifies its structure and function in response to changing demands and stresses. It then acquires a new but steady state and preserves its health. For example, the bulging muscles of a race horse result from **cellular adaptations**. The increase in muscle mass is due to an increase in the size of the individual muscle fibres. The workload is thus shared by a greater mass of cellular components, and each muscle fibre is spared from excess work and therefore escapes injury. This adaptive response is called **hypertrophy**. Conversely, **atrophy** is a response in which there is a decrease in the size and function of cells. **Hyperplasia** and **metaplasia** are the other examples of adaptive responses. All these cellular adaptations are considered in detail in Chapter 7.

If the adaptive capability is exceeded, or in certain cases when adaptation is not possible, a sequence of regressive changes occurs, collectively known as **cell injury** (L. re, retro = back; gress = step, i.e., step back, go back, fall in health; also called retrogressive or degenerative changes). In classical or traditional pathology, these changes were termed "*degenerations*", but now they are called **cell injury**. Within certain limits, injury is reversible and cells return to a normal state, but with severe and persistent stress, the cell reaches a '**point of no return**', suffers **irreversible injury** and then **dies**. **Adaptation, reversible injury, irreversible injury**, and **cell death** are states of progressive encroachment on the cell's normal function and structure.

Cell death, the ultimate result of cell injury, is one of the most important events in pathology, affects every type of cell, and is the main result of ischaemia (lack of blood flow), infections, toxins, and immune reactions. There are two main patterns of cell death: **necrosis** and **apoptosis**.

Necrosis (typically **coagulative necrosis**) is the more common type of cell death, and occurs after a loss of blood supply or after an exposure to toxins. It is characterized by cellular swelling, denaturation and coagulation of cytoplasmic proteins, and breakdown of the organelles. **Apoptosis** occurs when a cell dies through activation of an **internally controlled 'suicide' programme**. After this, the dead cells are removed. Apoptosis is designed to eliminate unwanted cells during development of embryo and in various physiological processes. It also occurs under pathological conditions, where it is sometimes accompanied by necrosis.

Causes of Cell Injury

1. **Hypoxia**: Hypoxia (loss of oxygen supply) is an extremely important and common cause of cell injury and cell death. It **affects cells aerobic oxidative respiration. Hypoxia** should be differentiated from **ischaemia**, which is a loss of blood supply due to obstructed arterial flow or reduced venous drainage in a tissue. In contrast to hypoxia during which glycolytic energy production can continue, ischaemia affects the availability of metabolic substrates, including **glucose. For this reason, ischaemia injures tissues faster than**

hypoxia. Reduction in the oxygen-carrying capacity of the blood, as in anaemia, may also result in significant cell injury.

2. **Physical agents**: Physical agents include mechanical trauma, extremes of temperatures (burns and deep cold), radiation, electric shock, and sudden changes in atmospheric pressure.

3. **Chemical agents and drugs**: Virtually any chemical substance or drug can cause cell injury. Simple chemicals such as glucose or salt in hypertonic concentrations may cause cell injury directly, or by deranging their osmotic environment. Even oxygen, in high concentrations, is severely toxic. Agents commonly known as poisons cause severe damage at the cellular level, and can result in the death of the whole organism. Many of these chemicals or drugs cause changes by acting on some vital functions of the cell, such as membrane permeability, osmotic homeostasis, or the integrity of an enzyme or cofactor. Other potentially toxic agents include air pollutants, herbicides, carbon monoxide, and asbestos. Even therapeutic drugs can cause cell or tissue injury.

4. **Infectious agents**: These agents range from the submicroscopic viruses to the large tapeworms. In between are the bacteria, fungi, rickettsiae, chlamydiae, mycoplasma, protozoa, and higher forms of parasites. The ways by which infectious agents cause injury are wide-ranging and are discussed in Chapter 15.

5. **Immunological reactions**: Although the immune system serves in the defence against infectious agents, immune reactions may also cause cell injury. Examples include anaphylactic reaction to a foreign protein or a drug, and autoimmune diseases.

6. **Nutritional imbalances**: Nutritional deficiencies such as avitaminoses and others are important causes of cell injury. Ironically, excesses of nutrition are also important causes of morbidity and mortality. In humans, diets rich in animal fat, cause atherosclerosis and obesity.

7. **Genetic defects**: Genetic defects may cause cell injury. The genetic injury may result in a defect as gross as congenital malformations, or in as subtle a change as the single amino acid substitution in haemoglobin S in sickle cell anaemia. The several inborn errors of metabolism due to congenital enzymatic deficiencies are examples of cell damage due to alterations at the level of DNA.

General Considerations of Cell Injury

The biochemical mechanisms responsible for cell injury and cell death are complex. Injury to cells has many causes. Also, there are a number of pathways to cell death that interact with one another. Thus, to find out exact cause and effect may be difficult. All the same, there are certain principles that are applicable to most forms of cell injury.

1.   The **morphological changes** of cell injury become noticeable only after some critical biochemical system within the cell has been deranged. Thus, the **first lesion** to develop is **biochemical (molecular)** in nature. This, in turn, causes structural changes first at an electron microscopical level (**ultrastructural lesion**), then **light microscopic lesions** develop, and these, when extensive, produce **gross lesions**.

2.   The **cellular response** to injurious stimuli depends on the type of injury, its duration, and its severity. For example, low doses of toxins or brief periods of ischaemia may cause reversible injury, whereas larger toxin doses or more prolonged ischaemia may result in irreversible injury and cell death.

3.   The **results of an injurious stimulus** depend on the type, status, adaptability, and genetic make-up of the injured cell. The same injury has different result depending on the cell type. For example, striated skeletal muscle in the leg can tolerate complete ischaemia for 2-3 hours without irreversible injury, whereas cardiac muscle dies after only 20-30 minutes. Similarly, following loss of blood supply neurons die within 3-5 minutes; myocardium, hepatocytes and renal epithelium between 30 minutes to two hours; whereas fibroblasts, epidermis and skeletal muscles survive for many hours. The nutritional (or hormonal) status can also be important. For example, a liver cell full of glycogen will tolerate ischaemia much better than one that has just burned its last glucose molecule. Genetically determined variations in metabolic pathways can also be important. For example, exposure of two individuals to exactly the same concentrations of a toxin, such as carbon tetrachloride, may be without effect in one and may produce cell death in the other.

4.   Although the exact biochemical site of action for many injurious agents is difficult to determine, four intracellular systems are particularly exposed to attack (1) **Cell membrane**. It is on the maintenance of the integrity of cell membrane that the ionic and osmotic homeostasis of the cell and its organelles depends, (2)

Anaerobic respiration involving mitochondrial oxidative phosphorylation and production of adenosine triphosphate (ATP), (3) Synthesis of **enzymic and structural proteins**, and (4) **Preservation of the integrity of genetic apparatus of the cell**.

5. The **structural and biochemical components of a cell** are so closely inter-related that, whatever the exact point of initial attack, injury at one site leads to wide-ranging secondary effects. For example, impairment of aerobic respiration disrupts the energy-dependent sodium pump in the membrane that maintains the ionic and fluid balance of the cell, resulting in the alterations in the intracellular content of ions and water. As a result, the cell can rapidly swell and rupture.

Common Biochemical Mechanisms

With certain injurious agents, the biochemical mechanisms are well defined. For example, cyanide inactivates cytochrome oxidase in mitochondria and certain bacteria can produce phospholipases that attack phospholipids in cell membranes. However, with many injurious stimuli the exact pathogenic mechanisms that lead to cell death are incompletely understood. In spite of this, there are several **common biochemical pathways** in the mediation of cell injury and cell death, **whatever the causative agent**. These include:

1. **ATP depletion**: High-energy phosphate in the form of ATP is required for many processes within the cell. ATP is produced in two ways: (1) The major route is **oxidative phosphorylation** of ADP, a reaction that **requires oxygen**, and (2) the second is the **glycolytic pathway** that can generate ATP **in the absence of oxygen** using glucose obtained either from body fluids, or from hydrolysis of glycogen. ATP depletion and decreased ATP synthesis are common consequences of both ischaemic and toxic injury.

2. **Lack of oxygen or generation of oxygen-derived free radicals**: A lack of oxygen certainly underlies the pathogenesis of cell injury in ischaemia, **but partially reduced activated oxygen species are also important mediators of cell death** (Fig. 1). Cells generate energy by reducing molecular oxygen (O_2) to water. During this process, small amounts of **partially reduced reactive oxygen forms** are produced as an unavoidable by-product of mitochondrial respiration. **They are highly toxic molecules** that can damage lipids, proteins, and nucleic acids (discussed later). These molecules are referred to as **activated or reactive oxygen species**. Cells have defence

systems to prevent injuries caused by these products. An imbalance between free radical-generating and free radical-inactivating systems results in **oxidative stress**, a condition associated with **cell injury**.

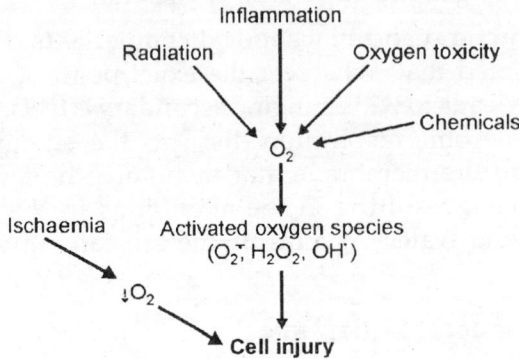

Fig.1. The role of oxygen in cell injury. Ischaemia causes cell injury by reducing its oxygen supply. Other stimuli, such as radiation, induce damage through **toxic activated oxygen species** (i.e., **free radicals**).

   3.   Loss of calcium homeostasis (stable state): Calcium (Ca^{++}) in cytosol is normally maintained at extremely low concentrations. (Cytosol is fluid portion of the cytoplasm). Concentration of calcium in cytosol is up to 10,000 times lower than the concentration of extracellular calcium, or of calcium sequestered (isolated) within mitochondria and endoplasmic reticulum. Normally, most of the intracellular calcium is sequestered in mitochondria and endoplasmic reticulum. Such gradients are maintained by membrane-associated, energy-dependent Ca^{++}, Mg^{++}-ATPases. **Ischaemia and toxins increase cytosolic calcium concentration** due to a net influx (entry) of extracellular calcium (Ca^{++}) through the plasma membrane, and also because of the release of Ca^{++} from mitochondria and endoplasmic reticulum (Fig. 2). Increased cytosolic calcium, in turn, activates a number of enzymes, with harmful cellular effects (Fig. 2). The enzymes activated by calcium include: (1) **phospholipases**, which cause membrane damage, (2) **proteases**, which break down structural and membrane proteins, (3) **ATPases**, which accelerate ATP depletion, and (4) **endonucleases**, which break down nuclear chromatin. Although cell injury results in increased intracellular calcium and this in turn causes a variety of harmful effects, **including cell death**, loss of calcium homeostasis is not always a necessary preceding event in irreversible cell injury.

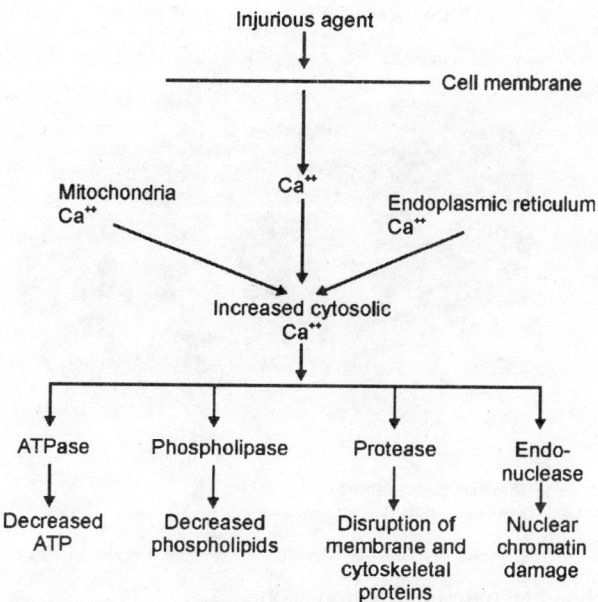

Fig. 2. Consequences of increased intracellular calcium in cell injury.

4. Defects in membrane permeability: The plasma membrane may be directly damaged by certain bacterial toxins, viral proteins, complement components, cytotoxic lymphocytes, and a number of physical or chemical agents. Changes in membrane permeability may also be secondary to a loss of ATP synthesis, or may result from calcium-mediated activation of phospholipases.

5. Mitochondrial damage: Since all cells depend on oxidative metabolism, mitochondrial integrity is most important for cell survival. **Irreparable damage to mitochondria will ultimately kill cells**. Mitochondria are almost always involved in most types of injury. They can be damaged by a variety of stimuli, such as increases of cytosolic calcium, by oxidative stress, and by breakdown of phospholipids through phospholipase A2 (discussed later). The damage ultimately results in the formation of **high-conductance channels** in the inner mitochondrial membrane. These channels are also called as **'mitochondrial permeability transitions'** (Fig. 3). Due to these pores, the proton gradient across the mitochondrial membrane disappears, **thereby preventing ATP generation**. Mitochondrial damage also results in the leakage of cytochrome c (an important soluble protein in the electron transport chain) into the cytosol (Fig. 3), **where it activates apoptotic death pathways** (i.e. cell death). (see 'Apoptosis' and Figs. 11 and 12).

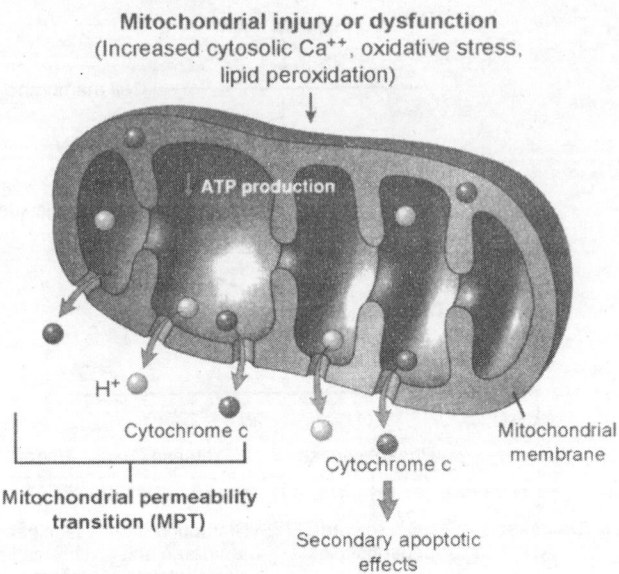

Fig. 3. Mitochondrial permeability transition.

Reversible and Irreversible Cell Injury

To trace the **sequence of events** in reversible and irreversible cell injury, we shall discuss two model systems (1) ischaemic and hypoxic injury, and (2) free radical-induced cell injury.

Ischaemic and Hypoxic Injury

This is the most common type of cell injury and has been studied extensively in humans, in experimental animals, and in culture systems (Fig.4). **Hypoxia** (loss of oxygen supply) must be differentiated from **ischaemia** which is a loss of blood supply. In contrast to hypoxia, during which glycolytic energy production can continue (although less efficiently than by oxidative pathways), iscahemia affects the delivery of substrates for glycolysis (e.g., glucose) supplied by the flowing blood. Therefore, in ischaemic tissues, anaerobic energy generation will stop after glycolytic substrates are exhausted. For this reason, **ischaemia injures tissues faster than hypoxia.**

Reversible Cell Injury

The first point of attack of hypoxia is the cell's aerobic respiration, that is, **oxidative phosphorylation** by mitochondria (Fig. 4). As the oxygen tension within the cell decreases, there is loss of oxidative

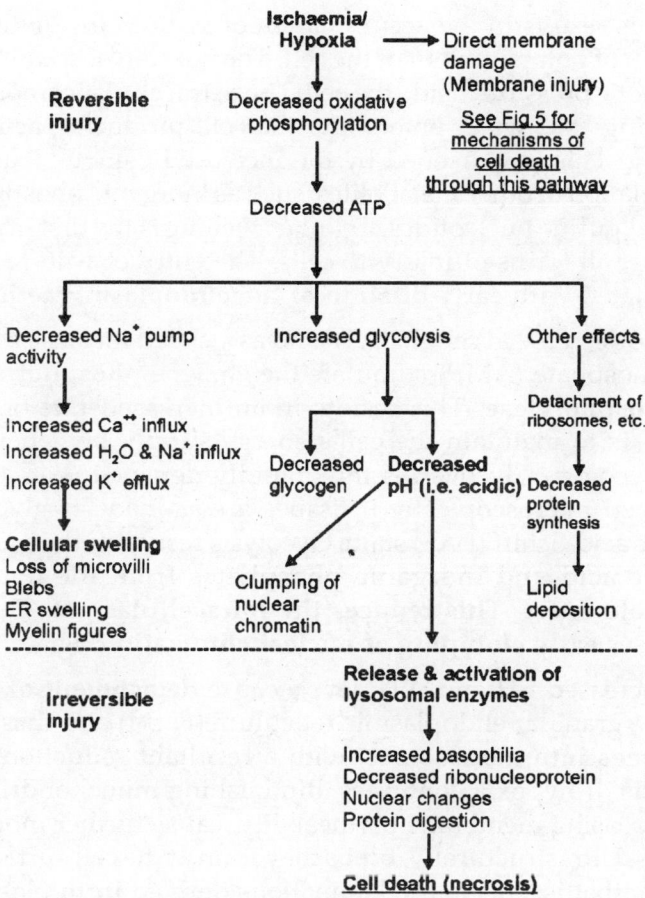

Fig. 4. Sequence of events in ischaemic injury.

phosphorylation and decreased generation of adenosine triphosphate (ATP). The depletion of ATP (the energy source) has widespread effects on many systems within the cell. As is known, a normal cell has a higher intracellular osmotic pressure exerted by a greater intracellular than extracellular concentration of proteins. To balance this, sodium is maintained at a higher concentration outside the cell than inside by an energy-dependent (ATP-driven) **"sodium pump"**, that is, by Na^+ and K^+-adenosine triphosphatase (ATPase) enzyme. This pump also keeps concentration of potassium significantly higher inside the cell than outside. The decreased ATP concentration, following acute hypoxia, reduces activity of the plasma membrane **"sodium pump"**, which then fails to regulate the active transport of ions. This results in the accumulation of sodium inside the cell, and diffusion of potassium out of the cell. The net gain of sodium increases the osmotic pressure inside the cell. The extracellular osmotic pressure now being low, water enters into the cell, producing **acute cellular swelling**. This is worsened by the increased osmotic load from the accumulation of other metabolites, such as inorganic phosphates, lactic acid, and purine nucleotides. Cellular swelling is the first manifestation of almost all forms of injury to cells. The entry of water into the cell is associated with **early dilation of the endoplasmic reticulum**.

The decrease in cellular ATP and associated increase in adenosine monophosphate (AMP) stimulate the enzyme **phosphofructokinase** and **phosphorylase**. This results in an increased rate of **anaerobic glycolysis** to maintain the cell's energy supply by generating ATP from glycogen. Glycogen is thus rapidly depleted (Fig. 4). This can be noticed microscopically if tissues are stained for glycogen with periodic acid-Schiff (PAS) stain. Gycolysis results in the accumulation of lactic acid and inorganic phosphates from the hydrolysis of phosphate esters. **This reduces the intracellular pH**. This reduced pH causes **early clumping of nuclear chromatin** (Fig. 4).

Decreased pH and ATP levels cause **detachment of ribosomes from the granular endoplasmic reticulum** (Fig. 4) and **dissociation of polysomes into monosomes**, with a resultant reduction in protein synthesis. If hypoxia continues, diminishing mitochondrial function and increasing membrane permeability, cause further morphological changes. Ultrastructurally, **blebs** may form at the cell surface. 'Myelin figures', that is, concentric laminations derived from plasma as well as organellar membranes, may be seen within the cytoplasm or extracellularly. At this time, mitochondria, endoplasmic reticulum, in fact the whole cell usually appears swollen due to a loss of osmotic regulation. However, all these changes are reversible if oxygen is restored. But if ischaemia persists, irreversible injury follows.

Irreversible Cell Injury

Irreversible injury is associated morphologically with severe swelling of mitochondria, extensive damage to plasma membranes, and swelling of lysosomes. Extracellular calcium enters into the cell. **Large, amorphous, calcium-rich densities accumulate in the mitochondrial matrix**. After this, there is continued loss of proteins, essential coenzymes, and ribonucleic acids from the hyperpermeable plasma membrane. The cells may also leak metabolites, which are vital for the reconstitution of ATP, thus further depleting net intracellular high-energy phosphates.

The **falling pH** (due to accumulation of lactic acid and inorganic phosphates) **causes injury to the lysosomal membranes**. This is followed by leakage of their lysosomal enzymes into the cytoplasm and activation of acid hydrolases. Lysosomes contain RNases, DNases, proteases, phosphatases, glucosidases, and cathepsins. Activation of these enzymes leads to enzymatic digestion of cytoplasmic and nuclear components (Fig. 4).

After death, cellular components are progressively digested by lysosomal hydrolases, and there is a leakage of potentially destructive cellular enzymes into the extracellular space, and entry of extracellular macromolecules into the dying cells. Finally, the dead cell may become replaced by large masses composed of phospholipids called **myelin figures**. These are then either phagocytosed by other cells, or degraded further into fatty acids. Calcification of such fatty acid residues may occur with the formation of calcium soaps.

Mechanisms of Irreversible Injury

The biochemical changes described so far are a continuous sequence of events from the onset of cell injury to ultimate digestion of the irreversibly damaged cell by lysosomal enzymes. But at what stage did the cell actually die? And what is the critical biochemical event responsible for the 'point of no return'? **Two phenomena** consistently **characterize irreversibility**. The **first** is the **inability to reverse mitochondrial dysfunction** (lack of oxidative phosphorylation and ATP generation) even after correction of the original injury (e.g., restoration of blood flow), and the **second** is the **development of profound disturbances in membrane function.**

Cell Membrane Damage

It is now clear that cell membrane damage is a central factor in the pathogenesis of irreversible cell injury. The **cell membrane** consists of a lipid-protein mosaic made up of bimolecular layer of **phospholipids** and globular proteins embedded within the lipid layer. **An intact plasma membrane is essential for the maintenance of normal cell permeability and volume.** There are several biochemical mechanisms that cause membrane damage (Fig. 5).

29

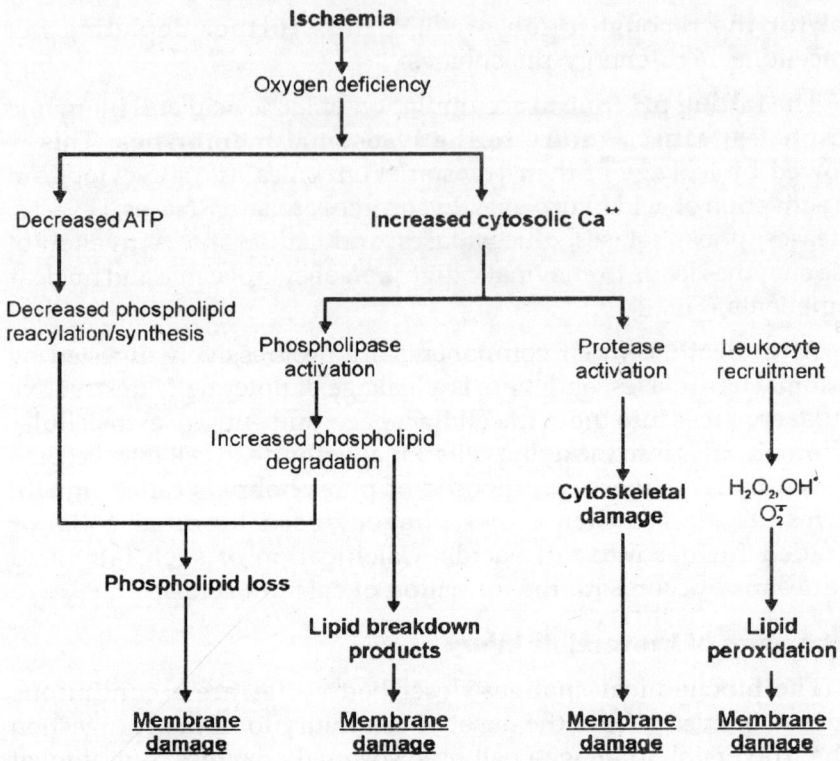

Fig. 5. Mechanisms of membrane damage in ischaemia.

1. **Progressive loss of membrane phospholipids**: Normally, the turnover of membrane phospholipids is associated with their re-synthesis so that the integrity of cell membrane is maintained. The normal intracellular calcium concentration is 10,000 times (10^{-7}M) lower than the concentration of calcium ions (Ca^{++}) in extracellular fluids (10^{-3}M), or of sequestered (isolated) mitochondrial and endoplasmic reticulum calcium. Moreover, the intracellular calcium is sequestered in mitochondria and endoplasmic reticulum. **Oxygen deprivation (hypoxia)** releases sequestered calcium from mitochondria and endoplasmic reticulum, **thus raising cytosolic calcium** (Fig. 5). The increased cytosolic calcium concentration induced by ischaemia, following acute hypoxic injury, **activates endogenous phospholipases**, whose activation is strongly calcium dependent. The phospholipases, in turn, cause **extensive cell membrane damage**. They do so by causing increased phospholipid degradation, and thus, phospholipid loss. Progressive phospholipid loss can also occur from decreased **de novo**

(fresh) synthesis of phospholipids, or decreased ATP-dependent reacylation (acylation is introduction of an acyl group).

Whatever the cause, following phospholipid degradation, **lipid breakdown products** (un-esterified free fatty acids, acyl carnitine, and lysophospholipids) accumulate within ischaemic cells, and cause further cell membrane damage and changes in permeability.

2. Mitochondrial dysfunction: Whatever the mechanism of cell injury, loss of membrane integrity causes further influx of calcium from the extracellular space, where it is present in high concentration, into the cells. Calcium is taken up greedily by mitochondria. Here it **activates mitochondrial phospholipases** and results in accumulation of free fatty acids. Phospholipases and free fatty acids together cause changes in the permeability of the inner mitochondrial membrane, such as **mitochondrial permeability transition**, as well as of the outer mitochondrial membrane (see Fig. 3).

3. Cytoskeletal abnormalities: Cytoskeletal filaments bind firmly plasma membrane to interior of the cell. **Activation of proteases** by increased intracellular calcium may cause damage to cytoskeleton (Fig. 5). In the presence of cell swelling, this damage results in **detachment of the cell membrane from the cytoskeleton, exposing it to stretching and rupture.**

4. Toxic oxygen radicals: As will be discussed in detail later, partially reduced oxygen free radicals are highly toxic molecules that cause injury to cell membranes and other cellular constituents (Fig. 5). Such oxygen radicals are increased in ischaemic tissues.

Whatever the mechanism of membrane damage, loss of membrane integrity causes massive influx (entry) of calcium into the cell from the extracellular space, where it is present in high concentration. Calcium is then readily taken up by mitochondria and permanently poisons them, inhibits cellular enzymes, denatures proteins, and causes the cytoplasmic changes characteristic of coagulative necrosis.

To summarize, hypoxia affects oxidative phosphorylation and hence the supply of vital ATP; membrane damage is a critical step in the development of lethal cell injury; and calcium is an important mediator of the biochemical and morphological alterations in cell death.

31

Free Radical-Induced Cell Injury

As mentioned in the discussion of **'cell membrane damage'**, injury induced by free radicals, particularly that induced by **activated oxygen species**, is an important mechanism of cell damage. It occurs in such widely different processes as chemical and radiation injury, oxygen and other gaseous toxicity, bacterial killing by phagocytic cells, inflammatory cell damage, cellular ageing, tumour destruction by macrophages, and other injurious processes. It is therefore extremely important that we understand this topic, as to what are free radicals. How do they mediate the cell injury, and once formed, how does the body get rid of them? For an easy understanding of this rather complicated topic, it would be helpful if we first briefly review certain basic facts of physical chemistry.

All matter in the universe is composed of the basic unit known as an **element**. There are 103 known elements. Elements are fundamental substances, that consist of atoms **of only one kind**, e.g., hydrogen, nitrogen, calcium, phosphorus, iron, etc. Although 103 elements are known, only a few play an important role in living organisms. In fact, just four elements, hydrogen, oxygen, carbon and nitrogen account for 96 percent of the body weight, and over 99 percent of the atoms in the body. **Atoms** are composed of three fundamental particles: **protons, neutrons**, and **electrons**. An atom has a central nucleus (containing protons and neutrons), and surrounding electrons. The **proton** has a positive charge, **electron** a negative, and **neutron** is electrically neutral. The electrons revolve (rotate) around the nucleus much as the planets revolve around the sun. The number of electrons, characteristic of an atom, is equal to the number of protons present in the nucleus. The **atomic number** of an element indicates the number of protons within the nucleus. For example, the atomic number of hydrogen is 1, therefore it has only a single proton in its nucleus; that of carbon is 4, so four protons, and that of oxygen is 8, it has 8 protons and so on.

Within an atom, the electrons are arranged within a series of shells or **orbitals** (orbits). Electrons in the orbitals are arranged **in pairs** and spin in opposite directions, thus cancelling each others physicochemical reactivity. The **inner (first) orbital** fills first, and for an atom to be stable, it must have two electrons (i.e., paired and the maximum number it can hold), otherwise it will be unstable and highly reactive. For example, an atom of hydrogen has only one electron in its orbital and is therefore unstable and highly reactive. It therefore reacts with another atom of hydrogen and, in combining, the two atoms share electrons so that the orbital has now two electrons, and form a molecule of hydrogen. Each pair of shared electrons is called a **covalent bond**, which 'holds' two adjacent atoms together. Thus, forming a covalent bond involves a sharing or an exchange of electrons between two atoms. The resultant stable group of two or more atoms, linked together by covalent bonds, is called a **molecule**. When atoms combine to form molecules, electrons in only the outer orbital are involved.

As per the **electronic theory of valency**, for an atom to be stable, the **outer orbital** must have a group of **8 electrons (octet)**. That is, **the most stable electron configuration is one in which the outer orbital contains maximum number of electrons**, otherwise the atom will be unstable and will react **until octet is formed**. For example, an atom of oxygen (atomic number 8) has only 6 electrons in the outer orbital (2 being in the inner orbital). It therefore combines with another atom of oxygen, shares electrons through covalent bonds, **fulfils its requirement of eight**, and forms a stable molecule; or it may react with two atoms of hydrogen, **achieve its electronic configuration of octet**, and thus form a stable molecule of water.

After this brief consideration of an atom and its electron configuration, it is now easy to understand what a free radical is. A free radical is an atom, or a group of atoms, that has one or more **unpaired electrons** in the outer orbital. In other words, **free radicals are chemical species that have a single unpaired electron in the outer orbital**. In such a state the free radical is **extremely reactive and unstable**, and enters into reactions in cells with inorganic or organic substances (proteins, lipids, carbohydrates), particularly with the key molecules in membranes and nucleic acids. A second feature of free radicals is that they initiate **autocatalytic reactions**. This means that the molecules that react with free radicals are themselves converted into free radicals, which in turn propagate the chain damage.

An unpaired electron can be associated with almost any atom, but **those derived from oxygen are the most important in cell injury**. However, **nitric oxide (NO)**, generated by many types of cells can act as a free radical, or can be converted into highly reactive **nitrite species. Oxygen-derived free radicals** are produced during normal metabolic processes in **reduction-oxidation (redox) reactions**. For example, during normal respiration molecular oxygen (O_2) is sequentially reduced in mitochondria by the addition of four electrons to generate water. In this process small amounts of toxic metabolites are produced. These include **superoxide radicals ($O_2^{\cdot-}$)** , **hydrogen peroxide (H_2O_2)**, and **hydroxyl radicals (OH$^{\cdot}$)**. These can be produced by the activity of a variety of **oxidative enzymes** in different sites of the cell, that is, endoplasmic reticulum (P-450, b5 oxidases), mitochondria (P-450, b5 oxidases), plasma membrane (NADPH oxidase), cytosol (xanthine oxidase, transition metals (Cu, Fe), peroxisomes (multiple oxidases), and lysosomes (in phagocytes - myeloperoxidase, NO synthase).

1. **Superoxide ($O_2^{\cdot-}$):** Superoxide is a molecule of oxygen that has 13 electrons in its outer orbital, instead of normal 12. **Because of the presence of an unpaired single electron in the outer orbital, it is extremely reactive.** Since it carries net negative charge (anion), it is a negative radical (oxide), and because it is extremely reactive (super), it is called a **'superoxide anion'**, termed simply as **superoxide**. It is generated either directly during auto-oxidation, or by the transfer of a single electron to O_2 in reactions catalyzed by cytoplasmic enzymes, such as cytochrome P450, xanthine oxidase, and the respiratory burst oxidase (NADPH oxidase) present in neutrophils.

$$O_2 + e^- \xrightarrow{\text{NADPH oxidase}} O_2^{\cdot-}$$

Rapid bursts of superoxide production occur in activated neutrophils during inflammation.

Once produced **($O_2^{\cdot-}$)** can be inactivated either spontaneously or more rapidly by the enzyme **superoxide dismutase (SOD)**, forming H_2O_2.

$$2O_2^{\cdot-} + 2H \xrightarrow{\text{SOD}} H_2O_2 + O_2$$

Superoxide dismutases are found in many types of cells. The group includes both manganese-superoxide dismutase, which is present in mitochondria and copper-zinc-superoxide dismutase, which is found in the cytosol.

2. **Hydrogen peroxide (H_2O_2):** H_2O_2 is produced either by the dismutation of **'superoxide'** as just mentioned, or directly by oxidases present in peroxisomes. Peroxisome is a cytoplasmic organelle containing enzymes, both for the production and degradation, of hydrogen peroxide.

· **Catalase**, present in peroxisomes, decomposes hydrogen

peroxide into oxygen and water.

$$2H_2O_2 \longrightarrow O_2 + 2H_2O$$

Being a free radical, hydrogen peroxide is an unstable compound.

Glutathione peroxidase (GSH-Px), an enzyme present in cytosol also protects against injury by catalyzing free radical breakdown.

$$H_2O_2 + 2GSH \longrightarrow GSSG + 2H_2O \text{ or } 2OH^\bullet$$
[reduced] [oxidized]

or

$$2OH^\bullet + 2GSH \longrightarrow 2H_2O + GSSG$$

The ratio of **oxidized glutathione** (GSSG) to **reduced glutathione** (GSH) within the cell indicates the oxidative state of the cell. It is an important aspect of the cell's ability to inactivate reactive oxygen species.

3. **Hydroxyl radicals (OH·)**: These are generated by:

(a) Hydroxyl radicals are produced by interaction with transition metals (e.g., iron, copper) in the **Fenton reaction**. In this reaction, iron and copper donate or accept free electrons during certain intracellular reactions and thereby catalyze free radical formation **(Fenton reaction)**.

$$Fe^{++} + H_2O_2 \longrightarrow Fe^{+++} + OH^\bullet + OH^-$$
[ferrous] [ferric]

Since most of the intracellular free iron is in the ferric (Fe^{+++}) state, it must first be reduced to the ferrous (Fe^{++}) form to participate in the **Fenton reaction**. This reduction step is catalyzed by superoxide. Thus, **iron and superoxide synergize** to produce maximal oxidative cell damage.

(b) Hydrolysis of water by ionizing radiation. This is due to the absorption of radiant energy (e.g., ultraviolet light, X-rays). Ionizing radiation can hydrolyze water into hydroxyl (OH·) and hydrogen (H·) free radicals.

$$H_2O \longrightarrow OH^\bullet + H^\bullet$$

Hydroxyl radical has only **seven electrons** in the outer orbital, **thus one is left unpaired. Hydroxyl radicals are the most reactive in inducing cell damage**.

4. **Singlet oxygen**: Singlet oxygen is a form of oxygen in which one electron is shifted into a high energy orbit. Because of its distorted

35

electron configuration, singlet oxygen is very unstable and reactive.

5. Nitric oxide (NO): NO is a soluble, free radical gas produced by endothelial cells, macrophages, neurons, and other cell types. It is an important chemical mediator (see Chapter 4). Apart from itself acting as a free radical, it can also be converted to highly reactive peroxynitrite anion ($ONOO^-$) as well as $NO2^{\cdot}$ (nitrogen dioxide) and $NO3^-$.

Mechanisms of Cell Injury

The effects of free radicals are wide-ranging. However, the following **three reactions** are most important in cell injury.

1. Lipid peroxidation of membranes: Free radicals in the presence of oxygen may cause **peroxidation of lipids** in plasma and organellar membranes. Oxidative damage begins when double bonds in unsaturated fatty acids of membrane lipids are attacked by oxygen-derived free radicals, particularly by **hydroxyl radicals (OH$^{\cdot}$).** Double bonds are vulnerable to attack by free radicals. **The lipid-radical interactions yield peroxides**, which are themselves unstable and reactive. Therefore, **an autocatalytic chain reaction follows** (called **propagation**), which can result in extensive membrane, organellar, and cellular damage. **Termination** takes place when the free radical is captured by a scavenger, such as **vitamin E,** embedded in the cell membrane. Also, **vitamin A, C** and **beta-carotene** either block the formation of free radicals or inactivate them once they are formed.

2. Cross-linking of proteins: Free radicals act on the **sulphydryl bonds** (-SH-HS-) of proteins. Cross-linking of proteins by the formation of **disulphide bonds** (-S-S-) in such labile amino acids as methionine, histidine, cystine, and lysine causes **extensive damage throughout the cell**. In particular, the free radicals inactivate the sulphydryl enzymes.

3. DNA fragmentation: Free radical reactions with **thymine** in nuclear and mitochondrial DNA produce single-stranded breaks. This induces mutations in the genetic code. Such DNA damage has been implicated **in both cell killing and malignant transformation of cells**.

To conclude, the final effects induced by free radicals depend on the net balance between free radical formation and termination.

Cellular Swelling

Cellular swelling (previously known as **cloudy swelling**, parenchymatous, or albuminous degeneration) is a disturbance of cellular metabolism in which cells swell and cytoplasm of the cell becomes more granular than normal. **Cellular swelling is the most common disturbance of cell metabolism and is the first reaction of a cell to injury**. It is caused by the mildest irritants and results from the shift of extracellular water into the cell, caused by mechanisms described earlier (see 'reversible injury'). The term **cloudy swelling** earlier referred to gross appearance of the affected organ, but is now outdated and no longer in use.

Aetiology: Since cellular swelling is caused by the mildest irritants, it can be produced by any factor that interferes with cellular metabolism. The **causes** include: (1) bacterial toxins (the most common cause). Cellular swelling occurs in infectious diseases. (2) a rise in body temperature (fever), (3) metabolic diseases (diabetes and acetonaemia), (4) organic or inorganic poisons (lead, arsenic, chloroform, and alcohol), and circulatory disturbances (anaemia, infarction, passive hyperaemia, and haemorrhage) when insufficient oxygen is brought to the cell.

Macroscopically, the affected organ (liver, kidney) is slightly enlarged, the edges are slightly rounded, and there is an increase in weight. The changes are due to an increased amount of fluid in the affected cells. The organ appears pale or anaemic, because the swollen cells compress the capillaries reducing the amount of blood in the organ. When incised, the cut surface bulges and its capsule draws back slightly. The cut surface is cloudy, slightly opaque, and appears as if it had been slightly scalded or cooked. **Microscopically**, cellular swelling is best observed in the liver, the convoluted tubules of the kidney, or in skeletal and cardiac muscle. The mechanism of cellular swelling has been discussed under reversible injury. Due to accumulation of fluid within the cells, the **cells become swollen**, and their edges become rounded. The cytoplasm stains slightly more intense with eosin. The internal structures of the cell are slightly hazy. **The cytoplasm of the cell is more granular than normal**. These granules are soluble in acetic acid, but not in lipid solvents such as chloroform. **Significance and result**: Cellular swelling is a reversible injury and indicates the cell has been exposed to a mild irritant, or that hypoxia has been present. As soon as the cause is removed, the granules disappear, the fluid leaves the cell, and the cell returns to normal.

Subcellular Responses to Injury

So far the changes described refer to either whole tissue, or the cell as a unit. However, certain conditions are associated with **changes involving only subcellular organelles and cytoplasmic proteins**. These include:

Lysosomal catabolism

Primary lysosomes are membrane-bound intracellular organelles containing a variety of hydrolytic enzymes. These fuse to form **secondary lysosomes** or **phagolysosomes** that contain material meant for digestion. Lysosomes break down the ingested materials in two ways: **heterophagy** and **autophagy**.

Heterophagy: In this, materials from external environment are taken up through the process of **endocytosis**. Uptake of particulate matter is called **phagocytosis** (G. phagein=to eat), and that of **soluble** macromolecules as **pinocytosis** (G. pinein=to drink). Endocytosed vacuoles and their contents ultimately fuse with a lysosome. This results in degradation of the engulfed material. Examples: bacteria are ingested and degraded by neutrophils, and macrophages engulf and degrade necrotic cells.

Autophagy: In this process, intracellular organelles are isolated from the cytoplasm in an **autophagic vacuole** formed from rough endoplasmic reticulum (RER). The autophagic vacuole then fuses with primary lysosomes to form an **autophagolysosome**. Autophagy is a common phenomenon and is involved in the removal of damaged or senescent (old) organelles and in the cellular remodelling associated with cellular differentiation. It is prominent in cells undergoing atrophy induced by nutrient or hormonal deprivation.

The **enzymes in lysosomes** can completely break down most proteins and carbohydrates, but some lipids remain undigested. Lysosomes with undigested debris may persist within cells as **residual bodies**, or may be thrown out. **Lipofuscin pigment** granules, discussed later, represent indigestible material that results from intracellular lipid peroxidation. Certain indigestible pigments, such as carbon particles, can persist in phagolysosomes of macrophages for decades.

Lysosomes are also places where cells isolate materials that cannot be completely metabolized. **Hereditary lysosomal storage disorders** caused by deficiencies of enzymes that break down various macromolecules, result in abnormal collections of intermediate metabolites in the lysosomes of cells all over the body, particularly neurons, leading to severe abnormalities.

Hypertrophy of Smooth Endoplasmic Reticulum

Prolonged use of barbiturates leads to increased tolerance. The patients are then said to have **'adapted'** to the medication. This adaptation is due to hypertrophy (increased volume) of liver cell smooth endoplasmic reticulum (SER). Barbiturates are metabolized in the liver through the P- 450 mixed-function oxidase system. The barbiturates stimulate the synthesis of more enzymes as well as more SER. In this manner, the cell is better equipped to detoxify the drugs and adapt to its altered environment. Cells adapted to one drug have increased capacity to metabolize other drugs.

Mitochondrial Alterations

As described earlier, mitochondrial dysfunction plays an important role in cell injury and death. In addition, various alterations in the number, size, shape, and function of mitochondria occur in some pathological conditions. For example, in **hypertrophy,** there is **an increase in the number of mitochondria in cells,** whereas mitochondria decrease in number during cell **atrophy**. Mitochondria may become extremely large and assume abnormal shapes (**megamitochondria**), as seen in hepatocytes in various nutritional deficiencies and alcoholic liver disease in humans. In certain inherited metabolic diseases of skeletal muscle, the **mitochondrial myopathies** are associated with increased numbers of unusually large mitochondria.

Cytoskeletal Abnormalities

The cytoskeleton consists of **actin** and **myosin filaments, microtubules**, and various classes of **intermediate filaments** that spread through the cytosol (the fluid portion of cytoplasm). The cytoskeleton is important in: (1) the transport of organelles and molecules inside the cell, (2) maintenance of basic cell architecture, (3) conveying cell-cell and cell-extracellular matrix signals to nucleus, (4) mechanical strength for tissue integrity, (5) cell locomotion (mobility), and (6) phagocytosis.

Abnormalities of the cytoskeleton occur in a variety of pathological conditions. Functioning microtubules are essential for various stages of leukocyte migration and phagocytosis. Functional deficiencies of the cytoskeleton cause certain defects in leukocyte movement towards an injurious stimulus (chemotaxis), or the ability of such cells to perform phagocytosis. For example, in **Chédiak-**

Higashi syndrome, a defect of microtubule polymerization causes delayed or decreased fusion of lysosomes with phagosomes in leukocytes, and this **impairs phagocytosis of bacteria.** Chédiak-Higashi syndrome has been described in **humans, cattle, cats,** and **rats.** Defects in the organization of **microtubules** can inhibit sperm motility and cause male sterility. Such defects of **microtubules** can immobilize cilia of the respiratory epithelium. This interferes with the ability of epithelium to clear inhaled bacteria and predisposes to respiratory tract infections, leading to **'immotile cilia syndrome'.** Accumulations of **intermediate filaments** may be seen in certain types of cell injury. The **Mallory body** is an eosinophilic, intracytoplasmic inclusion in liver cells that is characteristic of alcoholic liver disease in humans. It is composed mostly of intermediate filaments.

Heat Shock Proteins

One of the most important adaptive responses within the cell is formation of **stress proteins** after injurious stimuli. These were originally called **'heat shock proteins (HSPs)'** as they were observed after slight rises (4^0 to 5^0 C) in temperature in fruit fly larvae. It is now known that the same proteins are also found in all species in normal cell, and also in response to a wide variety of physical and chemical stimuli. Thus, **'heat shock protein'** is somewhat of a misnomer.

In a normal cell **newly synthesized polypeptide** chains of proteins made on ribosomes are arranged, either into alpha helices or beta sheets. Their proper arrangement (**protein folding**) is extremely important for the function of individual protein and its transport across the cell organelles. It is here that heat shock proteins play important roles in protein folding and in the transport of proteins into various intracellular organelles (**protein kinesis**). Thus, HSPs are also called **chaperones.** ('Chaperone' is a French word and means an older woman who looks after a girl. In the present context, chaperones (HSPs) look after proteins within the cell). For example, in the normal process of protein folding **partially folded intermediates** are formed (Fig. 6A) and these are very prone to form **intracellular aggregates** among themselves, or by involving other proteins. These intermediates are stabilized by a number of molecular chaperones that interact with proteins directly. **Thus, chaperones (HSPs) help in proper folding of proteins in their transport across the endoplasmic reticulum (ER), Golgi complex, and beyond** (Fig. 6B).

Some HSPs are produced **constitutively.** That is, their production is within the constitution or physical make-up of the cell, for example, **Hsp 60** and **Hsp 90** family members. The numbers are based on molecular weights. Others are induced by **cellular stress**. Stress causes protein aggregation and denaturation. Those formed after injurious stimuli (heat, UV or free radical injury, mutations, other factors), such as **Hsp 70** family members, protect (rescue) shock-stressed proteins from misfolding. **They handle the damaged (denatured) protein in two ways** (Fig. 6B): (1) **By re-folding the damaged proteins** to restore their function before they can cause **serious cell dysfunction or death**, and (2) When re-folding is not successful, **permanently damaged proteins** are bound to the **ubiquitin HSP molecule**. Ubiquitin binding makes these proteins as targets for intracellular degradation (destruction) by **proteasomes**, a particulate cluster of **non-lysosomal proteinases** (Fig. 6B).

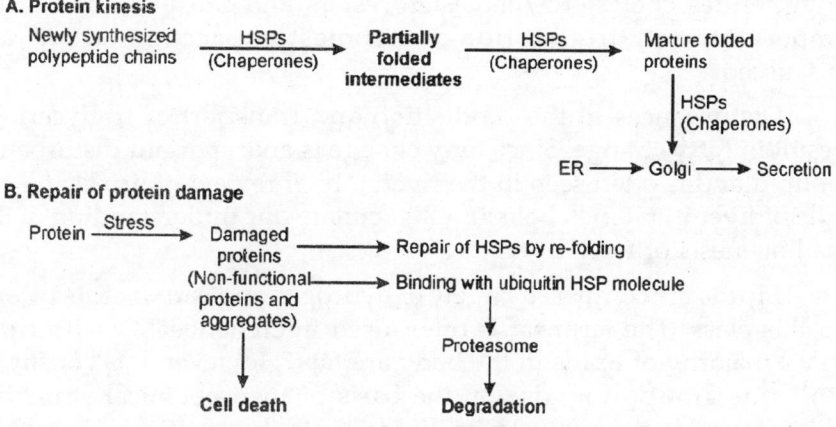

A. Protein kinesis

B. Repair of protein damage

Fig. 6. Role of heat shock proteins (HSPs, chaperones) in: (A) normal protein folding and transport into intracellular organelles, and (B) in repair of damaged proteins, either by re-folding, or by targeting for degradation through proteasomes. ER = endoplasmic reticulum

Intracellular Accumulations

Under some circumstances, cells may accumulate abnormal amounts of various substances. These may be harmless or may cause injury. The **location** of the substance may be either in the **cytoplasm**, within **organelles (lysosomes)**, or in the **nucleus**. The substance may be synthesized by the affected cells, or may be produced elsewhere. There are **three pathways** by which cells can accumulate abnormal substances.

41

1. **A normal substance** may be produced at a normal or an increased rate, but the metabolic rate is inadequate to remove it. An example of this type is **fatty change** in the liver (discussed later).

2. **A normal or an abnormal endogenous substance** accumulates because of genetic or acquired defect in its metabolism, transport, or secretion. Example: A genetic enzymatic defect in a specific metabolic pathway resulting in disorders called "**lysosomal storage diseases**".

3. **An abnormal outside substance** may accumulate because the cell has neither the enzymes to degrade the substance nor the ability to transport it to other sites. **Examples**: accumulations of carbon (**anthracosis**), or silica particles (**silicosis**) in the lungs.

Lipids

All major classes of lipids can accumulate within cells, that is, triglycerides, cholesterol/cholesterol esters, and phospholipids. Being important, only triglyceride and cholesterol accumulations are discussed.

Disturbances in the production and transport of triglycerides result in **fatty change**. Since fatty change is an important disturbance of lipid and is often seen in the **liver**, a brief review of lipids and the role of liver in fat metabolism will facilitate our understanding of the pathogenesis of **fatty liver**.

Lipids are composed largely of hydrogen and carbon. **Fats** belong to this class. The term **fat** is often used interchangeably with **lipid** since majority of lipids in the body are fats. However, fats constitute only one group of lipids. On the basis of their chemical structure, lipids found in the body **can be divided into three groups**: (1) **neutral fats**, (2) **phospholipids**, and (3) **steroids**. All have the common property that their molecules are relatively **insoluble in water**, but are soluble in organic solvents such as acetone, benzene, chloroform, or ether. Lipid molecules contain very few polar or ionic chemical groups, which accounts for their insolubility in water.

The **neutral fats** constitute majority of the lipids in body, and it is these that are generally referred to as **fat**. As is known, neutral fats consist of **fatty acids** and **glycerol**. When a **fatty acid** molecule contains a double bond, it is said to be **unsaturated**. If more than one double bond is present, the fatty acid is said to be **polyunsaturated**. For example, arachidonic acid present in the cell membrane phospholipids is a 20-carbon polyunsaturated fatty acid. Animal fats generally contain a high proportion of saturated fatty acids, whereas vegetable fats contain more polyunsaturated fatty acids.

The other component of the neutral fat is **glycerol** a three carbon molecule to which the fatty acids are attached. **Thus, a neutral fat molecule consists of three fatty acid chains joined through their carboxyl group to the three hydroxyl groups of glycerol by ester linkages.** It is referred to as a **triglyceride** because of the three fatty acids attached to the backbone of the glycerol molecule.

The **phospholipids** are also composed of glycerol and fatty acids, and are thus similar in structure to the neutral fats. However, they contain only two fatty acids, the third hydroxyl group of the glycerol is liked to a **phosphate group**. Phospholipids form a major component of the cell membrane. **Steroids** differ structurally from neutral fats and phospholipids. Steroids include such molecules as cholesterol, a structural component in cell membranes, and many of the hormones in the body (testosterone, oestrogen).

After this brief consideration of lipids, let us examine the **role of liver in fat metabolism**. Under normal conditions, lipids are transported to the liver from two sources: adipose tissue and the diet. From adipose tissue, lipids are released and transported in only one form - **free fatty acids** (i.e., fatty acids complexed with albumin). Dietary lipids on the other hand, are transported as either chylomicra (lipid particles consisting of triglycerides, phospholipids, and protein), or as free fatty acids. **Free fatty acids** enter the cell, and most are esterified to **triglycerides** (Fig. 7). Some are converted to **cholesterol**, incorporated into **phospholipids**, or oxidized in mitochondria to ketone bodies. Some fatty acids are synthesized from acetone as well, within the liver cells. In order to be secreted by the liver cells, intracellular triglycerides are first complexed with specific **apoprotein molecules** called 'lipid acceptor proteins' to form lipoproteins. **It is as lipoproteins that triglycerides are secreted from the liver** (Fig. 7). This step is required because triglycerides being water insoluble, lipoprotein formation makes triglycerides transportable in blood. Excessive accumulation of triglycerides within the liver (**fatty change**) may result from defects at any step from fatty acid entry to lipoprotein exit.

Fatty Change

Definition: Fatty change refers to any abnormal accumulation of **neutral fat (triglycerides)** within parenchymal cells. The appearance of fat vacuoles, whether small or large, represents **an absolute increase** in intracellular fat. It does not represent so-called unmasking (phanerosis) of the neutral fat content of cells.

The old concept of **fatty degeneration** and **fatty infiltration** has changed over the years. This is because neither a degenerative nor an infiltrative process is necessarily involved in the accumulation of fat within liver cells. The older terms fatty degeneration and fatty infiltration therefore have been replaced by the more non-committal term **fatty change**, which covers different mechanisms that may lead to accumulation of neutral fat within cells. Although itself a reversible alteration, fatty change is sometimes a precursor of cell death. In a severe form, fatty change may precede cell death, **but cells may die without undergoing fatty change**. In many situations, it is seen in cells adjacent to those that have died. Fatty change is mostly seen in liver, since it is the major organ involved in fat metabolism. But it also occurs in heart, skeletal muscle, kidney, and other organs.

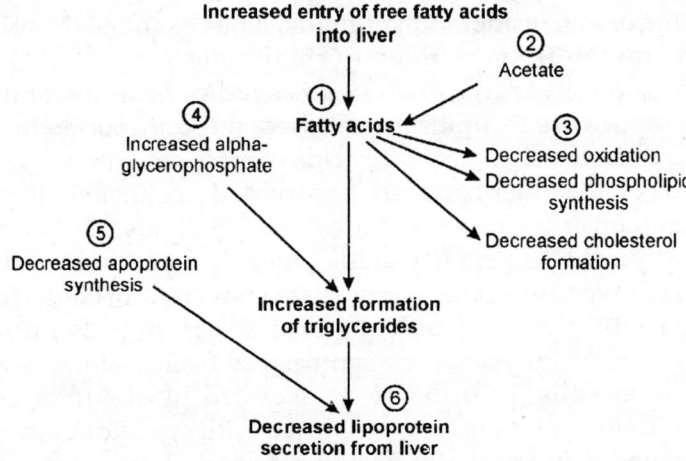

Fig. 7. Pathogenesis of fatty liver.

Aetiology: Fatty change is caused by a variety of irritants that are more severe than those which produce acute cellular swelling. The causes include:

1. Inadequate amounts of oxygen: This occurs in anaemia, following haemorrhage over a prolonged period as in ancylostomiasis, and in diseases like babesiosis when there is extensive destruction of erythrocytes. Circulatory disturbances like chronic passive hyperaemia,

44

which interfere with the transportation of oxygen to cells, also induce fatty change.

2. Hepatotoxins: Both organic and inorganic chemical substances cause fatty change. The list includes bacterial (salmonella) toxins, plants (Crotalaria); chemical poisons such as carbon tetrachloride, chloroform, tetrachloroethylene; and numerous inorganic substances like phosphorus, lead, and arsenic. In humans, alcohol is the most common cause of fatty liver. It is a hepatotoxin.

3. Metabolic diseases, such as diabetes mellitus and ketosis (acetonaemia).

4. Lipotropic factors: For transformation of neutral fats (triglycerides) to phospholipids, choline is needed and it is therefore called a **'lipotropic factor or agent'**. If choline is lacking in the diet, the conversion of neutral fat to phospholipid does not proceed normally, and neutral fat accumulates in the liver cells.

5. Miscellaneous: Protein malnutrition, corticosteroids, starvation, obesity, and certain chronic illnesses.

Pathogenesis: Abnormal accumulation of triglycerides within the liver may result from defects in any one of the events in the sequence from fatty acid entry to lipoprotein exit (Fig. 7). These include: (1) Excessive entry of fatty acids. For example, in starvation, adipose tissue fats are mobilized, and more fatty acids are brought to the liver, where they are synthesized into triglycerides. Corticosteroids also produce fat mobilization. (2) Increased fatty acid synthesis from acetate. (3) Decreased fatty acid oxidation. Both (2) and (3) result in increased esterification of fatty acids to triglycerides. (4) Increased esterification of fatty acids to triglycerides due to an increase in alpha-glycerophosphate, the carbohydrate backbone involved in such esterification. In humans, this occurs in alcohol poisoning. (5) Decreased apoprotein synthesis. As mentioned earlier, this protein is necessary for the conversion of triglycerides to lipoprotein for excretion. This mechanism is the cause of fatty change produced by carbon tetrachloride, phosphorus and protein malnutrition, and (6) Impaired lipoprotein secretion from the liver. It may be noted that an individual aetiological factor may act at more than one site within the complex process of fat metabolism.

Macroscopic appearance

Liver: Mild fatty change may not affect the gross appearance. With progressive accumulation of fat, the organ becomes increasingly

45

yellow. However, the colour of the organ will depend on the natural colour of the fat of that species of animal, and the amount of fat present. It is white in cat, yellow in cattle, and orange in horse. As the liver enlarges, its borders become rounded and are no longer angular. In consistency, it becomes soft and greasy, and the organ is less able to withstand mechanical forces. Fingers are easily forced into the liver. If a sudden rather severe mechanical force is applied, rupture of the organ occurs. When a sharp knife is used, the organ cuts with greater ease. The cut surface usually bulges and has a greasy appearance. Droplets of fat are visible on the surface of the knife blade used in incising the organ.

Heart: Lipid, as neutral fat, also occurs in heart muscle in the form of small droplets. It occurs in two patterns. **Moderate hypoxia** (e.g., in anaemia) induces a 'thrush breast' or 'tigered' effect. Here, the intracellular deposits of fat create bands of yellow myocardium, alternating with bands of darker, red-brown, uninvolved myocardium. In the other pattern, seen in **profound hypoxia**, the **cells are uniformly affected**.

Microscopic appearance: Fatty change begins with the development of minute, membrane-bound inclusions (**liposomes**) closely applied to the endoplasmic reticulum. With the light microscope, it is first manifested by the appearance of **small clear (fat) vacuoles** of varying size in the cytoplasm around the nucleus. When the fat droplets are very small they indicate a recent injury; if large, a disturbance that has existed for a long period of time. As the process progresses, the **vacuoles coalesce** to create cleared spaces that displace the nucleus to the periphery of the cell, until it is elongated and barely visible. Adjoining cells may rupture, and the enclosed fat globules coalesce to produce so-called **fatty cysts**. The fat droplets are very small and numerous in phosphorus poisoning. In diabetes, most of the droplets are large. Cells with fatty change stain poorly with haematoxylin-eosin stain. When paraffin-embedding techniques are used, fat is removed from the droplets leaving a vacuole.

Intracellular accumulation of **water** or **glycogen** may also produce clear vacuoles, and it becomes necessary to use special techniques to differentiate these three types of clear vacuoles. The identification of **fat** requires that the fat solvents commonly used in paraffin embedding for routine haematoxylin-eosin stain, be avoided. Further, to identify the fat, it is necessary to prepare frozen tissue sections. If frozen

46

techniques are used the droplets will retain fat which can be stained with various fat stains. The sections may then be stained with oil Red-O or Sudan IV, both of which impart an orange-red colour to the contained fat. The periodic acid Schiff (PAS) reaction is used to identify glycogen. When neither fat nor glycogen can be demonstrated within a clear vacuole, it is presumed to contain water or fluid with low protein content.

Significance: The significance of fatty change depends on the cause and severity of accumulation. It may have no effect on cellular function when mild. More severe fatty change may damage cellular function, but unless some vital intracellular process is irreversibly impaired (as in carbon tetrachloride poisoning), **fatty change in itself is reversible**. For example, the liver in the alcoholic may become extremely enlarged, leading to a progressive form of fibrosis of the liver termed **cirrhosis**. However, if an alcoholic who has not developed fibrosis, gives up drinking, the enlarged liver returns to normal. As a severe form of injury therefore fatty change may be forerunner of cell death. **If the cause is not removed and the irritant is severe, the cell eventually dies. However, it is emphasized that cells may die without undergoing fatty change**.

An organ undergoing fatty change does not have the ability to resist the mechanical strains. Any sudden violent mechanical force may result in rupture of an organ. This is observed in hens when they jump from the roost to the floor. The impact of striking the floor ruptures the liver, causing fatal haemorrhage into the peritoneal cavity.

Obesity

The excessive accumulation of fat in the body is known as **obesity**, or less commonly as **adiposity** or **lipomatosis**. It is associated with excessive intake of fats and carbohydrates. Calories consumed in excess of the body's requirements are stored mainly as fat, since fat is the most efficient form of stored energy. One gram of fat provides nine calories, while one gram of carbohydrate or protein provides only four. Decreased rate of metabolism associated with endocrine disorders of thyroid, pituitary, testis and ovary also cause obesity. Obesity is not desirable, and in humans, increases the risk for a number of conditions, such as diabetes, hypertension, atherosclerosis, cholelithiasis and several others.

47

Cholesterol and Cholesteryl Esters

Cholesterol and cholesteryl esters accumulate within the cells in a variety of diseases. **Macrophages**, whenever in contact with the lipid debris of necrotic cells or abnormal forms of plasma lipids, may become stuffed with lipid because of their phagocytic activities. They become filled with minute vacuoles of lipids that impart a foaminess to their cytoplasm (**foam cells**). Thus, foamy macrophages occur in foci of cell injury and inflammation. In atherosclerosis, **macrophages** and also **smooth muscle cells** within the intimal layer of the aorta, are filled with lipid vacuoles composed of cholesterol and cholesteryl esters. Aggregates of such cells produce the cholesterol-laden atheromas. In certain acquired or hereditary conditions associated with elevation of plasma cholesterol (hyperlipidaemia, hypercholesterolaemia), **macrophages** are laden with cholesterol and cholesteryl esters. Their localized accumulation in the skin produces tumourous masses known as **xanthomas**.

Proteins

Accumulation of proteins within the cells, seen as droplets, occurs in the renal epithelial cells of the proximal convoluted tubules, and in plasma cells. The former is seen in the kidney diseases associated with protein loss in the urine (**proteinuria**). When protein leaks across the glomerular filter, it is reabsorbed by the epithelial cells of the proximal tubule through pinocytosis. Pinocytotic vesicles fuse with lysosomes to produce phagolysosomes, which appear as pink hyaline droplets within the cytoplasm of the tubular cells. However, these aggregations do not impair cellular function. If the cause of proteinuria is controlled, the protein is metabolized and the droplets disappear.

Plasma cells engaged in active synthesis of immunoglobulins may become overloaded with them to produce large, homogeneous, eosinophilic inclusions called **Russell bodies**. With electron microscope, they are found to be in the cisternae of the endoplasmic reticulum, where protein synthesis occurs.

Glycogen

Excessive intracellular deposits of glycogen are associated with an abnormality with either glucose or glycogen metabolism. It is important in humans. **In animals**, glycogen infiltration has been observed in some rapidly growing **tumours**, in cells in areas of inflammation, and around areas of dead tissues. **In suppurative**

inflammation, the **neutrophils** in the general circulation and in pus contain many tiny droplets of glycogen. The presence of glycogen in tissues is of minor importance in veterinary medicine. **In humans**, it occurs in diabetes mellitus, where glycogen is found in the epithelial cells of the proximal convoluted tubules, as well as in liver cells, beta cells of the islets of Langerhans, and heart muscle cells. Glycogen also accumulates within the cells in a group of closely related genetic diseases called "**glycogen storage diseases or glycogenoses**" (see Chapter 13). In these diseases, glycogen cannot be metabolized, and massive accumulation within cells causes secondary injury and cell death.

Macroscopically, it is difficult to recognize glycogen infiltration. **Microscopically**, glycogen masses appear as clear vacuoles within the cytoplasm. **Glycogen is the only carbohydrate that can be seen under the microscope**. However, the tissues must be fixed immediately after death otherwise glycogen is quickly converted into glucose which is not stainable. **Therefore, glycogen is best preserved in non-aqueous fixatives**. Furthermore, special techniques are required to preserve and stain it. When the usual methods of making sections are employed, glycogen is dissolved in water and vacuoles appear in its place. It is then not possible to decide whether glycogen or fat was present in the cells. Therefore, to demonstrate glycogen, tissues must be obtained immediately after death **and fixed in absolute alcohol**. The glycogen is then made visible by special stains. Iodine stains it reddish brown, and Best's carmine and periodic acid-Schiff, bright red.

Pigments

Pigments are coloured substances. They are either **endogenous**, synthesized within the body, or **exogenous**, coming from outside. **Endogenous pigments** include melanin, lipofuscin, and certain derivatives of haemoglobin. The most common **exogenous pigment** is carbon or coal dust.

(A) Endogenous Pigments

(i) Melanin

Melanin (G. melas = black) is a brown-black pigment formed by melanocytes when the enzyme tyrosinase catalyzes oxidation of amino acid tyrosine to dihydroxyphenylalanine. Melanocytes are present in the basal layer of the epidermis. Melanin appears as a black, brown, or red pigment depending on the amount and its distribution in the

49

skin and other structures. Melanin protects the skin against harmful ultraviolet rays in sunlight. Actually very little pigment is present in an individual. It has been stated that the darkest African Negro contains less than one gram of melanin.

Microscopically, melanin appears as very minute, uniformly regular dirty-brown, spherical granules. The **dopa reaction** can be used to determine if certain cells in the skin or other tissues contain tyrosinase to produce melanin. The biological preparation is flooded with dihydroxyphenolalanine that is converted by the cell tyrosinase to a black pigment, which is similar to melanin.

Pigmented moles (naevus) and **freckles** are skin defects commonly observed in humans, but less commonly seen in domestic animals. Focal accumulations of melanin occur in the mammary glands and surrounding fat of gilts and sows. During the development of an animal, foci of melanocytes become located in various internal organs. As a result, focal areas of pigment are found in the intestine, heart, lungs, kidneys, and other organs. The condition is known as **melanosis**. Melanosis of cornea may cause blindness in some breeds of dogs. Pathological amounts of melanin are most frequently observed in association with the **tumour melanoma** (malignant melanoma, melanocarcinoma). There is a high incidence of these neoplasms in grey horses and heavily pigmented breeds of dogs. **Acanthosis nigricans**, an increased amount of melanin within the skin, is frequently observed in the dog. Destruction of the adrenal gland causes hyperpigmentation of the skin, commonly observed in human beings.

Albinism is the complete absence of melanin within an individual. The melanocytes are present but no melanin pigment is produced because of their inability to synthesize melanin due to an inherited deficiency of tyrosinase. The lack of pigmentation of skin, hair, sclera, or iris permits light to pour through the unpigmented iris or sclera, causing retinal injury. Its absence in the skin makes these patients vulnerable to skin cancer, including malignant melanoma. In **leukoderma**, there is local loss of the pigment. It is commonly observed in areas where there have been collar, saddle, or harness injuries. **Vitiligo** is a disorder characterized by partial or complete loss of melanocytes in the epidermis.

The pigment itself is not harmful. The importance of melanosis depends on the alterations, such as adrenal diseases, hormonal imbalances and neoplasia, which caused the disease.

(ii) **Lipofuscin**

Lipofuscin (L. fuscus = brown) is an insoluble brownish-yellow pigment. It is also known as **lipochrome** and **'wear-and-tear'** or **aging pigment**. It is seen in cells undergoing slow, regressive changes, and is prominent in liver and heart of aging patients, or in patients with severe malnutrition and in cancer cachexia.

Lipofuscin represents complexes of lipid and protein that are derived from the free radical-catalyzed peroxidation of polyunsaturated lipids of subcellular membranes. Gradually, lipofuscin loses its lipid characteristics and staining with Sudan dyes. It is not injurious to the cell, **but is an important marker that indicates whether the cell has suffered free radical injury**. Lipofuscin represents the indigestible residue of autophagic vacuoles (**residual bodies**) formed during aging or atrophy. When present in sufficient amounts, they impart a brown discoloration to the tissue (**brown atrophy**).

(iii) **Derivatives of Haemoglobin**

The average life of an erythrocyte is approximately 120 days, which means that almost 1% of the total erythrocytes in the body are destroyed everyday. The physiological destruction of old and worn-out (senescent) red cells takes place within the mononuclear phagocytic cells of the spleen, liver, and bone marrow, lining the blood vessels or lying close to them, and haemoglobin is released. The phagocytes ingest and destroy the erythrocytes by breaking down their large complex molecules with enzymes. Three components are formed in the disintegration of haemoglobin: **globin**, **iron**, and **haeme** (see Fig. 8). Globin is soluble in the tissue fluids and is removed from the area by the blood and lymph.

The total body iron is divided into two compartments: **functional** and **storage**. About 80% of the functional iron is found in haemoglobin, myoglobin and iron-containing enzymes such as catalase, and the cytochromes contain the rest. The storage pool represented by ferritin and haemosiderin contains about 15% to 20% of total body iron. As erythrocytes are destroyed, iron released from haemoglobin is returned to these compartments. **In cells, iron is normally stored in association with a protein, apoferritin, to form ferritin micelles** (L. small particles). Thus, **ferritin** is essentially a **protein-iron complex** that is found in all tissues, but particularly in liver, spleen, bone marrow, and skeletal muscles. In the liver, ferritin is stored within the parenchymal cells, whereas in spleen and bone marrow, it is in the mononuclear phagocytic cells. Within the cells, ferritin is located both in the fluid portion of the cytoplasm (cytosol) and in lysosomes. With the electron microscope, **ferritin** is seen as closely packed dense particles (6 nm in radius) arranged in tetrads (groups of four). When there is a local or systemic excess of iron, **ferritin forms haemosiderin granules**, which are easily seen with the light microscope. **Thus, haemosiderin pigment represents large aggregates of ferritin micelles**.

(a) **Haemosiderin**

Haemosiderin is a haemoglobin-derived, golden-yellow to brown granular or crystalline pigment in which form iron is stored in cells. Under normal conditions, small amounts of haemosiderin can be seen in mononuclear phagocytes of the bone marrow, spleen, and liver. It is greatest in spleen of the **horse** and least in the **dog**. Excess of iron causes haemosiderin to accumulate within cells, either as a **localized process or** as a **systemic derangement**.

Local accumulation of haemosiderin results from haemorrhage. The best example of **localized haemosiderosis** is the common **bruise**. Following local haemorrhage, the area is first red-blue. With lysis of erythrocytes, the haemoglobin is transformed to haemosiderin. Local macrophages phagocytose the red cell debris, and then lysosomal enzymes convert the haemoglobin, through a sequence of pigments, into haemosiderin. The play of colours through which the bruise passes reflects these changes. The original red-blue colour of haemoglobin is transformed to green-blue, indicating the local formation of **biliverdin** (green bile), then **bilirubin** (red bile), and thereafter iron moiety of haemoglobin is deposited as golden-yellow **haemosiderin**. Haemosiderin is observed in scars.

In the **systemic derangement**, haemosiderin is deposited in many organs and tissues, a condition called **haemosiderosis**. It is associated with increased absorption of dietary iron, impaired utilization of iron, haemolytic anaemia, and transfusion. The transfused red cells constitute an exogenous load of iron. In most cases, the pigment does not damage the parenchymal cells or impair organ functions. However, the more extreme accumulation of iron in a disease called **haemochromatosis**, in humans, is associated with liver fibrosis and diabetes mellitus. Haemochromatosis is an iron overload disorder. The total body iron pool ranges from 2-6 gm in normal human adults. In haemochromatosis the iron pool, mainly in the form of ferritin and haemosiderin, may reach 50 to 60 gm.

Large amounts of haemosiderin are found **in animals** that have absorbed excessive amounts of iron from feed, or have had iron compounds injected into them for the prevention of anaemia. The deposition of haemosiderin in the kidneys may occur in animals suffering from diseases associated with intravascular haemolysis, such as in equine infectious anaemia. The haemosiderin accumulates in the epithelial cells of the tubules and interferes with their excretory functions. Haemosiderin is occasionally observed in the lungs of animals that had chronic passive hyperaemia as the result of a cardiac lesion. Chronic passive hyperaemia causes numerous minute haemorrhages in the lung. Phagocytosis of extravasated erythrocytes results in the accumulation of large amounts of haemosiderin in phagocytes. Because of the increased amount of connective tissue deposited in the lung, the pulmonary change is known as **brown induration**. The haemosiderin-laden macrophages are known as **'heart-failure cells'**.

Microscopically, haemosiderin appears as coarse, golden, granular pigment lying within the cell's cytoplasm. It is insoluble in tissue fluids. Due to iron (ferric ions) in the ferritin micelles, haemosiderin can be identified by a histochemical procedure - the **Prussian blue reaction**. In this reaction, which can be applied to both gross and histological sections of tissues colourless potassium ferrocyanide reacts with iron (ferric) and is converted to an **insoluble blue-black ferric ferrocyanide**. This reaction helps to differentiate haemosiderin from lipofuscin, and can exclude non-iron-containing melanin. Although haemosiderin is normally not injurious to the cell, the fact that it is contained within the macrophages indicates that it is slightly irritating, and the mononuclear phagocyte system treats it as a foreign body.

(b) Porphyria

Porphyria refers to a group of uncommon inborn or acquired disturbances of porphyrin metabolism. **Porphyrins are pigments** normally present in haemoglobin, myoglobin, and cytochromes. A brown, black pigmentation of the bones called **osteohaemachromatosis**, has been observed in **cattle** and **pigs**. This condition is believed to be a misnomer, and the bones are discoloured by an iron-containing blood pigment, basically a disease of porphyrin metabolism (**congenital porphyria**).

(c) Bilirubin

Bilirubin is derived from haemoglobin, but contains no iron. It is the major pigment of bile. When bilirubin is raised in the blood and deposited in tissues, it results in the clinical disorder known as **jaundice**. A brief review of bilirubin formation and secretion (excretion) will help in the understanding of jaundice, and significance of bilirubin in its diagnosis. Bile production can be divided into: (1) bilirubin formation, (2) transport in the blood, (3) uptake and intracellular transport, (4) glucuronidation, and (5) secretion into the canaliculus (Fig. 8).

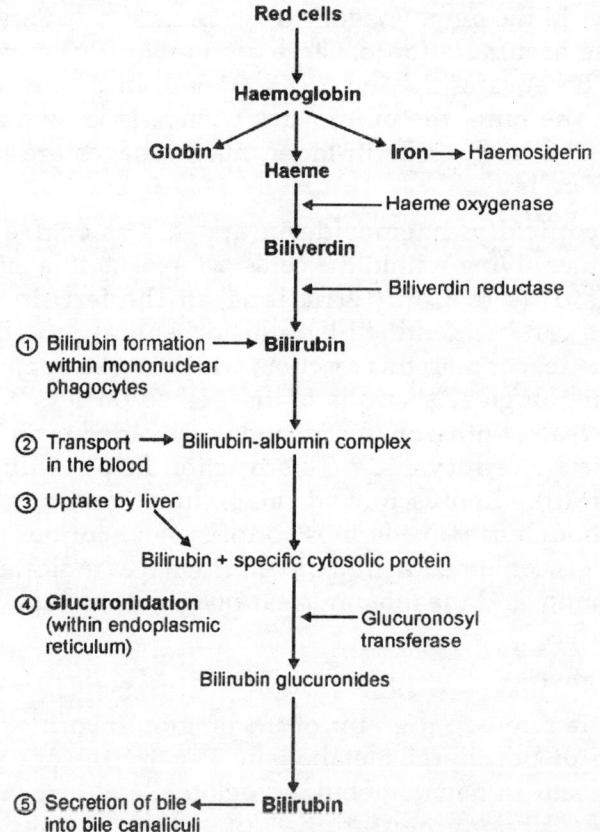

Fig. 8 . Bilirubin metabolism

Bilirubin formation involves cleavage of the haeme ring. About 70% of the bile is derived from the breakdown of senescent (old and

54

worn-out) erythrocytes in cells of the mononuclear phagocyte system (MPS) in the spleen, liver, and bone marrow. The remaining 30% bilirubin is derived mainly from the turnover of non-haemoglobin haeme proteins (haemoproteins) in the liver and from premature destruction of newly formed erythrocytes in the bone marrow. Whatever the source, the **haeme pigment** formed from the breakdown of haemoglobin is oxidized to **biliverdin** by the enzyme **haeme oxygenase**, and then reduced to **bilirubin** by the enzyme **bilirubin reductase** (Fig. 8). **The conversion occurs within the mononuclear phagocytes, mainly in the spleen. Birds** secrete only biliverdin because they lack biliverdin reductase. **Transport of bilirubin** in the blood from its site of formation to the liver requires that it is **bound tightly to albumin**, because this unconjugated bilirubin (explained later) is insoluble in water at pH of blood. The **uptake of bilirubin** is carrier-mediated at the sinusoidal membrane. Once across the plasma membrane, the bilirubin is bound to a specific cytosolic protein and is **transported** to the endoplasmic reticulum for further metabolism. **Glucuronidation** is required to convert water insoluble bilirubin into a water soluble, non-toxic pigment that can be secreted by the liver cell. It occurs in the endoplasmic reticulum. First, bilirubin is esterified with one molecule of **glucuronic acid** by the enzyme **glucuronosyl transferase** to form **bilirubin monoglucuronides**. Most (80-90%) is then converted into **diglucuronides**; the remainder persists as monoglucuronides. **Secretion of bilirubin** into bile canaliculi involves transfer of the glucuronides from the endoplasmic reticulum into the lumen of the bile canaliculus. Once in the canaliculus, bilirubin flows in the bile and reaches intestines. Here glucuronides are split and the bilirubin converted by bacterial action into **urobilinogens**, most of which are excreted in the faeces. About 20% of the **urobilinogens** formed are reabsorbed and returned to the liver to be again excreted into the bile. A small amount that escapes this enterohepatic circulation reaches the kidneys and is excreted in urine.

There are important differences between **unconjugated (indirect)** and **conjugated (direct) bilirubin. Unconjugated** bilirubin is not soluble in water at physiological pH, but is soluble in lipids, is toxic to tissues and is **tightly bound** to serum albumin. As such, it **cannot be excreted in the urine in jaundice**, even when the blood levels are high (**acholuric jaundice**). In contrast, **conjugated bilirubin** is water soluble, non-toxic, and only **loosely bound** to albumin. Because of its solubility and weak association with albumin, when present in excess in plasma (as in obstructive jaundice), **it is excreted**

in urine (bilirubinuria). After this brief consideration of bilirubin metabolism, let us examine jaundice.

Jaundice

Jaundice **(icterus)** is the yellow discoloration of skin and sclerae that occurs when bilirubin is increased in blood (hyperbilirubinaemia), and is deposited in tissues. Discoloration occurs only when bilirubin levels rise above 2.0 mg/dL, normal value being between 0.5 -1.0 mg/dL. The discoloration is particularly noticeable in the eyes because of the high scleral content of elastin, which has a specific affinity for bilirubin. The internal organs are also pigmented, except for the brain and spinal cord, which are usually not affected. Bile pigments may also be excreted in the urine and in the sweat; the tears, however, are not coloured, nor or the saliva and gastric juice.

The **normal serum bilirubin levels** are maintained because the rate of bilirubin production is equal to the rates of hepatic intake, conjugation, and biliary excretion. Jaundice occurs when equilibrium between bilirubin production and clearance is disturbed by one or more of the following mechanisms: (1) overproduction of bilirubin by increased breakdown of red cells, (2) reduced liver uptake from the blood due to intrahepatic lesions, (3) impaired conjugation either because of a genetic lack of glucuronosyl transferase, or some acquired disturbance in conjugation, (4) impaired intrahepatic secretion of bilirubin, and (5) impaired extrahepatic secretion of bilirubin. The first three mechanisms produce unconjugated hyperbilirubinaemia, the last two conjugated hyperbilirubinaemia (**cholestatic jaundice**).

More than one **mechanisms** operate to produce jaundice in some diseases, but in general, one mechanism predominates. Therefore, in a patient of jaundice, knowledge of the main type of plasma bilirubin (conjugated or unconjugated) is of great clinical value in arriving at the possible cause of hyperbilirubinaemia. For example, unconjugated hyperbilirubinaemia indicates excessive production of bilirubin as occurs in haemolytic anaemia, whereas the presence of conjugated bilirubin points to a cause away from the hepatic conjugating enzyme system. An example of the latter is biliary tract obstruction, which leads to regurgitation of conjugated bilirubin into blood. In this, the bilirubin is present in the urine, whereas in unconjugated hyperbilirubinaemia, it is not. Thus, depending on the location of the lesion responsible for hyperbilirubinaemia, **jaundice can be divided into three types:** (1) Haemolytic (prehepatic), (2) Toxic (intrahepatic), and Obstructive (posthepatic).

(1) Haemolytic (Prehepatic) Jaundice

In haemolytic jaundice, 80% or more of the **serum bilirubin** is **unconjugated** (unconjugated hyperbilirubinaemia). It is caused by three mechanisms.

(i) Overproduction of bilirubin: This occurs when there is increased destruction of erythrocytes. Various protozoan diseases (babesiosis, anaplasmosis, trypanosomiasis, haemobartonellosis) injure the erythrocytes and cause haemolysis. This type of jaundice also occurs in infectious viral equine anaemia. The toxins of *Clostridium haemolyticum* cause haemolysis of erythrocytes in **cattle** and subsequent jaundice. Haemolytic disease can be an important cause of excessive bilirubin production. For example, **mares** may become sensitized to the erythrocytes of the stallion to which they are bred. If the colt contains the same type of erythrocytes to which mare has been sensitized, he will develop jaundice 24-48 hours after obtaining antibodies from the colostrum of the mare. Similarly, a sow can be sensitized to the erythrocytes of the boar. Piglets that inherit erythrocytes of the type to which the sow has been sensitized are normal at birth, but develop a haemolytic anaemia a few hours after nursing. These conditions in domestic animals are comparable to the haemolytic anaemia and jaundice of newborn babies (erythroblastosis foetalis) which occurs when a mother is Rh-negative and develops antibodies against the foetus that is Rh-positive. **Unconjugated bilirubin**, because of its large molecular size (being tightly bound to albumin), **cannot pass the renal filter** and is therefore **not present in the urine (acholuric jaundice).**

(ii) Reduced hepatic uptake of bilirubin: This has been observed in humans after administration of certain drugs such as rifampin, an antitubercular drug.

(iii)   Impaired conjugation of bilirubin: As stated earlier, bilirubin is conjugated in the smooth endoplasmic reticulum of the hepatocytes through the action of glucuronosyl transferase. The activity of glucoronosyl transferase is low at birth and attains normal levels by about two weeks. Thus, almost every newborn develops transient and mild unconjugated hyperbilirubinaemia (**neonatal jaundice** or **physiological jaundice** of the newborns). Pathologically, however, there are several clinical conditions characterized by either hereditary, or acquired deficiency of glucuronosyl transferase. **Gilbert's syndrome** and **Crigler-Najjar syndrome** are characterized by a hereditary deficiency of this enzyme. In domestic animals, these conditions have been reported in **sheep**. Acquired deficiency may result from any cause of diffuse hepatocellular damage.

(2) Toxic (Intrahepatic) Jaundice

This results from injury to the hepatic cells and bile canaliculi, and is caused by any infectious or non-infectious agent that is capable of injuring hepatic cells. Various bacteria (salmonella, leptospira), viruses (infectious canine hepatitis), plant toxins (Crotalaria), inorganic poisons (phosphorus), and organic compounds can damage the liver cells. Since liver damage is associated with both acquired deficiency of glucuronosyl transferase and impaired secretion (excretion) of conjugated bilirubin into the bile canaliculi (intrahepatic cholestasis), **both unconjugated and conjugated bilirubins accumulate in the blood**. Thus, damage to liver cells may impair both conjugating and secretory mechanisms. Moreover, swelling and disorganization of liver cells can compress and block the canaliculi or cholangioles. Actually, transport of bile into the canaliculi is a rate-limiting step in bilirubin excretion, and therefore eventually the hyperbilirubinaemia of hepatocellular disease is mainly of the conjugated type.

(3) Obstructive (Posthepatic) Jaundice

This is characterized by **conjugated hyperbilirubinaemia**. It occurs when secretion (excretion) of conjugated bilirubin is impaired at any level within the excretory duct system (extrahepatic cholestasis). Thus, obstructive jaundice results from obstruction of the extrahepatic bile ducts. Parasites such liver flukes (*Fasciola hepatica*) in **cattle** and **sheep**, ascarids (*Ascaris lubricoides*) in **pigs**, and tapeworms in **sheep** are commonly found in the biliary ducts where they cause obstruction. **Gallstones** are a common cause of obstruction in humans, but are an uncommon cause in domestic animals. Tumours involving the bile duct or adjacent structures (pancreas and portal lymph nodes), inflammation of bile ducts (cholangitis) or the gallbladder (cholecystitis) or pancreas (pancreatitis), may also cause closure of the bile ducts.

When bile duct obstruction is complete, bile disappears from the faeces altogether. Stools lose their normal characteristic and become grey and putty-like. **However, the urine contains bilirubin because conjugated bilirubin is of small molecular size and is water soluble, and hence readily filtered by the kidney**. Since bile is necessary for the absorption of fats from the intestine, malabsorption of vitamin K predisposes the patient to haemorrhage. In obstructive jaundice, bilirubin and bile acids are regurgitated into the blood. Accumulated bile acids produce intense itching (pruritus). Cholestasis is also associated with elevation of plasma cholesterol, and this may lead to a localized accumulation of macrophages laden with cholesterol in the skin (**xanthomas**). Obstructive jaundice may also be accompanied by elevation of serum alkaline phosphatase value. However, alkaline phosphatase is also derived from a variety of sources (bone, kidneys, intestine). If conditions that affect other tissues rich in alkaline phosphatase can be excluded, then an increase in the level of this enzyme is very sensitive marker of impaired biliary excretion.

Icterus Index

In **domestic animals**, if jaundice is intense then there is no difficulty in diagnosis, but it is extremely difficult to decide slight or moderate degree of jaundice unless the colour of the serum or plasma is compared with a standard colour. An accurate evaluation of the degree of pigmentation in an animal can be made by means of the **icterus index**. This technique consists of a comparison of the colour of plasma or serum with the colour of standard solution of potassium dichromate. To use the icterus index with any degree of accuracy, a standard must be prepared for each species and breed of animal together with a correlating factor for the animal's age.

Van den Bergh Reaction

This reaction is used to determine **which type of bilirubin is present**. The test consists of mixing Ehrlich's reagent (diazotized sulphanilic acid) with plasma or serum. Bilirubin reacts with the reagent to form a coloured compound known as azobilirubin. The test is based on the observation that **unconjugated bilirubin gives a delayed reaction compared to the immediate reaction with conjugated bilirubin**. Depending on the colour and the rapidity with which it appears, three interpretations of the test are made. In the **direct reaction**, pink or purple colour develops immediately and reaches its maximum intensity in 1-2 minutes. Direct reaction indicates conjugated bilirubin and, thus, **obstructive jaundice**. The **indirect reaction** shows no colour change during the first two minutes. Within 10 minutes, a golden colour appears. This delayed reaction indicates the presence of unconjugated bilirubin and, thus, **haemolytic jaundice**. In the **biphasic reaction** a brownish-red colour appears during the first two minutes, rather than the typical pink or purple of the direct reaction. This reaction is observed in **toxic jaundice** when both conjugated and unconjugated bilirubins are present in the plasma or serum. Table 1 shows the differences to be considered in determining the type of jaundice.

Table 1. Comparison of the three types of jaundice

	Haemolytic jaundice	Toxic jaundice	Obstructive jaundice
Colour of tissues, plasma or serum	Slight to moderate yellow	Slight to moderate yellow	Intense yellow
Colour of the faeces	Intense yellow	Normal	Grey or clay-coloured
Consistency of the faeces	Normal	Normal	Greasy
Colour of urine	Light yellow	Intense yellow	Intense yellow
Icterus index	Low to moderate	Moderate	High
Van den Bergh reaction	Indirect	Biphasic	Direct

(B) Exogenous Pigments

Exogenous pigments come from outside the body. The lungs and their lymph nodes are the reservoir of various dust particles that are inhaled in the air. The dust particles act as mild irritants and induce slight increase in connective tissue (**fibrosis**) and an accumulation of **macrophages**. The condition is called **'pneumoconiosis'**. This term, originally applied to lung diseases caused by inhalation of dust, now includes all disorders caused by inhalation of any aerosol (i.e., fine solid or liquid particles). Since pneumoconioses are associated with certain occupations, they are considered as **occupational diseases**.

The **development of pneumoconiosis** depends on: (1) the amount of dust retained in the lung and airways, (2) the size and shape of the particles, and (3) their solubility and toxicity. The amount of dust retained in the lungs is determined by its concentration in the air, the duration of the exposure, and the effectiveness of clearance mechanisms. Most particles over **5 μm** in diameter are either filtered out in the vibrissae (stiff hairs) of the nares, or removed by the **mucociliary apparatus**. They are therefore unlikely to reach distal airways. Small particles, under **1μm** in diameter may remain suspended in the inspired air and are exhaled. That is, they tend to act like gases and move into and out of the alveoli, without significant deposition and injury. Thus, the most dangerous particles range from **1 to 5 μm** in diameter because they reach the terminal airways and airsacs and settle on their linings. However, here the **macrophage clearance mechanism** comes into play. Normally, there is a pool of intra-alveolar macrophages that is expanded by recruitment of more macrophages when dust reaches the alveoli. **Phagocytosis** of particles by pulmonary alveolar macrophages provides protection. However, this protection can be overcome by the large dust burden deposited in occupational exposures. The **solubility and cytotoxicity** of particles is influenced by its **size**. The smaller the particle, the more toxic it will be, depending, of course, on its solubility. Thus, finely divided dust may produce **exudative reaction**. On the other hand, larger particles resist dissolution and therefore persist within the lung parenchyma for years. They tend to induce **fibrosing collagenous pneumoconiosis**, such as is characteristic of silicosis. The **mechanism of lung injury and fibrosis** is as follows:

Most of the inhaled dust is trapped in the mucus and rapidly removed from the lung by ciliary movement. However, some of the particles become impacted at alveolar duct bifurcations, where **macrophages** accumulate and phagocytose the impacted particles. The more reactive particles, such as those of **silica**, **trigger macrophages to release a number of products that are toxic to the lung** (Fig. 9). **These products mediate an inflammatory response and initiate fibroblast proliferation and collagen deposition. The pulmonary alveolar macrophage is a key cell in the initiation and continuation of lung injury and fibrosis. Important mediators** released by macrophages include: (1) **Toxic factors (free radicals)**: reactive oxygen and reactive nitrogen species that induce lipid peroxidation of tissue damage, that is, **lung injury** (see 'free radicals'). (2) **Chemotactic factors (inflammatory factors)**: leukotriene B4 (LTB4), interleukin-8 (IL-8), IL-6, and tumour necrosis factor (TNF), which recruit and activate inflammatory cells, which in turn release damaging oxidants and proteases, and (3) **Fibrogenic cytokines**: IL-1, TNF, fibronectin, platelet-derived growth factor (PDGF), and insulin-like growth factor (IGF-1), **which recruit fibroblasts and induce collagen synthesis**, resulting eventually in **fibrosis**.

61

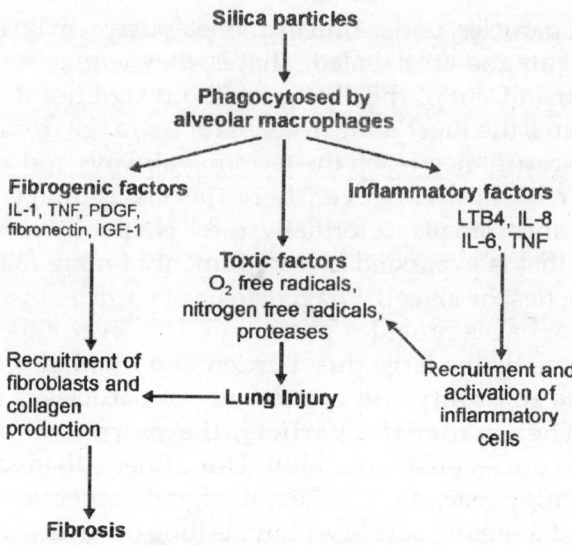

Fig. 9. Mechanisms involved in the pathogenesis of lung injury and fibrosis in pneumoconiosis.

(1) Anthracosis

Anthracosis is the **deposition of carbon** or **coal dust** in the lungs. It is seen in **horses** and **mules** used in coal mines. It also frequently occurs in **dogs** that live in industrial areas where coal dust, soot, and smoke pollute the air. **Tattooing** is a form of localized pigmentation of the skin. Carbon may be introduced through cutaneous abrasions. Various pigments in the form of tattooing inks are used to identify animals. The tattooing is usually done in the ear. The pigment is located in the macrophages in the dermis and subcutaneous tissue. Some of the pigment is carried to the regional lymph nodes.

Macroscopically, the carbon appears as black pigment in the tissues. Carbon in the lungs appears as focal accumulations or as a diffuse infiltration. Lungs are black in colour. The regional lymph nodes are also involved, pigment being present in the medulla. **The carbon is only mildly irritating.** As such only a **slight fibrosis** of lung occurs. When extensive fibrosis of lung is present, it indicates silicosis. **Silica (silicon) is extremely irritating to the lung and causes extensive fibrosis. Microscopically,** particles of carbon are contained **within macrophages.** The particles are just black in colour, extremely small and clustered together into globular masses. Since carbon is insoluble in tissue fluids, the pigmentation persists for the life of the animal. Extensive deposits in the lung may cause slight respiratory distress, but if silicon is also present, then a serious pulmonary disease may result.

(2) Siderosis

Siderosis is **deposition of iron** in the lungs and pigmentation and cellular reaction associated with it. It results from inhalation of iron dust, and occurs in **horses, mules**, and **dogs** working in and around iron mines, smelters, and foundries. **Macroscopically**, iron dust causes a brown or rusty red pigmentation, which is focal in the beginning due to the local accumulation of macrophages containing iron dust. The pigmentation becomes diffuse as more and more dust enters the lungs. **Iron is mildly irritating causing only slight fibrosis**. If silica (silicon) is also present in the dust, extensive fibrosis of the lung occurs. If tissues containing iron are placed in potassium ferrocyanide solution and hydrochloric acid (**Prussian blue test**), the tissues become blue in colour. **Microscopically**, the iron occurs as brown or black irregularly shaped granules (usually spherical masses) **within macrophages**. When **Prussian blue test** is applied, the granules become blue in colour. There is only mild fibrosis, unless silicon is also present with the iron dust. Since iron is only slightly soluble in the tissue fluids, it persists in the tissues for the life of the individual. Siderosis is usually of no clinical significance. When iron is present in large amounts or if silicon is also present, extensive chronic inflammation of the lungs results which may lead to chronic general passive hyperaemia.

(3) Silicosis

Silicosis is the **deposition of silicon** (silicon dioxide, i.e., **stone dust**) in the lungs. **It is more common and important in humans than in animals. In humans,** it is currently the most prevalent chronic occupational disease in the world, and presents itself as slowly progressing, nodular, fibrosing pneumoconiosis. Persons, especially sandblasters and those working in mines are at risk. Silica occurs in both crystalline and amorphous forms, but crystalline forms are most harmful. **Silica** is insoluble in body fluids and is a **powerful irritant**, causing **extensive fibrosis** which predisposes the lungs to tuberculosis. **Macroscopically**, lungs present small, discrete nodules. Fibrotic lesions may also occur in the regional lymph nodes and pleura. **Microscopically**, the nodular lesions consist of concentric layers of hyalinized collagen.

(4) Plumbism

Plumbism is pigmentation of tissues resulting from the presence of both **lead and hydrogen sulphide**. It occurs when the lead is ingested in the form of paint, and when water or food containing lead is consumed. Paint, especially in **calves**, is usual source of lead. Water passing through lead pipes may result in poisoning and pigmentation of tissues. **Macroscopically**, pigmentation occurs in only those areas where hydrogen sulphide is present. The lead in the tissue combines with hydrogen sulphide to form **lead sulphide,** which is a black pigment. Thus, pigmentation is seen at the gum line (**lead line**) where lead in the tissues comes in contact with hydrogen sulphide produced by putrefactive bacteria found around the teeth. Formation of lead sulphide in intestines turns the contents black. **Macroscopically**, no tissue reaction to the pigment occurs. Clinically, plumbism indicates the presence of lead. However, the discoloration produced must not be confused with almost identical colour which occurs with putrefaction when iron combines with hydrogen sulphide and forms iron sulphide, which is also a black pigment.

Other **miscellaneous exogenous pigmentations** include **asbestosis** if the dust particle consists of asbestos; **chalicosis** if the dust is calcium carbonate; and **argyrosis**, which results from the administration of excessive amounts of silver compounds. Asbestos is a family of crystalline hydrated silicates. **Asbestosis** is very important in humans, since occupational exposure to asbestos is linked to such conditions as parenchymal interstitial fibrosis, bronchogenic carcinoma, pleural effusions, mesotheliomas, and extrapulmonary neoplasms, including colon carcinomas. **Lipochromatosis** is the yellow, orange, and brown pigmentation of tissues, resulting from the ingestion of carotenes and xanthophylls. These pigments, common in grasses and some vegetables as carrots, are fat soluble, and therefore colour the adipose tissue of the body depot fat. Their presence indicates that carotenes and xanthophylls have been ingested.

Hydropic Degeneration

It is a change closely related to cellular swelling, in which cells take on clear fluid to such an extent that they swell and may burst.

Aetiology: The causes are similar to those of cellular swelling but are more severe, and include: (1) **Mechanical injuries** of a rubbing nature. Examples: skin of the hands of men exposed to the friction from a shovel or axe handle; ill fitting shoes cause friction of the

64

human foot and may lead to blister. (2) **Thermal injuries**, both heat and cold cause hydropic degeneration. Barn fires, hot water, hot oil, hot metal or flame produce blisters in animals. Skin injured by freezing temperatures also cause hydropic degeneration. (3) **Chemical injuries**: treatment of lameness by croton oil, cantharidin, red iodide of mercury, and oil of mustard, in **horses**, may lead to sharp blisters. (4) **Infectious agents**, particularly viruses, such as pox viruses produce blisters in stratified squamous epithelium. The viruses of foot-and-mouth disease in cattle and that of vesicular exanthema of swine, produce hydropic degeneration, and (5) **Neoplasms**, especially those of the cervix.

Macroscopically, it may be seen as a blister on the skin. Upon incision, fluid escapes and the blister collapses. If pyogenic bacteria enter the injured epithelium, suppurative inflammation may result. This is common in blisters produced by burns or pox virus. **Microscopically**, there is an increase in the size of the cells due to accumulation of fluid. Small clear vacuoles may be seen within the cytoplasm. These vacuoles presumably represent distended and pinched off or sequestered segments of the endoplasmic reticulum. The change is also sometimes called **vacuolar degeneration**. As more fluid is taken into the cells, they enlarge, the droplets coalesce and finally the cells become so distended that they burst. In the stratified squamous epithelium this leads to blister or vesicle formation. In the skin, the hydropic change occurs mainly in the prickle-cell layer. The hydropic fluid stains pink with eosin due to protein content. The identity of the vacuoles in the cells is usually determined by negative methods. The cells are stained for fat, glycogen, and mucin. If none of these can be demonstrated, it is assumed that the vacuoles in the cytoplasm of the cells contained hydropic fluid. **Significance and results**: An area of hydropic degeneration uncomplicated by bacterial invasion heals rapidly and leaves no scar or permanent injury. The invasion of the area by pathogenic bacteria, especially staphylococci and streptococci, may result in the abscess, septicaemia, or death.

Mucinous or Mucous Degeneration

Mucinous or mucous degeneration is the excessive accumulation of mucin in degenerating epithelial cells. Mucin, a glassy, viscid, stringy, slimy glycoprotein, is normally produced by columnar and cuboidal epithelial cells. In mucous membrane of the large intestine, the large mucin-producing cells are called goblet cells. When mucin is mixed with water or tissue fluid, it is known as **mucus**.

Aetiology: Mucinous or mucous degeneration occurs whenever a mild irritant is applied to a mucous membrane. The **causes** include mild mechanical injury to a mucous membrane; mild chemicals such as disinfectants and soaps used on mucous membranes during obstetrical procedures; irritating effect of moderate heat and cold; infectious agents, especially viral (canine distemper, viral diarrhoea of cattle); and neoplasms involving columnar epithelium, e.g., adenocarcinoma of the cattle stomach. **Macroscopically**, the mucous membrane is covered with a clear, white transparent material, which is stringy and slimy in consistency. The viscous and watery material flowing from the human nose during the course of common cold is an excellent example of its appearance. The mucous membrane is usually hyperaemic. A layer of mucus often encloses the faecal excrement of animals when they are constipated. Large amounts of mucus are produced by the genital tract during oestrus. Long strings of mucus are usually observed hanging from the vulva of cattle. Since it is a normal reaction, it is called physiological mucus. **Microscopically**, mucin first appears in the cytoplasm of the cell as a small droplet. As more droplets appear, they coalesce forming larger droplets. This displaces the nucleus to one side, which eventually gets compressed against the cell wall. With increasing accumulation of mucin the cell enlarges and ultimately ruptures. The ruptured cell dies and is desquamated. Mucin stains blue with haematoxylin and red when thionin, mucicarmine, and periodic acid-Schiff staining techniques are used. **Significance and results**: As soon as the causative agent is removed, overproduction of mucin stops and the lost epithelium is repaired by regeneration of the surviving cells. Therefore, no permanent damage occurs.

Mucoid or Myxomatous Degeneration

Mucoid degeneration is the appearance of glycoprotein similar to mucin in connective tissue, which is undergoing a disturbance in cell metabolism.

Aetiology: The connective tissue cells, in the foetus, produce mucin-like glycoprotein (Wharton's jelly in the umbilical cord), which is not normally present in the adult tissues. Sometimes this substance is found in the adult in mucoid degeneration, which is observed in: (1) connective tissue tumours known as myxomas and myxosarcomas, (2) myxoedema, a disease associated with thyroid deficiency with humans, and (3) in cachectic animals, as the result of starvation, parasitism, or chronic debilitating diseases. It is usually observed in the adipose tissue along the coronary band of the heart, inter- and intramuscular fat, and in the mesenteric, omental, and perirenal fat. **Macroscopically**, the tissue is shrunken, flaccid and flabby in consistency, and has a translucent, jelly-like appearance. When incised, a watery, slimy, stringy material exudes from the cut surface. **Microscopically**, the degenerating tissue stains more intensely blue with haematoxylin, the nuclei are hyperchromatic, and the fluid in the intercellular spaces has a slightly bluish tinge. **Significance and results**: How common mucoid degeneration is in the domestic animals has never been determined. Mucoid degeneration of the fat disappears as soon as the cause of cachexia is removed. Its presence in the tumours indicates that the tumour is quite embryonal, and suggests a more unfavourable prognosis.

Pseudomucin: It is the normal secretion of ovarian tissue and paraovarian cysts, observed in ovarian cystadenomas and cystadenocarcinomas. Since it resembles mucinous degeneration and could mislead, its characteristic must be recognized. It is not precipitated by acetic acid while mucin is precipitated. This glycoprotein stains pink with eosin instead of blue with haematoxylin, as does mucin. Pseudomucin is not harmful since it is a normal cell secretion.

Hyaline Change

The term **hyaline change is a descriptive histological term rather than a specific marker for cell injury**. It refers to any alteration within cells or in the extracellular space, which gives the tissue a homogeneous, glassy (L. hyaline = glassy), translucent, pink appearance in routine histological sections stained with haematoxylin and eosin. The affected cells and tissues lose their structural characteristics and fuse together into a homogeneous mass. The fusing of the tissues and cells probably represents a process of coagulation and dehydration of protein in the involved area. However, the physicochemical mechanism underlying this change is not clear. **It is the physical appearance of tissue rather than its chemical composition, that determines whether hyaline degeneration is present or not**. Hyaline degeneration therefore includes a group of tissue changes, involving many different organs, tissues, and cells. No specific cause for hyaline change can be stated since it is brought about by a variety of conditions that produce disturbances in protein metabolism. Hyalin is composed of protein of varying composition, and is of three major types:

67

Keratohyalin: Stratum corneum produced during the normal cornification of the skin is the best example of keratohyalin, but is physiological. Pathological amounts of keratohyalin appear in (1) excessive mechanical irritation of the skin produced by shoes in humans (corns and bunions), or by saddles or harnesses in the horses; also seen as calluses on the hands of workmen, (2) by the action of papilloma (wart) virus in cattle and dogs, (3) hyperkeratosis (chlorinated naphthalene poisoning) in cattle, (4) in squamous-cell carcinoma in all species of animals, keratohyalin appears in the form of epithelial pearls, and (5) in vitamin A deficiency as keratinization of epithelium in the digestive and upper respiratory tracts of the chicken. Keratohyalin may be a protection or hindrance. Calluses on the hands are beneficial, while corns and bunions are undesirable and may be very painful. When the cause is removed, excessive keratohyalin is desquamated and the epithelium returns to normal.

Cellular hyalin: This occurs in cells other than those found in stratified squamous epithelium and connective tissue. Cells in many organs are desquamated into a glandular lumen or cavity. There, they fuse into a homogeneous mass resembling starch or sand. These firm masses stain deeply with iodine. Because of this staining reaction, they were called **corpora amylacea** (L. starch bodies). They are so commonly observed in the prostate, that they are considered normal for that gland. They are observed in the alveoli of the lungs in pneumonia or following pulmonary infarction, in the mammary glands of cows 'dried off ' too quickly, and are commonly found in the ventricles of the brain and central canal of the spinal cord where they are known as **'brain sand'**. Cellular hyalin is also observed in the islets of Langerhans in individuals having diabetes; platelets in thrombi fuse together into homogeneous masses of hyalin; and cells desquamated from the renal tubular epithelium with albumin form hyaline casts in the renal tubules in nephritis. The presence of corpora amylacea is seldom of any pathological significance, and indicates an excessive rate of desquamation of epithelial cells.

Connective tissue hyalin: This is observed in old scars, in the degenerating stroma of tumours, in the lymph nodes draining areas of chronic inflammation, in the renal glomeruli in chronic nephritis, and in the intima and media of blood vessels in arteriosclerosis. The alteration is a permanent change and persists for the life of the individual.

To conclude, it is important to recognize the large number of mechanisms that produce hyaline change and implications of the changes when they are seen in different pathological conditions. It is obvious that the various forms of cellular derangements cover a wide spectrum, which range from the reversible to irreversible forms of cell injury. The tissue, however, usually dies before hyaline change takes place.

NECROSIS

Necrosis is the local death of tissue within the living individual. However, this simple definition needs to be understood. This is because **tissue placed immediately in fixative is dead but not necrotic.** Tissues or cells can be recognized as dead only after they have undergone certain changes. Therefore, to be more precise **necrosis refers to a sequence of morphological changes that follow cell death in living tissue or organ,** resulting from the progressively degradative action of enzymes on the irreversibly injured cell. Its most common manifestation is **coagulative necrosis**, characterized by denaturation of cytoplasmic proteins, breakdown of cell organelles, and cell swelling.

The **morphological appearance** of necrosis is the result of two concurrent processes: (1) enzymatic digestion of the cell, and (2) denaturation of proteins. The digestive enzymes are derived either from the lysosomes of the dead cells themselves, in which case the digestion is referred to as **autolysis**, or from the lysosomes of infiltrating leukocytes, termed **heterolysis**.

Aetiology

(1) **Poisons**: (a) **Chemical poisons**: These may be strong acids and alkalies, drugs, insecticides, fungicides, and other toxic chemicals like lead arsenate (an insecticide), phenol, mercuric chloride, uranium nitrate, and others. They cause cell death either by coagulation of proteins or by poisoning the enzymatic systems. (b) **Toxins of pathogenic organisms**: The toxins (harmful products) produced by bacteria, viruses, fungi, rickettsiae, protozoa, and metazoan parasites may cause necrosis. For example, bacteria of various types (Salmonella, Fusobacterium and Staphylococcus) commonly cause necrosis of tissues. (c) **Plant poisons**: Alkaloids produce necrosis. For example, plants of Senecio species in large amounts are hepatotoxic and produce necrosis of hepatic cells in cattle. Mushrooms contain a toxic glycoside, phallin, which causes renal tubular necrosis. Croton oil causes necrosis

69

of epithelium in the skin and mucous membrane. (d) **Animal poisons**: Cantharidin from beetles, and bee stings, cause focal necrosis of tissue. Parasites of many types (e.g., *Histomonas meleagridis* in chickens) also cause necrosis.

(2) **Disturbances in circulation**: (a) **Ischaemia or loss of blood supply** results in necrosis and infarction. It is produced by thrombus and embolism; compression of the artery by tumour, abscess, cyst, ligature, tourniquet; ergot poisoning which causes contraction of the smooth muscles of the arteries. (b) **Passive hyperaemia** causes necrosis when it persists. It is commonly observed in torsion, volvulus, and strangulation of the intestine. (c) **General anaemia** may result in necrosis (brain and liver) if the amount of oxygen and nutrient is not sufficient to maintain cellular metabolism.

(3) **Mechanical injuries** cause necrosis when tissues are crushed or when blood supply is injured or destroyed. (4) **Thermal changes**: Both heat and cold can coagulate protein and cause necrosis. The coagulation of tissues with a branding iron and freezing of extremities are common causes of necrosis. Frostbite causes thrombosis of blood vessels resulting in necrosis of the affected parts. (5) **Electric currents** produced by lightning or generators may coagulate or char tissues. High voltage electric currents cause coagulation of protoplasm. (6) **X-ray and nuclear fission substances** cause protoplasmic alterations that result in necrosis.

Macroscopic appearance: Areas of necrosis are white, grey, or yellow in colour. They appear as if the tissues were coagulated or cooked, and stand out distinctly from the surrounding normal tissue. Their borders are sharply demarcated and are usually surrounded by a red zone of inflammatory reaction. If pyogenic bacteria are present, abscesses may form; and when putrefactive bacteria enter, gangrene may occur which produces additional colour changes of green, orange, or black as a result of iron sulphide formation (see 'gangrene').

Microscopic appearance: The necrotic cells show **increased eosinophilia**. That is, they stain more intensely pink with eosin than normal cells. This is on account of two reasons: (1) in part to loss of normal basophilia imparted by RNA in the cytoplasm (basophilia is the blue staining from haematoxylin), and (2) in part to the increased binding of eosin to denatured intracytoplasmic proteins. Cell outlines are indistinct or absent. The cells may have a more glassy homogeneous appearance than normal cells, due mainly to the loss of glycogen particles. When lysosomal enzymes have digested the cytoplasmic organelles, the cytoplasm becomes vacuolated and appears moth-eaten. Finally, calcification of the necrotic cells may occur.

Nuclear changes appear in the form of **three patterns**, all due to non-specific breakdown of DNA. These include: (1) basophilia of the chromatin may fade (**karyolysis**), presumably due to the action of DNases of lysosomal origin. (2) second pattern is **pyknosis**, characterized by nuclear shrinkage and increased basophilia. The DNA condenses into a solid shrunken mass. (3) in the third pattern, **karyorrhexis**, the pyknotic nucleus undergoes fragmentation. In a day or two, nucleus in the necrotic cell completely disappears.

Types of Necrosis

Once the necrotic cells have undergone these early changes, the necrotic tissue may show distinctive morphological patterns, depending on whether **protein denaturation or enzymatic digestion** predominates. When denaturation is the primary pattern, **coagulative necrosis** develops. When enzymatic digestion is dominant, the result is **liquefactive necrosis**. In special circumstances, **caseous necrosis** and **fat necrosis** may develop.

(1) **Coagulative necrosis: This is the most common type of necrosis**. It is characterized by preservation of the basic structural outline of the coagulated cells or tissue, for at least some days. The nucleus, however, is usually lost, but the basic cellular shape is preserved permitting recognition of the cell outlines and tissue architecture. In other words, **the architectural detail of the area persists, but the cellular detail is lost**. This pattern results from denaturation, not only of structural proteins, but also of enzymic proteins due to cell injury, or from the subsequent increase in intracellular acidosis. **The denaturation of structural and enzymic proteins of the cytoplasm blocks the proteolysis (dissolution or digestion) of the cell, and thus the tissue architecture is preserved**. Coagulative necrosis results most commonly from sudden severe ischaemia, that is, **hypoxic death of cells** in such organs as the heart, kidney, and adrenal gland. Thus, infarcts are the best example (see 'infarction'). The process of coagulative necrosis, with preservation of the general tissue architecture, is characteristic of hypoxic death of cells **in all tissues, except the brain**.

71

Fusobacterium necrophorum (previously *Sphaerophorus necrophorus*) is a common cause of coagulative necrosis in the livers of cattle. Other examples include muscular dystrophy in cattle and sheep associated with vitamin E deficiency; renal tubular epithelium in mercury, thalium, or uranium poisoning; in skin, mucous membrane or wound following application of concentrated phenol.

Macroscopically, the necrotic area is firm and rather dry in consistency. It has a homogeneous, opaque, cooked appearance, and is grey, white, or tan. **Microscopically**, the architectural outline of the tissue or organ is maintained but the cellular details are lost. **Result**: The area does not attract much neutrophils. As the autolytic enzymes are destroyed and leukocytes appear slowly, the dead material remains in the area for a long period of time. Ultimately, the necrotic cells are removed by fragmentation and phagocytosis of the cellular debris by the action of proteolytic lysosomal enzymes of leukocytes.

(2) **Liquefactive necrosis**: This type of necrosis is characterized by transformation of the tissue into a liquid mass in which cellular and architectural detail is lost. Whatever the pathogenesis, liquefaction completely digests the dead cells. It results from the action of powerful lysosomal enzymes. Liquefactive necrosis is characteristic of focal bacterial infections, because these agents constitute powerful stimuli to the accumulation of neutrophils. Enzymes of bacterial and leukocytic origin contribute to the digestion of dead cells. A few chemicals, such as turpentine, cause accumulation of neutrophils and the resulting liquefactive necrosis. This is the type of necrosis observed in abscesses and suppurative wound infections.

For reasons unknown, hypoxic death of cells in all tissues produces coagulative necrosis, **but in brain it produces liquefactive necrosis**. Brain tissue undergoing liquefactive necrosis is ultimately converted into a cystic structure filled with debris and fluid. In the central nervous system, liquefactive necrosis occurs in areas of infarction and traumatic injury. It is also associated with hypoxia; carbon monoxide and cyanide poisoning; thiamine deficiency in cat; vitamin E deficiency in chickens; and mouldy maize poisoning in horses. Nervous tissue is normally very soft, has little structural support, and has a very high lipid and water content. Perhaps on this account the autolytic (lysosomal) enzymes in the brain cells convert these cells into a liquid or semi-liquid mass.

Macroscopically, the tissue in the area of necrosis is liquefied; and may be watery, tenacious or semisolid in consistency. The colour

72

is usually white, yellow, or red. If the necrosis is of long standing, a connective tissue wall may be formed around the necrotic mass. **Microscopically, no architectural or cellular detail is visible in the area of necrosis**. The dead tissue is homogeneous and stains pink with eosin. If bacteria are present, neutrophils in varying degrees of disintegration are found. The entire necrotic mass is surrounded by a zone of acute or chronic inflammation depending on the length of time necrosis has been present. Necrotic tissue in the central nervous system does not contain neutrophils, unless pyogenic bacteria are present.

(3) **Caseous necrosis**: Caseous necrosis is characterized by the **conversion of dead tissue into a homogeneous granular mass resembling cheese, and by the absence of both architectural and cellular detail**. The term **'caseous'** means cheesy (L. caseus = cheese) and is derived from the white and cheesy appearance of the area of necrosis. Caseous necrosis is encountered mainly with tuberculosis in animals, and caseous lymphadenitis in sheep. The cheesy appearance in tuberculosis has been attributed to the capsule of the tuberculous bacillus *Mycobacterium tuberculosis*, which contains lipopolysaccharides, but the exact relationship of this material with dead cells is not well understood. Oesophagostomiasis in sheep produces multiple focal areas of caseous necrosis.

Macroscopically, the area of necrosis is a granular amorphous material resembling cheese. The mass is dry but creamy in consistency. It is soft, friable, and white-grey in colour. Calcium salts are frequently deposited in the dead tissue. The caseous mass is enclosed within a connective tissue capsule. **Microscopically**, the necrotic focus is composed of structureless, amorphous granular debris enclosed within a distinctive ring of granulomatous inflammation (see 'granulomatous inflammation'). Neither architectural nor cellular detail is present. Calcification commonly occurs in the necrotic areas, especially in **sheep** and **cattle**.

(4) **Fat necrosis**: Fat necrosis is the **death of adipose tissue** within the living individual. There are **three types**: **pancreatic, traumatic,** and **nutritional**.

Pancreatic fat necrosis is the death of adipose tissue in the vicinity of the pancreas due to the action of **lipases**. It is caused by some injury to the pancreas or its duct. Acute pancreatitis is the most common cause in the **dog, pig,** and **sheep**. Primary or secondary tumours of the pancreas may also induce this necrosis. Powerful lipases released from the pancreas destroy not only the pancreatic substance itself, but also the adipose tissue in and around the pancreas and throughout the peritoneal cavity. The activated pancreatic enzymes liquefy fat cell membranes and hydrolyze the triglyceride esters contained within them. The released fatty acids combine with calcium to produce grossly visible chalky white areas (**fat saponification**).

Macroscopically, the necrotic fat appears as white or yellowish white, chalky, opaque masses in the interstitial adipose tissue of the pancreas and the peripancreatic fat. A zone of acute or chronic inflammation appears around the necrotic areas. The connective tissue may undergo metaplasia and produce **bone**, seen in the abdominal fat of the **pig** and **cattle**. Antemortem fat necrosis must be differentiated from the postmortem fat autolysis and putrefaction. In the postmortem change, inflammation and calcification are absent which can occur only in the living individual. **Microscopically**, only shadowy outlines of necrotic fat cells may be seen, with basophilic calcium deposits, and a surrounding inflammatory reaction.

Traumatic fat necrosis is the death of adipose tissue in an area of mechanical injury. It commonly occurs in subcutaneous adipose tissue due to mechanical injuries during working, fighting, or exercising. Examples: in canine from dog bites, in backs of fat pigs from injury produced by erysipelas, perivaginal fat in cattle from mechanical injury during parturition, breast adipose tissue in humans from trauma. **Macroscopically**, the pancreatic fat appears as firm, opaque, chalky mass in the area of injury, surrounded by a zone of acute or chronic inflammatory reaction. An area of fat necrosis should not be mistaken for an abscess or a wound infection.

Nutritional fat necrosis is a necrobiotic alteration in fat that is associated with extreme emaciation and debility. This form of fat necrosis occurs in starving or debilitated animals, usually observed in **cattle** and **sheep** in tuberculosis and Johne's disease (paratuberculosis). The necrosis may occur throughout the body but is most common in the abdominal fat (mesenteric, omental, and perirenal). **Macroscopically**, the fat is opaque, chalky white, and usually firm. It may undergo calcification. Such a change in mesenteric fat may immobilize the intestinal tract, and interfere with the passage of ingesta. **Microscopically**, the adipose cells contain a pale pink (H & E stain) slightly granular material in which numerous clefts and crystals are seen. The clefts are the site of fatty acid crystals, derived from the breakdown of fat to fatty acids and glycerol. Glycerol being soluble in body fluids disappears. The fatty acid crystals dissolve in the fat solvents used in histopathology, and thus leave the clefts. When calcification occurs, the small spherical masses present stain blue with haematoxylin. A chronic inflammatory reaction occurs at the junction of the necrotic and living tissue. Nutritional fat necrosis must be differentiated from fat autolysis and putrefaction. In the latter, both hyperaemia and calcification are absent which can occur only in the living individual.

APOPTOSIS

Apoptosis is a distinctive and important method of cell death. This pattern of cell death is **different from necrosis**, although it does share some features (see Table 2).

Apoptosis was first recognized in 1972 by its characteristic morphology, and was named after the Greek word **'apoptosis'** meaning **'a falling away from'** (G. apo = away from; G. ptosis = falling). **Apoptosis** (pronounced with a silent 'p', as **'apotosis'**) is a form of cell death designed to eliminate unwanted host cells through activation of a coordinated, internally programmed, series of events brought about by a set of gene products. It is responsible for the **programmed cell death** in several important **physiological as well as pathological processes**. These include:

(1) The programmed destruction of cells **during embryogenesis** (development of an embryo), as occurs in **organogenesis** (development of organs).

(2) Hormone-dependent physiological involution, such as involution of the endometrium during menstrual cycle in humans, or the lactating breast (mammary gland in animals) after weaning, or pathological atrophy, as in the prostate after castration in humans.

(3) Cell deletion in proliferating populations, such as intestinal crypt epithelium, or cell death in tumours.

(4) Death of neutrophils during an acute inflammatory response.

(5) Deletion of autoreactive B- and T-cells: More than 95% of B-cells die in the bursa of Fabricius in the chicken (bone marrow in mammals) and thymocytes in the thymus during maturation! (see 'Immunological tolerance'). Other examples from immunology include cell death induced by cytotoxic T-cells, and cell death of cytokine-starved lymphocytes (both B- and T-cells).

(6) A variety of injurious stimuli that produce necrosis, but when given in low doses (i.e., mild stimuli) produce apoptosis. For example, heat, radiation, cytotoxic anti-cancer drugs, and hypoxia can induce apoptosis **if the irritant is mild**, but large doses of the same stimuli result in necrosis. **The mild injurious stimuli cause irreparable DNA damage**. This, in turn, triggers cell suicide pathway, for example, through the tumour suppressor protein TP53 (discussed later).

Failure of cells to undergo physiological apoptosis may result in abnormal development, unhindered tumour proliferation, or autoimmune disease (see 'Neoplasia' and 'autoimmune diseases').

Before the **mechanisms of apoptosis** are discussed, it would be better if first we get familiar with the **morphological changes** characteristic of this process.

Morphological Features

Apoptosis usually involves **single cells or small clusters of cells** that appear in H & E stained sections as round or oval masses with intensely eosinophilic cytoplasm. The following morphological features characterize cells undergoing apoptosis. **They are best seen with the electron microscope** (Fig. 10).

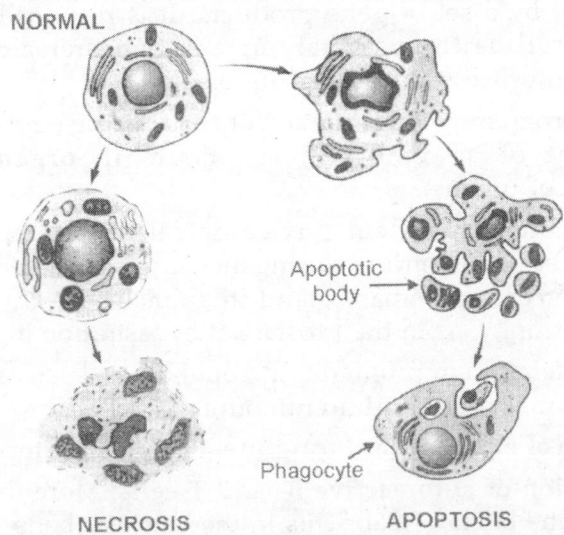

Fig. 10. The sequential ultrastructural (electronmicroscopic) changes seen in coagulative necrosis (left) and apoptosis (right). In apoptosis, the changes consist of nuclear chromatin condensation and fragmentation, followed by cytoplasmic budding and phagocytosis of the thrown out **apoptotic bodies**. Changes in coagulative necrosis include chromatin clumping, organellar swelling, and membrane damage.

(1) **Cell shrinkage**: The cell is smaller in size. The cytoplasm is dense, and the organelles are more tightly packed.

(2) **Chromatin condensation: This is the most characteristic feature of apoptosis.** The nuclear chromatin is condensed, and it aggregates peripherally, under the nuclear membrane, into well-defined dense masses of various shapes and sizes. The nucleus itself may break up, producing two or more fragments. The karyorrhexis (fragmentation) occurs at a molecular level. It is reflected as fragmentation of DNA into nucleosome-sized pieces, through the activation of **endonucleases**. (A **nucleosome** is a repeating subunit of chromatin that consists of a complex of DNA and histone).

(3) **Formation of cytoplasmic blebs (buds) and apoptotic bodies**: The apoptotic cells rapidly shrink, then show extensive surface blebbing (bud formation), and finally undergo fragmentation into a number of membrane-bound apoptotic bodies (vesicles) composed of cytosol (fluid portion of the cytoplasm) and tightly packed organelles, with or without nuclear fragments (Fig. 10).

(4) **Phagocytosis of apoptotic cells or bodies** by nearby healthy cells, either parenchymal cells or macrophages (Fig. 10). Because apoptotic bodies are quickly extruded (thrown out) and phagocytosed and degraded within lysosomes, **even significant apoptosis may be microscopically not visible**. Also, the nearby cells migrate or proliferate to replace the space earlier occupied by the apoptotic cell. **Moreover, apoptosis, in contrast to necrosis, does not produce inflammation**. This makes it more difficult to detect apoptosis microscopically.

Table 2 shows the differences between necrosis and apoptosis.

Table 2. Differences between coagulative necrosis and apoptosis

	Coagulative necrosis	Apoptosis
1. Stimuli	Hypoxia, toxins	Physiological and pathological factors
2. Microscopic appearance	Cellular swelling, coagulative necrosis, disruption of organelles	Single cells, chromatin condensation, apoptotic bodies
3. DNA breakdown	Random, diffuse	Inter-nucleosomal
4. Mechanisms	ATP depletion, membrane injury, free radical damage	Gene activation, endonucleases, proteases
5. Tissue reaction	Inflammation	No inflammation, phagocytosis of apoptotic bodies

Mechanisms of Apoptosis

This aspect of apoptosis is the subject of intense investigation. The basic process involves **four components**.

(1) **Signalling**: Apoptosis may be triggered (initiated) by **a variety of stimuli**. These range from intrinsic embryonic signals (e.g., during development), selected injurious stimuli (e.g., radiation), a lack of growth factor, specific receptor-ligand interaction, or release of granzymes from cytotoxic T-cells (see Fig. 11). These apoptotic stimuli generate **signals** that are transmitted through the plasma membrane. The **transmembrane signals** may either suppress already existing death programme, or initiate a death cascade (i.e., a sequence of events leading to death). The most important of this latter group which initiate death cascade are those that belong to the tumour necrosis factor receptor (TNFR) superfamily of plasma membrane molecules (discussed later). These include FAS and TNF surface receptor molecules. These plasma membrane receptors share a **'death domain'** protein sequence present within the cell. When this protein sequence is reduced to a few units (oligomerized), usually into three units (trimerized), **it leads to activation of initiator caspases and a cascade of enzyme activation culminating in cell death** (Fig. 11) (discussed next).

(2) **Control and integration**: This is performed by **specific proteins**. These proteins connect the original death signals (described under signalling) with the execution programme (death programme). These proteins are important because their actions may result in either success or failure of original death signals. There are **two broad pathways** of their action: (1) **Direct transmission** of death signals by specific **adapter proteins** to the execution mechanism. Examples: Fas-Fas ligand model and target cell killing by cytotoxic T-lymphocytes (discussed later). (A ligand is a specific chemical group or molecule that binds to its **receptor,** i.e., receiver. A receptor is the chemical group or molecule on the cell surface (or in the cell interior) that receives ligand), and (2) **Second pathway** of apoptotic death involves members of the *BCL-2* **family of proteins** (Fig. 11). These proteins play a major role in apoptosis **by regulating mitochondrial permeability.** *BCL-2* **is situated in the outer mitochondrial membrane** (Fig. 12). Its function is regulated by other family members. These other related proteins, by binding to *BCL-2*, can alter *BCL-2*'s activity. These proteins either promote apoptosis (cell death), e.g., *BAX, BAD,* or inhibit cell death, e.g., *BCL-X$_L$* (Fig. 11). *BCL-2* **suppresses apoptosis**

in two ways: (1) By its direct action on mitochondria. **It prevents increased mitochondrial permeability**. (2) By effects mediated through interactions with other proteins.

However, first, let us examine the significance of **mitochondrial permeability**. It was discussed earlier under cell injury (see 'mitochondrial damage') that a variety of stimuli (Ca^{++}, free radicals, etc.) can damage mitochondria by forming channels (pores) known as **'mitochondrial permeability transitions'**. Formation of these pores in the inner mitochondrial membrane reduces membrane potential, resulting in diminished ATP production and mitochondrial swelling. **The signals also cause increased permeability of outer mitochondrial membranes releasing the apoptotic trigger (initiator), cytochrome c, from mitochondria into cytosol** (fluid portion of the cytoplasm) (Fig. 12). Cytochrome c is located between inner and outer mitochondrial membrane.

Let us now understand how *BCL-2* mediates its effects through interactions with other proteins. Apart from its direct action on mitochondria, *BCL-2* can also suppress apoptosis by binding proteins from the cytosol and segregating them on the mitochondrial membrane. Important among the *BCL-2* binding protein is the **'pro-apoptotic protease-activating factor or Apaf-1'**. When cytochrome c is released from mitochondria by death signals, it binds to certain cytosolic proteins, **mainly Apaf-1, and activates them** (Fig. 12A). **This event first triggers activation of initiator caspases and then execution caspases, and sets in motion the proteolytic events that kill cell** (discussed next) (Fig. 12A). Thus, *BCL-2* **binding protects** because it segretes Apaf-1 and inhibits its caspase-triggering function, **so that caspase activation does not occur, even if cytochrome c has leaked out of mitochondria** (Fig. 12B). Also, *BCL-2* prevents increased mitochondrial permeability. **It is thought that mitochondrial permeability is determined by the ratio of pro-apoptotic and anti-apoptotic members of the *BCL-2* family in the mitochondrial membrane.**

The **two ways of the anti-apoptotic actions of *BCL-2***: (1) direct prevention of cytochrome c release, and (2) inhibition of Apaf-induced caspase activation despite cytochrome release, **are not mutually exclusive**. Moreover, other important proteins are also involved in apoptotic regulation, one of the most important being TP53 (p53) protein.

(3) **Execution (Death):** The final pathway of apoptosis is characterized by certain distinctive biochemical changes. These changes underlie the structural alterations described earlier. Some of these events may be seen in necrosis, but other alterations are more specific of apoptosis. These events result from the **synthesis and/or activation of a number of cytosolic catabolic (destructive) enzymes.** The final execution (death) pathways are:

(i) **Protein cleavage (breakup):** A specific feature of apoptosis is **protein hydrolysis.** This is brought about by a newly discovered family of **cysteine proteases,** called **'caspases'.** The term **'caspase'** is based on two properties of this family. The **'c',** indicates a cysteine protease mechanism, that is, they all have the amino acid cysteine in their active site, and **'aspase'** refers to their unique ability to cleave (split) after aspartic acid residues. The **caspase family** can be divided functionally into **two basic groups:** (1) **Initiator caspases,** and (2) **Execution caspases** (see Fig. 11). **Initiator caspases** include caspase 9 which binds to Apaf-1, and caspase 8 which is triggered by Fas-Fas ligand interactions (discussed later). After an initiator caspase is triggered, the enzymic death programme is set in motion. **Execution caspases** cleave the nuclear structure and cytoskeletal proteins, and this forms the basis for the characteristic nuclear and cytoplasmic changes seen in apoptotic cells.

Over-expression of any of the caspases results in apoptosis, suggesting that under normal circumstances they must be tightly controlled. Activation of one or more of such caspase enzymes leads to activation of **other proteases,** ultimately resulting in **cell death (cell suicide).** For example, **endonuclease activation** results in the characteristic DNA fragmentation (Fig. 11). (**Endonuclease** is an enzyme that breaks down a nucleotide chain (of nucleic acid) into two or more shorter chains).

$\longrightarrow$

Fig. 11. Events in apoptosis. A variety of stimuli (1-5) can induce apoptosis. Some stimuli (such as cytotoxic T-cells) directly activate execution caspases (5). Others act through adapter proteins and initiator caspases (4), or through mitochondrial release of cytochrome c (3). Regulatory proteins of the BCL-2 family can either inhibit or promote cell death. Execution caspases activate latent cytoplasmic endonucleases and proteases that degrade cytoskeletal and nuclear proteins. This results in a cascade of intracellular degradation, including breakdown of the cytoskeleton and endonuclease-mediated fragmentation of nuclear chromatin. The end result is the formation of apoptotic bodies containing various intracellular organelles and other cytosolic constituents. These bodies express new ligands that mediate phagocytic cell binding and uptake.

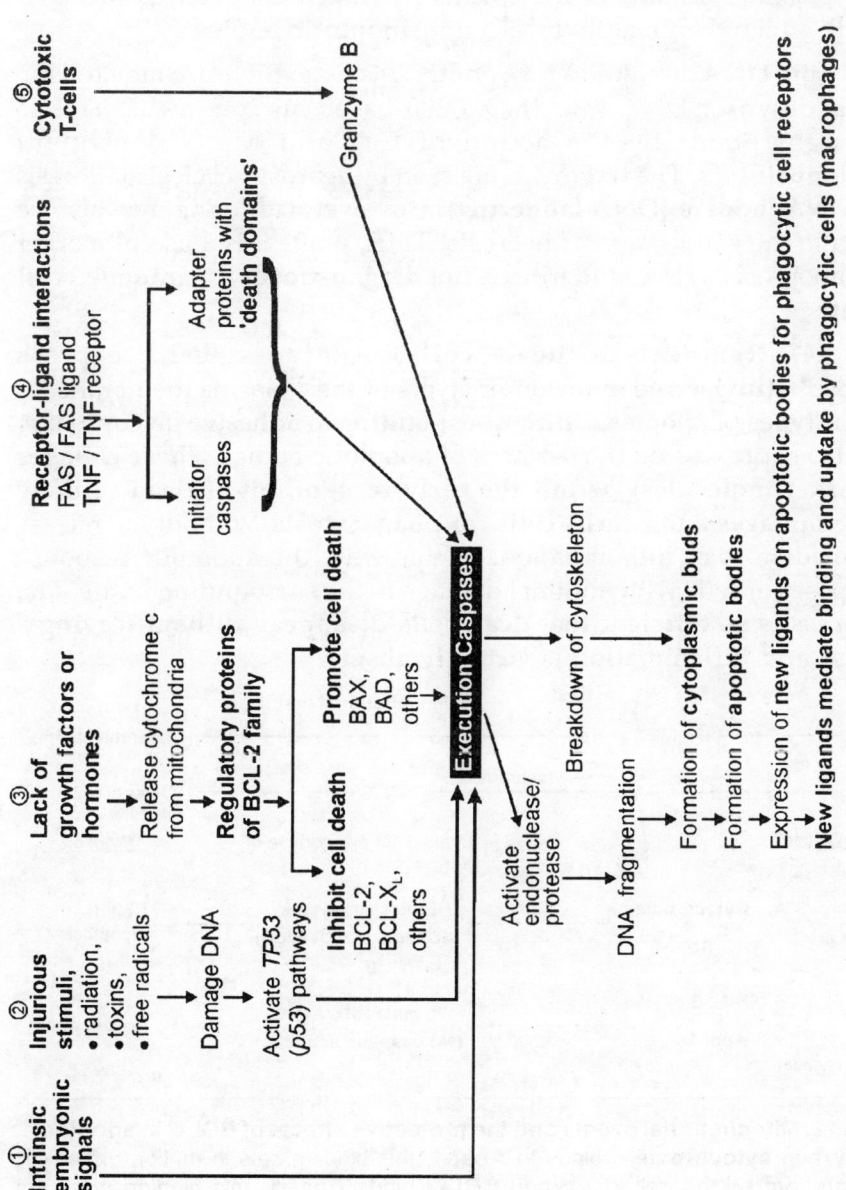

Fig. 11

(ii) **Protein cross-linking**: Extensive protein cross-linking brought about by **transglutaminase activation** converts soluble cytoplasmic proteins into a covalently linked condensed shrunken shell, which then readily breaks into **apoptotic bodies**.

(iii) **DNA breakdown**: Apoptotic cells exhibit a characteristic breakdown of DNA into 180 to 200 base pair fragments. This is brought about by the action of Ca^{++} and Mg^{++}- dependent **endonucleases**. The fragments are seen by agarose gel electrophoresis as **DNA ladders (DNA laddering)**. However, laddering may also be seen in the early stages of **necrosis**. Thus, while it is a useful marker for apoptosis, **DNA laddering is not diagnostic for programmed cell death.**

(4) **Removal of dead cells**: Apoptotic cells express **phosphatidylserine** in the outer layers of their plasma membrane. In some types of apoptosis, **thrombospondin**, an adhesive glycoprotein, is also expressed on the surfaces of apoptotic bodies. **These changes (marker molecules) permit the early recognition of dead cells by macrophages and nearby cells for phagocytosis**, without the release of mediators of inflammation. In this way, the apoptotic response disposes of cells with minimal damage to the surrounding tissue. **The process is so efficient that dead cells disappear without leaving a trace, and inflammation is virtually absent.**

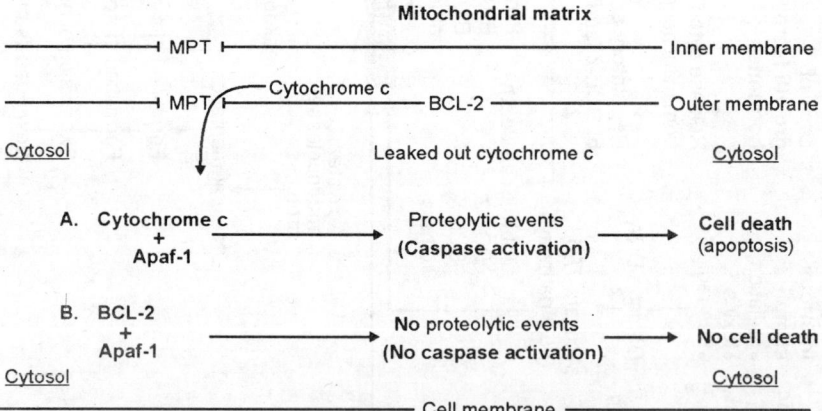

Fig. 12. Mitochondrial events and the protective effects of BCL-2 in apoptosis. (A) When **cytochrome c** binds to **Apaf-1**, this binding sets in motion proteolytic events that kill the cell. (B) When **BCL-2** binds **Apaf-1**, this binding does not trigger proteolytic events, and **there is no cell death, even if cytochrome c has leaked out of mitochondria. MPT** = mitochondrial permeability transition. **Apaf-1** = Pro-apoptotic protein-activating factor.

Specific examples of apoptosis

1. **Signalling by tumour necrosis factor (TNF) family of receptors**: The TNFR family includes members that bind not only the important cytokine TNF, but other significant ligands as well. Some initiate apoptosis, some cell proliferation, and others initiate both. The important members of the sub-family of TNFR include **Fas** and **TNFR**. Both exhibit exactly similar **'death recognition domains'**. Two important examples of cell death are mediated by this sub-family. Death signalling in both requires binding of receptors with cytoplasmic **'adapter proteins'** (see Fig. 11) that show corresponding 'death domains', that is, **FADD** (or Fas-associated proteins with a death domain) in the case of Fas, and **TRADD** (TNFR-adapter protein with a death domain) in the case of TNFR (i.e., TNF receptor). These adapter proteins through separate **'death effector domains'**, in turn, bind to corresponding domains in initiator caspases. **This triggers the executive phase**. The **two examples** of such cell death are:

(i) **Fas-Fas ligand-mediated apoptosis**: This type of apoptosis is caused by a cell surface receptor called **Fas** (CD95). A membrane-bound ligand, called **Fas ligand** (FasL or CD95L), produced by cells of the immune system, **binds to Fas on T-cells and activates a death programme**. This system is important in eliminating lymphocytes from an immune reaction, thereby limiting the host response (see Chapter 9).

(ii) **TNF-induced apoptosis**: Activation of one of the **TNF receptors (TNFR)** by the cytokine **TNF** can lead to apoptosis by causing association of receptor with the adapter protein **TRADD**. As with Fas-Fas ligand system, TRADD, in turn, binds to FADD and leads to apoptosis through caspase activation, as discussed.

2. **Cytotoxic T-lymphocyte-stimulated apoptosis**: CTLs recognize foreign antigens on the surface of host cells. **On recognition, they express Fas ligand on their surfaces and kill target cells by ligation (binding) of Fas receptors**, as described earlier. Alternatively, CTLs cause apoptosis of target cells by secreting **perforin**, a transmembrane pore-forming molecule, and the release of cytoplasmic granules into target cells. These granules contain the important enzyme serine protease **granzyme B**. **This enzyme is able to directly activate execution caspases** (Fig. 11). **In this way, the cytotoxic T-lymphocyte kills target cells by directly inducing the effector phase of apoptosis**, without the upstream signalling events (see 'T-cell-mediated cytotoxicity', Chapter 9).

3. **Apoptosis after growth factor withdrawal**: Survival of many cells depends on the supply of cytokines or growth factors. **In the absence of growth factor, the cells undergo apoptosis** (Fig. 11). On withdrawal of growth factor, pro-apoptotic members of the BCL-2 family of proteins move from the cytosol to the outer mitochondrial membrane and change the ratio of pro-apoptotic and anti-apoptotic members of the BCL-2 family at this site. **This change causes increased permeability of the membrane, leakage of cytochrome c, and activation of the proteolytic cascade**, as described earlier.

4. **DNA damage-mediated apoptosis**: Exposure of cells to radiation, or chemotherapeutic agents, induces apoptosis by damaging DNA (**genotoxic stress**) and activating tumour suppressor gene *TP53* (previously *p53*). *TP53* accumulates when DNA is damaged and arrests the cell cycle (at G1 phase) to allow additional time for repair (see Chapter 5 and 8). **However, if the repair process fails, *TP53* triggers apoptosis** (Fig. 11). Thus, *TP53* normally stimulates apoptosis, but when it is mutated or absent, as it is in certain cancers, it favours cell survival. Thus, *TP53* seems to serve as a critical **'life or death switch'** in the case of **genotoxic stress**. The DNA damage induces apoptosis through execution caspases (Fig. 11).

To end this discussion of apoptosis, recently a concept of **dysregulated apoptosis ('too little or too much')** has emerged to explain a wide range of diseases. (1) **Disorders associated with inhibited apoptosis and increased cell survival**: Here, a low rate of apoptosis may prolong survival of abnormal cells. These accumulated cells can give rise to: (i) Cancers, especially those carcinomas with *TP53* mutations, and (ii) **Autoimmune disorders**, which could arise if autoreactive lymphocytes are not removed after an immune response (see Chapter 9). (2) **Disorders associated with increased apoptosis and excessive cell death**: These disorders are characterized by a great loss of normal or protective cells and include(i) **neurodegenerative diseases** manifested by loss of specific sets of neurons, (ii) **ischaemic injury**, such as in myocardial infarction and stroke, and (iii) **virus-induced lymphocyte depletion**, such as occurs in acquired immunodeficiency syndrome (AIDS) in humans (Chapter 9).

To summarize, apoptosis is a distinctive form of cell death manifested by **characteristic chromatin condensation and DNA fragmentation**. Its function is the deletion of cells in the normal development, organogenesis, immune function, and tissue growth, but it can also be induced by pathological stimuli. The mechanism of apoptosis has **several key stages**; (1) There are **many pathways of cell death**. (2) There is a **control stage**, in which the apoptotic level is established by the relative expression and activity of different **positive and negative regulators, including the BCL-2 family of proteins**. (3) There is an **execution stage**, involving the activation of caspases that perform the **terminal proteolysis. Apoptotic bodies are then engulfed by macrophages by receptor-mediated phagocytosis**. Dysregulation of this process may contribute to a variety of disease states.

GANGRENE

Gangrene is the invasion and putrefaction of necrotic tissue by saprophytic bacteria. Aetiology: Gangrene is seen most often in the lungs, intestine, mammary gland, heavy muscles of the thigh and shoulder, and the extremities. (1) **Lungs**: Gangrene occurs most commonly from **faulty drenching of medicines**. The medicine is often quite irritating and injures the lung. In addition, it carries bacteria with it into the lungs. As a result of the lung injury and invasion of the necrotic tissue by saprophytic organisms, gangrene occurs. Pulmonary gangrene can also be caused by **improper insertion of a stomach tube**, in which case medicines are poured into the lungs rather than the stomach. In paralysis and infectious diseases of the throat, food may pass into the trachea and produce gangrene. (2) **Intestine: In the horse** infarction results from **a verminous thrombus** in the **anterior mesenteric artery**, or the acute local passive hyperaemia associated with a malposition of the viscera (torsion, volvulus, or intussusception) may cause gangrene of the intestinal tract. The vascular disturbance causes necrosis of the intestinal wall, and the necrotic tissue is then invaded with saprophytic bacteria found in the intestinal contents. (3) **Extremities**: Gangrene of the leg, ear, tail, wattle, or comb is associated with freezing. Freezing temperatures cause coagulative necrosis of tissue that is later invaded with saprophytic bacteria. Certain drugs or plants (ergot and mould on fescue grass) contain active principles which cause arterial spasms and restrict the blood flow. Because of the ischaemia, necrosis of the extremities occurs, and later the tissues are invaded with bacteria. **Senile gangrene** may occur in humans in old age from arteriosclerosis which causes ischaemia. Diabetic gangrene also occurs from narrowing of arteries. Bacteria grow well in the tissue due to their high sugar content.

85

Gangrene is of two types: **dry gangrene** and **moist gangrene**. Whether dry occurs or moist, depends on the **amount of moisture** as well as the **temperature of the tissue**. When the coagulative necrosis is dominant, the process is dry gangrene, and when the liquefactive necrosis is more pronounced, it is moist or wet gangrene.

Dry Gangrene

Dry gangrene is usually observed in the extremities. When necrosis occurs, circulation is no longer maintained. The necrotic tissue then gets dehydrated by evaporation and becomes dry. Since bacteria require **moisture** for growth, invasion and spread of bacteria in the area are slow. Besides moisture, the second determining factor for dry gangrene is **temperature** of the extremity. When the tissue is dead and circulation absent, the part becomes cool. The growth of bacteria is suppressed. Invasion and spread of bacteria through the necrotic tissue are therefore slow.

Macroscopically, the area is dry, shrivelled and appears mummified as a result of dehydration. It is reddish brown, green, grey or black in colour. The colour depends on the amount of iron sulphide formed. The disintegrating erythrocytes liberate haemoglobin. Bacterial putrefaction of the dead tissue produces hydrogen sulphide. When hydrogen sulphide comes in contact with iron of haemoglobin, **iron sulphide** (a black pigment) **is produced**. Since it produces black discoloration of false melanin, the change is called **pseudomelanosis**. The area also has a very putrid odour due to hydrogen sulphide. The gangrene extends in the direction of the body until a point is reached where sufficient circulation is present to keep the part alive. At this point, the dead tissue is demarcated sharply from the living by a line of severe inflammatory reaction. This is an attempt by the body's defences to prevent the bacteria from spreading. In addition, the defence line also tries to prevent the entrance of toxins formed in the dead tissue from being absorbed by the living tissue. The neutrophils and macrophages in the inflammatory zone digest the necrotic tissue by their hydrolytic enzymes. The gap is then repaired by granulation tissue formation. **Microscopically**, a structureless necrotic area, stained pink, is seen with numerous bacteria. A few gas bubbles are evident by clear spaces. An acute inflammatory reaction is present at the junction of the living and dead tissue.

Moist Gangrene

Moist gangrene occurs in the internal organs where there is an abundance of moisture and the temperature is higher. With optimum conditions of moisture and warmth, the growth and spread of saprophytic bacteria are very rapid. The spread is particularly important when moist gangrene involves the intestinal tract, because numerous bacteria capable of invading the intestinal wall are contained within the contents of the intestine. When the intestinal wall gets necrotic, rupture occurs and the faecal contents are discharged into the peritoneal cavity, spreading microorganisms throughout the viscera. The course of events is extremely rapid, and death occurs from septicaemia, toxaemia, and shock.

Macroscopically, the gangrenous tissue is moist; and red, green, grey or black in colour as a result of iron sulphide formation. The odour is extremely offensive because of the abundance of hydrogen sulphide and other decomposition products associated with putrefaction. The putrefaction process produces gas, and numerous gas bubbles are present within the tissues. The intestine is distended with large quantities of gas. There is no sharp line of demarcation between the living and dead tissue.

Gas Gangrene, Malignant Oedema and Blackquarter (Blackleg)

These are specific types of moist gangrene frequently observed in humans and animals, and are due to invasion of the tissue by various clostridial organisms (*Clostridium perfringens* (previously *C. welchii*), *C. chauvoei*, *C. septicum*, and *C. novyi*). These organisms are inhabitants of the soil and the digestive tract. They enter into the wounds of various types, e.g., shearing, castration, docking, and ear notching. The injury to tissue results in necrosis, and in this necrotic tissue these organisms grow and multiply. They produce toxins that kill the surrounding tissue. They then invade the necrotic tissue, spread throughout the body and bring about the death. The same series of events occurs in blackquarter and malignant oedema in cattle and sheep. Cattle and sheep are injured by other animals by kicks, horn thrusts, or bunts (head thrusts). Blackquarter and malignant oedema are described in detail elsewhere.

In humans, gas gangrene usually begins in large traumatic wounds with pyogenic infections. *C. perfringens*, the agent of gas gangrene, literally digests host tissues, including the relatively resistant collagens by its **collagenases**. This helps in the spread of infection. The **clostridial lecithinases** attack cell membranes. Thus, gas gangrene is characterized by marked oedema and enzymatic necrosis of involved muscle cells. Gas bubbles caused by fermentative reactions appear early in the gangrenous tissues. Numerous bacteria are present within the exudate.

Results of Necrosis and Gangrene

Necrosis may terminate in several ways:

1. **Liquefaction and removal** by the neutrophils, lymph, and blood occur when the area of necrosis is small. When the area is large, removal is achieved as described below in No. 2.

2. **Liquefaction of the tissue and formation of a cyst** occur when the area of necrosis is large, and the necrotic tissue is converted into fluid by cellular enzymes. Since the fluid is irritating, a protective wall of connective tissue is formed around it.

3. **Liquefaction, abscessation, and discharge** of the necrotic material occur when pyogenic bacteria invade the necrotic tissue.

4. **Encapsulation without liquefaction** occurs when tissue and cellular enzymes capable of liquefying the necrotic area are not present (coagulative and caseous necrosis). Since necrotic tissue acts as an irritant, a connective tissue capsule is formed around the mass.

5. **Sloughing and desquamation** of the connective tissue may occur if the external surfaces are involved. This may occur in digestive tract, or when burns involve the skin.

6. **Organization of the necrotic tissue** occurs when it is invaded by new blood vessels, fibroblasts, and macrophages. Macrophages digest necrotic tissue, and the area is replaced by new vascular fibrous tissue, leaving a scar. This is known as **organization**.

7. **Calcification** of the necrotic material may occur. For the mechanisms involved, refer to dystrophic calcification.

8. **Metaplasia** may occur in the necrotic tissue. Appearance of bone is seen in fat necrosis, especially in the abdominal fat of pigs.

9. **Death of the individual** is the usual result if the moist gangrene is present. Death may or may not occur if dry gangrene is present. Death or survival with different types of necrosis will depend on the organ involved, location of the lesion within the organ, and the extent of damage. If a vital organ like heart, brain or lung is involved, death will be most likely outcome.

Postmortem Changes

As soon as an animal dies certain changes occur which are known as **postmortem changes**. It is important to know these changes because every animal that dies shows some of these alterations. **One should therefore be able to differentiate postmortem changes from lesions found in disease**. Moreover, the changes become more advanced with the passage of time. But before we discuss these changes, let us first consider the factors which influence the rapidity of their onset. These include: (1) **Environmental temperature**: Since increased summer temperatures increase the rate of enzymatic and bacterial activity, animals decompose very rapidly in the summer. Animals can be preserved for long periods with modern refrigeration. (2) **Size of the animal**: The larger the animal, the more rapidly will postmortem changes occur. This is because the large animals require a longer period of time before the body heat is dissipated. (3) **External insulation**: Thick cutaneous coverings of fur, feathers, hair, or wool prevent heat dissipation. As such, sheep decompose very rapidly because of insulating wool. (4) **Nutritional state of the animal**: Fat is an insulating substance. The fatter the animal the slower will be the loss of heat and the more rapid will be the rate of decomposition. Rigor mortis occurs more rapidly in fat animals than in emaciated animals. (5) **Species of animal**: Apart from the size and insulation, the species of animal also determines the character of the flesh. Pig flesh is soft, moist, and contains fat. Therefore, the rate of decomposition is rapid. On the other hand, horse flesh is dry and rather firm. Therefore, the decomposition is relatively slow.

The postmortem changes include:

1. **Autolysis** is the digestion of tissues by their own cellular enzymes. When tissue is fixed or embalmed cellular enzymes are inactivated by formalin or alcohol and autolysis is prevented.

2. **Putrefaction** is the decomposition of tissues by enzymes of saprophytic bacteria. After death, bacteria from the digestive tract and body surfaces invade, multiply and eventually digest the tissue with their enzymes.

3. **Rigor mortis** is the shortening and contraction of muscles that occur after death, and result in stiffness and immobilization of the body. It begins in the anterior portion and progresses in a posterior direction (head, neck, trunk, and limbs). It usually appears 1 to 8 hours after death. Its appearance is quickened by high external temperatures (summer), violent exercise (racing, fighting, or

struggling), or when violent muscular contractions have occurred as in tetanus or strychnine poisoning. It is retarded by low temperatures (winter). In emaciated animals, it appears slowly, it is never very pronounced, and may not appear at all.

Rigor mortis disappears in the same order it appeared (head, neck, trunk, and limbs). The muscular immobility usually disappears 20 to 30 hours after death. Once it disappears, it does not return. The rapidity with which it appears and disappears is used to estimate the length of time the animal has been dead. **This is of great importance in medico-legal (forensic) cases.**

4. **Postmortem clotting of blood** is the coagulation of blood in vessels after death. In dead animals the endothelial cells begin to degenerate and liberate thromboplastin which then clots the blood within the heart, arteries, and veins. In anthrax, however, no clotting occurs because fibrinolysin produced by the bacteria liquefies fibrin. In sweet clover poisoning also clotting does not occur since prothrombin activity is inhibited.

5. **Imbibition with haemoglobin** is the staining of tissue with haemoglobin. After death, the erythrocytes are haemolysed by cellular and bacterial enzymes, and haemoglobin in liberated. Being soluble in body fluid, it diffuses into the surrounding tissues and stains them red.

6. **Hypostatic congestion** is the accumulation of blood in the ventral portion of organs and the entire carcass due to the influence of gravity (see Chapter 6).

7. **Pseudomelanosis** is the appearance of grey, green, or black pigment in the tissues after death. Hydrogen sulphide produced during putrefaction combines with the iron to form iron sulphide, a black pigment. The concentration of this pigment and its combination with other tissue pigments result in a variety of shades of green, grey, and black.

8. **Imbibition with bile** is the yellow pigmentation of tissue occurring near the gallbladder when bile pigments diffuse into the surrounding tissue.

9. **Postmortem emphysema** is the accumulation of gas in tissues as the result of bacterial fermentation.

10. **Rupture of organs and tissues** occurs when gases produced cause progressive distension of body structures until they burst. This

usually occurs in stomach, intestine, diaphragm, and ventral abdominal wall.

11. **Displacement of organs** occurs when the dead animal is rolled over or moved. The intestine is usually displaced. This must be differentiated from antemortem malposition of the viscera (volvulus and torsion). Displaced intestine will show no passive hyperaemia while the displacements occurring during life will show acute local passive hyperaemia. A loop of intestine may also pass through a tear in the diaphragm into the thoracic cavity. If the ventral abdominal wall ruptures, portions of viscera may pass through the rent (tear) and appear externally.

Pathological Calcification

Pathological calcification is a common process in a wide variety of disease states. The amount of calcium in bones, tissues, cells, and fluids of the body changes constantly. Its concentration in the blood fluctuates within rather narrow limits and in general averages about 10 mg per 100 ml of blood (10 mg percent). Calcium exists in the blood in a supersaturated solution to meet rapid and sudden body requirements. The amount of calcium in the blood is associated with parathyroid activity. When it is low, there is increased parathyroid activity that causes calcium to be removed from the skeleton to restore blood calcium to a normal amount. When calcium content of the blood decreases to 8 mg percent, excitability occurs, when to 6 mg percent, the animal goes into tetany, and when it reaches 3 mg percent, the animal dies. On the other hand, if the calcium rises to 12 mg percent or higher, the excess precipitates in various tissues.

Definition: Pathological calcification is the abnormal deposition of calcium salts, together with smaller amounts of iron, magnesium, and other minerals, in tissues other than the bone. It is of **two types**: (1) **Dystrophic** (or **local**), and (2) **Metastatic** (or **general**).

Dystrophic or Local Calcification

When the deposition occurs in dead (necrotic) or dying tissues, it is called dystrophic calcification (G. dys + trophe = faulty nutrition). It occurs in a **focal area of the body**. Dystrophic calcification may occur despite normal serum levels of calcium, and in the absence of derangements in calcium metabolism.

Pathogenesis: The pathogenesis of dystrophic calcification ultimately leads to the formation of crystalline **calcium phosphate**.

91

This occurs in **two phases**: **initiation** (or **nucleation**) and **propagation** (or **extension**), both of which may occur either within the cells or extracellularly. **Initiation in extracellular sites** occurs in membrane-bound vesicles about 200 nm in diameter. In normal cartilage and bone, they are known as **matrix vesicles**, and **in pathological calcification they are derived from degenerating cells**. It is thought that calcium is initially concentrated in these vesicles by its affinity for membrane lipids, while phosphates accumulate from the action of membrane-bound phosphatases. **Initiation of intracellular calcification** occurs in the mitochondria of dead or dying cells that have lost their ability to regulate intracellular calcium. After initiation in either location, **propagation of crystal formation occurs.** This is dependent on the concentration of Ca^{++} and PO_4^- in the extracellular spaces, the presence of mineral inhibitors, and the degree of collagenization. Collagen increases the rate of crystal growth, but other proteins such as **osteopontin** (an acidic, calcium-binding phosphoprotein) are also involved.

Site of deposition: Dystrophic calcification is associated with many diseases, and occurs in **areas of necrosis** whether coagulative, caseous, or liquefactive type, and also in foci of enzymic necrosis of fat. One of the most common causes is **tuberculosis**. Calcium is deposited in the caseous tissue of the tuberculous lesion. Sometimes, a tuberculous lymph node is virtually converted to stone. Calcification is almost inevitable in the atheromas of advanced atherosclerosis, which are focal intimal injuries in the aorta and larger arteries characterized by the accumulation of lipids. Other sites include old abscesses, degenerative and necrotic portions of tumours, dead parasites, and parasitic lesions (**Trichinella, Oesophagostoma, Sarcosporidia,** and **Onchocerca**), necrotic ganglion cells, necrotic renal tubules (in bichloride of mercury poisoning), areas of infarction, foot pads of old dogs, and thrombi. In humans, it also commonly develops in aging or damaged heart valves, further hampering their function.

Macroscopically, the calcium salts appear as fine, white granules, or as yellowish-white or grey chalky masses within the tissue, **often felt as gritty deposits.** Calcified tissue has a firm consistency, and when cut with a knife, a definite grit can be detected against the knife blade. **Calcification is especially common in cattle, sheep, and rabbit. Microscopically**, with the usual H & E stain, calcium salts appear as deep blue (basophilic) granules or masses. They can be intracellular, extracellular, or in both locations. A more specific staining

92

technique is Von Kossa's silver nitrate stain that stains the calcium salts as black spheres or masses within the tissue. In time, **bone** may be formed in the focus of calcification.

Metastatic or General Calcification

Metastatic calcification is deposition of calcium salts in many tissues throughout the body. In contrast to dystrophic calcification, **deposition of calcium salts can occur in normal tissue**, and it almost always indicates some derangement of calcium metabolism, resulting in **hypercalcaemia**. Obviously, hypercalcaemia also aggravates dystrophic calcification.

Aetiology: Metastatic calcification occurs whenever there is a **hypercalcaemia** (more than 12 mg percent). The **four major causes of hypercalcaemia are**: (1) **increased secretion of parathyroid hormone (hyperparathyroidism)** (discussed later), (2) **destruction of bone** due to tumours (e.g., increased bone catabolism associated with diffuse skeletal metastases), (3) **vitamin D-related disorders**, including vitamin D intoxication, and (4) **renal failure**, in which phosphate retention leads to **secondary hyperparathyroidism**.

Hyperparathyroidism is associated with a parathyroid neoplasm. The increased parathyroid activity removes calcium from the bones that become rarefied, and large cyst-like spaces appear within them. The resultant hypercalcaemia leads to metastatic calcification. Likewise, myeloid tumours in the bone marrow and metastatic cancer cause demineralization of the skeleton, and the bloodstream is flooded with calcium. Hypercalcaemia may also arise in renal diseases, particularly in advanced renal failure. This leads to retention of phosphorus, which in turn, causes increased activity of parathyroid gland (**secondary hyperparathyroidism**). This results in demineralization of the bones, hypercalcaemia, and metastatic calcification, as described above. The deposition of calcium salts may occur in organs throughout the body, especially in those **that secrete or excrete acid substances** such as the **stomach** (hydrochloric acid), **kidney** (hippuric acid, and **lungs** (carbon dioxide). **Morphologically** the calcium salts in all these sites, resemble those described in dystrophic calcification. **Significance and results**: Calcification in itself is usually not harmful and causes no clinical dysfunction. Occasionally, it may impair organ's motility. Massive deposits in kidney (nephrocalcinosis) may in time cause renal damage. Calcium disappears from the tissue when the primary cause is removed.

GOUT

Gout is a disorder of uric acid metabolism characterized by deposition of urate crystals in tissues. Deposition is due to an increase in the concentration of uric acid in blood (**hyperuricaemia**) and body fluids. Gout is mainly a disease of **humans and birds**, and has not been clearly established in other species. Clinically, the disease in humans is characterized by recurrent episodes of painful acute arthritis.

Gout is usually divided into **primary** and **secondary forms**. The term **primary gout** is used to indicate cases in which the basic cause is unknown, or when the cause is an inborn metabolic abnormality characterized by hyperuricaemia and gout. In the **secondary gout**, cause of the hyperuricaemia is known.

Pathogenesis in humans: An increase in the level of **serum uric acid** may result from **overproduction** or **reduced excretion** of uric acid, **or** from **both**. Uric acid is the end product of purine metabolism. Increased synthesis of uric acid, a common feature of primary gout, results from some abnormality in the production of purine nucleotides.

Most cases of gout are characterized by an overproduction of uric acid with or without excessive excretion of uric acid. **In most such cases, the cause of overproduction is not known.** Although the cause of excessive uric acid production is unknown, some patients have **known enzyme defects**. Less commonly, uric acid is produced at normal rates, and hyperuricaemia occurs **because of decreased excretion of urate by the kidneys.**

Whatever the cause increased levels of uric acid in the blood and other body fluids (e.g., synovium) lead to **precipitation of monosodium urate crystals**. Precipitation of the crystals, in turn, triggers a chain of events that end in **joint injury**. The released crystals are chemotactic and also activate complement. This results in the generation of C3a and C5a, which induce accumulation of neutrophils and macrophages in the joints and synovial membranes. Phagocytosis of crystals causes release of **toxic free radicals** and **leukotrienes**, particularly B4. Death of the neutrophils releases destructive lysosomal enzymes. Macrophages also participate in joint injury. After ingestion of urate crystals, **macrophages secrete a variety of pro-inflammatory mediators**, such as interleukin-1, IL-6, IL-8, and tumour necrosis factor (TNF). These not only intensify the inflammatory response, but also activate synovial cells and cartilage cells to release proteases (e.g., **collagenases**) that cause the tissue injury. This is how develops an **acute arthritis**.

Typical cases of acute gouty arthritis are accompanied by the formation of large crystalline aggregates in joints, termed **tophi**. They result from precipitation of **monosodium urate crystals** from supersaturated body fluids into the tissues.

Gout In Poultry

Uric acid is produced in the liver and is the end product of nitrogen metabolism in birds, unlike mammals. In mammals, the end product of nitrogen metabolism is urea. Therefore, birds can develop gout following an abnormal accumulation of urates. **Thus, in poultry gout should not be considered as a disease entity, but a clinical sign of severe renal dysfunction that causes hyperuricaemia.**

Usually gout is classified as **visceral gout** if the urates are deposited in the viscera and as **articular gout** if the urates are deposited around the joints. However, recent studies have revealed that **this classification is incorrect. This is because gout occurs as two different syndromes - visceral and articular gout. These two syndromes differ in respect of their aetiology, morphology, and pathogenesis.**

Pathogenesis: Birds are prone to gout because they are **uricotelic**. That is, in them, the waste product of protein metabolism (i.e., excretion of nitrogen) is mainly in the form of **uric acid**. This is because they lack the enzyme **uricase**, which converts uric acid into allantoin. Moreover, uric acid is **water insoluble**. Therefore, any injury or damage to bird's kidney, from whatever cause, interferes with elimination of uric acid, which then accumulates in the blood (**hyperuricaemia**) and leads to visceral gout, that is, deposition of urate crystals on the surfaces of internal organs.

Mammals, on the other hand, are **ureotelic**. That is, in them the waste product of protein metabolism is mainly in the form of **urea**, and therefore mammals are not prone to gout like birds. Also, **urea is water soluble**.

Visceral gout (visceral urate deposit): Visceral gout is a common finding during necropsy of poultry. It is characterized by precipitation (deposition) of **urates** in the kidneys and on serous surfaces of the heart, liver, mesentery, airsacs, or peritoneum. In severe cases synovial sheaths of tendons and joints and surfaces of muscles may be involved,

95

and precipitation may occur within the liver, spleen, and other organs. **Microscopically**, the deposits on serous surfaces appear as **white chalky coating,** and those within viscera may be recognized only microscopically. **Microscopically**, the clusters of urate crystals appear as pale, elongated, needle-shaped structures in tissue sections. The crystals are surrounded by an inflammatory reaction of macrophages, lymphocytes, fibroblasts, and foreign-body giant cells. The crystals are usually not observed in paraffin-embedded tissue sections, but the clefts in which the urates were present can be seen.

Causes: Visceral urate deposition is usually due to a failure of urinary excretion. This may be due to obstruction of ureters, renal damage, or dehydration. **Dehydration due to water deprivation is a common cause of visceral gout in poultry. Other causes** include vitamin A deficiency, mycotoxins such as oosporein, secondary to urolithiasis, and treatment with sodium bicarbonate. It is not clear whether the kidney necrosis seen in visceral gout is primary or secondary to hyperuricaemia and urate deposition. Recent studies indicate that one of the first changes observed in birds treated with high concentration of sodium bicarbonate is **metabolic alkalosis** and **hyperuricaemia**. It has been suggested that a state of **alkalosis** induces breakdown and turnover of nucleoprotein, causing hyperuricaemia. This leads to precipitation and crystallization of urates. However, the mechanism for urate crystal precipitation in certain sites is still not known. **Significance**: Visceral gout is seen only at necropsy. It is difficult to say whether any affected birds recover. Even if the birds survive, they are no longer profitable.

Articular gout: Unlike visceral gout, **articular gout is a sporadic problem of not much economic importance in poultry**. Clinically, it is characterized by leg shifting, lameness, and inability to bend the toes. Articular gout is characterized by **tophi.** These are deposits of urates around joints, particularly those of the feet. The joints are enlarged, and the feet appear deformed. When these joints are opened, the periarticular tissue is white due to urate deposition. **White semi-fluid deposits of urates** may be found within the joints. **The white appearance of urate deposits should not be confused with pus. In chronic cases**, urate precipitates can be observed in the comb, wattles, and trachea.

AMYLOIDOSIS

Amyloidosis is deposition of amyloid in the interstitial tissues in a wide variety of clinical disorders. **Amyloid is a generic term.**

That is, it is not a specific term, but a term used for a variety of proteinaceous materials, collectively called, **amyloid**. At one time, amyloid was thought to be starch-like, hence the name **'amyloid'** (L. amylum = starch; amyloid = starch-like). **But it is now known to be composed mainly of protein**. With H & E stain, **amyloid appears as an amorphous (shapeless), eosinophilic, hyaline (homogeneous and translucent) extracellular substance. It is deposited between cells** in various tissues and organs of the body, usually **between** the capillary endothelium and the adjacent cells.

Amyloid resembles starch in some of its chemical reactions. The name amyloid was derived from its reaction with **iodine**. The test may be applied to gross specimens, as well as tissue sections. When cut surface of affected organs is painted with an iodine solution, amyloid stains yellow-red. This colour is transformed into blue or violet after the application of dilute sulphuric acid. This technique was first used by Rudolph Virchow over a century ago, and he interpreted the result to be **starch-like**, hence the name amyloid. As stated, amyloid is now known to be composed mainly of protein. To differentiate amyloid from hyaline deposits (see 'hyaline change') a number of histochemical techniques are used. Most commonly used is the **Congo red stain**, which imparts amyloid a pink or red colour. Recent studies have revealed that even more specific is the **yellow-green birefringence** of the Congo red stained amyloid when observed **by polarizing microscopy**. Yellow-green birefringence is the characteristic image obtained from refraction (splitting) of light in two different directions.

Despite the striking morphological uniformity of amyloid in all cases, **amyloid is not a single chemical entity.** Two major and several biochemical forms exist. They are all deposited by different pathogenic mechanisms. Therefore, **amyloidosis is not a single disease, but rather a group of diseases that share deposition of similar-looking proteins.** It is now known that the uniform morphological appearance and staining characteristics are due to the remarkably constant physical organization of amyloid protein. Let us therefore first consider the physical nature of amyloid. This is followed by a discussion of its chemical nature.

Physical nature of amyloid: By electron microscopy, amyloid appears to be made up of non-branching fibrils of indefinite length, and 7.5 to 10 nm in width. Studies using other sophisticated techniques have demonstrated that the fibrils have a characteristic pattern, which has been described as **"beta-pleated sheet structure"** (Fig. 13). The amyloid fibrils are unique in that they are the only fibrillar proteins to show this pattern. This means that this conformation (organization) is always seen, regardless of the clinical disorder or the chemical composition, and is responsible for the characteristic staining and optical properties of amyloid. **In other words, any fibrillar protein deposited in tissues that yields a beta-pleated sheet will be seen as amyloid**. In addition to the fibrils, a non-fibrillar glycoprotein (**P component**) and **proteoglycans** are minor components of all amyloid deposits. About 95% of any amyloid deposition consists of fibril proteins, with the remaining 5% being the P component and other glycoproteins.

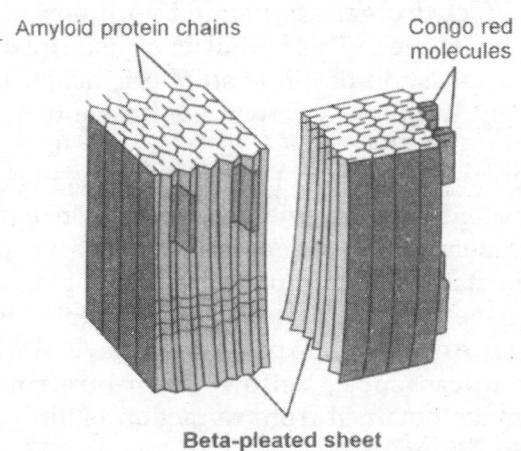

Fig. 13. Beta-pleated sheet structure of amyloid and binding sites for the Congo red dye.

Chemical nature of amyloid: Of the 15 biochemically different forms of amyloid proteins that have been identified, **two are more common**: (1) **AL (amyloid light chain)** derived from plasma cells and contains **immunoglobulin light chains**, and (2) **AA (amyloid-associated)** is a non-immunoglobulin protein synthesized by the liver. Both these proteins are antigenically distinct, and are deposited in different clinical conditions. The **AL protein** is made up of either complete immunoglobulin light chains, or their fragments, or both. The AL amyloid protein is produced by immunoglobulin-secreting cells, and its deposition is associated with some form of monoclonal B-cell proliferation. The **AA amyloid fibril** is composed of a protein that does not have structural similarity with immunoglobulins. AA proteins are typically deposited during **chronic inflammatory diseases**. They are derived from a larger serum precursor protein synthesized in the liver **called SAA (serum amyloid-associated) protein**.

Occurrence: Amyloidosis is most common in humans, but it **also occurs in all species of domestic animals**. It is common in the **dog, cattle, horse, and chicken**. Amyloidosis may affect any tissue. It may be restricted to a single organ, or be generalized. Most common sites are **spleen, liver, and kidneys**. Lymph nodes and adrenals are also commonly involved.

Classification: Amyloidosis may be **systemic** (generalized), involving several organs, or it may be **localized**, when deposits are limited to a single organ. On clinical grounds, the systemic pattern is further classified, both in humans and animals, into: (1) **Primary amyloidosis** when associated with some immunological disorder (immunocyte dyscrasia), and (2) **secondary amyloidosis** when it occurs as a complication of an underlying **chronic inflammatory or tissue destructive process**.

Aetiology: The term **primary amyloidosis**, in animals, is used to describe amyloid deposition in patients that did not have any detectable underlying disease. That is, it occurred independently of any disease. **Secondary amyloidosis** occurred in association with some chronic inflammatory diseases, especially long-standing infections such as **tuberculosis and chronic suppurative processes like osteomyelitis**. For example, amyloidosis is very common in the chicken affected with tuberculosis. Amyloidosis is also associated with various **neoplasms**, especially multiple myeloma (a malignant neoplasm of plasma cells) and lymphoma.

In the past, circumstantial evidence indicated that amyloid was a precipitate resulting from an antigen-antibody reaction. Experimental amyloidosis was accompanied by hyperglobulinaemia. Amyloidosis often occurred in **horses** that were used in the production of antiserum and antitoxins for certain infectious diseases of humans, e.g., diphtheria and tetanus antitoxins. Also, amyloidosis could be produced experimentally by repeated injections of antigenic materials such as casein, and certain drugs, into **rabbits.**

However, **in domestic animals and birds**, mechanisms responsible for amyloid formation and the pathogenesis of amyloidosis, are still largely unknown. On the other hand, a lot of

99

information is available in **humans**. Let us therefore examine these recent advances, and see if they could correlate with animal settings.

In **humans, primary amyloidosis** is also known as **immunocyte dyscrasias with amyloidosis**, since it is associated with some **immunocyte dyscrasia**, that is, an abnormal condition of immunoglobulin-secreting cells. It results from deposition of **immunoglobulin light chains (AL), or their fragments, or both,** and is associated with some form of monoclonal cell proliferation. This is the most common form of amyloidosis in humans. The best example is the amyloidosis associated with **multiple myeloma**, a malignant neoplasm of plasma cells. The **malignant B-cells** are monoclonal (i.e., originating from a single cell) and therefore synthesize abnormal amounts of a **single** specific immunoglobulin, (**monoclonal gammopathy**), producing an **M (myeloma) protein** spike on serum electrophoresis. In addition to whole immunoglobulin molecules, plasma cells also synthesize and secrete only the lambda or kappa light chains. The two light chains are known as **Bence Jones proteins**. By virtue of their small molecular size, they are often excreted in the urine. These are present in the serum of patients with multiple myeloma, but only a few patients who have free light chains develop amyloidosis. Clearly, **the presence of Bence Jones proteins, although necessary, is by itself not enough to produce amyloidosis.** Other factors, such as the type of light chain produced, that is **amyloidogenic potential**, and the subsequent degradation of these chains influence the deposition of Bence Jones proteins. **In animals also**, patients of multiple myeloma show Bence Jones proteins in the serum and this may help explain primary amyloidosis in them. An extramedullary plasmacytoma (a plasma cell neoplasm) in a **cat** has been found associated with **monoclonal gammopathy** and with **systemic AL amyloidosis**.

In **secondary amyloidosis** (also known as **reactive systemic amyloidosis**) the amyloid deposits are also systemic in distribution, **but are composed of AA protein.** This type is called "secondary" because it is secondary to a **chronic inflammatory condition.** The underlying cause in a wide range of infectious and non-infectious chronic inflammatory conditions is the **long-standing cell injury.** **Tuberculosis, bronchiectasis, and chronic osteomyelitis** are the most common causes, but secondary amyloidosis is also seen in chronic infections caused by autoimmune diseases (e.g., rheumatoid arthritis). Rheumatoid arthritis is particularly amyloidogenic.

Pathogenesis: **In secondary amyloidosis**, long-standing tissue injury and inflammation lead to **increased SAA levels** (Fig. 14). SAA is synthesized by the liver cells under the influence of cytokines such as interleukin-1 and IL-6. In **chronic inflammation**, there is activation of macrophages that, in turn, produce cytokines IL-1 and IL-6. However, increased production of SAA by itself is not sufficient for the deposition of amyloid. This is because in many inflammatory conditions, a rise in serum SSA is common but in most cases this does not lead to amyloidosis. It is believed that SAA is **normally** broken down to **soluble end products** by the action of monocyte-derived enzymes. **Individuals who develop amyloidosis have an enzyme defect**. This results in the **incomplete breakdown (limited proteolysis) of SAA**, thus generating **insoluble AA molecules** (Fig. 14).

In the case of **primary amyloidosis**, the source of the precursor protein is **immunoglobulin light chain**. Amyloid material can be produced *in vitro* by proteolysis of immunoglobulin light chains. However, it is still not known why only a few persons (or animals) that have circulating Bence Jones proteins develop amyloidosis. It is believed that **defective proteolytic breakdown (limited proteolysis) of soluble immunoglobulin light chains to insoluble AL protein leads to amyloidosis** (Fig. 14).

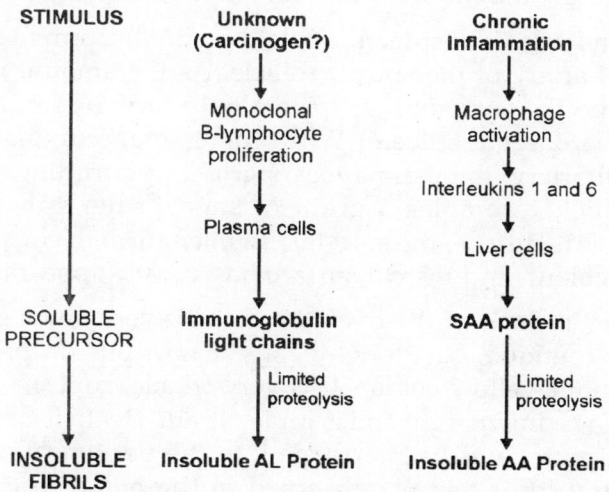

Fig. 14. Scheme for the pathogenesis of two major forms of amyloid.

Harmful effects: Regardless of the organ involved, deposition of the amyloid occurs in the perivascular tissue between the blood vessel and the adjacent cells. The mass of amyloid around the blood vessel gradually enlarges, producing larger and larger cuffs as more and more is deposited. With progressive accumulation, **three important changes** occur: (1) The extracellular amyloid encroaches on, and produces **pressure atrophy** of adjacent cells. (2) The deposited amyloid is quite impervious (impenetrable) to fluids and gases. As a result, exchange of gases, nutrients and waste material between the blood vessel and adjacent cells cannot occur. This results in **degeneration and necrosis** of the surrounding cells. (3) Further, as the mass of amyloid enlarges, it presses upon the vessel and causes **stenosis** (narrowing). This restricts the flow of blood through the vessel and causes **ischaemia** in a portion of the involved organ.

Macroscopic appearance: **Deposition** of the amyloid may be **local or general** in distribution. It is found in all organs, but is more common in some than others. The incidence in organs varies with the species. In the **horse**, it occurs in spleen, liver, adrenal, and kidney. In the **cattle**, it is seen in kidney, adrenal, spleen, and liver, and in the **dog**, usually in the kidney, but sometimes also in the spleen, liver, and adrenal. Amyloidosis is a prominent lesion in the spleens of **chickens** having tuberculosis. The kidney, liver, spleen, lymph nodes, adrenal, and thyroid are the common sites for amyloid deposition in **humans**.

In **amyloidosis of spleen**, amyloid gradually forms a cuff around the central artery of the splenic follicle. As the amount increases, it extends into the surrounding splenic pulp forming large, sheet-like deposits ('**lardaceous spleen**'). With progressive accumulation around the central artery, the mass appears grossly protruding, waxy, grey focus, which resembles a grain of sago ('**sago spleen**'). When amyloidosis is diffuse, the spleen is swollen, firm in consistency, has a greyish colour, and the cut surface has a waxy appearance.

In **amyloidosis of the liver**, the organ is very much enlarged, its edges are rounded, has doughy consistency, pits on pressure, and has a cyanotic yellow colour. It is very friable, ruptures easily, and the capsule is drawn tight and is under strain. Death is usually due to hepatic rupture, and haemorrhage into the peritoneal cavity. **Fatal hepatic rupture is usually observed in the horse**. The amyloid in liver is deposited between the endothelium of the sinusoids and cells of the hepatic cords. With its progressive accumulation, the blood flow is hindered. The hepatic cells are compressed, and undergo pressure and nutritional atrophy. Fatty change occurs from hypoxia and inadequate nutrition. This gives the organ its cyanotic-yellow colour. Death is due to rupture and massive haemorrhage into the peritoneal cavity.

Amyloidosis of the kidney occurs in the glomeruli. The amyloid is deposited between the capillary endothelium and the epithelium of the glomeruli. Most of the renal damage is due to obliteration (disappearance) of the glomerular circulation. With progressive accumulation, the glomerular capillaries are stenosed (narrowed), and finally obliterated (destroyed). Since part of the vascular circulation to the tubules depends on the glomeruli, obliteration of the glomeruli results in ischaemia of the portions of the nephron below the glomeruli. The ischaemia leads to atrophy, fatty change, and coagulation necrosis. The kidney is swollen, has a bulging cut surface, and a mottled (marked with coloured spots) red and yellow appearance. The kidneys are especially large in the **cattle**. Uraemia and death occur before extensive fibrosis and scarring.

Amyloidosis of the pancreas occurs in islets of Langerhans. The amyloid is deposited between the capillaries and the islet cells. The destruction of the islet cells causes **diabetes**. Amyloid deposition is sometimes observed in the conjunctiva of **horse,** and may lead to blindness. Amyloidosis of the respiratory passages and skin (dermis, subcutaneous connective tissue) is also occasionally observed in horses.

Microscopic appearance: Large amounts of amyloid can be detected just with H & E stain only. However, with small amounts and their unusual location, special staining is required. **Amyloid stains pink with eosin**. However, to differentiate amyloid from collagen, a connective tissue stain such as Van Gieson technique must be used. With this amyloid stains **yellow**, while collagen and connective tissue red.

Methyl violet, methyl green, crystal violet, and thionin **stain** amyloid **red** and the surrounding tissue blue or green. These dyes are aniline dyes, and their reaction is called metachromatic staining reaction. **Congo red** is rapidly absorbed by amyloid, and gives it a red colour.

Amyloid appears as a homogeneous perivascular mass. It may occur as sheets, masses, or globules, depending on the stage of deposition when it is observed. It should not be confused with collagen. Amyloid mass has an irregular border, contains few nuclei, and does not contain any connective tissue fibres.

To summarize, histologically, the deposition always begins between cells. The histological diagnosis of amyloid is based on its staining characteristics. **The most common dye used is Congo red,** which under ordinary light imparts a **pink or red colour** to amyloid deposits. Under polarized light, the Congo-red stained amyloid shows a green birefringence. This reaction is shared by all forms of amyloid, and is caused by the crossed beta-pleated configuration (arrangement) of amyloid fibrils. Confirmation can be obtained by electron microscopy, which reveals amorphous non-oriented thin fibrils.

Significance and results: Amyloidosis may be an unsuspected finding at necropsy. Most cases are encountered incidental to other diseases. **Amyloid deposition is a permanent change, and persists for the life of the individual**. Amyloid stops depositing if the inciting cause is removed. However, what has been already deposited remains in tissues. It is especially serious in the kidney (uraemia), pancreas (diabetes), and liver (hepatic rupture).

Chapter 4

Inflammation

General Features

The same stimuli that cause cell injury also produce **a complex reaction in the vascularized connective tissue called inflammation.** Basically, it is the **reaction of blood vessels leading to accumulation of fluid and leukocytes in extravascular tissues.**

The **inflammatory response is closely interwoven with the process of repair.** Repair begins during the early phase of inflammation. Healing, which is the end result of inflammation, is a part of the dynamic process and not a separate entity.

Inflammation is fundamental to the survival of the organism. Without it, there could be neither protection against the effects of noxious external stimuli, nor repair of the damaged tissue. **Inflammation serves to destroy, dilute, or otherwise neutralize harmful agents (microbes, toxins), and repair the damaged tissues. It is basically a protective response.** Without inflammation, infections would go unchecked, wounds would never heal, and injured organs might remain permanent festering sores. However, under certain circumstances, inflammation may wander away from its beneficial path and may become considerably more harmful to the body as in life-threatening hypersensitivity reactions to insect bites, drugs, and toxins as well as some chronic diseases such as rheumatoid arthritis, atherosclerosis, and lung fibrosis.

As inflammation is the most basic and the most common response, its understanding forms the very backbone of pathology. Most diseases at some time in their course are examples of inflammation.

Types

Inflammation is of two types: **acute** and **chronic**. Acute inflammation is of relatively short duration lasting for a few minutes, several hours, or a few days; and its main characteristics are the exudation of fluid and plasma proteins (oedema) and the emigration of leukocytes, mainly neutrophils. **Chronic inflammation**, on the other hand, is of longer duration and is associated histologically with the presence of lymphocytes and macrophages, and with the proliferation of blood vessels, fibrosis, and tissue necrosis.

Acute Inflammation

Since acute inflammation is the immediate and early response to an injurious agent, we shall first discuss acute inflammation and begin with its causes.

Aetiology (Causes)

Acute inflammation can be provoked by any noxious stimulus - called an **irritant**. The causes of acute inflammation include:

1. Infectious agents: These include bacteria, viruses, fungi, chlamydiae, rickettsiae, mycoplasma, protozoa, helminths, and even arthropods (insects).

2. Chemical agents: These are of endless variety and include toxins, acids, alkalies, and other caustic substances.

3. Physical agents: These include burns, electricity, radiation, excessive cold, and trauma.

4. Immunological reactions: Inflammation is associated with all types of tissue damaging antigen-antibody interactions that occur under certain circumstances. These include various hypersensitivity reactions and autoimmune diseases.

5. Nutritional imbalances: These include deficiencies in specific vitamins.

6. Necrotic tissue: Certain stimuli, such as toxins, bacteria, and ischaemia, cause cell necrosis directly, and the necrotic tissue, in turn, can trigger the release of inflammatory mediators.

The Cardinal Signs

The local signs that characterize inflammation are **redness, swelling, heat, pain, and loss of function.** They are known as the cardinal (chief, principal) signs of inflammation. The first four signs were described by Cornelius Celsus, a Roman writer of the first century AD (AD 35). The **fifth sign, loss of function,** was added much later in AD 1858 by the famous German pathologist Rudolph Virchow, and not by the Greek physician Claudius Galen (AD 130-200), as is traditionally believed.

1. Redness (L. rubor): This is due to a great increase of blood in the inflamed area as a result of hyperaemia.

2. Swelling (L. tumor): This is partly due to hyperaemia that results in increased blood flow. Blood has volume and therefore the part becomes larger than normal. Secondly, there is outpouring of protein-rich fluid containing blood cells into the extravascular tissues (called '**exudate**'). This is the major cause of swelling.

3. Heat (L. calor): An increase in heat at the site of inflammation results from increased blood flow through the area that carries warmth to the periphery from the higher interior temperature of the body. Also, as the rate of metabolism is increased at the inflamed site, there is greater production of heat.

4. Pain (L. dolor): The inflamed area is painful. Pain occurs partly from increased pressure on sensory nerve endings, and by stretching of tissues from accumulation of exudate. Also, chemical mediators are released following injury and produce pain. Important among these are 5-hydroxytryptamine (serotonin), kinins (bradykinin), and prostaglandins. **Histamine** plays a relatively minor role in producing pain, and **has mostly the itching effect.** The potassium ions that escape from the injured cells and acetylcholine liberated by nervous stimuli, may also cause pain.

5. Loss of function (L. functio-laesa): This is due to a combination of pain, swelling and destruction of tissues.

Tissue Alterations in Acute Inflammation

These can be placed into two groups - the **vascular changes** and the **cellular events**.

VASCULAR CHANGES

Julius Cohnheim (1839-1884) was the first to describe vascular changes in 1877. He spread the mesentery of a curarized frog (anaesthetized by curare) across the stage of a microscope and observed the flow of blood through the vessels, following the application of a drop of dilute acetic acid. Cohnheim's original description is still fully applicable. Based on his observations, the vascular changes are:

1. Changes in the Blood Vessels

(a) Momentary constriction: Immediately upon application of the irritant, the arterioles are constricted. The constriction is very short-lived (seconds), and is therefore of not much importance. The mechanism of vasoconstriction is unknown. It may well be neurogenic, or possibly due to the action of chemical mediators.

(b) Vasodilation: The momentary constriction of vessels is quickly followed by their dilation that involves first arterioles and then results in the opening of new capillary beds in the area. Normally, a number of capillaries remain dormant or collapsed. The opening of new vascular beds results in increased vascularity of the area. Dilation is caused by the action of chemical substances released locally. These substances are known as **chemical mediators of inflammation.** Vasodilation leads to hyperaemia and increased blood flow, the cause of heat and redness.

2. Changes in the Rate of Flow

The early vasodilation results in increased blood flow, but is soon followed by **slowing of the circulation.** The **slowing** is brought about by **increased permeability of the microvasculature** (venules, small veins, and capillaries), and leads to the outpouring of protein-rich fluid into the extravascular tissues. This results in concentration of red cells in small vessels and increased viscosity of the blood. In tissue sections, this is seen as dilated small vessels packed with red cells - a condition termed **stasis.**

(i) Increased vascular permeability (vascular leakage): The endothelial wall of capillaries and venules forms a semi-permeable barrier that allows free movement of water and small molecules, and is only slightly permeable to plasma proteins. **A characteristic feature of acute inflammation is the striking increase in permeability of the vessels to proteins.** Plasma proteins, namely, albumin, the globulins, and fibrinogen, leave the leaky vessels. This is roughly proportional to their concentration in blood and inversely proportional to their molecular size. **The loss of protein from plasma reduces the intravascular osmotic pressure of the interstitial fluid.** Together with the increased hydrostatic pressure due to vasodilation, they cause a marked **outflow** of fluid and its accumulation in the interstitial tissue. This net increase of extravascular fluid is called **inflammatory oedema.**

Mechanisms of Increased Vascular Permeability

How does the normal intact endothelium become leaky in inflammation? The following mechanisms have been proposed.

(a) Formation of endothelial gaps in venules: Normally, the endothelial cells of blood vessels are fused by tight intercellular junctions. In inflammation, these are loosened to permit outflow of fluid and protein. **Most chemical mediators of inflammation cause an increase in vascular permeability by opening inter-endothelial junctions.** The endothelial cells contain a network of microtubules and fibrils, and a contractile protein **actomyosin** (actin + myosin) that induce cell contraction. The inter-endothelial gaps (0.5 - 1.0 μm wide) are produced by contraction of endothelial cells, which results in widening of the junction. **This is the most common mechanism of vascular leakage, and is produced by histamine, bradykinin, leukotrienes, and many other types of chemical mediators.** It occurs rapidly, is reversible, and short-lived (15 to 30 minutes). It is therefore called the '**immediate transient response'.** This type of leakage affects **only venules** (20 to 60 mm in diameter); **endothelium in capillaries and arterioles is unaffected.** This is due to **a greater density of receptors** for the relevant chemical mediators. Many of the later leukocyte events in inflammation (adhesion and emigration) also occur in the venules in most organs.

(b) **Endothelial cell retraction:** In this mechanism, there is a structural reorganization of the endothelial cytoskeleton. As a result cells retract (draw back) from each other, **which leads to the formation of endothelial gaps**. Cytokine mediators, such as interleukin-1, tumour necrosis factor and interferon-gamma, induce endothelial cell retraction. In contrast to the histamine effect, endothelial retraction takes 4-6 hours to develop and persists for 24 hours or more.

(c) **Direct endothelial injury:** This results in vascular leakage from endothelial cell necrosis and detachment. It is usually seen after **severe injuries** (burns or infections). Leakage begins immediately after injury and persists for several hours (or days) until the damaged vessels are thrombosed or repaired. The reaction is known as the **immediate sustained response. Venules, capillaries, and arterioles can all be affected.**

(d) **Delayed prolonged leakage:** Direct injury to endothelial cells may also cause delayed prolonged leakage. It begins after 2 to 12 hours, lasts for several hours or even days, and involves venules and capillaries. Examples: mild-to-moderate thermal injury, certain bacterial toxins, x-radiation or ultraviolet radiation.

(e) **Leukocyte-dependent endothelial injury:** This occurs from leukocyte accumulation during inflammation. Such leukocytes may release toxic oxygen species and proteolytic enzymes that cause endothelial injury and detachment - resulting in increased vascular permeability. This form of injury is usually seen in those vascular sites (venules and pulmonary capillaries) where leukocytes can adhere to the endothelium.

(f) Increased transcytosis through an intercellular vesicular pathway (i.e., across the endothelial cytoplasm) increases vascular permeability. Transcytosis occurs across channels formed by fusion of uncoated vesicles. Certain mediators, e.g., **vascular endothelial growth factor (VEGF)** cause increased transcytosis.

(g) Leakage from new blood vessels: Tissue repair involves new blood vessel formation (angiogenesis). **New vessel sprouts remain leaky** until endothelial cells differentiate and form intercellular junctions. New endothelial cells also have increased expression of receptors for vasoactive mediators and certain angiogenic factors (e.g., vascular endothelial growth factor).

Estimation of Increased Vascular Permeability

Increased vascular permeability can be demonstrated or quantitated, experimentally, in several ways: **(1) dye technique (gross or macroscopic method)**, and **(2) colloidal carbon technique (microscopic method)**.

In the **dye technique**, a vital dye such as Evans blue or pontamine sky blue is injected into the blood where it becomes immediately bound to serum albumin. Wherever there is a leak, the **dye-albumin complex** comes out and forms **a blue patch** indicating an increase in vascular permeability. Increased vascular permeability can then be assessed by measuring size of the blue patch and the intensity of its colour. Also, the exuded dye can be extracted chemically and measured spectrophotometrically. **Thus, an increase in vascular permeability can be quantitated.**

The dye technique, whereas it demonstrates an increase in vascular permeability, it does not identify the leaky vessels. **Colloidal carbon technique**, in contrast, **identifies the particular vessels through which the protein has been leaking during inflammation.** In this technique, a colloidal suspension of carbon, which contains particles 25-30 nm in diameter, is injected intravenously. In the leaky vessels, the carbon particles are trapped between the endothelium and the basement membrane. **Thus, the blood vessels showing an increase in permeability are "labelled" with carbon** (Fig. 15). Normal blood vessels are not labelled. The vascular labelling can then be studied under the light microscope in tissue sections and also in cleared preparations. The carbon labelling of vessels can be scored on an arbitrary scale of 0 to ++++. The labelled vessels can also be examined by electron microscopy.

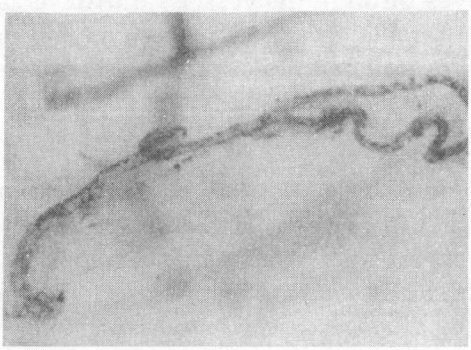

Fig. 15. Carbon labelling of a tortuous venule of the chicken skin immediately after intradermal turpentine.

The term capillary is applied to blood vessels of 4-6 μm in diameter. Vessels larger than 7 μm but less than 100 μm in diameter, and histologically of a venous character, are classified as venules. It is not known why chemical mediators act exclusively on venules. Some evidence suggests that venular endothelium has a higher concentration of high-affinity binding sites **(receptors)** for histamine 1-type mediators than does arteriolar and capillary endothelium.

(ii) Slowing of the circulation: As mentioned, the early vasodilation results in increased blood flow, but is soon followed by slowing of the circulation. This change is essential for emigration of the leukocytes. Retardation is achieved in four ways: **(i) by increasing the capillary bed in the area.** When a large number of so far collapsed capillaries are suddenly opened, and when blood has to flow through them, the rate of blood flow naturally decreases, **(ii) by swelling of the endothelial cells** lining the capillaries. As the endothelial cells swell and increase in their diameter, they project into the lumen, offer resistance to the flow of blood, and so the rate is decreased, **(iii) haemoconcentration** that occurs following passage of plasma out of the blood vessels, increases viscosity of blood, and this leads to further retardation of the flow, **(iv) margination of the leukocytes.** Following a marked reduction in the flow, leukocytes adhere to the endothelial wall **(leukocytic margination)**, narrow the lumen, and their presence in the vessel increases roughness of the endothelial surface. This increases the peripheral resistance of the blood vessel and thereby

111

further retards the rate of flow.

(iii) Stasis: When the above factors markedly reduce the flow, blood barely moves through the vessels, and **stasis** is produced. This situation is ideal for the escape of molecular and cellular elements essential for the formation of inflammatory exudate.

3. Changes in the Bloodstream

The main change consists of a **redistribution** of the cellular elements of the bloodstream. Normally in the bloodstream of a vessel, two distinct zones can be seen. In the centre are found the cellular elements (erythrocytes and leukocytes). This part is called the **axial stream.** The cellular elements are held in the centre by the centripetal force of the flowing blood. External to the axial stream is the **plasmatic stream,** a clear zone consisting mainly of plasma, which is in contact with the wall of the vessel. As the blood flow slows, the centripetal force of the bloodstream is overcome by the centrifugal force and the leukocytes fall out of the axial stream. Here, they have a better opportunity to interact with the lining endothelial cells. This process of leukocyte adhesion at the periphery of vessels is called **margination.** Afterwards, leukocytes tumble (roll over and over) slowly along the endothelial surface and adhere transiently. This process of **brief, loose sticking of leukocytes** to the endothelium is called **rolling.** Finally, leukocytes come to rest at some point where they adhere firmly. This **firm sticking** of leukocytes to the endothelium is called **adhesion.** In time, the endothelium is virtually lined by white cells. This appearance is called **pavementing** (see 'cellular events').

4. Exudation of Plasma

Following increased vascular permeability, fluid part of the blood escapes into the inflamed area. This is known as **exudation.** The accumulated plasma outside the vessel is known as an **inflammatory exudate.**

5. Emigration of Leukocytes

This is the process by which leukocytes come out of the blood vessels into the extravascular space. It will be discussed under 'cellular events'.

6. Diapedesis of Erythrocytes

Red cells may also leave the intact blood vessels. However, they have no power of movement and are pushed out of the vessel passively by the intravascular pressure following emigration of leukocytes. This

112

is called **diapedesis**. In severe injuries, red cells may also enter the tissue **by rhexis** (break) of the vessel wall.

Chemical Mediators of Inflammation

Although injury brings about the inflammatory response, **released chemicals** mediate it. Their existence was long suspected for two reasons:

(i) Regardless of the nature of injury, the inflammatory changes that followed constituted a fairly uniform, almost stereotyped reactions, and

(ii) Inflammation developed in tissues deprived of their nervous connections.

In 1927, Sir Thomas Lewis described the **'triple response'**. He demonstrated that when the skin is firmly stroked, three separate changes can be observed. **First**, within seconds, a dull red line **(erythema)** develops along the line of the stroke. **Second**, a bright red halo **(the flare)** appears around the stroke mark. **Third**, swelling of the stroke mark **(the weal)** appears. Neither the red stroke mark nor the weal, could be abolished by cutting local sensory nerves. He thus postulated the release of a humoral histamine-like substance **(H-substance)** by injured tissue as the cause of erythema; and suggested that the erythema was brought about by vasodilation and the weal by increased vascular permeability. **Thus, Lewis's experiments were the first to suggest the action of chemical mediators in inflammation.** In other words, **he established the concept that chemical mediators, locally produced by injury, mediate the vascular changes of inflammation.** However, soon it became clear that histamine alone could not account for all features of inflammation. The active search for other mediators since has revealed a large number of factors, and the list ever increases. We shall discuss only the more important mediators.

Mediators can originate either from **cells**, or from **plasma** (Fig. 16). **Cell-derived mediators** are either already formed **(preformed)** (e.g., histamine in mast cells), or are **synthesized** *de novo* (i.e., newly synthesized; e.g., prostaglandins) in response to stimulus. **Plasma-derived mediators** are present in **inactive or precursor forms that must be activated to acquire their biological properties.**

Vasoactive Amines

Histamine: Histamine is the principal mediator of **the immediate**

phase of increased vascular permeability. It is widely distributed in tissues and stored mainly in the granules of **mast cells**, but also in circulating **basophils** and **platelets.** Histamine causes dilation of the arterioles and increased vascular permeability of the venules. It induces venular endothelial contraction and formation of inter-endothelial gaps. Histamine acts on the venules mainly through H1 receptors. Soon after its release, histamine is inactivated by the enzyme histaminase.

Histamine is formed from the amino acid histidine by the enzyme histidine decarboxylase. A variety of stimuli release **preformed histamine** from mast cells by causing their degranulation. These include: (1) physical injury such as trauma, cold, or heat, (2) immune reactions involving binding of IgE antibodies to Fc receptors on mast cells, (3) fragments of complement called anaphylatoxins (C3a and C5a) , (4) histamine-releasing proteins derived from neutrophils, (5) certain cytokines (IL-1 and IL-8), and neuropeptides (substance P).

Histamine can be isolated from the early inflammatory exudate. The early inflammatory response induced by mild injury is also suppressed by H1 histamine antagonists. However, the histamine content of the exudate falls within an hour, and antihistamines have no effect on the delayed permeability responses. **Thus, histamine is important mainly in the early inflammatory responses,** and in immediate IgE-mediated hypersensitivity reactions.

5-Hydroxytryptamine (5-HT, Serotonin): 5-HT is the second preformed vasoactive amine, and it also mediates the immediate phase of increased vascular permeability. However, it is present in the **mast cells of rat and mouse only. Its presence in the chicken mast cell is suspected.** It is also present in platelets. Although 5HT induces effects similar to those of histamine, its role as an inflammatory mediator in animals and humans is not established.

Arachidonic Acid Metabolites: Prostaglandins, Leukotrienes, Lipoxins

Products derived from the metabolism of arachidonic acid (AA) **affect inflammation.** They are **short-range hormones (autocoids) that act locally** at the site of formation, and then decay either spontaneously, or are destroyed enzymatically.

Arachidonic acid is a 20-carbon polyunsaturated fatty acid (four double bonds) derived primarily from dietary linoleic acid. In the

114

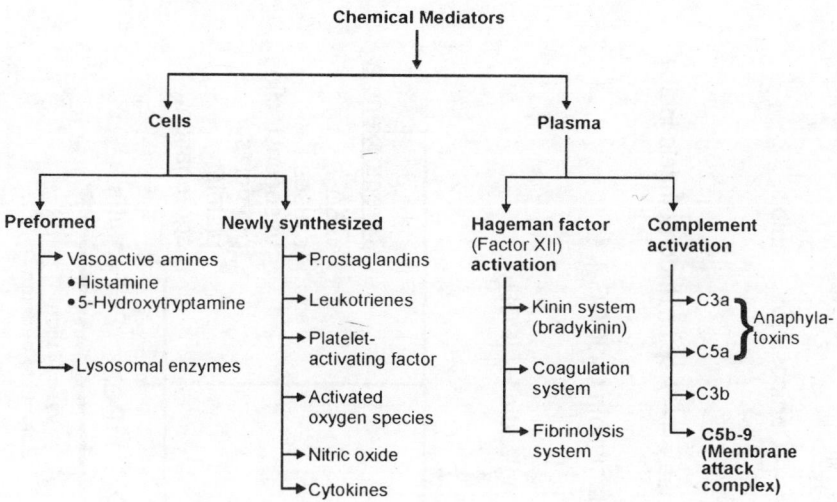

Fig. 16. Chemical mediators of inflammation

body, it does not occur free, but is present mainly in its esterified form **as a component of the cell membrane phospholipids.** It is released from membrane phospholipids through the activation of cellular phospholipases (e.g., phospholipase A2) by mechanical, chemical, or physical stimuli, or by inflammatory mediators such as C5a (Fig. 17). Following activation of phospholipases, **AA metabolism takes place by two major classes of enzymes: (1) cyclooxygenases,** which synthesize **prostaglandins** and **thromboxanes,** and **(2) lipoxygenases,** which synthesize **leukotrienes** and **lipoxins** (Fig. 17). **AA metabolites** (also called **eicosanoids) can mediate virtually every step of inflammation.** Their synthesis is increased at sites of inflammatory response and they are found in inflammatory exudates. Agents that inhibit their synthesis also reduce inflammation.

(1) **Cyclooxygenase pathway:** Cyclooxygenases (COX-1 and COX-2) transform arachidonic acid into **prostaglandin endoperoxide (PGG$_2$),** which is then converted into **prostaglandin H$_2$** by peroxidase (Fig. 17). PGH$_2$ is highly unstable and is converted enzymatically into **three products: (1) thromboxane A$_2$ (TXA$_2$)** is found in platelets, since only platelets contain the enzyme **thromboxane synthase.** TXA$_2$ is a platelet-aggregating agent and vasoconstrictor. **(2) prostacylin (PGI$_2$)** is formed in vascular endothelium, since it contains the enzyme **prostacyclin synthase.** (Endothelium lacks thromboxane synthase enzyme). PGI$_2$ is a vasodilator and an inhibitor

115

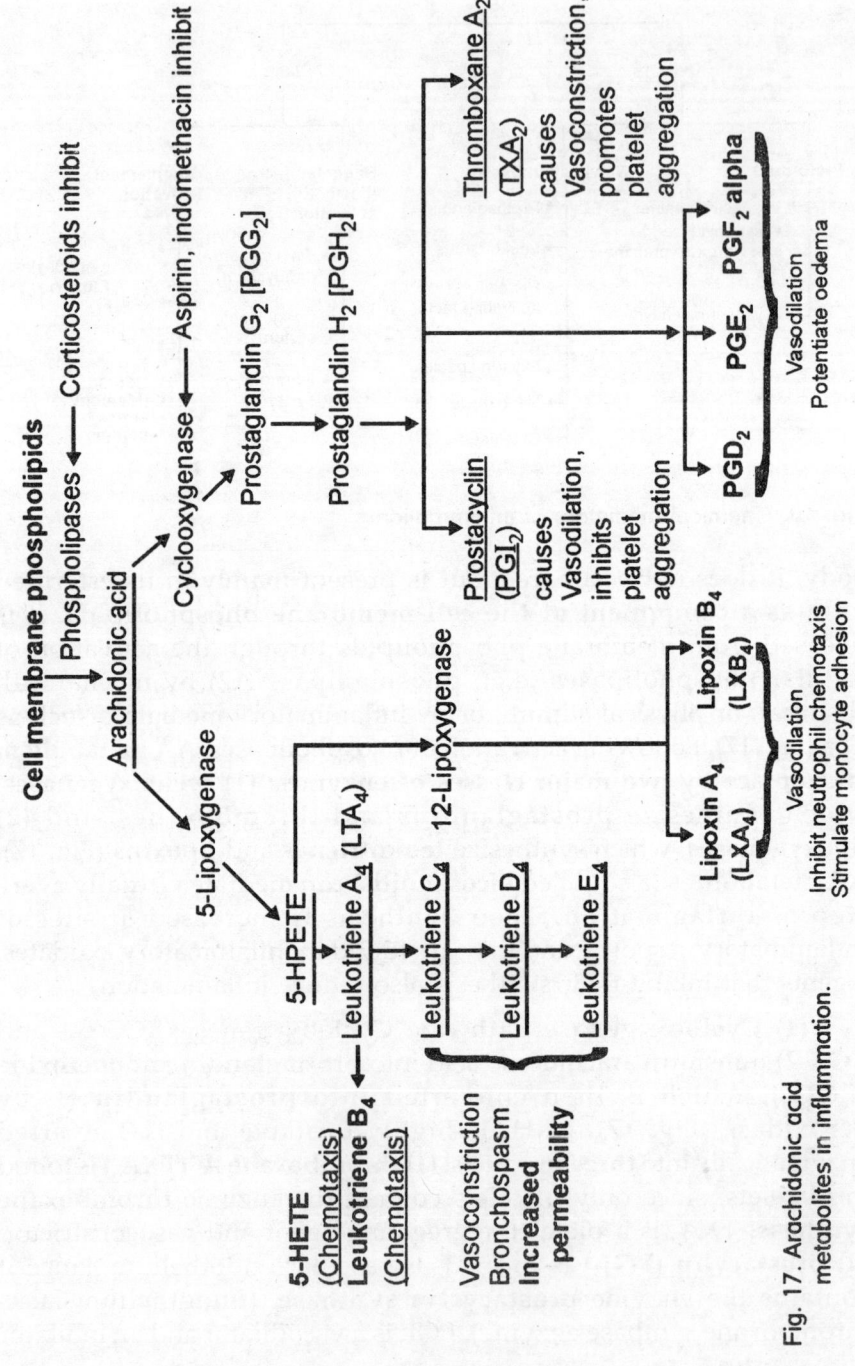

Fig. 17. Arachidonic acid metabolites in inflammation.

of platelet aggregation. The opposing roles of TXA_2 and PGI_2 in haemostasis are further discussed under thrombosis. PGI_2 also markedly potentiates the permeability-increasing and chemotactic effects of other mediators. **(3)** more stable **prostaglandins (PGs)** - PGE_2, PGD_2 and PGF_2-alpha are formed in many other cells, since they contain the enzyme **prostaglandin synthase.** PGD_2 is the major AA metabolite in **mast cells.** PGE_2 and PGF_2 **alpha** are more widely distributed. PGD_2, along with PGE_2 and PGF_2-alpha, causes **vasodilation** and **potentiates oedema formation.** The prostaglandins are also involved in the pathogenesis of **pain** and **fever** in inflammation. PGE_2 increases pain sensitivity to a variety of other stimuli and interacts with cytokines to cause **fever.** Aspirin and non-steroidal anti-inflammatory agents, such as indomethacin and ibuprofen inhibit synthesis of cyclooxygenase and therefore reduce inflammation. **Lipoxygenase is not affected.**

(2) **Lipoxygenase pathway:** The enzyme 5-lipoxygenase converts arachidonic acid (eicosatetraenoic acid) into hydroperoxy derivatives (hydroperoxyeicosatetraenoic acid, 5-HPETE), **by adding hydroperoxy group to AA** (Fig. 17). **5-Lipoxygenase** is the main enzyme in neutrophils. Its product 5-HPETE (5-hydroperoxy derivative of AA) is quite unstable and is either reduced to **5-HETE** (hydroxyeicosatetraenoic acid), which is chemotactic for neutrophils, or converted into a family of compounds collectively called **leukotrienes.** Lekotrienes were so called because they were first isolated from **leukocytes** and also because they contained **triene chain** (i.e., three double bonds). The first leukotriene produced from 5-HPETE is called **leukotriene A₄ (LTA₄),** which is then converted to **leukotriene B₄ (LTB₄)** by enzymatic hydrolysis, or to **leukotriene C₄ (LT C₄)** by addition of glutathione. LTC_4 is converted to leukotriene D_4 **(LTD₄),** and finally to **leukotriene E₄ (LTE₄)** (Fig.17). LTB_4 is a potent chemotactic agent and causes aggregation of neutrophils. LTC_4, LTD_4 and LTE_4 cause vasoconstriction, bronchospasm, and **increased vascular permeability.** LTs, like histamine, increase vascular permeability **only in venules, but their potency is about 1000 times greater than that of histamine.**

(3) **Lipoxins:** Lipoxins are the most recent addition to the family of products formed from arachidonic acid (AA). Lipoxins are synthesized by transcellular pathways, that is, **cell-cell interaction. They are formed by platelets, but platelets alone cannot form lipoxins.** However, when platelets interact with neutrophils, they form lipoxins from neutrophil-derived **LTA₄.** Neutrophils can generate leukotrienes

only up to LTB_4 from AA, but cannot form LTC_4 because they lack the enzyme LTC_4-synthase. In contrast, although platelets cannot form LTC_4 on their own, platelets can generate both LTC_4 and **lipoxins** from neutrophil **LTA_4**, because they possess the necessary enzyme **platelet 12-lipoxygenase.** This enzyme acts on **LTA_4** and produces **lipoxins A4** and **B_4 (LXA_4** and **LXB_4)** within platelets (Fig.17). **Lipoxins have both pro- and anti-inflammatory actions.** For example, LXA_4 causes vasodilation and antagonizes LTC_4-stimulated vasoconstriction. Lipoxins inhibit neutrophil chemotaxis and adhesion, but stimulate monocyte adhesion. Thus, there is an inverse relationship between lipoxins and leukotrienes, which suggests that **lipoxins may be the natural negative regulators of leuktriene actions.**

Table 3. Action of AA metabolites in inflammation

Action	AA Metabolite
Vasoconstriction	Thromboxane A_2. leukotrienes C_4, D_4, E_4
Vasodilation	Prostacyclin (PGI_2), PGE_1, PGE_2, PGD_2, lipoxins
Increased vascular permeability	Leukotrienes C_4, D_4, E_4
Chemotaxis and leukocyte adhesion	Leukotriene B_4, lipoxins

PG = Prostaglandin

To summarize, prostaglandins and leukotrienes can mediate virtually every step of acute inflammation (Table 3). Both are found in inflammatory exudate. Anti-inflammatory drugs such as **aspirin** and **indomethacin** inhibit biosynthesis of prostaglandins by acting on cyclooxygenase; whereas **corticosteroids** by blocking the synthesis of AA through its action on phospholipases, effectively prevent the generation of both prostaglandins and leukotrienes. PGE_2 and PGI_2 are important mediators of vasodilation. They do no increase vascular permeability but potentiate the effect of histamine and bradykinin. **LTC_4, LTD_4,** and **LTE_4** (also known as **slow-reacting substance of anaphylaxis, SRS-A)** are at least 1000 times as potent as histamine in increasing vascular permeability. LTB_4 causes marked aggregation and adhesion of leukocytes to vascular endothelium and is a powerful chemotactic agent. The PGs are also involved in the production of pain and fever during inflammation. **Lipoxins** are the most recently known products generated from arachidonic acid metabolism. They have both pro- and anti-inflammatory actions. They have an inverse relationship with leukotrienes, which suggests that lipoxins may be the natural negative regulators of leukotrienes.

Lysosomal Constituents

The **lysosomal granules of neutrophils and monocytes contain many molecules that can mediate acute inflammation.** These may be released after cell death, by leakage during formation of the phagocytic vacuole, or by **frustrated phagocytosis** against large, indigestible surfaces (described later). Neutrophils exhibit two main types of granules - the smaller **specific** (or secondary) **granules** and large **azurophil** (or primary) **granules**. The **specific granules** contain lysozyme, collagenase, alkaline phosphatase, lactoferrin, plasminogen activator, and histaminase. The **azurophil granules** contain myeloperoxidase, bactericidal factors (lysozyme, defensins), acid hydrolases, and a variety of neutral proteases (elastase, cathepsin G, non-specific collagenases, proteinase 3). **Acid proteases** degrade bacteria at an acid pH **within** the phagolysosomes, whereas **neutral proteases** degrade various **extracellular** components and cause destructive tissue injury by degrading elastin, collagen, basement membrane, and other matrix proteins. **Neutral proteases** can also cleave C3 and C5 directly to generate C3a and C5a **anaphylatoxins** and promote the generation of bradykinin-like peptides from kininogen. Thus, if the initial leukocyte infiltration is left unchecked, it can lead to further increases in vascular permeability, chemotaxis, and tissue damage. These harmful proteases, however, are held in check by a system of **antiproteases** in the serum and tissue fluids. The most important of these is **alpha-1-antitrypsin,** which is the major inhibitor of neutrophil elastase.

Platelet Activating Factor (PAF)

PAF, like prostaglandins and leukotrienes, is a phospholipid-derived mediator. It was so named because of its ability to aggregate platelets and cause degranulation. However, it is now known to have **many inflammatory effects.** PAF is not stored as a preformed mediator, but is generated from the membrane phospholipids of a variety of cell types, including neutrophils, monocytes, basophils, endothelium, and platelets by the action of **phospholipase A2.** Chemically, PAF is **acetyl glycerol ether phosphocholine (AGEPC).** Besides platelet stimulation, PAF causes **vasoconstriction,** and at extremely low concentrations, it induces **vasodilation and increased**

119

vascular (venular) permeability with a potency 100 to 10,000 times greater than that of histamine. PAF also causes increased leukocyte adhesion to endothelium, chemotaxis, degranulation, and the oxidative burst. **Thus, PAF can produce most of the changes of inflammation.**

Oxygen-Derived Free Radicals

Oxygen-derived free radicals may be released extracellularly from **neutrophils** and **macrophages** after exposure to chemotactic agents, immune complexes, or following phagocytic activity. Their production is dependent, as we have seen, on activation of the NADPH oxidative system (see 'free radical-induced cell injury'). Superoxide $(O_2^{\bullet-})$, hydrogen peroxide (H_2O_2), and hydroxyl radical $(OH^{\bullet})$ are the major species produced within the cell, and these metabolites can combine with nitric oxide (NO) to form other **reactive nitrogen intermediates** (i.e., **toxic NO derivatives**). **At low levels**, these reactive oxygen species can increase chemokine, cytokine, and adhesion molecule expression, thus amplifying the effects of inflammatory mediators. **At high levels**, these short-lived molecules are involved in a variety of tissue injury mechanisms. They cause endothelial cell damage, which results in increased vascular permeability.

Nitric Oxide

Nitric oxide (NO) is a short-lived, soluble, **free radical gas** produced by a variety of cells. Apart from its effect on the inflammatory response, NO is capable of mediating a vast number of effector functions. When produced by endothelium (where it was first discovered and named **'endothelium-derived relaxation factor'**), it causes smooth muscle relaxation (**vasodilation**).

Since the half-life of NO is in seconds, the gas acts only on those cells near the source where it is generated. NO is synthesized from the amino acid **arginine, molecular oxygen, and NADPH** by the enzyme **nitric oxide synthase (NOS)** (Fig. 18). There are **three different types of NOS,** with different tissue distribution: (1) **Type I (nNOS)** is a constitutively expressed neuronal NOS. That is, it is present in the constitution, or physiological make-up of neurons. (2) **Type II (eNOS)** is also a **constitutively** synthesized NOS found mainly within endothelium. (3) **Type III (iNOS)** is an inducible enzyme. That is, it is produced when cells are activated by cytokines (TNF-alpha, IFN-gamma) or other agents. This enzyme is present in many cell types, which include macrophages, endothelium, smooth muscle cells, hepatocytes, cardiac myocytes, and respiratory epithelium. It is induced by a number of inflammatory cytokines and mediators, mainly IL-1, TNF-alpha, and interferon-gamma, and by lipopolysaccharide (LPS) present in the cell walls of Gram-negative bacteria.

Nitric oxide plays many roles in inflammation. It is a **potent vasodilator.** In addition, NO **reduces platelet and leukocyte adhesion.** Nitric oxide free radicals also act as a **microbicidal agent in activated macrophages.**

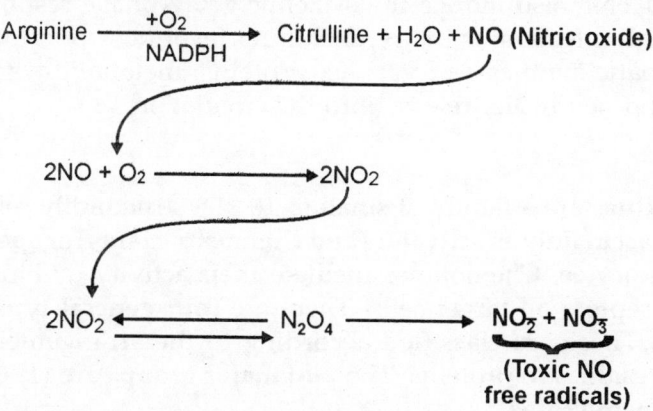

Fig. 18. Production of nitric oxide from arginine, a major antimicrobial system in macrophages.

Cytokines

Cytokines are **proteins** produced by many cells, mainly **activated lymphocytes** and **macrophages** that modulate (regulate) the function of other cell types. Those secreted from lymphocytes are called **'lymphokines'**, and from monocytes as **'monokines'**. Collectively, they are all known as **'cytokines'**. Cytokines have long been known to be involved in cellular immune responses, but they also **play an important role in both acute and chronic inflammation.**

The **two most important cytokines** that mediate inflammation are (1) **interleukin-1 (IL-1),** and (2) **tumour necrosis factor (TNF).** IL-1 and TNF share many biological properties. **IL-1 and TNF are produced by activated macrophages** (see 'macrophages'). Their secretion is stimulated by endotoxins, immune complexes, toxins,

121

physical injury, or a variety of inflammatory mediators. Their most important actions are their effects on endothelium, leukocytes, and fibroblasts; and induction of the systemic acute-phase reactions. Both IL-1 and TNF induce **endothelial activation** that causes increased expression of **adhesion molecules** that mediate leukocyte sticking (see 'cellular events'), secretion of additional cytokines and growth factors, and production of arachidonic acid (AA) metabolites, and nitric oxide. TNF also causes aggregation and activation of neutrophils and release of proteolytic enzymes, thus contributing to **tissue damage**. Both the cytokines activate fibroblasts, resulting in fibrosis.

IL-1 and TNF also induce the systemic **acute-phase responses** associated with infection or injury, including fever, loss of appetite, lethargy, hepatic synthesis of various proteins, metabolic wasting (**cachexia**), and neutrophil release into the circulation.

Chemokines

Chemokines are a family of small (8-10 kD) structurally related **proteins** that **act mainly as activators and chemoattractants for specific types of leukocytes.** Chemokines mediate their activity by binding to specific receptors on target cells. There are **four general types of chemokines.** These are classified according to the arrangement of cysteine (C) residues in proteins. The **two major groups are** (1) **CXC**, and (2) **CC chemokines.**

CXC chemokines act mainly on **neutrophils.** Interleukin-8 (IL-8) is typical of this group. It is produced by **activated macrophages**, endothelium, or fibroblasts, mainly in response to IL-1 and TNF. **CC chemokines** include **monocyte chemoattractant protein-1 (MCP-1),** and **macrophage inflammatory protein-1 alpha (MIP-1 alpha).** Both are chemotactic mainly for **monocytes. To conclude, chemokines play a role in regulating leukocyte recruitment and activation during inflammation.**

Plasma Proteases

Three inter-related systems - the kinin, clotting/fibrinolytic, and complement systems - come under this category (Fig. 19). They mediate many of the effects of inflammation. The kinins are highly vasoactive, whereas complement components are both vasoactive and chemotactic.

The kinin, clotting, and fibrinolytic systems are all linked to the initial activation of **Hageman factor** (Fig. 19). Hageman factor (factor

XII of the intrinsic coagulation pathway) is a protein synthesized by the liver that circulates in an **inactive form.** It gets activated when it comes in contact with collagen, basement membrane, or activated platelets at the site of endothelial injury.

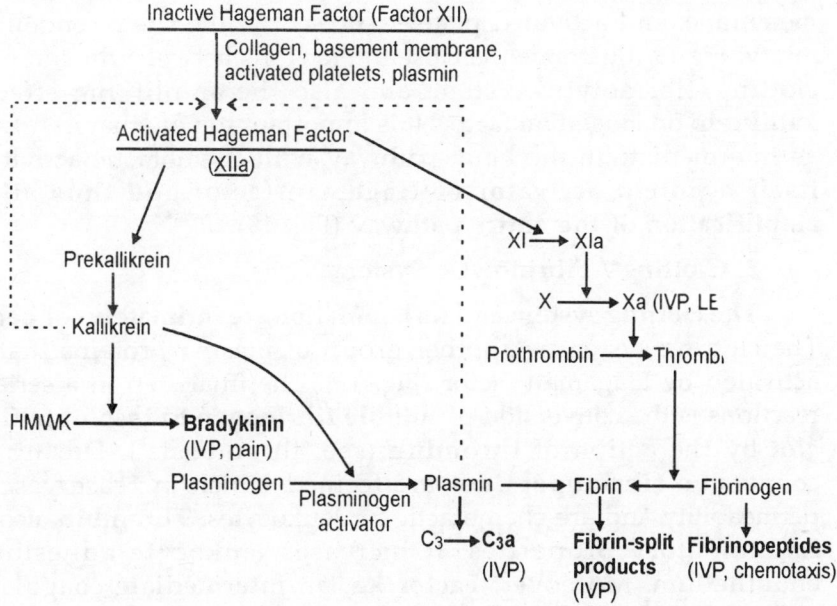

Fig. 19. Inter-relationships between kinin, clotting, and fibrinolytic systems and their role in inflammation. IVP = increased vascular permeability; LE = leukocyte emigration

1. Kinin System

The **kinin system** is one of the three systems triggered by the activation of Hageman factor. Activation of the kinin system leads to the formation of **bradykinin** (Fig. 19). Like histamine, **bradykinin causes increased vascular permeability and arteriolar dilation.** It also causes contraction of smooth muscle, and **pain.** The action of bradykinin is short-lived because it is quickly inactivated by an enzyme called **kininase** present in plasma and tissues. **The role of bradykinin is limited to the early phase of increased vascular permeability.**

Bradykinin is a vasoactive nonapeptide (i.e., has nine amino acids) derived from plasma, where it is present in a glycoprotein-

123

precursor form called **high-molecular-weight kininogen (HMWK)**. This precursor glycoprotein is cleaved (split) by a proteolytic enzyme, **kallikrein**. Kallikrein is activated from its own precursor, **prekallikrein** by activated factor XII of the clotting system (**Hageman factor**). As already mentioned, Hageman factor gets activated on contact with the injured tissues, especially collagen, basement membrane, and activated platelets present at the site of endothelial injury. Fig.19 illustrates the close interactions between the kinin and clotting/fibrinolytic system, and also the amplifying effect of **kallikrein** on Hageman factor. It is important to note that **kallikrein**, an intermediate in the kinin pathway with chemotactic activity, **is itself a potent activator of Hageman factor and thus allows amplification of the entire pathway** (Fig. 19).

2. Clotting / Fibrinolytic System

The clotting system and inflammation are intimately connected. The clotting system is another group of plasma proteins that are activated by Hageman factor (Fig. 19). The final step in a series of reactions is the conversion of **soluble fibrinogen** to **insoluble fibrin clot** by the action of **thrombin** (see 'thrombosis'). During this conversion **fibrinopeptides** are formed which increase vascular permeability and are chemotactic for leukocytes. **Thrombin** also has inflammatory properties. It increases leukocyte adhesion to endothelium. Moreover, **Factor Xa,** an intermediate coagulation protease in the clotting cascade (pathway), causes increased vascular permeability and leukocyte emigration.

While activated Hageman factor is producing clotting, at the same time it also activates the **fibrinolytic system.** This mechanism exists to control clotting, by breaking fibrin, thereby solubilizing the fibrin clot (i.e., **fibrinolysis**). Without fibrinolysis, activation of the clotting system, even by insignificant injury, would lead to continuous and uncontrollable clotting of the entire vascular system. **Plasminogen activator** (released from endothelium, leukocytes, and other tissues) and **kallikrein,** cleave (split) **plasminogen**, a plasma protein, to produce a protease known as **plasmin**. Plasmin is important in lysing (dissolving) fibrin clots, but has several actions on inflammation: (1) **It activates Hageman factor (XII),** thereby it amplifies the entire set of responses (Fig.19). (2) **It splits C3**, the third component of complement, to produce **C3a,** resulting in vasodilation and increased vascular permeability. (3) **It degrades fibrin** to form **fibrin split products** (fibrin degradation products), which increase vascular permeability (Fig.19).

3. Complement System

The **complement system** consists of a group of serum proteins (20) that play an important role in both immunity and inflammation. Complement is an essential part of the body's defences. In immunity, this system acts for defence against bacteria. Complement proteins ultimately produce a **pore-like membrane attack complex (MAC)** (discussed later) that punches holes in the membrane of invading bacteria. In the process of producing MAC, a number of complement fragments are produced, including **C3b opsonins** as well as **fragments that contribute to the inflammatory response by increasing vascular permeability and leukocyte chemotaxis.**

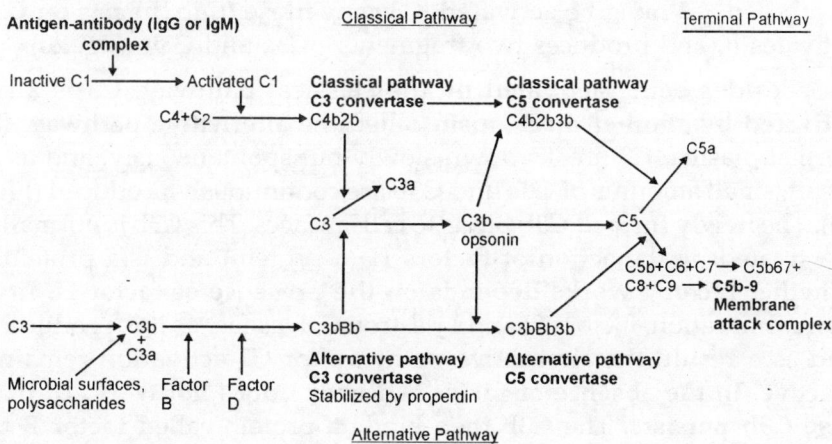

Fig. 20. Complement activation pathways.

Complement components (numbered C1 to C9) are present in **inactive forms** in serum. They are activated in two major ways: (1) by **classical pathway**, and (2) by **alternative pathway** (Fig. 20). However, **the most important of these is the classical pathway.** By classical pathway, activation occurs rapidly and efficiently, whereas with the alternative pathway, it occurs more slowly. The **classical pathway** is initiated by the fixation of C1 to antigen-antibody complexes, whereas the **alternative pathway** by a variety of non-immunological stimuli, such as microbial surfaces (e.g., endotoxins), complex polysaccharides, or aggregated IgA. As a result of activation, **cleavage products** are produced which **have profound effects on inflammation.** Both pathways converge into the **common terminal**

pathway (Fig. 20).

Briefly, the classical pathway is initiated by fixation (binding) of C1 to antigen-antibody (IgG or IgM) complexes. The **activated C1** then acts on C4 and C2. Although the complement components are numbered, they do not act in numerical order. Interactions between C4 and C2 first generate the complex **C4b2** and afterwards **C4b2b**. C4b2b is a potent protease, which acts on its substrate **C3**. **C4b2b** is therefore called **classical C3 convertase. C3 is the most important of the complement components**, and its activation is the most critical step in the production of the biological functions of complement. C3 is synthesized by liver cells and macrophages, and is the complement component of highest concentration in serum. For further reactions to proceed, **C3 must be activated. C3 convertase (C4b2b)** acts on C3, activates it, and produces two fragments - **C3a** and **C3b** (Fig. 20).

Besides being activated by the classical pathway, **C3 is also activated by another mechanism** called the **alternative pathway.** In normal plasma, C3 breaks down slowly but spontaneously, and as a result, small amounts of **C3a** and **C3b** are continuously produced (Fig. 20). The **newly formed C3b** binds to cell surfaces. This C3b is normally inactivated by the action of **factors H** (a protein) and **I** (a protein). **Whether factor I works depends on the presence of factor H.** In a normal situation, factors H and I destroy C3b as fast as it is produced, and as a result, the alternative pathway for C3 activation remains inactive. **In the absence of factor H, factor I does not work. In that case C3b persists**. The C3b then binds a protein called **factor B** to form a complex called **C3bB**. The bound factor B is then split by another protease, **factor D**, into Ba and **C3bBb**. The complex **C3bBb** is a potent **C3 convertase of the alternative pathway** (Fig. 20). (Remember the classical C3 convertase is C4b2b). The **alternative C3 convertase (C3bBb)** can split **C3** to generate **C3b**, but C3bBb's half-life is of only 5 minutes. If a protein called **factor P** (or **properdin**) binds to C3bBb to form C3bBbP, its half-life is extended to 30 minutes. C3b can also be produced by other proteases acting on C3, for example, proteases from activated macrophages. **As a result, C3b is produced at sites of inflammation.**

The **terminal pathway** is initiated by the binding of surface-bound **C3b to C5**. When **C3b** is bound to **C5**, C5 becomes susceptible to either **C4b2b** (classical C3 convertase), **or C3bBb** (alternative C3 convertase). Thus, these enzymes are also **C5 convertase (C4b2b3b** of classical pathway and **C3bBb3b** of alternative pathway) (Fig. 20). Once

126

C5 binds to C3b, **C4b2b3b** or **C3bBb3b** splits off a small fragment from **C5** called **C5a**, and the part of C5 molecule remaining attached to **C3b**, is called **C5b**. This split exposes a site on C5b that binds C6 and C7 to form **C5b67**. The **C5b67 complex** can detach from **C3b** and insert itself into the nearby cell or microbial membranes. Once inserted in these membranes, the complex incorporates one **C8** and many **C9** molecules. C9 is a protein of the perforin family. 12 to 19 C9 molecules come together with the **C5b678** complex to form **C5b-9**, a tubular transmembrane ring-shaped structure called the **membrane attack complex (MAC, C5b-9).** The MAC inserts itself into a cell membrane and forms a cylindrical transmembrane channel. **If sufficient MACs are formed on the cell membrane, osmotic lysis (death) of the target cell occurs.**

Complement-derived factors exert a variety of effects on inflammation. These include:

1. Vascular effects: **C3a** and **C5a** (also called **anaphylatoxins**) **increase vascular permeability** and **vasodilation**, mainly by releasing **histamine** from mast cells. **C5a** also activates the lipoxygenase pathway of arachidonic acid (AA) metabolism in neutrophils and monocytes, causing further release of inflammatory mediators.

2. Leukocyte activation, adhesion, and chemotaxis: **C5a** activates leukocytes and increases the affinity of their integrins (discussed later), thereby increasing adhesion to endothelium. It is also **a potent chemotactic agent** for neutrophils, monocytes, eosinophils, and basophils.

3. Phagocytosis: **C3b** and **C3bi**, when fixed to the bacterial cell wall, act as **opsonins** and favour phagocytosis by neutrophils and macrophages, which bear cell surface receptors for C3b.

Among the complement components, C3 and C5 are the most important inflammatory mediators. Their significance is further increased by the fact that they **can also be activated by proteolytic enzymes present within the inflammatory exudate.** These include **lysosomal enzymes released from neutrophils**, as well as **plasmin**. Thus, the chemotactic effect of complement and the complement activating effects of neutrophils, can set up **a self-perpetuating cycle of neutrophil emigration**.

From this discussion of the plasma proteases, **a few general conclusions** can be drawn:

1. **Activated Hageman factor (factor XIIa)** initiates **four systems**

involved in the inflammatory response: (i) **kinin system,** producing vasoactive kinins, (ii) **clotting system,** inducing activation of thrombin, fibrinopeptides, and factor X, all with inflammatory properties, (iii) **fibrinolytic system,** producing plasmin and degrading thrombin, and (iv) **complement system,** producing anaphylatoxins C3a and C5a.

2. **Bradykinin, C3a, and C5a** are major mediators of increased vascular permeability.

3. **C5a** is a major mediator of chemotaxis.

4. **Thrombin** has significant effects on many cells and pathways, such as leukocyte adhesion, vascular permeability, and chemotaxis.

5. Many of the products of the pathway, for example, **kallikrein** and **plasmin**, can amplify the system by feedback activation of Hageman factor (see Fig. 20).

Summary of the Chemical Mediators of Acute Inflammation

Table 4 summarizes the major actions of the principal mediators. **Vasodilation** is mainly regulated by the prostaglandins PGI_2 and TXA_2 and by NO, while **increased vascular permeability** is mediated through histamine, anaphylatoxins (C3a and C5a), kinins, PAF, and leukotrienes C, D, and E. Cytokines (IL-1, TNF) and prostaglandins also play a major role in **leukocyte and endothelial activation** as well as in the systemic manifestations of acute inflammation (**fever, pain**). Finally, **tissue damage** is mainly due to the effects of NO, oxygen-derived free radicals, and leukocyte lysosomal enzymes. A point of great significance is that with all these mediators there seems to be a system of checks and balances. Life, otherwise, would be impossible.

Regarding chemical mediation of the acute inflammation in **domestic animals and birds,** role of histamine, kinins and anaphylatoxins (C3a, C5a) has been established. Participation of other mediators/factors, though strongly suspected is, at present, not well defined.

CELLULAR EVENTS

The cellular events in inflammation were clarified by the Russian biologist Elie Metchnikoff, in 1884. He inserted rose thorns into the larvae of a starfish and next day observed a grey zone around the thorns. The grey zone turned out to be an accumulation of large cells. Because the cells were large and possessed phagocytic properties, he named them **macrophages** (G. macro = large; phagein = to eat) in

Table 4. Most likely mediators in inflammation

Vasodilation

Prostaglandins

Nitric oxide

Increased vascular permeability

Vasoactive amines (histamine, 5-hydroxytryptamine)

C3a and C5a (by causing release of vasoactive amines)

Bradykinin

Leukotrienes C_4, D_4, E_4

Platelet-activating factor

Chemotaxis, leukocyte activation

C5a

Leukotriene B_4

Bacterial products

Chemokines (interleukin-8)

Fever

IL-1, IL-6, tumour necrosis factor

Prostaglandins

Pain

Prostaglandins

Bradykinin

Tissue damage

Neutrophil and macrophage lysosomal enzymes

Oxygen metabolites

Nitric oxide

contrast to the small phagocytic cell, the **neutrophil**, which was called **microphage** (G. micro = small).

Thus, **the most important function of inflammation is delivery of leukocytes, particularly neutrophils and monocytes, to the site of injury.** Leukocytes engulf and kill bacteria and degrade necrotic tissue and immune complexes. In addition, their lysosomal enzymes also contribute to the defensive response. Unfortunately, during these defensive reactions, leukocytes may themselves prolong inflammation and induce tissue damage by releasing lysosomal enzymes, chemical mediators, and toxic oxygen radicals.

The sequence of events in the journey of leukocytes from the lumen of blood vessels into the extravascular space is called **extravasation**. These events can be divided into: (1) margination, (2) adhesion, (3) emigration (transmigration), (4) phagocytosis, and (5) release of leukocyte products.

(1) **Margination**: In normally flowing blood in venules, the red and white cells are confined to the **central axial column**, leaving a relatively cell-free layer of plasma in contact with the vessel wall. As blood flow slows early in inflammation (as a result of increased vascular permeability), white cells fall out of the central column. Here, they have a better opportunity to interact with lining endothelial cells. This process of leukocyte accumulation at the periphery of vessels is called **margination**. Afterwards, leukocytes tumble (roll over and over) slowly along the endothelial surface and adhere transiently. This process of **brief, loose sticking** of leukocytes to the endothelium is called **rolling**.

2. **Adhesion**: Finally, leukocytes come to rest at some point where they adhere firmly. This **firm sticking (attachment)** of leukocytes to the endothelium is called **adhesion**. Leukocytes can be compared with pebbles over which a stream runs without disturbing them. In time, the endothelium is virtually lined by white cells. This appearance is called **pavementing.**

3. **Emigration (transmigration)**: After **firm adhesion**, leukocytes insert their pseudopods into the inter-endothelial junctions. Then, they squeeze through these gaps and occupy a position between the endothelial cell and the basement membrane. Finally, they crawl through the basement membrane and escape into the extravascular space. This process by which leukocytes come out of the blood vessels into the extravascular space is called **emigration**. It is also known by two other names - **transmigration** and **diapedesis**. Neutrophils, **monocytes, lymphocytes, eosinophils, and basophils all use the same pathway.**

Molecular Mechanisms of Rolling, Adhesion, and Emigration

It is now clear that **leukocyte adhesion and emigration in inflammation involve binding of complementary 'adhesion molecules' present on the surfaces of leukocytes and endothelial cells, like a key and lock.** It is also now clear that **chemical mediators (chemoattractants and certain cytokines) affect these processes by regulating the surface expression or affinity of such adhesion**

molecules. The adhesion molecules involved belong to the following three molecular families (Table 5).

1. **Selectins**: **Selectins are receptors** expressed on leukocytes and endothelium. These consist of: (i) **E-selectin** (previously **ELAM-1**). It is confined to endothelium; (ii) **P-selectin,** present on endothelium and platelets; and (iii) **L-selectin** (previously LAM-1), present on most leukocytes. **E- and P-selectins** bind to their receptors **sialyl-Lewis-X modified glycoprotein** present on leukocytes, while **L-selectin on leukocytes** binds to its **L-selectin ligand** present on endothelium (see Table 5, Fig. 21B-2).

2. **Immunoglobulins**: The immunoglobulin molecules include **two endothelial adhesion molecules** (i) **ICAM-1** (intercellular adhesion molecule-1), and (ii) **VCAM-1** (vascular cell adhesion molecule-1). Both of these molecules interact with **integrins** (discussed next) found on leukocytes (Table 5).

3. **Integrins**: These are glycoproteins. The main integrin receptors for **ICAM-1** are the integrins **LFA-1** and **MAC-1**, and that for **VCAM-1** is the integrin **VLA-4** (Table 5).

How are these molecules regulated (governed) to induce leukocyte adhesion in inflammation? There are **three important mechanisms.**

1. **Redistribution of adhesion molecules**: **P-selectin** is normally present in intracellular **Weibel-Palade bodies** in non-activated endothelial cells. However, within minutes of exposure to mediators such as **histamine, thrombin, platelet activating factor** (PAF), P-selectin is rapidly re-distributed to the cell surface, where it can bind to leukocytes.

2. **Induction of adhesion molecules on endothelium**: Some inflammatory molecules, particularly **cytokines (IL-1** and **TNF)** induce synthesis and surface expression of adhesion molecules on endothelium. The process requires **new protein synthesis** and begins after 1 or 2 hours. **E-selectin,** which is not present on normal endothelium, is induced after stimulation by **IL-1 and TNF** and mediates the adhesion of neutrophils, monocytes, and certain lymphocytes by binding to its receptors. The same cytokines also increase the expression of **ICAM-1 and VCAM-1**, which are present at low levels in normal endothelium.

3. **Increased binding affinity**: This mechanism is most important in the binding of **integrins**. For example, **LFA-1** is present on

Table 5. Endothelial and leukocyte adhesion molecules

Endothelial molecule	Leukocyte molecule	Major role
P-Selectin	Sialyl-Lewis X-modified protein	**Rolling** (neutrophils, monocytes, lymphocytes)
GlyCam-1, CD34	L-selectin	**Rolling** (neutrophils, monocytes)
E-Selectin	Sialyl-Lewis X-modified protein	**Rolling and adhesion** (neutrophils, monocytes, T-lymphocytes)
VCAM-1 (immunoglobulin family)	VLA-4 integrin	**Adhesion** (eosinophils, monocytes, lymphocytes)
ICAM-1 (immunoglobulin family)	LFA-1, Mac-1 (CD11/CD18 integrins)	**Adhesion, arrest, emigration** (neutrophils monocytes, lymphocytes)
PECAM-1 (CD31)	PECAM-1 (CD31)	**Arrest, emigration** (neutrophils, monocytes, lymphocytes)

ICAM-1 = Intercellular adhesion molecule-1

PECAM-1 = Platelet endothelial cell adhesion molecule-1

VCAM-1 = Vascular cell adhesion molecule-1

leukocytes (neutrophils, monocytes, lymphocytes) but does not attach to its ligand ICAM-1 on endothelium. To become firmly attached the neutrophil has to be activated in such a way that **LAF-1** is converted from a state of **low-affinity binding to high-affinity binding** toward **ICAM-1**. The main agents which cause such leukocyte activation are **chemotactic agents**, such as C5a and LTB4 (including **chemokines**, discussed earlier). **During inflammation**, the increased affinity of **LFA-1** on the activated leukocytes, accompanied by increased ICAM-1 expression on endothelium caused by cytokines, brings about **strong LFA-1/ICAM-1 binding. The LFA-1/ICAM-1 interaction causes firm adhesion** to the endothelium and is also necessary for subsequent emigration across the endothelium.

Molecules mediating endothelial-neutrophil interactions

The following steps are involved in **neutrophil adhesion and emigration** in acute inflammation (see Fig. 21).

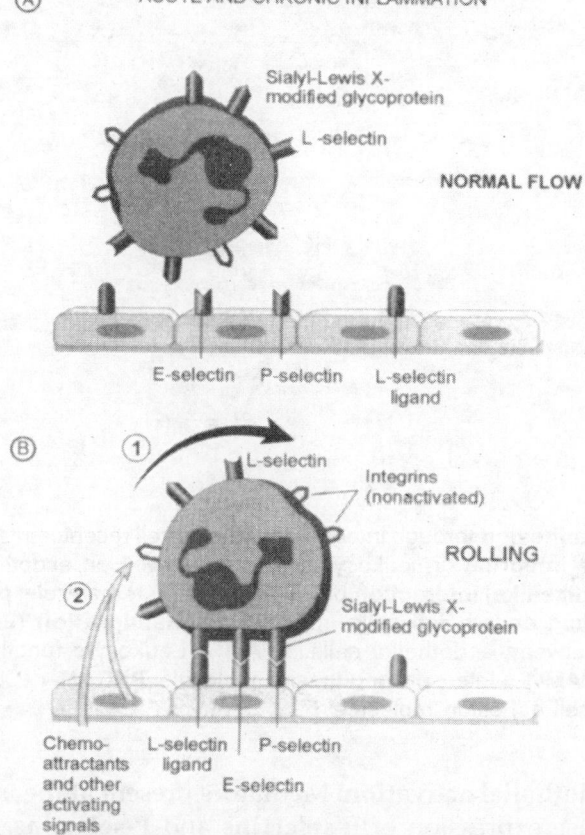

Fig. 21. Molecules that mediate endothelial-neutrophil interactions. (A) Normal flow (B) Rolling (1) Initial adhesion. At the inflammatory sites, **E** and **P-selectins** are increasingly synthesized on endothelial cells by specific mediators. **E** and **P-selectins** bind **sialyl-Lewis X-modified glycoproteins** on leukocytes, while **L-selectins** on leukocytes bind **L-selectin ligands** on endothelial cell. **(2) Activation of leukocytes** by chemokine mediators increases strength of **integrin** affinity.

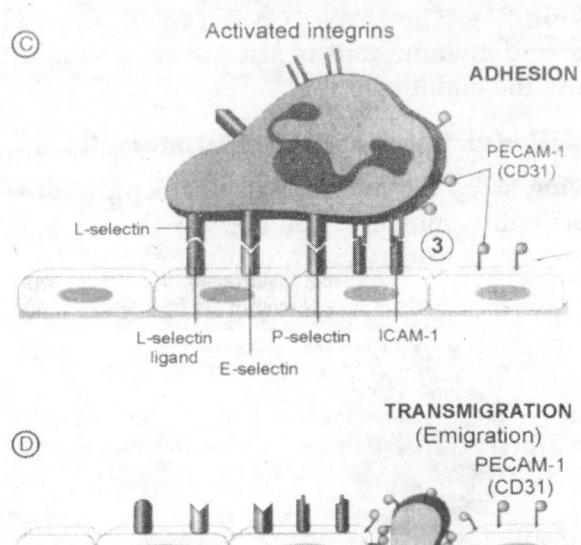

(C) (3) Firm adhesion through integrin-endothelial cell receptor interactions. **LFA-1** and **Mac-1 integrins** on leukocytes bind to **ICAM-1** on endothelial cells. **(D)** **Homotypic (like-like) interaction** of **PECAM-1** (CD31) molecule, present on both leukocytes and endothelial cells, mediates **transmigration (emigration)** of neutrophil between endothelial cells. **LFA-1** = Leukocyte function-associated antigen-1; **ICAM-1** = Intercellular adhesion molecule; **PECAM-1** (CD31) = Platelet endothelial cell adhesion molecule 1

1. **Endothelial activation**: Mediators present at the inflammatory sites increase expression of E-**selectins** and **P-selectins**.

2. **Leukocyte rolling**: This is a **loose adhesion**, resulting from interactions between selectins and their ligands (Fig. 21B).

134

3. **Firm adhesion**: The leukocytes are then activated by **chemokines**, or other agents, **to increase the affinity of their integrins** (Fig. 21C-3)

4. **Emigration (transmigration)**: This is mediated by interactions between **PECAM-1** (platelet endothelial cell adhesion molecule-1) (CD31) **present on both leukocytes and endothelial cells** (Fig. 21D). This is called **homotypic or homophilic interaction**, that is, like-like interaction. In other words, interaction between similar adhesion molecules **that bind to each other.**

The proof of the importance of adhesion molecules has come from a genetic deficiency in the leukocyte adhesion glycoproteins called **leukocyte adhesion deficiency (LAD)**, which is characterized by defective leukocyte adhesion and recurrent bacterial infections. In **LAD type-1**, there is a defect in the biosynthesis of the beta chain shared by **LFA-1** and **Mac-1 integrins** that mediate leukocyte-endothelial adhesion (see Table 5). LAD type-2 is caused by the absence of **sialyl-Lewis X**, the ligand for **E-selectin,** due to a generalized defect in fucose metabolism.

Although passage through the endothelial cell cytoplasm (intracellular) has been described, **emigration of leukocytes occurs mainly through the intercellular junctions.** Certain homophilic (homotypic) adhesion molecules, present in the intercellular junction of endothelium, are involved. One of these is a member of the immunoglobulin family and is **PECAM-1** (platelet endothelial cell adhesion molecule) or **CD31.** After travelling through the endothelium, leukocytes are temporarily slowed down in their journey by the continuous basement membrane. But, ultimately, they pierce by secreting enzymes **collagenases** that degrade (destroy) the basement membrane.

It is now clear that **increased vascular permeability is not the cause of leukocyte emigration** and that both are separate phenomena, that is, they are independent of each other.

In most forms of acute inflammation, **neutrophils emigrate first and monocytes later.** Neutrophils predominate during the first 6 to 24 hours in most inflammatory infiltrates. However, between 24 to 48 hours, they are replaced by monocytes, owing to two factors: (1) neutrophils are short-lived. They undergo apoptosis (die) and disappear after 24 to 48 hours, whereas monocytes survive much longer and may persist for long periods as tissue macrophages. (2) different adhesion molecules or specific chemotactic factors for neutrophils and monocytes are activated at different times of the inflammatory response. However, there are exceptions to this pattern of cellular emigration. In **Pseudomonas** infection, neutrophils predominate over 2 to 4 days; in viral infections, lymphocytes may be the first cells to arrive; in some hypersensitivity reactions, eosinophils may be the main cell type.

CHEMOTAXIS

After escape from blood, leukocytes migrate in tissues towards the site of injury by a process called **chemotaxis**. Chemotaxis is the force that attracts leukocytes into the inflamed tissue. (**Chemotaxis** is a Greek word and means **chemical attraction**). Leukocytes migrate along a chemical gradient. That is, towards an increasing amount of the chemical attractant. Thus, **chemotaxis is defined as the unidirectional migration of cells towards a chemical attractant.** The term should be differentiated from **chemokinesis**, which is an accelerated random movement of cells.

Chemotaxis can be clearly demonstrated by Boyden's micropore filter technique. In this technique, leukocytes are placed in one compartment of a chamber, and separated by a porous filter membrane from a second compartment in which the chemotactic substance is placed. If a chemotactic influence is present, leukocytes crawl across the pores of the filter. By counting the cells in the second chamber, quantitation of chemotaxis can be done. **Some chemotactic factors act only on the neutrophils, others only on monocytes, and some affect both.**

Both **exogenous** and **endogenous substances** can act as chemotactic agents (i.e., chemoattractant) for leukocytes. The most common **exogenous agents** are **soluble bacterial products,** particularly peptides that possess an N-formyl-methionine terminal amino acid. Others are lipid in nature. **Endogenous chemical mediators** include: (1) **components of the complement system,** particularly C5a, (2) **products of the lipoxygenase pathway,** mainly leukotriene B_4 (LTB$_4$), and (3) **cytokines,** particularly those of the chemokine family, for example, interleukin-8 (IL-8). **Among these, the most important attractants for neutrophils are bacterial products, C5a, and LTB$_4$.**

But how do these diverse chemotactic agents actually induce directed cell movement (i.e., chemotaxis)? Not all the answers are known, but several important steps and second messengers are recognized (Fig. 22).

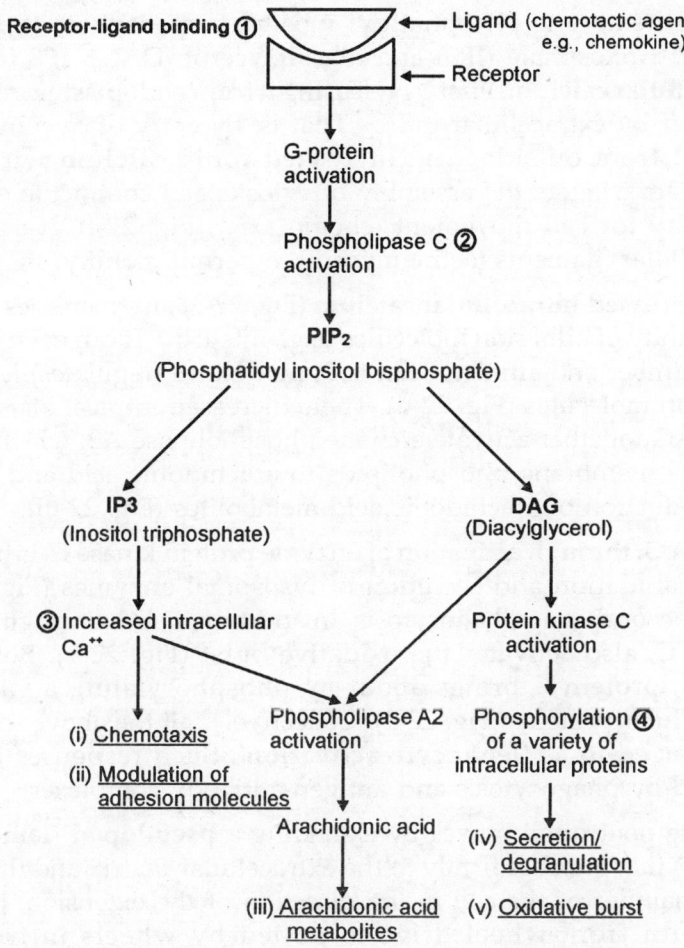

Fig. 22. Biochemical events in leukocyte activation. The key events are: (1) receptor-ligand binding, (2) phospholipase C activation, (3) increased intracellular calcium, and (4) activation of protein kinase C, resulting in protein phosphorylation. **The biological activities that result from leukocyte activation include**: (i) chemotaxis, (ii) modulation of adhesion molecules, (iii) elaboration of arachidonic acid metabolites, (iv) secretion/degranulation, and (v) the oxidative burst.

First, chemotactic agents bind to specific receptors on the cell membranes of leukocytes. **Receptor-ligand binding** results in activation of the membrane-associated G-protein, from its inactive form (Fig. 22-1). Active G-protein causes **activation of enzyme phospholipase C** (Fig. 22-2). Phospholipase, in turn, hydrolyzes (splits) membrane phosphatidyl inositol bisphosphate (PIP2) into inositol triphosphate (IP3) and diacylglycerol (DAG). **IP3 increases intracellular calcium.** First by releasing it from endoplasmic reticulum and later by extracellular influx. That is, by entry of calcium within the cell from outside. The **increased ionic calcium within the cytoplasm** triggers the assembly of cytoskeletal contractile elements necessary for cell movement (chemotaxis) (Fig. 22-i). It assembles intracellular filaments (actin, myosin) to permit motility, chemotaxis.

Increased intracellular calcium (Fig. 22-3) also increases number and affinity of adhesion molecules (e.g., integrin). It can even increase their number and affinity. That is, it modulates (regulates) leukocyte adhesion molecules (Fig. 22-ii). Then, increased intracellular calcium and DAG together activate enzyme phospholipase A2, which in turn converts membrane phospholipids to arachidonic acid and triggers the production of arachidonic acid metabolites (Fig. 22-iii).

DAG, through activation of enzyme protein kinase C, is involved in degranulation and secretion of lysosomal enzymes (Fig. 22-iv), which occur during phagocytosis. In addition, DAG, through **protein kinase C**, also activates the oxidative burst (Fig. 22-v). Both these actions, protein C brings about by phosphorylating a variety of intracellular proteins (Fig. 22-4). Collectively, all the above responses are referred to as **'leukocyte activation'.** Such responses are also induced by phagocytosis and antigen-antibody complexes.

The neutrophil moves by extending a **pseudopod (lamellipod)** (Fig. 23) that attaches firmly to the extracellular matrix and then pulls the remainder of the cell in the direction of the extension, just as a jeep with front-wheel drive is pulled by wheels in front. (L. 'pseudopod' = false foot; and 'lamellipod' means a foot having the form of a thin layer). The inside of the pseudopod consists of a branching network of filaments composed of **actin** and the contractile protein **myosin**. Locomotion involves rapid assembly of actin monomers into linear polymers at the pseudopod's leading edge. In other words, actin monomers are polymerized into long filaments. At the same time, actin filaments away from the leading edge get disassembled to allow flow in the direction of the extending pseudopod. The direction of such movement is controlled by a high density of receptor-chemotactic ligand interactions, on the leading edge of the cell. These complex events, in turn, are controlled by the action of calcium ions and phosphoinositol on a number of actin-regulating proteins, such as **filamin, gelsolin, prolifin,** and **calmodulin**. These components interact with actin and myosin in the pseudopod to produce contraction.

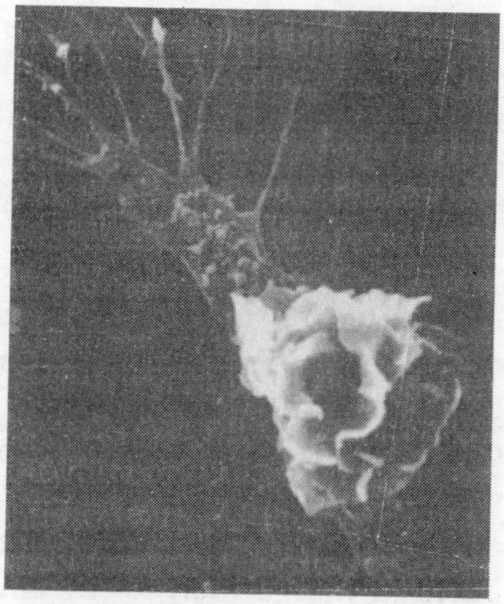

Fig. 23. Scanning electron micrograph of a moving neutrophil showing a pseudopod (lamellipod) (upper left), and a trailing tail.

4. Phagocytosis

As already mentioned, the most beneficial function of inflammation is the delivery of neutrophils and monocytes to the site of injury and killing and degradation of the ingested material, mostly bacteria. The process of taking particulate matter in the cytoplasm by cells is known as **phagocytosis**, and that of the fluid as **pinocytosis**.

The process of phagocytosis was discovered by Metchnikoff, in 1884. He observed ingestion of bacteria by mammalian leukocytes, and concluded that the purpose of inflammation was to bring phagocytic cells to the injured area to engulf invading bacteria. At that time, he contradicted the prevailing theory developed by Paul Ehrlich that the purpose of inflammation was to bring factors from the serum to neutralize the infectious agents. However, it soon became clear, as we shall see, that both cellular (**phagocytosis**) and serum factors (**antibodies**) were essential defence against microorganisms. In recognition of this, both Metchnikoff and Paul Ehrlich shared the Nobel Prize in 1908.

Phagocytosis involves three different but inter-related steps (Fig. 24): (i) first is **recognition** and **attachment** of the particle to the surface of the neutrophil, (ii) second is its **engulfment** with subsequent formation of a phagocytic vacuole, and (iii) third is **killing and degradation** of the ingested material.

(i) Recognition and Attachment

Most microorganisms (bacteria) are not recognized by neutrophils and macrophages until they are coated by certain naturally occurring serum proteins called **opsonins** (Fig. 24). Opsonins bind specific molecules on bacteria and facilitate their binding with specific **opsonin receptors on leukocytes (neutrophils)**. Thus, opsonization of particles such as bacteria greatly increases the effectiveness of phagocytosis.

The most important opsonins are: (1) **immunoglobulin G (IgG) molecules**, specifically their **Fc portions** (Fig. 24). IgG is the naturally occurring antibody against the ingested particle, (2) **C3b** fragment of complement (Fig. 24), the so-called **opsonic component of C3** generated by activation of complement by immune or non-immune mechanisms, and (3) plasma carbohydrate-binding lectins called **collectins**, which bind to bacterial cell wall sugar groups. Opsonized bacteria then attach to the **corresponding receptors** on the surface of neutrophils and macrophages. These receptors are (1) **Fc receptor (FcR)**, which recognizes the Fc fragment of IgG, (2) **complement receptors 1, 2, and 3** (CR1, 2, and 3) which interact with complement fragment C3b and C3bi, and (3) **C1q receptors** that bind to collectins.

(ii) Engulfment

Binding of the opsonized particle to the Fc receptor (FcR) is sufficient to trigger **engulfment,** which is greatly increased in the presence of complement receptors. Binding to the C3 receptors alone is not followed by engulfment. IgG binding to FcR induces cellular activation that increases degradation of ingested bacteria.

During engulfment, extensions of the cytoplasm (pseudopods) flow around the particle and eventually enclose the particle within a **phagocytic vacuole (phagosome)**, created by the cytoplasmic membrane of the cell (Fig. 24). This process of engulfment is known as **endocytosis**. The membrane of the phagocytic vacuole then fuses with the membrane of a lysosomal granule, resulting in discharge of the granule's content into the **phagolysosome** (Fig. 24). In the course of this process, neutrophil gets degranulated. During degranulation there is some leakage of hydrolytic enzymes and metabolic products (such as hydrogen peroxide) from the neutrophil into the external medium. This process is termed **'regurgitation during feeding'.** The process is important because some of the leaked enzymes have proteolytic activity and may cause tissue damage.

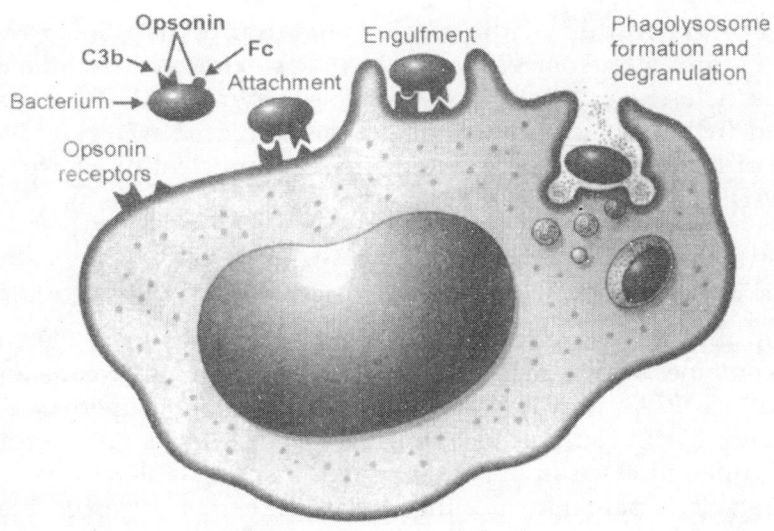

Fig. 24. Phagocytosis of a bacterium. It involves: (1) attachment and binding of opsonins (C3b, Fc) to receptors on the leukocyte surface, followed by (2) engulfment, and (3) fusion of the phagocytic vacuole with granules (lysosomes) and degranulation.

Many of the biochemical events involved in phagocytosis and degranulation are similar to those described for chemotaxis (see Fig. 22). The process is associated with receptor-ligand binding, phospholipase C activation, DAG and IP3 production, protein kinase C activation, and increased concentration of cytoplasmic calcium. The last two changes act as second messengers to initiate the cellular events.

(iii) Killing and Degradation

The final step in phagocytosis of bacteria is **killing and degradation.** Bacterial killing is achieved largely by **reactive oxygen species.** Two types of bactericidal mechanisms are recognized: (a) oxygen-dependent, and (b) oxygen-independent.

(a) Oxygen-Dependent Bactericidal Mechanisms

Phagocytosis is an energy dependent phenomenon and stimulates numerous intracellular events. Following phagocytosis, there is a burst (a sudden increase) in oxygen consumption (**oxidative burst**), glycogenolysis (breakdown of glycogen to glucose), increased glucose

141

oxidation via the hexose-monophosphate shunt, and production of reactive oxygen metabolites.

The generation of the **oxygen metabolites** is due to rapid activation of a leukocyte enzyme **NADPH oxidase.** Attachment of the particle to neutrophil activates the enzyme NADPH oxidase, present in the cell membrane. This enzyme oxidizes NADPH (reduced form of NADP, i.e., nicotinamide adenine dinucleotide phosphate) to NADP (i.e., oxidized form).

$$2O_2 + NADPH \xrightarrow{\text{NAPDH oxidase}} 2O_2^{\cdot -} + NADP^+ + H^+$$
$$\text{(reduced form)} \qquad \text{(superoxide)} \quad \text{(oxidized form)} \quad \text{(hydrogen ion)}$$

In this process, electrons are released. One of these electrons first combines with a molecule of oxygen to form superoxide anion (or ion) $(O_2^{\cdot -})$. As already described under Chapter 3, superoxide is a molecule of oxygen that has an extra electron in its outer orbital. **This unpaired electron makes superoxide an unstable free radical.** To be stable, superoxide can either donate the extra electron or receive one to convert the unpaired electron into pair. **It is therefore highly reactive (super); hence the name.**

The NADP generated by NADPH oxidase accelerates the hexose-monophosphate shunt, a metabolic pathway that converts glucose to a pentose and CO_2, **and releases energy for use by the cell.**

Superoxide is then converted into **hydrogen peroxide (H_2O_2),** mostly by spontaneous dismutation, as follows:

$$O_2^{\cdot -} + 2H^+ \longrightarrow H_2O_2$$

Or, is converted into H_2O_2 by the enzyme **SOD (superoxide dismutase),** gaining a second electron and reacting with hydrogen ions to form hydrogen peroxide.

$$2O_2^{\cdot -} + 2H \xrightarrow{\text{SOD}} H_2O_2 + O_2$$

Fortunately, NADPH oxidase is active only after the transfer of its cytoplasmic subunit to the membrane of the phagolysosome. Therefore, the reactive end products are generated only within phagolysosome. **Thus, the hydrogen peroxide is produced within the lysosome. These oxygen metabolites are the principal killers of bacteria.** However, the quantities of H_2O_2 produced in the phagolysosome are insufficient to kill bacteria (although superoxide and hydroxyl radical formation may be sufficient to do so). Therefore, one of the following two bactericidal pathways, operate.

(A1) Myeloperoxidase-Dependent Killing (The H_2O_2-MPO-Halide System)

The lysosomes of neutrophils (called **azurophilic granules**) contain the enzyme **myeloperoxidase (MPO)**. In the presence of a halide such as Cl^- (chloride), myeloperoxidase converts H_2O_2 to $HOCl^{\bullet}$ (hypochlorous radical), as follows:

$$H_2O_2 + Cl^- \xrightarrow{\quad MPO \quad} HOCl^{\bullet} + H_2O$$
$$\text{(hypochlorous radical)}$$

$HOCl^{\bullet}$ is a powerful oxidant and antimicrobial agent that kills bacteria by halogenation (covalent binding of halide), or by oxidation of proteins and lipids (i.e., lipid peroxidation). **The H_2O_2-MPO-halide system is the most efficient bactericidal system in neutrophils.** A similar mechanism is also effective against fungi, viruses, protozoa, and helminths.

After oxygen burst, most of the H_2O_2 is broken down by **catalase** present in peroxisome (a cytoplasmic cell organelle) into H_2O and O_2, as follows. The other reactive oxygen species are also degraded.

$$2H_2O_2 \xrightarrow{\quad Catalase \quad} 2H_2O + O_2$$

Some H_2O_2 is destroyed by the action of **glutathione peroxidase.**

$$H_2O_2 + 2GSH \longrightarrow 2H_2O + GSSG$$
$$\text{(reduced}$$
$$\text{glutathione)}$$

The dead microorganisms are then destroyed by the action of lysosomal acid hydrolases.

Blood monocytes also contain MPO granules and use the H_2O_2-MPO-halide system for bacterial killing.

The most important evidence regarding the presence of H_2O_2-myeloperoxidase system came from a **chronic granulomatous disease (CGD) of childhood in humans.** The disease is characterized by a **genetic deficiency** in one of the several components of the **NADPH oxidase** responsible for generating superoxide (see earlier). In these patients, engulfment of bacteria does not result in activation of oxygen-dependent killing mechanisms, despite the fact that myeloperoxidase activity of neutrophils is normal. This results in the failure of H_2O_2 production during phagocytosis. Inactivation of H_2O_2-myeloperoxidase-halide killing system makes the patient very susceptible to recurrent bacterial infections.

143

(A2) Myeloperoxidase-Independent Killing

The H_2O_2-myeloperoxidase-halide system is the most efficient bacterial system in neutrophils. But myeloperoxidase-deficient neutrophils are also capable of killing bacteria, although more slowly than normal neutrophils. This MPO-independent killing also requires oxygen. Extremely reactive superoxide, hydroxyl radicals, and singlet oxygen are involved in such killing. The superoxide ions react with H_2O_2. This reaction generates hydroxyl radicals ($OH^\bullet$) and singlet oxygen ($\bullet O_2$).

$$H_2O_2 + O_2^{-} \longrightarrow 2OH^\bullet + \bullet O_2$$

Or

$$H_2O_2 + O_2^{-} \longrightarrow OH^\bullet + OH^- + O_2$$

(This is Haber-Weiss reaction)

The hydroxyl radical is very unstable and reacts with lipids to form bactericidal hydroperoxides. Singlet oxygen is a form of oxygen in which one electron is shifted into a high energy orbit. Because of its distorted electron shell, singlet oxygen is very unstable and also reacts with bacterial lipids to form toxic hydroperoxides.

Activated macrophages also produce H_2O_2 but do not contain MPO. They may kill bacteria by producing sufficient quantities of H_2O_2, or other toxic radicals such as hydroxyl radicals.

(b) Oxygen-Independent Bactericidal Mechanisms

Bacterial killing can also occur in the absence of oxidation burst by substances present in eosinophil granules. These include:

1. Bactericidal permeability increasing protein (BPI): It causes phospholipase activation, membrane phospholipid degradation, and increases permeability in the outer membrane of bacteria.

2. Lysozyme: This enzyme hydrolyzes the muramic acid-N-acetyl-glucosamine bond, found in the glycopeptide coat of all bacteria.

3. Lactoferrin: It is an iron-binding protein present in specific granules. Lactoferrin adsorbs iron molecules, and thus prevents bacterial proliferation and invasion.

4. Major basic protein (MBP): It is an important cationic protein of eosinophil granules. It has limited bactericidal activity but is cytotoxic to many parasites.

5. Defensins: These are cationic arginine-rich granules peptides that are cytotoxic to bacteria. They kill bacteria by forming holes in their membranes.

After killing, acid hydrolases found in azurophil granules degrade the bacteria within phagolysosomes. **The pH in the phagolysosome drops to between 4 and 5 after phagocytosis,** which is the optimal (most favourable) pH for the action of these enzymes.

Although most organisms are readily killed by neutrophils, some are sufficiently virulent to destroy them. Others, such as the tubercle bacillus, survive within the phagocyte. They are thus protected against the action of antibacterial drugs and body's other defence mechanisms. Moreover, when phagocytes migrate through the lymphatics, infection may be spread. Thus, persistence of organisms within the phagocytes poses a serious problem in the eradication of infections like tuberculosis.

5. Release of leukocyte products and leukocyte-induced tissue injury

The metabolic and membrane disturbances that occur in leukocytes during chemotaxis, activation, and phagocytosis result in the release of products not only within the phagolysosome, **but also into the extracellular space.** The most important of these substance in **neutrophils** are: (i) **lysosomal enzymes**, present in the granules; (ii) **oxygen-derived active metabolites** (i. e., free radicals), and (iii) **products of arachidonic acid metabolism**, including prostaglandins and leukotrienes. Besides amplifying effects of the initial inflammatory stimulus, these products are also powerful mediators of endothelial injury and tissue damage. Thus, if persistent and unchecked, leukocytes themselves become offender and inflict tissue injury. This occurs in many acute and chronic diseases. The release of lysosomal granules and enzymes may occur in four ways:

(i) **Regurgitation during feeding**: This occurs when the phagocytic vacuole remains briefly open to the outside before complete closure of the phagolysosome. This permits escape of lysosomal hydrolases.

(ii) **Frustrated phagocytosis (reverse endocytosis)**: This occurs when neutrophils are exposed to indigestible materials, such as immune complexes, on flat surfaces (e.g., glomerular basement membrane). Attachment of immune complexes to the neutrophil triggers membrane movement, but because of the flat surface, phagocytosis does not occur, and lysosomal enzymes are released

145

outside, hence the name **'frustrated phagocytosis'**. It occurs in certain forms of immune-complex induced glomerular injury.

(iii) **Surface phagocytosis**: Lysosomal hydrolases may also be released during surface phagocytosis. It is a mechanism by which phagocytes facilitate ingestion of bacteria, and other foreign material by trapping them against a resistant surface.

(iv) **Cytotoxic release**: This occurs when neutrophil dies and its lysosomal enzymes are released into the extracellular space. Neutrophil may die after phagocytosis of potentially membranolytic substances (i.e., substances which destroy the cell membrane), such as urate crystals. In addition, certain granules, particularly the specific (secondary) granules of neutrophils, may be directly secreted by **exocytosis**. After phagocytosis neutrophils rapidly undergo **apoptotic cell death** (see 'apoptosis') and are either ingested by macrophages or are cleared by lymphatics. Such phagocytosis-induced cell death is dependent on the presence of integrin Mac-1 (CD11b) on the surface of neutrophils. It points to the important role this molecule has in acute inflammation.

6. Defects in leukocyte function

As we have seen, neutrophils play a central role in host defence. Therefore, defects in leukocyte function, both genetic and acquired, lead to increased susceptibility to infections. Defects in almost every phase of leukocyte function - from adherence to vascular endothelium, emigration, chemotaxis, phagoctosis to killing and degradation of bacteria - have been identified. Although rare, the most important defects are:

(i) **Defects in leukocyte adhesion**: The classical example is that of **leukocyte adhesion deficiency (LAD)** of humans, already described under adhesion. **In LAD type 1**, there is defective synthesis of the CD18 beta subunit of the leukocyte integrins LFA-1 and Mac-1 that mediate leukocyte-endothelial adhesion. **This leads to defective neutrophil adhesion**, phagocytosis, and generation of the oxidative burst. The deficiency is characterized by recurrent bacterial infections and defective wound healing. **LAD type 2** is caused by a general defect in fucose metabolism resulting in the absence of sialyl-Lewis X, the carbohydrate ligand on neutrophil that binds to selectins expressed by cytokine-activated endothelium. This deficiency is milder than type 1, but is also characterized by recurrent bacterial infections. Among animals, leukocyte adhesion deficiency has been reported in

dogs and **cattle**.

(ii) **Defects in phagocytosis:** One such disorder is **Chédiak-Higashi syndrome of humans** characterized by neutropaenia (decreased number of neutrophils), defective degranulation, and delayed bacterial killing. The neutrophils have **giant granules**, which can be readily seen in blood smears. These are thought to result from abnormal intracellular fusion of organelles, ultimately impairing transfer of lysosomal enzymes into phagocytic vacuoles (phagolysosomes). This results in susceptibility to infections. Chédiak-Higashi syndrome has been reported in **cattle, cat, and rat.**

(iii) **Defects in microbicidal activity:** An example is **chronic granulomatous disease (CGD)** of childhood in humans (discussed earlier). It is a congenital disorder in bacterial killing, which renders patients susceptible to recurrent bacterial infections. The disease results from **a genetic deficiency** in one of the several components of the **NADPH oxidase** responsible for generating superoxide. In these patients, engulfment of bacteria does not result in activation of oxygen-dependent killing mechanisms, despite the fact that myeloperoxidase activity of neutrophils is normal. Chronic granulomatous disease has not been reported yet to occur in domestic animals, although it undoubtedly does.

To summarize the cellular events, the leukocytes, initially mainly neutrophils, first adhere to the endothelium through adhesion molecules. They then leave the microvasculature (i.e., minute vessels - venules and capillaries) and migrate to the site of injury under the influence of chemotactic agents. Phagocytosis of bacteria occurs, which may lead to the death of pathogenic microorganisms. During chemotaxis and pinocytosis, activated neutrophils may release toxic metabolites and proteases extracellularly, causing tissue damage.

Cells of Acute Inflammation

We may now discuss briefly various cells involved in inflammation.

1. Neutrophils

These are also known as **polymorphs, polymorphonuclear leukocytes,** and **granulocytes**. The mature polymorphonuclear leukocyte has a characteristic multi-lobed nucleus, from which its name is derived. These cells spend less than 48 hours in circulation before they migrate into the tissues. In tissues, they may engulf foreign

147

material and eventually die. The term **heterophil** is used to describe functional counterpart of the neutrophil in certain species such as rabbit, guinea pigs, and the domestic fowl (chicken), in which granules of the cells are eosinophilic.

As already discussed, neutrophils are actively amoeboid and phagocytic. The neutrophil granules are lysosomes and contain a host of digestive enzymes, which enable neutrophils to destroy bacteria through phagocytosis. On this account, neutrophils are also called **microphages** of Metchnikoff, being smaller than **macrophages**. Most bacteria are killed following phagocytosis. Neutrophilic granules also release endogenous pyrogens (fever-inducing substances), which produce fever (see 'fever').

Neutrophils show two major types of granules. The smaller **specific (or secondary) granules** contain lysozyme, collagenase, gelatinase, lactoferrin, plasminogen activator, histaminase, and alkaline phosphatase. The large **azurophil (or primary) granules** contain myeloperoxidase, bactericidal factors (lysozyme, defensins), acid hydrolases, and a variety of neutral proteases (elastase, cathepsin G, non-specific collagenases, proteinase 3). Both types of granules can empty into phagocytic vacuoles that form around engulfed material, or the contents can be released after cell death. **There are, however, differences in the mobilization of specific and azurophil granules.** The **specific granules** are secreted **extracellularly** more readily, while the more destructive **azurophil granules** release their contents mainly **within the phagosome.**

The neutrophils are highly chemotactic and are usually the first to arrive at the site of inflammation. They are therefore called the **first line of cellular defence.** Neutrophils cannot multiply and are drawn from the bone marrow where they are in great store. Neutrophils are the characteristic feature of acute inflammation, and are the main component of the purulent exudate (**pus**). They constitute the **pus cells** in purulent exudates. An increase in the number of leukocytes in blood is known as **leukocytosis**; if neutrophils, then as **neutrophilia. Schilling index** helps in determining the immature (juvenile) forms of neutrophils in the blood, and an increase in their number is known as **'shift to the left'.**

An increase in the number of neutrophils is believed to be due to an increased production of a humoral mediator (a glycoprotein hormone) known as **granulocyte colony-stimulating factor (G-CSF).** It is produced by a variety of cells. It stimulates mitotic activity in neutrophil precursors in the bone marrow.

Even after neutrophils are destroyed, they are useful since they liberate proteolytic enzymes that are helpful in the digestion and liquefaction of dead material and thus help in its removal, paving way for regeneration and repair.

2. Eosinophils

In domestic animals, eosinophils in blood are normally between 1-7 percent. They are very short-lived, and are found more in tissue fluid than in blood. They also occur in significant numbers in epithelial lining of the intestine, the respiratory tract, and skin. They are motile and appear early in an area of inflammation, by their amoeboid movement. Eosinophils are characteristic of inflammations associated with **parasitic infestations** and immune reactions mediated by IgE, typically those of **allergies**. The finding of an increased number of eosinophils in the blood (**eosinophilia**) is an indication of **parasitism** or **allergy**.

Emigration of eosinophils is controlled by adhesion molecules, similar to those used by neutrophils. However, eosinophils are mainly recruited by specific **chemokines** derived from leukocytes or epithelial cells, the most important being **eotaxin**. **Eotaxin** is unusual among the class of chemokines in that it binds to only one receptor (CCR-3) **that is expressed only by eosinophils.** Eotaxin has the ability to prime eosinophils selectively for chemotaxis, and to direct their migration.

The accumulated eosinophils exert a variety of effects. Their range of mediators is as extensive as that of mast cells. Eosinophil specific granules contain: (i) **major basic protein**, a highly charged cationic protein that is **toxic to parasites** but also causes lysis of epithelial cells. They may thus be of benefit in parasitic infections but contribute to tissue damage in immune reactions; (ii) **eosinophil cationic protein (ECP)**, which is directly toxic to the epithelial cells; (iii) **eosinophil peroxidase** causes tissue damage through oxidative stress. **Activated eosinophils** are also a rich source of **leukotrienes**, especially **leukotriene C$_4$**, as well as of **platelet-activating factor. Thus, eosinophils can amplify and sustain the inflammatory response without additional exposure to the triggering antigen.**

3. Basophils

Basophils are few in blood, making up to only 0.5 to 1.0 percent of leukocytes. They are not phagocytic. Like other granulocytes, they can be recruited to inflammatory sites. Basophils are similar to **mast cells** in many respects, including the presence of cell- surface IgE Fc receptors as well as cytoplasmic granules. While both are bone marrow derived, mast cells are not present in blood but are widely distributed in connective tissues throughout the body. They are most numerous around the blood vessels, and in serous membranes and sub-epithelial sites.

Both basophils and mast cells contain a large number of basophilic membrane-bound granules that posses a variety of biologically active mediators. These are histamine, eosinophil chemotactic factor (ECF), neutrophil chemotactic factor (NCF), and granule matrix-derived mediators such as heparin and neutral proteases, like tryptase. Neutral proteases generate kinin and cleave (split) complement components to produce additional chemotactic and inflammatory factors (e.g., C3a). In addition, they also synthesize and release secondary mediators such as arachidonic acid metabolites (leukotrienes B_4, C_4, D_4, prostaglandin D_2, platelet-activating factor, cytokines (TNF, IL-1, IL-4, IL-5, and IL-6), and chemokines.

The **function of basophils and mast cells** are similar because of the similarities in their biochemical constituents. The most important function is production of type I hypersensitivity. Basophils and mast cells are **'armed'** with IgE to certain antigens. When these antigens are subsequently encountered, the pre-armed basophils and mast cells are activated by antigens by cross-linking IgE bound to their surface by high-affinity Fc receptors (see Fig. 67; 'type I hypersensitivity'). These cells then release histamine and AA metabolites (leukotrienes, prostaglandins) **that produce early vascular changes of acute inflammation.**

4. Lymphocytes, Monocytes (Macrophages), Plasma Cells

These cells appear late in inflammation and are the important cells of **chronic inflammation** (see 'cells of chronic inflammation').

The Inflammatory Exudate

As already mentioned, the escape of fluid, proteins, and blood cells from the vascular system into the interstitial tissues or body cavities is known as **exudation**, and the accumulated protein-rich extravascular fluid as the **inflammatory exudate**. The exudate is composed of five major components: (1) the irritant, (2) injured tissue cells, (3) leukocytes (also macrophages and plasma cells), (4) plasma constituents (water, protein, fibrin, and antibodies), and (5) erythrocytes. These components give the exudate a very characteristic appearance and composition that differentiate it from **transudate**. Table 6 lists the main characteristics of an exudate and a transudate.

Table 6. Comparison of an exudates and a transudate

Exudate	Transudate
1. Cloudy	1. Clear
2. Thick, creamy, and contains tissue fragments	2. Thin, watery, resembles lymph, and contains no tissue fragments
3. May have an odour	3. No odour
4. Acidic	4. Alkaline
5. Colour - white, yellow or red	5. Colour - like water or pale yellow depending on the normal plasma colour of the animal
6. Specific gravity - 1.020 or higher	6. Specific gravity - 1.012 or lower
7. High protein content (mainly albumin) - more than 4 percent	7. Low protein content (mainly albumin) - less than 3 percent
8. Coagulates *in vivo* and *in vitro*	8. Does not coagulate or contains only a few fibrin strands
9. High cell count - many leukocytes and erythrocytes	9. Low cell count - none or few leukocytes and erythrocytes
10. High enzyme content	10. Low enzyme content
11. Bacteria may be present	11. No bacteria are present
12. Associated with inflammation	12. No association with inflammation

Exudate is beneficial to the body. Its **functions** include:

1. **It dilutes the irritant**. The irritant is thus changed from severe to mild, and therefore less damage is caused to the tissues. Moreover, irritants like bacteria are dispersed and therefore better phagocytized.

2. The exudate also mechanically **carries the irritant away**, especially to the outside in the case of cutaneous or mucous surfaces. This helps in getting rid of the irritant from the body.

3. It **brings phagocytes** (neutrophils, macrophages) to the site of inflammation to destroy the irritant.

4. Exudate also **brings fibrin** to the area. Fibrin is formed from fibrinogen that leaves the vessels following increased permeability.

Fibrin performs several useful functions (a) it **traps the irritant** and thus slows down its spread. This facilitates their phagocytosis, (b) it **forms a kind of layer around the cells,** which protects them from the damaging effect of irritant, (c) it **seals lumen of the lymphatics** effectively. This prevents irritant like bacteria from entering into them, thus stopping their spread to the regional lymph nodes, (d) **fibrin helps in healing and repair.** It does so by forming a kind of scaffold (framework) for fibroblasts and endothelial cells to work, (e) fibrin also has a **stimulating effect on proliferation of fibroblasts.** This further helps in healing, and finally, (f) **for the movement of leukocytes, fibrin is required**. It acts as a scaffold, since leukocytes cannot move in a fluid medium.

5. The **exudate brings antibodies** to the area of inflammation, which are most effective against bacteria and viruses.

6. Finally, exudate brings to the area of inflammation **more nutrients and oxygen** that are so much needed by the tissues in their increased activity in defending the body, as well as for regeneration and repair. Exudate also drains the area of products of tissue destruction and altered metabolism, which are acidic in nature. The optimum (best possible) H-ion concentration for phagocytosis of the irritant is thus maintained. Exudate also provides a suitable medium for the working of phagocytes, enzymes, and antibodies under optimum conditions.

In the early stages of inflammation, fibrin may be useful as the adhesions formed by it limit the area of inflammation. But later, when fibrin is not completely removed, but gets organized, the parts involved are constricted by contraction of the granulation tissue. **This affects function of the organ,** example being constrictive pericarditis.

The proteolytic enzymes of neutrophils liquefy fibrin. Since pus contains a large number of neutrophils that liquefy the clot, **pus does not clot.**

Classification of Inflammation

Inflammation is variously classified. It can be mild or severe depending on the nature of irritant. According to its duration, inflammation may be **peracute, acute, subacute,** or **chronic** in its course. The duration depends on whether the irritant is severe, or of low intensity. **Acute inflammation** is comparatively of a short duration, whereas the **chronic inflammation** is of a relatively **long duration** and is accompanied by marked proliferation of connective

152

tissue, blood vessels, and epithelium.

The acute inflammation, which is always accompanied by exudate formation, is further classified as follows, **based on the main component of the exudate.**

1. Catarrhal or Mucous Inflammation

This is present when the main component of exudate is **mucus.** Catarrhal inflammation occurs in only those areas where cells capable of producing mucin are present. It is therefore limited to mucous membranes. Catarrhal inflammation is produced by **irritants** that are **mild in nature**, such as mildly irritating chemicals (formalin, phenol, detergents), irritating foods in the digestive tract, inhaled dust, cold air, bacterial and viral infections of low virulence in respiratory tract. The term catarrhal inflammation is also applied to inflammation of epithelium lining the ducts and tubules (e.g., uriniferous tubules).

In catarrhal inflammation, there is proliferation of epithelium, which is desquamated into the exudate. The exudate consists of desquamated cells, neutrophils, and mucus. Mucus is a clear, transparent, glistening slimy material containing water and mucin. **Microscopically**, mucus stains blue with haematoxylin. The secretion becomes mucopurulent following infection by pyogenic organisms.

In result, if the cause is removed recovery occurs quickly. But if it persists, it may progress to a chronic stage when epithelium of the mucosa is denuded and its wall becomes thickened due to fibrosis.

2. Serous Inflammation

This is present when the main component of exudate is **plasma** derived from blood, **or a clear watery fluid** derived from secretions of the mesothelial cells lining the peritoneal, pleural, and pericardial cavities.

Serous inflammation is caused by, **moderately severe irritants.** Various chemical irritants when applied to the skin cause blisters. Traumatic injuries of rubbing nature and second-degree burns also form blisters on the skin. Certain viruses (foot-and-mouth, vascular stomatitis) also produce blisters in skin or mucous membrane. Serous inflammation is common in the serous membranes (pericardium, pleura, peritoneum) and in joint spaces. **It is often the first stage in many inflammatory processes.** In some cases of inflammation of serous membranes, the exudate may contain enough fibrin, which gives a frosted glass or shaggy (rough) appearance to the smooth surface.

Microscopically, in haematoxylin and eosin stained sections, the exudate appears as a homogeneous to finely granular material which stains pink with eosin; the intensity of eosin-staining depending on the amount of protein present.

Serous inflammation being mild, **the outcome is favourable.** The fluid is promptly absorbed if the cause is overcome. If it persists, because the number of neutrophils that could remove the exudate by autolysis is very low, exudate usually gets **organized** and **adhesions** may form.

3. Fibrinous Inflammation

This is present when the main component of exudate is **fibrin.** This type of inflammation is caused by **a more violent type of injury.** The resulting marked increase in vascular permeability enables fibrinogen to escape into the surrounding tissue. Fibrinous inflammation is seen in various viral diseases, such as infectious feline enteritis and malignant catarrhal fever, and when mucous membranes are invaded by *Corynebacterium diphtheriae*, various salmonella, or *Fusobacterium necrophorum* (previously *Sphaerophorus necrophorus*).

The organ is firmer and tenser than normal. It is especially seen when fibrin accumulates in the alveoli of lungs in pneumonia. The lung then acquires both consistency and appearance of liver (hepatization). On epithelial surfaces (mucous, serous or cutaneous) fibrin is seen as stringy (long and thin, like strings), yellowish, net-like material. At such places, it traps desquamated epithelium and foreign material. In tubular organs, it forms cast of the organ.

Fibrinous inflammation commonly occurs in body cavities, such as pleural and peritoneal sac. In fibrinous pericarditis, the space may become filled with large masses of rubbery fibrin loosely gluing the parietal and visceral epithelium (**'bread and butter' pericarditis**).

Masses of fibrin on epithelial surface may either form a **pseudomembrane (croupous membrane)** when it is easily peeled away, or a **diphtheritic membrane** when it is quite firmly attached to the underlying tissue. The latter is the result of epithelium having undergone coagulative necrosis. If the necrotic, denuded epithelial cells are also included in the mass, it is a **'true membrane'**, otherwise, without epithelial cells it is called a **'false membrane'**. The best examples of diphtheritic membrane formation are pharynx in calf diphtheria, and intestinal tract in swine fever. Fibrin stains dirty pink with eosin. **In result**, in this type of inflammation tissue destruction is so much that the animal may not survive.

In body cavities, fibrinous exudate is often reabsorbed by fibrinolysis (enzymatic breakdown of fibrin) and removal by phagocytes, a process referred to as **resolution of the exudate.** However, it may also invite ingrowth of fibroblasts and capillary buds, which transform the proteinaceous precipitate into vascularized connective tissue, a process referred to as **organization of the exudate**. Organization of the fibrinous pericarditis or pleurisy may obliterate these serosal cavities, and hamper function of the organ due to **adhesions** with the surrounding structures. In peritoneal cavity also, it may result in adhesions that interfere with intestinal motility and create further complications.

4. Suppurative or Purulent Inflammation

This form of inflammation is characterized by the production of **pus** or **purulent exudate**, which results from softening and liquefaction of the tissues. The purulent exudate consists of liquefied tissue, neutrophils, and organisms.

For suppuration (pus formation) to occur three factors are essential, and if any one of these is absent, suppuration will not occur. These are: (a) necrosis, (b) presence of sufficient number of neutrophils, and (c) digestion of necrotic material by proteolytic enzymes. The presence of neutrophils alone does not constitute suppuration. **Hence, any irritant causing positive chemotaxis and necrosis will produce suppuration**.

The main **causes** of suppurative inflammation are:

1. Pyogenic (pus-producing) bacteria: Examples: staphylococci, streptococci, and members of the Coli group.

2. Specific organisms like *Corynebacterium pyogenes*, *Pseudomonas mallei* (previously *Malleomyces mallei*), *Actinomyces bovis*, etc.

3. Chemicals - turpentine, zinc chloride, mercuric chloride, croton oil etc.

The proteolytic enzymes are produced mostly by leukocytes, and to a lesser extent, by the infecting bacteria and the necrosed tissue cells themselves. Serum contains an antienzyme that tends to inhibit the action of proteases of the leukocytes. The rabbit serum is particularly rich in the antienzyme and poor in leukocytes, and therefore it is not common to see suppurative conditions in this animal in infections caused by pyogenic organisms. The antienzyme is lipid in character. It is rich in unsaturated fatty acids. Caseous material in tuberculosis is also rich in unsaturated fatty acids and so acts as an antienzyme. As such, suppuration is not encountered in tuberculosis.

Pus is composed of necrotic neutrophils, necrotic tissue cells (more or less liquefied), and minor amounts of other constituents of inflammatory exudate, including serum. Pus, which is alkaline, is usually of creamy colour. It may be white, yellow, green, red, black or blue depending on the species of the animal, and the aetiological agent present. Streptococci and staphylococci produce **white or yellow** pus. Corynebacteria, particularly in cattle, produce **greenish** pus; **blue-green** colour comes from the pigment-forming pyocyaneus bacillus; and **black** colour comes from disintegrating hoof material (iron sulphide). Pus is **red** when there is haemorrhage. Consistency may vary from thin and watery to creamy, thick, viscid (sticky, gluey), or granular depending on the species of animal, amount of necrotic material, and dehydration of the exudate. Pus is liquid because of the proteolytic enzymes of the neutrophils. **Lysosomal enzymes are present in pus, and the extent of proteolysis that they produce determines the viscosity of pus. Canine pus** is thin and watery due to extremely proteolytic neutrophilic enzymes. **Bovine pus** is rather viscid. **Avian pus** has a dry, caseous consistency due to the presence of antienzymes. The pus serum, **liquor puris**, does not coagulate because the exudate gets digested by the proteolytic enzymes of the leukocytes.

Cellulitis (phlegmon) is a diffusely spreading suppurative inflammation of connective tissue caused by streptococci, and has red raised margins.

Abscess: Collection of pus locally within a closed cavity in an organ or tissue is called an **abscess**. When pyogenic organisms enter an organ, an acute inflammation results with death of cells in the centre. This dead material is liquefied by the proteolytic enzymes mainly from the neutrophils, resulting in pus in a cavity. The neighbouring tissue, partly damaged and partly living, constitutes the wall of this cavity, and at this wall, active warfare goes on to limit the spread of infection. Therefore, dead tissue and dead inflammatory cells are continually shed into the cavity from this zone. This increases the quantity of pus, and thus the abscess becomes enlarged. The limiting zone is therefore called the **pyogenic (producing pus) membrane**. In time, the abscess may become walled off by connective tissue that serves as a barrier and limits its further spread. Or, the abscess may become bigger and bigger till it reaches the surface (skin or mucous membrane) points and opens, discharging the pus. The discontinuity of skin or mucous membrane that results by the opening of an abscess on the surface is called an **ulcer** and the base lies in the subcutaneous tissue. Ulcer may also form from direct action of the irritant on skin or mucosa.

Sinus: It is a tract in the tissues communicating with an epithelial surface, discharging pus from an abscess.

Fistula is a tract that connects two epithelial surfaces - skin and mucous membrane, for the discharge of pus from an abscess.

Boil (furuncle): This is a small suppurative inflammation in the skin that involves a hair follicle or a sebaceous gland, and is caused by *Staphylococcus aureus*.

Pustule: It is a circumscribed cavity in the epidermis containing pus.

Microscopically, in suppurative inflammation, the main cell of the exudate is neutrophil in various stages of disintegration. **In significance**, the presence of pus indicates the presence of bacteria in the area of inflammation. If an abscess persists for a long time, bacteria are destroyed and it would yield no organism on culture (**sterile abscess**). Persistence of confined pus can lead to toxaemia.

5. Haemorrhagic Inflammation

This is present when the main component of exudate is **erythrocyte**. It is caused by **a violet type of irritant,** that causes serious damage to blood vessels. Bacterial, viral and protozoal diseases (blackquarter, anthrax, haemorrhagic septicaemia, infectious laryngotracheitis, coccidiosis) may cause so severe injury that haemorrhage occurs. The result of haemorrhagic inflammation is extremely unfavourable. Due to severe haemorrhage, the animal may die from anaemia, as in coccidiosis in the chicken.

Terminology of Inflammation

Inflammation of an organ or tissue is designated by adding suffix 'itis', after its name in Latin or Greek. As shown in Table 7, the term **acute diffuse serofibrinous peritonitis** indicates an acute inflammation of the entire peritoneum characterized by serofibrinous exudate. The term **chronic diffuse suppurative interstitial hepatitis** signifies chronic inflammation of the interstitial tissue of the liver characterized

157

by pus formation.

To describe combination of exudate, **the least important component of the exudate is placed first**. For example, the term **serofibrinous** would mean that fibrin is the main component. The term **mucopurulent** would mean more pus in the exudate than mucus.

Table 7. Terminology of inflammation

Time	Extent	Exudate	Position in organ	Anatomy	Suffix
Acute	Focal	Serous	Parenchymatous	Nephr-	-itis
Chronic	Diffuse	Fibrinous	Interstitial	Hepat-	-itis
		Catarrhal		Rhin-	-itis
		Suppurative		Periton-	-itis
		Haemorrhagic		Enter-	-itis

Lymphatics and Lymph Nodes in Acute Inflammation

The system of lymphatics and lymph nodes filters the extravascular fluids. **Together with the mononuclear phagocyte system, it constitutes a secondary line of defence** that comes into operation whenever a local inflammatory reaction fails to contain and neutralize injury.

Lymphatics are extremely delicate channels and are difficult to visualize in tissue sections, because they readily collapse. During inflammation, lymph flow increases and helps in the drainage of oedema fluid, from the extravascular space. Not only fluid, leukocytes and cell debris may also find their way into the lymph. **Thus, these vessels are important in the resolution of inflammation.**

Unfortunately, lymphatic drainage also provides channels for spread of the injurious agent, bacteria or even chemicals. Lymphatics themselves may then become inflamed (**lymphangitis**), as also the draining lymph nodes (**lymphadenitis**). The painful enlargement is caused by hyperplasia of the lymphoid follicles and also by hyperplasia of the phagocytic cells lining the sinuses of the lymph nodes. The histological changes constitute **reactive or inflammatory lymphadenitis**. If lymph nodes are unable to contain the spread of infection, the infectious organisms drain through larger lymphatics and gain access to the vascular circulation, resulting in **bacteraemia**. The phagocytic cells of the liver, spleen and bone marrow constitute the next line of defence. But in massive infections, bacteria seed distant tissues of the body, such as kidneys, heart valves, meninges, and even joints.

CHRONIC INFLAMMATION

Chronic inflammation is an inflammation of prolonged duration (weeks, months, or even years) **in which active inflammation, tissue destruction, and healing proceed simultaneously**. In contrast to acute inflammation, which is characterized by vascular changes, oedema and neutrophilic infiltration, chronic infiltration is characterized by **infiltration with mononuclear cells, tissue destruction and repair, involving new vessel proliferation and fibrosis.**

Acute inflammation may end up either in:

1. **Complete resolution** with restoration of the site of acute inflammation to normal. This is the usual outcome when injury is mild, e.g., a superficial burn or limited trauma, or when there is little tissue destruction, or in

2. **Healing by scarring:** This occurs after substantial tissue destruction, or when inflammation occurs in tissues that do not regenerate, or when there is abundant fibrin exudation, or in

3. **Abscess formation:** This occurs particularly in infections with pyogenic organisms, or may

4. **Progress to chronic inflammation.**

Thus, chronic inflammation may occur as follows:

1. **It may follow an acute inflammation.** When the body is unable to remove and destroy irritant, it continues to persist in the area, interferes with the normal process of healing, and causes constant irritation. Persistence of the injurious agent then leads to chronic inflammation. Even persistence of the necrotic tissue in the area, by acting as a foreign body, may cause chronic inflammation.

2. **The response may be chronic from the outset.** If the irritant is of low intensity, it fails to stimulate body defences to cause its destruction and removal, and chronic inflammation occurs. In these cases chronic inflammation is initiated as a primary process. This is because the injurious agents are less toxic than those that lead to acute inflammation. Examples comprise two major groups:

(a) In **persistent infections** by certain intracellular microorganisms, such as tuberculosis, Johne's disease, actinomycosis, actinobacillosis and also certain fungal diseases. These organisms are of low toxicity and evoke an immune reaction called delayed hypersensitivity.

159

(b) In **prolonged exposure to potentially toxic agents**. Examples include asbestos and silica particles. After being inhaled for a prolonged period these particles set up a chronic inflammatory response in the lungs called asbestosis and silicosis, respectively.

In general, the irritants causing chronic inflammation are:

(i) **Bacteria** causing acute septicaemic diseases, but have later on become attenuated and localized, for example, *Pasteurella aviseptica* (liver) and *Erysipelothrix rhusiopathiae* (heart valves - vegetation, and in joints).

(ii) **Phytotoxins** of certain plants, belonging to the genus **Crotalaria** and **Senecio**, produce lesions in the liver of horses.

(iii) **Foreign bodies**, e.g., sharp objects as in traumatic reticulitis and pericarditis in cattle; dust in pneumoconiosis; encysted larvae in trichinosis. Inert material that is difficult to be phagocytosed (splinters, thorns, suture material, dead parasites, necrotic tissue) persists in the tissue and induces a proliferating type of reaction.

(iv) **Constant and repeated mechanical irritation (trauma)** to a wound, by preventing or delaying healing, causes chronic inflammation. Examples include saddle and collar galls, and kennel granuloma in the dog.

Cells of Chronic Inflammation

The characteristic **microscopic features** of chronic inflammation are (1) **infiltration with mononuclear cells (chronic inflammatory cells)**. These include macrophages, lymphocytes, and plasma cells. Their presence indicates persistent reaction to injury. (2) **tissue destruction.** This is mainly caused by the inflammatory cells. (3) **repair**. This is achieved by proliferation of small vessels (**angiogenesis**) and, in particular, **fibrosis**. Fibrosis involves proliferation of fibroblasts and deposition of extracellular matrix by these cells.

Macrophages

Macrophages are the main components of chronic inflammation. They are tissue cells and are derived at sites of inflammation from blood. In blood, monocytes comprise 1 to 5 percent of the total leukocytes. The **half-life** of **blood monocytes** is about **1 day**, whereas the **life-span of tissue macrophages** is **several months**. Monocytes begin to emigrate relatively early in acute inflammation, and within 48 hours they constitute the main cell type. Emigration of monocytes is controlled by the same factors that are involved in neutrophil emigration. After monocyte comes out of the blood vessel, in tissues it undergoes transformation into a large phagocytic cell, the **macrophage**.

Monocytes and macrophages belong to the **mononuclear phagocyte system (MPS)**. The scattered collections of macrophages in the body were previously grouped under the term 'reticulo-endothelial system (RES)'. This name is no longer applicable, and has now been replaced by a more appropriate term MPS. This is because neither reticulin (collagen fibrils found in connective tissue), nor endothelium (cells lining blood vessels or lymphatics), are concerned with phagocytosis. Apart from several other functions, MPS is concerned mainly with cellular defence in microbial infections.

Macrophages are just one component of MPS. The others are closely related cells of bone marrow origin, including blood monocytes and tissue macrophages. Tissue macrophages (histiocytes or resident macrophages) are diffusely scattered in connective tissues, or grouped in organs such as liver (Kupffer cells); spleen and lymph nodes (sinus histiocytes); lungs (alveolar macrophages); central nervous system (microglial cells); adrenal cortex (sinusoidal cells); and bone marrow (osteoclasts); or in serous cavities (pleural and peritoneal macrophages). All arise from a common precursor in bone marrow, which gives rise to blood monocytes.

Macrophages are highly specialized for the function of phagocytosis and intracellular digestion. As indicated earlier, the uptake of particles is carried out due to the presence on the macrophage surface of **Fc receptor (FcR)** which recognizes the **Fc fragment of IgG** and the **complement receptors 1, 2, and 3** that interact with complement fragment C3b and C3bi. Macrophages are the cells that eventually complete destruction of the irritant through their powerful enzymes, and remove the necrotic tissue from the area. On this account, they are called the **second line of cellular defence**. Macrophages are involved mainly in chronic inflammation, and are particularly abundant in certain chronic inflammatory diseases like tuberculosis and Johne's disease.

Besides performing phagocytosis, macrophages have the potential (latent capacity) of getting **activated**. This process results in an increase in their size, increased levels of lysosomal enzymes, more active metabolism, and greater ability to phagocytose and kill ingested bacteria. Activation signals include: (i) **cytokines**, mainly interferon-

161

gamma secreted by sensitized T-lymphocytes (type1 helper T-cells), or (ii) **non-immunological stimuli,** such as bacterial endotoxins, other chemical mediators, and extracellular matrix proteins such as fibronectin (Fig. 25). **Following activation, macrophages secrete a wide variety of biologically active products that, if unchecked, result in tissue injury and fibrosis characteristic of chronic inflammation.**

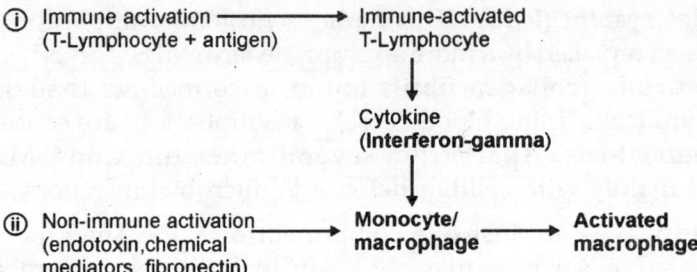

Fig. 25. Two stimuli for macrophage activation (i) cytokines (mainly **interferon-gamma)** from immune-activated T-lymphocytes, and **(ii)** non-immunological stimuli such as endotoxin.

The biologically active products secreted by activated macrophages include:

1. Enzymes

Neutral proteases

Elastase

Collagenase

Plasminogen activator

Acid hydrolases

Phosphatases

Lipases

2. Plasma proteins

Complement components (C1 to C5, properdin)

Coagulation factors (factors V, VIII, tissue factor)

3. Reactive metabolites of oxygen

4. Arachidonic acid (AA) metabolites (leukotrienes, prostaglandins)

162

5. Cytokines, chemokines (IL-1, TNF, IL-8)

6. Growth factors (PDGF, FGF, TGF-beta), and

7. Nitric oxide (NO)

1. Enzymes: These include both neutral and acid proteases. Neutral proteases, such as elastase and collagenase, act as mediators of tissue damage in acute inflammation. Others, such as plasminogen activator, trigger production of the fibrinolytic agent, **plasmin**. Proteases are toxic to extracellular matrix.

2. Plasma proteins: These include **complement proteins** C1 to C5 and properdin; coagulation factors V and VIII; and tissue factor. Although liver is the major source of these proteins in plasma, **activated macrophages** may release significant amounts of these proteins into the extracellular matrix.

3. Reactive metabolites of oxygen: These are toxic to cells.

4. Arachidonic acid metabolites: These include leukotrienes and prostaglandins.

5. Cytokines and chemokines (chemotactic factors): These include interleukin -1 (IL-1) and tumour necrosis factor (TNF). Chemokines cause influx of other cell types. Interferon-gamma (IFN-gamma) and interleukin-4 (IL-4) can also cause macrophages to fuse into large, multi-nucleated cells called **giant cells** (see 'giant cells').

6. Growth factors: These include platelet-derived growth factor (PDGF), epidermal growth factor (EGF), fibroblast growth factor (FGF), and transforming growth factor (TGF). These growth factors cause proliferation of fibroblasts, smooth muscle cells, and angiogenesis (i.e., formation and differentiation of blood vessels). In addition, they also play an important role in healing and repair through production of extracellular matrix (collagen deposition).

In chronic inflammation, accumulation of macrophages occurs in three ways: (i) **continued recruitment of monocytes from circulation.** This occurs from a continuous expression of adhesion molecules and chemotactic factors. **This is the most important source for macrophages.** Chemotactic stimuli for macrophages include C5a; chemokines produced by activated macrophages, lymphocytes, and other cell types (e.g., MCP-1, i.e., monocyte chemoattractant protein-1; see 'chemokines'); certain growth factors (PDGF, TGF-beta); fragments from the breakdown of collagen and fibronectin; and fibrinopeptides. Each of these plays a role under specific circumstances.

For example, chemokines are involved in delayed hypersensitivity immune reactions. (ii) **local proliferation of macrophages** by mitosis, after their emigration from the bloodstream. This is a rare source of macrophages. (iii) **immobilization of macrophages** in the area of inflammation. Certain cytokines (macrophage inhibitory factor) and oxidized lipids can cause such immobilization.

Thus, **macrophage is the central figure in chronic inflammation** because of the great number of substances activated macrophages can produce. However, it is important to note that whereas various mediators, enzymes and other factors make macrophages powerful cells in defending the body against infectious agents, the very same weapons can also inflict considerable tissue damage when macrophages are inappropriately activated (Fig. 26). Thus, **tissue destruction is one of the characteristic features of chronic inflammation.**

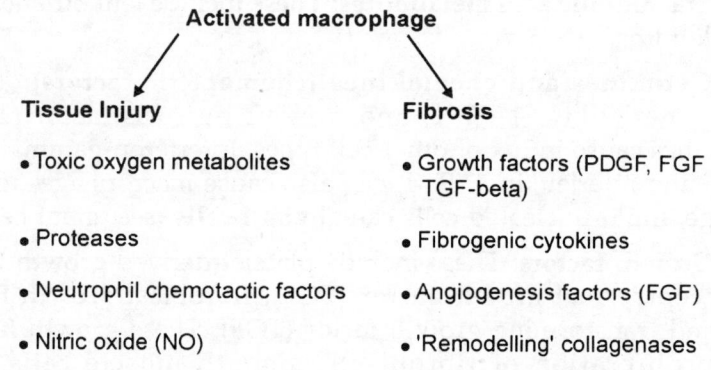

Activated macrophage

Tissue Injury
- Toxic oxygen metabolites
- Proteases
- Neutrophil chemotactic factors
- Nitric oxide (NO)

Fibrosis
- Growth factors (PDGF, FGF TGF-beta)
- Fibrogenic cytokines
- Angiogenesis factors (FGF)
- 'Remodelling' collagenases

Fig. 26. Macrophage products involved in tissue destruction and fibrosis.

Other types of cells present in chronic inflammation are **lymphocytes, plasma cells, eosinophils, mast cells,** and **giant cells.**

Lymphocytes

Lymphocytes comprise 40 to 60 percent of the total blood leukocytes. They are not phagocytic and possess only limited power of amoeboid movement. At best, they succeed in getting just outside the blood vessel, constituting perivascular lymphocytic infiltration known as **'perivascular cuffing'.** They usually appear late in inflammation and **are the important cells in chronic inflammation.**

Lymphocytes arise from stem cells in the bone marrow. There

164

are two populations of lymphocytes - one dependent on thymus for its development called 'T-lymphocytes' and the other on bursa of Fabricius (bone marrow in mammals) called B-lymphocytes. Most of the lymphocytes present in blood are T-lymphocytes (60% -70%), B-lymphocytes being 10%-20%, the rest (10%-15%) are natural killer (NK) cells. B-lymphocytes further differentiate into plasma cells that synthesize antibodies (immunoglobulins). In contrast, T-lymphocytes are responsible for cell-mediated immunological reactions; they do not form immunoglobulins. Natural killer cells are also lymphocytes. They are the first line of defence against infectious agents (see 'natural killer cells'). Lymphocytes are mainly found in chronic inflammation like tuberculosis and in certain viral infections.

Both T- and B-lymphocytes migrate into inflammatory sites. They use the same adhesion molecules and chemokines that recruit monocytes. Lymphocytes are mobilized in both antibody-mediated and cell-mediated immune reactions, and for reasons unknown, in non-immune-mediated inflammation. T-lymphocytes have a reciprocal relationship to macrophages in chronic inflammation (Fig. 27).

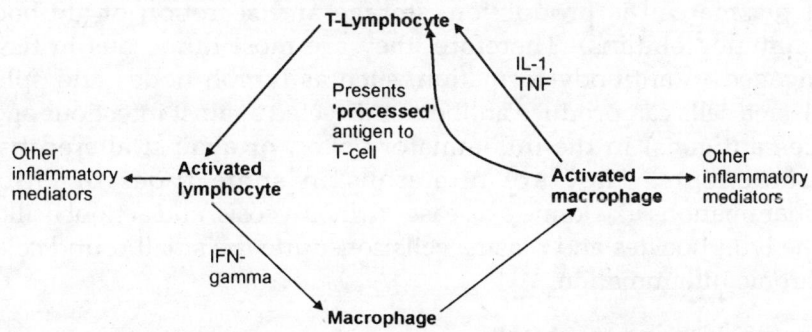

Fig. 27. Macrophage-lymphocyte interactions in chronic inflammation. IL-1 = interleukin-1, TNF = tumour necrosis factor, IFN-gamma = interferon-gamma

T-lymphocytes can be activated by contact with antigen (e.g., infectious agents). This occurs when macrophages present to them 'processed' antigen fragments (see Chapter 9). Activated lymphocytes then produce cytokines, and one of these, interferon-gamma (IFN-gamma) is a major stimulator of monocytes and macrophages. Activated macrophages, in turn, release cytokines, including interleukin-1 (IL-1) and tumour necrosis factor (TNF) that further activate lymphocytes. Activated lymphocytes themselves also produce inflammatory mediators. These types of macrophage-lymphocyte interactions, where macrophages and T-lymphocytes stimulate one another, are responsible for persistence of the inflammatory response until the triggering agent is removed.

Plasma Cells

Plasma cells are not found in blood, but are present in tissues. They are an important component of **many chronic inflammatory reactions.** Plasma cells possess more cytoplasm than lymphocytes and are therefore larger. They are recognized by their characteristic morphological features. The nucleus is eccentrically placed in the cell (i.e., away from the centre) and is spherical. The arrangement of chromatin granules along the nuclear membrane imparts it a clock-face or cart-wheel appearance. The cytoplasm is highly basophilic; basophilia is due to a complex endoplasmic reticulum, which is rich in RNA.

Plasma cells do not undergo mitosis. They originate from B-lymphocytes in response to antigenic stimulation, and are the terminally differentiated end product of B-cell activation. The function of plasma cell is production, storage and secretion of antibodies (immunoglobulins). Therefore, they are most numerous in tissues engaged in antibody formation, such as lymph nodes and spleen. Plasma cells can produce antibodies directed against infectious agents (i.e., antigens) in the inflammatory sites, or against altered tissue components. They are numerous in some types of chronic inflammations like Johne's disease, actinomycosis, and actinobacillosis. The lymphocytes and plasma cells constitute the small round cells of chronic inflammation.

Eosinophils and Mast Cells

These have been discussed under **'Cells of acute inflammation'.**

Giant Cells

When macrophages fuse to form a large phagocytic cell, the cell so formed is called a **giant cell.** It has multiple nuclei (i.e., multi-nucleated) and has abundant cytoplasm. Giant cells are of two basic types (i) **foreign-body type giant cells,** and (ii) **tumour giant cells.** The first type is produced by the fusion of macrophages and is formed in response to foreign material present in tissues. It is now known that macrophages fuse under the influence of certain cytokines, **mainly interferon-gamma** (but also interleukin-4), to form giant cells.

Interferon-gamma is derived from activated type 1 helper T-lymphocytes (CD4+ Th1 cells; see Chapter 9).

Foreign body giant cells contain multiple nuclei - 50, 100 or more, and may attain a diameter of 40 to 50 μm. Nuclei may be arranged around the periphery of the cell (creating a horseshoe pattern), or grouped at one or both poles of the cell, or scattered throughout the cytoplasm. A good example of the foreign-body giant cell is **Langhans' giant cell** of tuberculosis. They are also seen in Johne's disease, actinomycosis, and blastomycosis. Giant cells are also formed in the presence of large amounts of indigestible material, and they often collect around a foreign body, hence the name **foreign-body giant cell. Tumour giant cells** are much larger than their neighbouring cell and possess either one very large nucleus, or several nuclei.

Finally, proliferation of fibroblasts at the site of injury and deposition of extracellular matrix by these cells, that is, **fibrosis**, is an important feature of chronic inflammation. The mechanisms of fibrosis are similar to those that occur during repair, and are discussed in Chapter 5.

Acute Chronic Inflammation

Although neutrophils are characteristic of acute inflammation, many forms of chronic inflammation show large numbers of neutrophils (and even pus), caused by either, persistent bacteria or by the mediators produced by macrophages or necrotic cells. Examples include actinomycosis and chronic osteomyelitis. In actinomycosis, centre of the lesion remains full of neutrophils months or years after the initial infection. **This, then, is an example where chronic and acute responses co-exist.** This is sometimes called 'acute chronic infammation'. On the other hand, presence of lymphocytes does not always mean that inflammation is chronic. This is especially true in viral infections.

Granulomatous Inflammation

Some agents produce a different type of chronic inflammation called **granulomatous inflammation.** This inflammation is characterized by accumulation of **activated macrophages** that assume an epithelial cell-like (**epithelioid**) appearance. Activated macrophages become large, flat, and eosinophilic. Such cells are called '**epithelioid cells'** (epithelium-like). The epithelioid cells sometimes fuse under the influence of certain cytokines (mainly **interferon-gamma**) to form

167

multi-nucleated giant cells. **Interferon-gamma is also important in transforming macrophages into epithelioid cells.** An accumulation of epithelioid cells, surrounded by a collar (rim) of lymphocytes, is called a **granuloma**. Granulomas are small, 0.5 to 2 mm in size. Tuberculosis, Johne's disease, actinomycosis, actinobacillosis, schistosomiasis, leprosy, and deep fungal infections are the classical examples of granulomatous disease.

Granulomas form in the presence of **persistent T-cell responses** to certain microbes, such as *Mycobacterium tuberculosis*, where T-cell-derived cytokines are responsible for persistent macrophage activation. In tuberculosis, a combination of hypoxia (a deficiency of oxygen reaching the tissues) and free radical injury leads to a central zone of necrosis. Grossly, necrosis has a granular cheesy appearance, and is therefore called **'caseous necrosis'**. In tuberculosis, granuloma is called **tubercle** and is characterized by the presence of central caseous necrosis. In contrast, caseous necrosis is rare in other granulomatous diseases. Granulomas may also develop in response to relatively inert foreign bodies (e.g., suture, splinter), forming what are known as **foreign body granulomas,**

Granuloma formation does not always lead to removal of the causal agent, which is usually resistant to killing. Nevertheless, formation of a granuloma effectively 'walls off' the infectious agent and is therefore a useful defence mechanism.

The differences between acute and chronic inflammation can be summarized as follows (see Table 8).

Table 8. Comparison of acute and chronic inflammation

Acute inflammation	Chronic inflammation
1. Short duration	1. Long duration
2. Irritant is severe	2. Irritant is of low intensity
3. Marked vascular changes	3. Vascular changes are less prominent
4. Profuse exudation	4. Exudation scanty
5. Soft consistency	5. Firm consistency
6. No, or only slight, proliferation of connective tissue, blood vessels, and epithelium	6. Proliferation of connective tissue, blood vessels, and epithelium

Systemic Effects of Inflammation

The systemic effects of inflammation are collectively called **acute-phase reactions**. **Fever** is one of the most prominent of these systemic effects.

Acute-Phase Reactions

(A) **Fever**

Fever, the abnormal rise of body temperature, is one of the most prominent systemic manifestations, especially when inflammation is associated with infection.

In generalized inflammatory diseases, there is an increased metabolic rate, and as a result, the body temperature rises. Body temperature is normally maintained by a complex series of feedback reactions that control the dissipation and production of body heat. Heat is normally lost by radiation, conduction, evaporation of sweat, pulmonary ventilation, and by the loss of heat when excretory (urine) or secretory (milk) substances are eliminated from the body. In very severe inflammatory reactions, these processes of heat dissipation are not able to keep pace with the increased metabolic rate, and fever occurs. Or, it may so happen that the heat-regulating centre in the hypothalamus is injured by the irritants and so heat regulation cannot be properly controlled, again resulting in fever.

Fever is a syndrome in which there is, besides rise of body temperature (**pyrexia**), an alteration in metabolism and various functional disturbances such as increased pulse rate, anorexia (loss of appetite), nausea, vomiting, constipation, increased thirst, scanty urine, and dehydration.

Hyperpyrexia is merely an increase in the body temperature due to heat storage without systemic disturbances, and hence differs from fever or pyrexia.

Causes of Fever

Among the most common causes of fever are **bacteria**. Most of the known pyrogenic (fever-producing) agents are derived from microbes, or their products. In fact, all infections, whether bacterial, viral, protozoal, fungal or rickettsial, may cause fever. **Thus, fever may be produced by:**

1. Endotoxins of Gram-negative bacteria: These are bacterial pyrogens. They form part of the cell wall of Gram-negative bacteria.

169

They are present in all Gram-negative organisms (both rough and smooth forms), but Gram-positive bacteria and other microorganisms lack them. The endotoxins are macromolecular complexes, and are chemically **lipopolysaccharide (LPS).**

2. Gram-positive bacteria: A fundamental difference between Gram-positive and Gram-negative bacteria is that Gram-positive bacteria do not possess the pyrogenic lipopolysaccharide endotoxins present in cell walls of Gram-negative bacteria. Therefore, the fever-producing activities of Gram-negative and Gram-positive bacteria are markedly different; the former being more potent as fever-producers. Fever resulting from Gram-positive bacteria appears to be due to multiple causes.

3. Viruses: The pyrogenic function is closely associated with the viral particle. However, little is known at present about the specific factors in viruses that cause fever.

4. Protozoa: Examples include trypanosomes, piroplasma, and anaplasma.

5. Fungi and rickettsiae.

6. Hypersensitivity: The mechanism of fever has been studied in several types of delayed hypersensitivity. The basic mechanism is the formation of antigen-antibody complexes that act as a stimulus for pyrogen release.

7. Mechanical injuries such as severe crushing, and extensive surgical operations.

8. Vascular disorders producing infarcts, such as myocardial infarction.

9. Neoplasms: Most of the malignant tumours may cause fever due to their undergoing degenerative and necrotic changes.

Mechanism of Fever

It is now known that the various factors mentioned above do not themselves produce fever, but they act indirectly by releasing **'endogenous pyrogens (EPs)'** from the leukocytes.

Cytokines play a key role in producing fever. Interleukin-1 (IL-1), interleukin-6 (IL-6), and tumour necrosis factor-alpha (TNF-alpha) are involved. These are produced by **leukocytes**, and also by other cells in response to infectious agents, or immunological and toxic reactions, and are released into the circulation. Among the cytokines,

IL-1, IL-6, TNF-alpha and the **interferons** can cause fever. Thus, they function as **'endogenous pyrogens'**. They reach the brain and interact with **vascular receptors in** the **thermoregulatory centre of the hypothalamus.** Then through local production of **prostaglandin E (PGE),** information is transmitted from hypothalamus to the **vascular centre.** This results in stimulation of sympathetic nerves, vasoconstriction of the skin vessels, decrease in heat dissipation, and fever (Fig. 28).

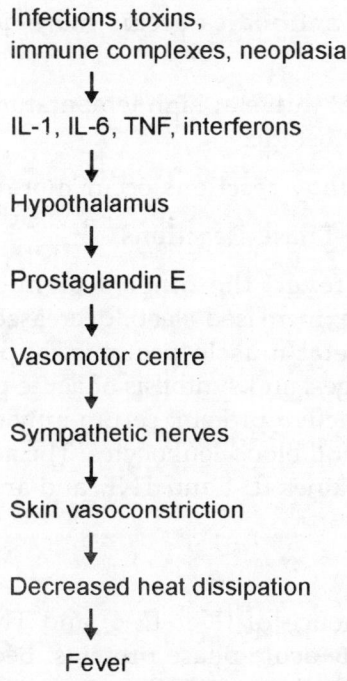

Infections, toxins,
immune complexes, neoplasia
↓
IL-1, IL-6, TNF, interferons
↓
Hypothalamus
↓
Prostaglandin E
↓
Vasomotor centre
↓
Sympathetic nerves
↓
Skin vasoconstriction
↓
Decreased heat dissipation
↓
Fever

Fig. 28. Mechanism of fever.

Interleukin-6 stimulates synthesis by liver of several plasma proteins, most important being fibrinogen. Increased fibrinogen levels cause red cells to agglutinate more readily. Fibrinogen reduces the charge on the surface of red cells and therefore the cells agglutinate. This explains **why inflammation is associated with higher erythrocyte sedimentation rate.**

Functions of Fever

These are beneficial and include:

1. **Increased phagocytosis**: Even a moderate rise in temperature improves the killing efficiency of neutrophils and interferes with multiplication of many pathogenic microorganisms.

2. Increased production of **neutrophils**.

3. Distribution of leukocytes is accelerated due to increased viscosity of blood.

4. Formation of **antibodies** occurs more quickly and in larger quantities.

5. Bacteria cannot thrive at high temperature and so to a certain extent **fever is bacteriostatic.**

6. **Antigen-antibody reactions** occur more quickly.

(B) Other Acute-Phase Reactions

In addition to fever, the other systemic manifestations of inflammation include: increased sleep, decreased appetite, increased degradation of skeletal muscle proteins, hypotension and other haemodynamic changes, and synthesis of acute phase proteins by the liver, including C-reactive protein, serum amyloid A, and a variety of changes in peripheral blood leukocytes. The **acute-phase reactions** are mediated by cytokines IL-1 and TNF, and are summarized below (Fig. 29).

Acute-Phase Proteins

Under the influence of IL-1, IL-6, and TNF-alpha, liver cells synthesize and secrete acute-phase proteins. Because their synthesis accompanies acute infections and inflammation and also because their concentrations rise very rapidly, they are known as 'acute-phase proteins'. They are synthesized within a few hours of injury and subside within 24 to 48 hours. Almost all of them help in controlling infections **and are therefore beneficial to the body.** The three most important acute-phase proteins are: (1) C-reactive protein (CRP), (2) serum amyloid P (SAP), and serum amyloid A (SAA). The **various acute-phase proteins** associated with inflammation are shown in Table 9.

1. Major proteins: The levels of CRP, SAA, and SAP in the blood **may rise a thousand-fold** following bacterial infections and tissue

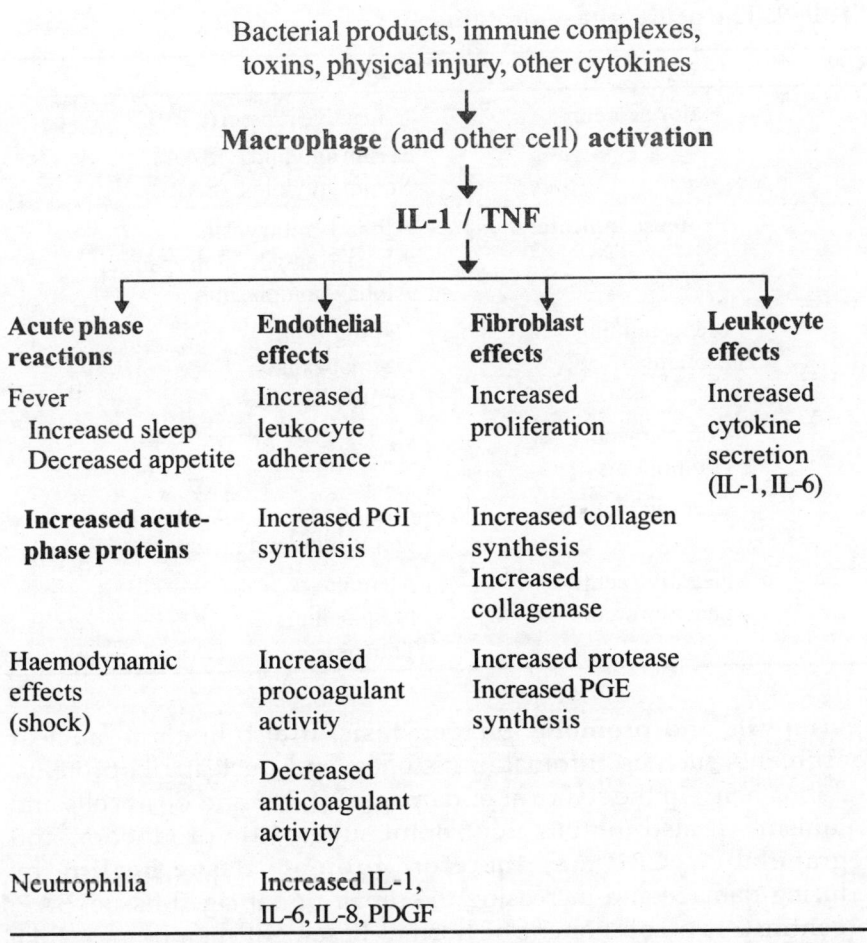

Bacterial products, immune complexes,
toxins, physical injury, other cytokines

↓

Macrophage (and other cell) **activation**

↓

IL-1 / TNF

↓

Acute phase reactions	Endothelial effects	Fibroblast effects	Leukocyte effects

Fever
  Increased sleep
  Decreased appetite
	Increased leukocyte adherence	Increased proliferation	Increased cytokine secretion (IL-1, IL-6)

Increased acute-phase proteins	Increased PGI synthesis	Increased collagen synthesis Increased collagenase	
Haemodynamic effects (shock)	Increased procoagulant activity	Increased protease Increased PGE synthesis	
	Decreased anticoagulant activity		
Neutrophilia	Increased IL-1, IL-6, IL-8, PDGF		

Fig. 29. Major effects of interleukin-1 (IL-1), and tumour necrosis factor (TNF) in inflammation. PDGF = platelet-derived growth factor, PGE = prostaglandin E, PGI = prostaglandin I.

damage. **CRP and SAP are closely related both structurally and functionally.** However, **only one of the two (CRP or SAP), rises in a given species.** For example, **CRP** is the major acute-phase protein in **humans, monkeys, pigs, rabbits** and **dogs**, whereas SAP is the major protein in **mice.** CRP is not an acute-phase protein in **cattle** or **horses**, even though it is found in normal serum. CRP binds to bacterial cell walls and may act as opsonin by binding to phagocyte Fc receptor, where it activates the classical complement pathway. **CRP binds to**

Table 9. The acute-phase proteins

S. No.	Group	Name
1.	**Major proteins**	C-reactive protein (CRP)
		Serum amyloid A (SAA)
		Serum amyloid P (SAP)
2.	**Protease inhibitors**	Alpha 1-antitrypsin
		Alpha 1-antichymotrypsin
		Alpha-2 antiplasmin
3.	Metal-binding proteins	Haptoglobin
		Haemopexin
		Ceruloplasmin
4.	Complement components	C2, C3, C4, C5
5.	Clotting factors	Fibrinogen
		von Willebrand factor
6.	Negative acute-phase proteins	Albumin
		Pre-albumin
		Transferrin

neutrophils and promotes phagocytosis. It also binds to nuclear constituents such as chromatin, histones, and nuclear riboproteins, and thus helps in the removal of damaged, dying and dead cells and organisms. It also inhibits neutrophil superoxide production and degranulation. **CRP may therefore promote tissue healing** by reducing damage and increasing the repair of damaged tissue. **SAP,** in contrast, is a component of normal basement membranes. Like CRP, it can bind nuclear constituents such as DNA, chromatin and histones, and can also bind and activate the first component of the complement system.

SAA proteins are found in high concentrations in the serum of patients undergoing chronic antigenic stimulation, as in tuberculosis or rheumatoid arthritis. In **dogs,** SAA increases up to twenty-fold after bacterial infection. Since SAA proteins are strongly immunosuppressive, it is believed that **SAA normally controls the immune response. SAA is strongly chemoattractive for neutrophils, monocytes, and T-cells.**

2. Protease inhibitors: This group of acute-phase proteins increase their concentrations 2-3 fold, and include protease inhibitors, such as alpha 1-antitrypsin, alpha 1-antichymotrypsin, and alpha-2 macroglobulin. **All of these inhibit tissue damage caused by neutrophil proteases** in sites of acute inflammation.

3. Metal-binding proteins: This group includes iron-binding proteins **haptoglobin** and **haemopexin**. **Both bind iron molecules** and make them unavailable to invading bacteria. Thus, they **inhibit bacterial proliferation and invasion**. Unfortunately, haptoglobin also reduces availability of iron for the production of red blood cells. Therefore, **anaemia** is usually associated with severe or chronic infections. **Haptoglobin** is a major acute-phase protein in **ruminants**.

4. Complement components: Rise in the third component of complement (C3) increases anti-microbial resistance.

5. Negative acute-phase proteins: Some proteins are negative acute-phase proteins. They are so named because their levels fall during acute inflammation and include albumin, pre-albumin, and transferrin.

(C) Changes in Peripheral Blood Leukocytes

Leukocytosis (increased white blood cell count) is a common feature of inflammatory reactions, especially in those caused by bacterial infections. It is usually due to an absolute increase in the number of neutrophils **(neutrophilia)**. The leukocyte count usually rises to 15,000 or 20,000 cells per µL (normal = 4000 to 10,000 cells per µL), but sometimes may rise to as high as 40,000 to 100,000 cells per µL. These extreme elevations are referred to as **leukaemoid reactions,** because they are similar to the white cell counts obtained in leukaemia. Leukocytosis initially occurs because of **accelerated release of white cells** from the bone marrow reserve pool (caused by IL-1 and TNF); and is associated with a rise in the number of relatively immature neutrophils in the blood ('**left-shift'**). However, prolonged infection also induces proliferation of precursors in the bone marrow caused by increased production of **colony-stimulating factors (CSFs)**. Increased production of CSFs is also mediated by IL-1 and TNF.

Most bacterial infections cause a selective increase in polymorphonuclear cells **(neutrophilia)**, while allergic and parasitic infections are accompanied by an absolute increase in the number of eosinophils **(eosinophilia)**. On the other hand, certain infections, for example infections caused by most viruses and certain protozoa, are associated with a decreased number of circulating white cells **(leukopaenia)**.

To conclude, the purpose of inflammation is to rid the body of the irritant, and to restore the tissues to their normal condition. This is achieved by the vascular and cellular responses. If the irritant is mild and not too abundant, then the vascular and cellular responses are adequate to destroy and remove the pathogen, before it causes much damage. The dead tissue is removed partly through phagocytosis by macrophages, and partly by lymphatics after it is liquefied by the proteolytic enzymes. The inflammatory cells that have infiltrated into the area wander away, the blood vessels return to normal, and thus the whole tissue regains it normal state. The process is called **resolution.**

The **repair** of injury begins almost as soon as the inflammatory changes have started, and thus constitutes a sequence of events as important as that of inflammation. Repair involves several processes, including cell proliferation, differentiation, and extracellular matrix deposition, and is dealt with in the next chapter.

AVIAN INFLAMMATION

Information on avian inflammation is scanty. Studies carried out on the comparative pathology of inflammation in the sheep have shown clear differences between species (Vegad, 1979). Based on Vegad and Katiyar's review (1995), this section briefly describes the work carried out in the chicken **and highlights differences of the inflammatory mechanisms from those in mammals.**

As in mammals, **two main events** take place **in avian inflammation,** namely, **increased vascular permeability** and **leukocyte emigration** (see 'Inflammation').

Increased Vascular Permeability

A cardinal feature of avian inflammation is a **marked increase in the permeability of blood vessels** to plasma proteins, mainly **albumin.** **Three different types of techniques** have been used in the chicken to estimate an increase in vascular permeability. These included: **(1)** the radioactive albumin technique, **(2)** the dye technique, and **(3)** the colloidal carbon technique (see Fig. 30, 31). Based on these techniques, studies have revealed that a **biphasic pattern of increased vascular permeability** (i.e., having two phases) occurs in the chicken following acute inflammation induced by various stimuli. These included chemical injury, thermal injury, bacterial injury, parasitic injury, traumatic injury (wounding); and immunological injury, such as

176

anaphylactic reaction, Arthus reaction, and delayed hypersensitivity reaction. The **biphasic pattern** comprised an **immediate transient** (short-lived) and a **delayed more prolonged** increase in vascular permeability. **A striking feature of avian inflammation is that the permeability response at all stages is confined to venules only** (Fig. 30, 31). It is now established that the action of known mediators of inflammation (mainly laboratory animal work) is restricted to venules and small veins only. Similarly, **in the chicken**, intradermal histamine, 5-h y d r o x y t r p t a m i n e (serotonin) and bradykinin have been found to induce **an increase in vascular permeability in the venules only**. In addition, use of antihistamines in

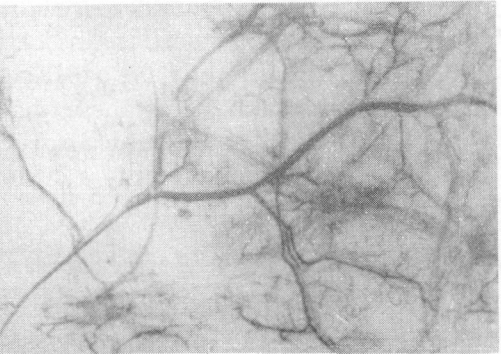

Fig. 30. Carbon labelling of vessels (venules) of the chicken skin immediately after intradermal turpentine.

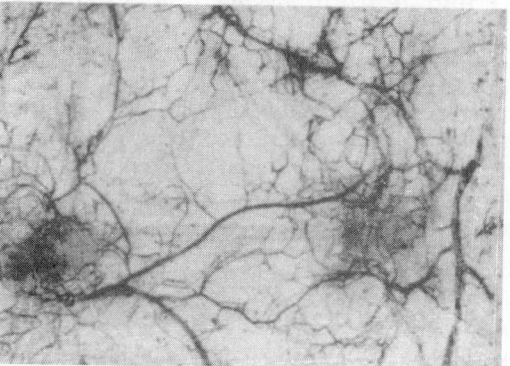

Fig. 31. Carbon labelling of vessels (venules) of the chicken skin immediately after thermal injury.

avian inflammation has demonstrated **involvement of histamine**. Thus, it is concluded that the **venular response in avian inflammation appears to be a mediated response,** as in mammals, rather than the result of direct injury to vessel.

Chemical Mediation

Little information is available at present on chemical mediation of increased vascular permeability in avian inflammation. Various studies have indicated that the **permeability response is biphasic** and that **the early phase is mediated by histamine**. Role of histamine in increasing vascular permeability in the early phase of avian inflammation appears similar to that in mammals. However, in marked contrast to mammals, there are indications that **5-hydroxytryptamine (5-HT, serotonin) may also play an important role in avian inflammation**. All the same, these findings need further investigation. Unlike mammals, **bradykinin appears to be unimportant in birds and prostaglandins have only a minor role in delayed phase of the avian inflammatory reaction**.

Increased Vascular Permeability *vis-a-vis* Leukocyte Emigration

Vascular permeability in vessels in the chicken starts almost immediately following inflammatory stimuli, whereas leukocyte emigration occurs after one hour. **Thus, increased vascular permeability to protein is dissociated in time from leukocyte emigration**. It is now well established that the two phenomena are similarly dissociated in mammalian inflammation, and leukocytes can emigrate from vessels, which have normal permeability.

Leukocyte Emigration

Standard histological methods have been used to study cellular changes. **Tissue leukocytosis** in lesions was assessed qualitatively by counting the number of different cells. In addition to the routine microscopic study, histopathology has been used together with a colloidal carbon technique to examine vascular and cellular changes simultaneously in the same tissue section.

In the chicken, the **leukocytic sequence appears to be of the same type qualitatively regardless of the nature of inflammatory stimulus**. The **initial emigration** of cells comprises **heterophils and monocytes**. Heterophils are the predominant granular leukocyte in acute inflammatory response of the chicken. This is soon **followed by emigration of basophils**, with **lymphocytes appearing much later**. Thus, a **mixed cellular exudate** occurs in the **early stages** of avian inflammation. It is now well established that **concurrent emigration of heterophils** and **monocytoid cells**, and participation of **basophils** appear to be the **characteristic features** of the early inflammatory reaction **in the chicken**. In mammals, however, there is controversy about the sequence of emigration of leukocytes.

Basophils

In avian inflammation, basophils are seen in significant numbers showing degranulation during the early phase. In mammals, basophils do not appear to play any significant role in the development of acute inflammatory reaction. These studies suggest that basophils may be playing a specific role in the chicken, presumably through the release of histamine **and possibly also 5-hydroxytryptamine (serotonin). In mammals,** basophils and mast cells contain only histamine. **5-hydroxytryptamine is absent.** However, further work is required to clarify functional significance of the basophilic leukocyte in avian inflammation.

Mast Cells

Marked degranulation and disruption of **mast cells,** accompanied by a significant decrease in their numbers in avian inflammation, suggest **their active participation in the early phase of the acute inflammatory reaction.** Mast cell response occurs in mammalian inflammation, but except in the rat and mouse, mast cells in other mammalian species lack 5-hydroxytrptamine, **whereas 5-HT appears to play a role in avian inflammation together with histamine.** Several other studies strongly indicate the role of 5-HT in avian inflammation. It then appears that the chicken mast cell may contain 5-HT. **Thus, vasoactive amines, histamine and possibly also 5-HT, released from the degranulated mast cells and basophils, may initiate the vascular changes in avian inflammation.** However, the significance of chicken mast cell and basophil must await further studies on the biochemical nature of these cells and chemical mediation of the avian inflammatory response.

Eosinophils

In the chicken, eosinophils do not participate in the local inflammatory reaction. It is interesting that all the methods used successfully in mammals have failed to evoke eosinophil responses in birds. In the immunological inflammation also, **eosinophils are absent,** which suggests that avian eosinophils do not respond to immunological inflammatory stimuli in the same manner as mammalian eosinophils. **It is concluded that eosinophils in the chicken behave differently than in mammals, and are not commonly found even in allergic and parasitic inflammation.**

Giant Cell

Giant cell formation occurs in the later stages of acute inflammation in the chicken following different inflammatory stimuli. In mammalian species, they are generally seen in chronic inflammation. **It appears that formation of giant cells may be a characteristic feature** of avian inflammation. Other studies indicate that **giant cell formation may also accompany tissue repair in the chicken. This is in marked contrast to the situation occurring in mammals, where giant cell formation does not seem to occur during the healing process**. However, further studies are required to establish clearly the exact nature of giant cells in the chicken and the role of macrophages in their formation.

Phagocytosis

Heterophils

Chicken heterophils are **highly phagocytic** and are capable of a broad-spectrum of antimicrobial activity. They are the predominant leukocyte in the acute inflammatory response. **The avian heterophil lacks myeloperoxidase** and depends mainly on non-oxidative mechanisms for antimicrobial activity. The **beta-defensins** found in heterophil granules can kill a wide variety of bacterial pathogens and are a major component of the heterophil antimicrobial weapons. Heterophils form the **first line of cellular defence** against invading microbial pathogens **in the lungs and airsacs**, where resident macrophages are lacking.

Monocytes

As in mammals, **the chicken monocyte is phagocytic**. This has been clearly demonstrated in avian inflammation.

Basophils

The basophil in mammals is not phagocytic. **In contrast, avian basophils may share a phagocytic property with other cells under immunological stimulus, and may play a dual function in certain types of inflammation through phagocytic and pharmacological mechanisms.**

Thrombocytes

In view of the **considerable phagocytic activity** in the chicken thrombocytes, and the fact that they possess lysosomal structures, it appears that **thrombocytes play a useful role in helping to clear the blood of foreign materials.**

Perivascular Lymphoid Aggregations

The occurrence of **perivascular lymphoid aggregation appears**

180

to be a common feature of avian inflammation induced by a wide variety of stimuli. Little is known, however, of their functional significance. It has been suggested that they form an integral part of the defensive response, or that they may have a similar function to mammalian lymph nodes. Their functional significance in inflammation therefore warrants further attention.

Healing and Repair

Studies on healing and repair carried out in the chicken have revealed that proliferation of fibroblasts and angiogenesis occur by 18 hours and 3 days, respectively. This conforms to the general pattern of healing described for mammals. **Mast cells in mammals** participate in the acute inflammatory response and **are found in great numbers in the granulation tissue during healing**. It is speculated that mast cells may play an important role in the development of new blood vessels in mammals. **In contrast, mast cells are not seen in granulation tissue in the chicken**. This suggests an **important species difference** and underlines the possibility that the mechanisms involved in angiogenesis during healing in the chicken may not depend on involvement of mast cells.

To conclude, in wound healing in the chicken, inflammatory and reparative processes run together and are closely interwoven. This is similar to that in the mammals. However, several studies suggest that **there could be significant differences in the inflammatory-reparative response between avian and mammalian species**, and thus underlie the necessity of further investigations.

Conclusions

There are similarities and differences between the avian and mammalian inflammatory reaction. Work in the chicken suggests that **a few generalizations of the inflammatory reaction may be made between birds and mammals**.

1. The biphasic increase in vascular permeability appears common to both and that histamine and/or 5-hydroxytryptamine appear to mediate the early response, whereas mediation of the late phase is very complex.

2. However, **there are clear differences between mammalian and avian inflammation**, and there are some peculiarities in the acute inflammatory response of chickens.

3. Because inter-species differences may be wide and basic, **it must not be assumed that results obtained in one species necessarily apply to another**. Extensive work is required to categorize mechanisms in the chicken.

1. Vegad, J.L. (1979) The acute inflammatory response in the sheep. *Veterinary Bulletin*, **49**, 555-561

2. Vegad, J.L. and Katiyar, A. K. (1995) The acute inflammatory response in the chicken. *Veterinary Bulletin*, **45**, 399-409

Chapter 5

Tissue Repair (Healing)

As we have seen, the primary objective of the inflammatory process is to destroy and remove the irritant from an area. After the injurious agent has been overcome, repair of the damaged tissues takes place. **Tissue repair (healing) is the process whereby the body restores the injured part to as near its previous normal condition as possible**. Body's ability to replace dead cells and to repair the damaged tissues is critical to survival.

Repair therefore is closely associated with inflammation, and **begins very early in the process of inflammation**. In fact, the two processes are inseparable, and occur simultaneously. It is often impossible to determine where inflammation stops and repair begins.

Tissue repair is a fundamental process in nature. The lower an animal in involution, the greater are the powers of repair. For example, when an earthworm is cut, a new part grows in its place. Similarly, the tail of a salamander (a lizard-like amphibian) or the limb of an amphibian, will grow when amputated. Also, in young goats a remarkable regeneration of the rumen and reticulum takes place after their complete removal.

Tissue or organ involved also influences the process of repair. If the tissue or organ is very highly specialized, it has less ability to regenerate. For example, in brain and spinal cord the lost nerve cells cannot be replaced. Similarly, the **age of an animal** also influences repair. The younger the animal, the more rapid and complete is repair.

Before tissue repair can take place, the products of inflammation, such as exudate and dead cells, have to be removed from the area. This is accomplished by liquefaction of dead tissue. This, in turn, is achieved by the autolytic enzymes of the dead tissue itself (**autolysis**), and also by the enzymes derived from inflammatory leukocytes (**heterolysis**). The liquefied material (fluid) is then readily absorbed into lymph and blood, and paves the way for repair.

Repair involves two distinct processes: (1) **repair by regeneration**. In this, the lost cells are replaced **by cells of the same type**, and (2) **replacement by connective tissue** (called **fibroplasia** or **fibrosis**), which leaves a permanent **scar**. In most cases, both processes

183

contribute to repair. This chapter describes healing of the skin wounds as a basic model (prototype) of the repair process of inflammation. But before proceeding further, let us understand some of the general features of cell regeneration.

Proliferative Potential of Different Cell Types

The cells of the body are divided into **three groups on the basis of their regenerative capacity,** and their relationship to the cell cycle: labile, stable, and **permanent cells** (see Fig. 33).

1. Labile cells: These are **continuously dividing cells.** They proliferate throughout the life to replace cells that are continuously dying. Regeneration occurs from a **population of stem cells** that have virtually an unlimited capacity to proliferate. When a **stem cell** divides, one daughter cell retains the ability to proliferate (**self-renewal**), while the other differentiates into non-mitotic cells, which carry on the normal function of the tissue. **Labile cells include** surface epithelia, such as stratified squamous epithelium of the skin, oral cavity, vagina, and cervix; the cuboidal epithelium of the ducts draining exocrine glands (salivary glands, pancreas, biliary tract); the columnar epithelium of the gastrointestinal tract, uterus, and Fallopian tubes; the transitional epithelium of the urinary tract; and haematopoietic cells in the bone marrow.

2. Stable (or quiescent) cells: These cells are quiescent, and have only a low-level of proliferative capacity in their normal state. However, these cells are capable of undergoing rapid division in response to injury. They constitute the **parenchyma of glands,** such as liver, kidney, and pancreas; endothelial cells lining blood vessels; and the fibroblasts and smooth muscle (mesenchymal) cells as well as chondrocytes and osteocytes. All proliferate in response to injury. However, **proliferation of fibroblasts and smooth muscle cells is particularly important in response to injury and wound healing.**

For labile and stable cells to reconstitute normal structure, it is essential that **the underlying supporting stroma of the parenchymal cells - particularly intact basement membranes - must be present to permit orderly regeneration.** The basement membranes **(BMs)** form a scaffold for accurate regeneration of parenchymal cells. When BMs are disrupted, cells proliferate in a haphazard fashion and produce disorganized masses of cells with no resemblance to the original arrangement, or scarring (fibrosis) may occur. For example, in liver, the hepatitis virus destroys only parenchymal cells without injuring the more resistant connective tissue cells, or framework of the liver lobule. Thus, after viral hepatitis, regeneration of liver cells completely reconstitutes the liver lobule. On the other hand, the liver abscess that destroys both hepatocytes and the connective tissue framework is followed by scarring (fibrosis).

3. Permanent (or non-dividing cells): These cells are terminally differentiated and **cannot undergo mitotic division in postnatal life.** To this group belong most neurons and the skeletal and cardiac muscle cells. **Neurons** destroyed in the central nervous system are permanently lost. They are replaced by proliferation of glial cells. Thus, injury to brain or heart is irreversible and results in only scar, since the tissues cannot proliferate. Although skeletal muscle is usually classed as a permanent cell type, satellite cells attached to the endomysial sheath do give some regenerative capacity. There is also some evidence that heart muscle cells may proliferate after myocardial necrosis.

Except for the tissues composed primarily of non-dividing cells (cardiac muscle and nerve), most mature tissues contain varying proportions of continuously dividing cells, quiescent cells, and non-dividing cells.

Apart from their **regenerative capacity**, division of cells into the above three groups is also based on their relationship to the **cell cycle**. The cell cycle is divided into **four phases** (Fig. 32): (1) the pre-synthetic **growth phase 1 or G1**, (2) a DNA-**synthetic phase or S**, (3) the pre-mitotic **growth phase 2 or G2**, and (4) the **mitotic phase or M**. G1 is the time of 'gap' between the end of mitosis and the start of DNA synthesis, and S is the period of DNA synthesis and the beginning of mitosis. In a cell with a cycle of 16 hours G1 = 5 hours, S = 7 hours, G2 = 3 hours, and mitosis = 1 hour. **Thus, mitosis represents only a small part of the life cycle of a cell** (about 1 hour in most cells). **The cell spends most of its lifetime in interphase** (i.e., G1 + S + G2 phases combined together), the period during which it replicates DNA and doubles its size. The most variable period is G1. Depending on the type of cell, it may last days, months, or years. Cells that stop proliferating become arrested at G1 and remain withdrawn from the cell cycle in the Go state (Fig. 32, 33).

With this background, we may now consider the relationship of labile, stable, and permanent cells to the cell cycle (see Fig. 33). Constantly dividing **labile cells** continuously cycle from one mitosis

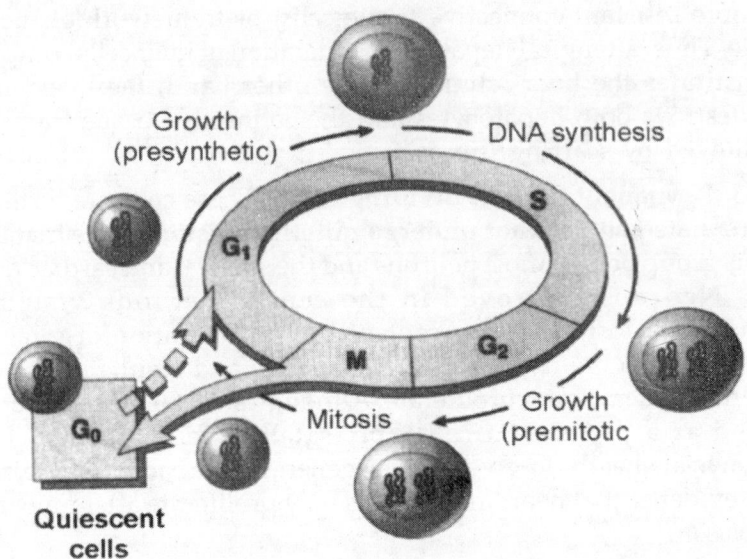

Fig. 32. Stages of the cell cycle. G1 (presynthetic) and S (synthetic) stages take most of the time of the cell cycle. **M (mitotic) phase is typically brief.** Note that while some cell populations continuously cycle and proliferate, most cells in the body are quiescent and are in stage Go.

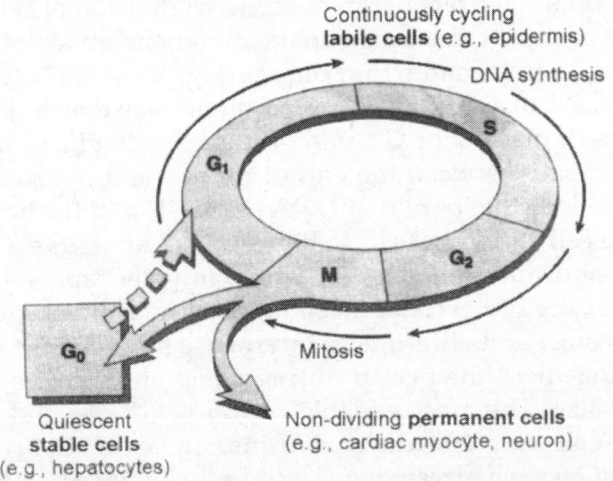

Fig. 33. Cell populations and cell cycle phases. Constantly dividing **labile cells** continuously cycle from one mitosis to the next. Non-dividing **permanent cells** have left the cycle and would die without further division. Quiescent **stable cells** in Go are neither cycling nor dying, and can be made to re-enter the cycle by appropriate stimulus.

to the next. Non-dividing **permanent cells** have left the cycle and are destined to die without further division. Quiescent **stable cells** in **Go** are neither cycling nor dying and can be **induced** to re-enter the cycle by an appropriate stimulus.

Repair by Regeneration

This type of repair is governed by the fact whether the cells possess the capacity to proliferate or not. If the cells have lost this capacity, they cannot repair themselves by regeneration. The power of regeneration differs widely with different cells. In tissues where the cells have retained their powers to proliferate, healing occurs by regeneration, but in tissues where the cells have lost this capacity, the place of such cells is filled by less specialized **connective tissue**.

Repair by Connective Tissue (Fibrosis)

Repair by connective tissue involves **four important steps**: (1) formation of new blood vessels (**angiogenesis**), (2) migration and proliferation of fibroblasts, (3) deposition of extracellular matrix (ECM), and (4) maturation and reorganization of the fibrous tissue (**remodelling**).

Repair begins early in inflammation. Sometimes as early as 24 hours after injury, fibroblasts and vascular endothelial cells begin to proliferate to form, by 3-5 days, a specialized type of tissue that is characteristic of healing, called 'granulation tissue'. The term 'granulation tissue' derives from its pink, soft, **granular gross appearance** on the surface of wounds. The loops of new vessels, when viewed from the surface, have a **granular appearance**. It is this appearance that accounts for the name granulation tissue. However, it is the histological features that are characteristic: (i) formation of new small blood vessels (**angiogenesis** or **neovascularization**), and (ii) **proliferation of fibroblasts**. Granulation tissue then gradually accumulates connective tissue, eventually resulting in dense fibrosis (scarring) that may further remodel over time.

Let us now discuss the three important steps of repair by connective tissue, namely: (i) **angiogenesis**, (ii) **fibrosis**, and (iii) **scar remodelling**, at some detail.

1. Angiogenesis or neovascularization: In this, pre-existing vessels send out capillary buds or sprouts **to produce new vessels**. Angiogenesis is an important process. Besides healing, it is also involved in the growth of tumours. **Four steps** are involved in the

187

development of a new capillary vessel: (1) enzymatic degradation of the basement membrane (BM) of the parent vessel to allow formation of a capillary sprout, (2) migration of the endothelial cells from the original capillary towards an angiogenic stimulus, (3) proliferation of the endothelial cells behind the leading edge of migrating cells, and (4) maturation of endothelial cells. This includes inhibition of growth and organization into capillary tubes. These new vessels are leaky because of the incompletely formed inter-endothelial junctions, and allow the passage of proteins and red cells into the extravascular space. **Therefore, new granulation tissue is often oedematous.** This leakiness also accounts for much of the oedema that persists in healing wounds long after the acute inflammatory response has subsided.

Several factors induce angiogenesis, but most important are **basic fibroblast growth factor (bFGF),** and **vascular endothelial growth factor (VEGF)** (discussed later). Both are secreted by a variety of cells. bFGF can bind to proteoglycans in the BM, to be released when such structures are damaged. Although these angiogenic factors are produced by many cell types, **the receptors** (all with intrinsic kinase activity) **are restricted to endothelial cells**. Besides causing proliferation, they induce endothelial cells to secrete **proteinases** to degrade the basement membrane and direct (along with laminin) vascular tube formation from the remaining endothelial cell population.

2. Fibrosis (fibroplasia, scar formation): Fibrosis, fibroplasia, or scar formation occurs within the granulation tissue framework of new blood vessels and loose extravascular matrix (ECM) that form early at the repair site. The process of fibrosis occurs in **two steps** (1) **migration and proliferation of fibroblasts into the site of injury,** and (2) **deposition of ECM by these cells. Migration** of fibroblasts to the site of injury and their **proliferation** are caused by **growth factors**, described later. These include **platelet-derived growth factor (PDGF), basic fibroblast growth factor (bFGF),** and **transforming growth factor-beta (TGF-beta).** The sources of these factors include platelets, inflammatory cells, and activated endothelium. **Macrophages**, in particular, are important cellular components of granulation tissue. Besides clearing cellular debris, fibrin, and other foreign material at the site of injury, **they produce many growth factors** (TGF-beta, PDGF, bFGF) that induce fibroblast migration and proliferation and ECM production (see 'growth factors'). Sites of inflammation are also rich in **mast cells**, and if the appropriate chemotactic stimuli are present, **lymphocytes** and **eosinophils** may also be present. Each of these can contribute directly or indirectly to fibroblast migration and proliferation. Of the growth factors involved in fibrosis, **TGF-beta is the most important because it favours fibrous tissue deposition.**

As healing (repair) progresses, the number of new vessels and proliferating fibroblasts decreases. However, the **fibroblasts now become more synthetic and deposit increased amounts of ECM. Collagen synthesis** is particularly important for the development of strength in healing wounds. As described later, **collagen synthesis by fibroblasts begins early in wound healing (days 3 to 5)** and continues for several weeks. **Many of the same growth factors** that regulate fibroblast growth proliferation also stimulate ECM synthesis. For example, collagen synthesis is induced by growth factors PDGF, bFGF, and TGF-beta, and cytokines interleukin-1 (IL-1) and tumour necrosis factor (TNF) secreted by leukocytes and fibroblasts in healing wounds. **Net collagen accumulation, however, depends not only on increased synthesis, but also on reduced collagen degradation** (discussed later). In the end, the granulation tissue becomes a scar composed of largely inactive spindle-shaped fibroblasts. **As the scar matures, disappearance of vessels eventually transforms the highly vascularized granulation tissue into a pale, avascular scar.**

(3) Scar Remodelling

The replacement of granulation tissue with a scar involves changes in the composition of ECM. **Even after its synthesis and deposition, ECM in the scar continues to be modified and remodelled.** So far we have discussed the cells and factors that regulate ECM **synthesis.** The **degradation** of collagen and other ECM components is achieved by a family of **metalloproteinases,** so called because they are dependent on **zinc ions** for their activity. (A metalloenzyme is an enzyme that contains tightly bound metal atoms.) The net result of **ECM synthesis versus degradation** results in **remodelling** of the connective tissue framework, an important feature of wound repair. The metalloproteinases should be differentiated from neutrophil elastase, cathepsin G, plasmin, and other serine proteinases that can also degrade ECM, **but are not metalloenzymes. Metalloproteinases** include **interstitial collagenases** which cleave (split) the fibrillar collagen types I, II, and III; **gelatinases** (or **type IV collagenases**), which degrade amorphous (shapeless) collagen and fibronectin; and **stromelysins** which degrade a variety of ECM components, including proteoglycans, fibronectin, and amorphous collagen.

189

These enzymes are produced by a variety of cell types (fibroblasts, macrophages, neutrophils, synovial cells, and some epithelial cells). Their synthesis and secretion are regulated by growth factors (PDGF, FGF), cytokines (IL-1, TNF-alpha), phagocytosis, and even physical stress. Their synthesis is inhibited by transforming growth factor-beta (TGF-beta) and corticosteroids. Looking at their potential to do great damage in tissues, **the activity of the metalloproteinases is tightly controlled.** Thus, they are secreted as inactive precursors that must be first activated. This is achieved by certain chemicals (e.g., HOCl·, hypochlorite ion produced during the oxidation burst of neutrophils), or proteases (e.g., plasmin) likely to be present only at sites of injury. **In addition, activated metalloproteinases can be rapidly inhibited by** a family of specific **tissue inhibitors of metalloproteinases (TIMPs)** which are produced by most mesenchymal cells. This prevents uncontrolled action of these proteinases.

Growth Factors in Cell Regeneration and Fibrosis

Although there is a long list of growth factors and new ones are constantly being discovered, only the most important are presented here. That is, those which have a broad target action, **or are specifically involved in healing.** These growth factors play a role in angiogenesis, recruitment of cells to sites of healing, fibroblast proliferation, and collagen deposition or remodelling. Note that although there are usually many sources for these growth factors at sites of healing, **activated macrophages are the most important.** Growth factors are **polypeptides.**

1. Epidermal growth factor (EGF) is **mitogenic** (i.e., causes mitosis/proliferation) **for a variety of epithelial cells and fibroblasts.** It stimulates cell division by binding to a **tyrosine kinase receptor** on the cell membrane (ERB B-1), followed by phosphorylation and other activation events, described later under 'molecular events in cell growth'. **Transforming growth factor-alpha** (TGF-alpha) is similar to EGF. It **binds to EGF receptor**, and has biological activities similar to those of EGF.

2. Platelet-derived growth factor (PDGF): PDGF is a family of several closely related **dimers** consisting of **two chains A and B.** All three combinations (AA, AB, and BB) are secreted and are biologically active. PDGF is stored **in the platelet alpha granules,** and released on platelet activation. It is produced by **activated macrophages,**

endothelial and smooth muscle cells, and a variety of tumours. **PDGF causes both migration and proliferation of fibroblasts, smooth muscle cells, and monocytes.** PDGF exerts its effect by binding to two types of cell surface receptors (**alpha** and **beta**) that have different ligand specificities with intrinsic **protein kinase** activity.

3. Fibroblast growth factors (FGFs): These are **a family of polypeptides** that bind tightly to heparin and other anionic (i.e., negatively charged) molecules. Therefore, they have a strong affinity for basement membrane, and in addition to growth stimulation, exhibit a number of other activities. FGF is recognized by a family of cell surface receptors, that have intrinsic **tyrosine kinase** activity after ligand-induced activation. **Beta-FGF recruits macrophages and fibroblasts to wound sites and has the ability to produce all the steps necessary for angiogenesis** (discussed earlier). It is secreted by **activated macrophages,** and other cells.

4. Transforming growth factor-beta (TGF-beta): TGF-beta has many and often **opposite effects.** It is produced in an inactive form by platelets, endothelium, T-cells, and activated macrophages, and it must be enzymatically cleaved (e.g., by plasmin) to become functional. **TGF-beta functions both as an inhibitor and a stimulator factor**. It stimulates fibroblast chemotaxis and the production of collagen and fibronectin by cells, while at the same time it inhibits degradation of the extracellular matrix by metalloproteinases. **All these factors favour fibrogenesis,** and it is now believed that **TGF-beta is involved in the development of fibrosis in a variety of chronic inflammatory conditions.**

5. Vascular endothelial growth factor (VEGF): VEGF is a family of glycoproteins with some similarity to PDGF. **It promotes blood vessel formation in early development (vasculogenesis) and has a central role in the growth of new blood vessels (angiogenesis).** VEGF promotes angiogenesis in healing wounds, in cancer, and in chronic inflammatory conditions, and is responsible for a marked increase in vascular permeability. The **receptors** for VEGF are expressed only **on endothelial cells.** Therefore, effects on other cell types are all indirect.

6. Cytokines: Discussed in Chapter 4 as mediators of inflammation, cytokines also act in many cases as growth factors. **Interleukin-1 (IL-1) and tumour necrosis factor (TNF) induce fibroblast proliferation.** They are also chemotactic for fibroblasts and stimulate synthesis of collagen and collagenase by these cells. **The net results of their actions tend to be fibrogenic** (i.e., produce fibrosis).

Wound Healing

Wound healing is a complex, but orderly process. Here, particularly, **wound healing in the skin** is described to illustrate the general principles of healing that apply to all tissues. Wound healing in the skin involves both **epithelial regeneration** and the **formation of connective tissue scar**. However, each different tissue in the body has specific cells that provide some organ specificity to the healing response (see 'healing of some special tissues').

Healing by First Intention (Primary Union)

The wound caused by surgeon's sterile scalpel and aseptically sutured is the best example of a **clean closed wound**. When there is no infection and the wound is not open, wound healing takes place without interference. This is known as **healing by first intention or by primary union.** Thus, healing of a clean uninfected surgical incision approximated by surgical sutures is the best example of healing by first intention. It occurs in a closed wound where there is minimal loss of tissue, very slight bleeding, and no contamination. As a result, epithelial regeneration predominates, over fibrosis. The narrow incisional space immediately fills with clotted blood, containing fibrin and blood cells. Dehydration of the surface clot produces a scab to cover and protect the wound.

Within 24 hours, neutrophils appear at the margins of the incision and migrate toward the fibrin clot. Basal cells at the cut edges of the epidermis begin to exhibit increased mitotic activity. Within 24-48 hours, epithelial cells from both edges begin to migrate and proliferate along the dermis. They deposit basement membrane components as they grow. The cells fuse in the midline beneath the surface scab, thus producing a thin but continuous epithelial layer.

By day 3, neutrophils get largely replaced by **macrophages**. **Granulation tissue** gradually fills the incision space. Collagen fibres are now seen at the margin of the incision, but in the beginning these are vertically oriented and do not bridge the incision. Epithelial cell proliferation continues, thickening the epidermal covering layer.

By day 5, the increased space is filled with granulation tissue. Angiogenesis (neovascularization) is minimal. Collagen fibrils become more abundant and begin to bridge the incision. The epidermis recovers its normal thickness, and differentiation of surface cells produces a mature epidermal architecture with surface keratinization.

During the second week, there is continued accumulation of collagen and proliferation of fibroblasts. The leukocytic infiltration, oedema, and increased vascularity are greatly reduced. There is increasing collagen deposition within the incisional scar and disappearance of vascular channels.

By the end of first month, the scar (cicatrix) is composed of cellular connective tissue devoid of inflammatory cells and covered by a normal epidermis. However, dermal appendages (hair, sebaceous glands, sweat glands) destroyed in the incision are permanently lost. Tensile strength of the wound increases thereafter, but it may take months for the wounded area to obtain its maximal strength (see 'wound strength').

Healing by Second Intention (Secondary Union)

When cell or tissue loss is more extensive, as in inflammatory ulceration, abscess formation, or even just **large wounds**, the reparative process (healing) is more complicated. **The common thing in all these situations is a large tissue defect that must be filled.** Regeneration of parenchymal cells alone cannot restore the original architecture. As a result, **extensive granulation tissue** grows inward from the wound margin to complete repair, followed by accumulation of ECM and scarring. This form of healing is referred to as **healing by second intention or secondary union.** This secondary healing differs from primary healing in several ways:

1. Large tissue defects have **more fibrin and more necrotic debris and exudate** that must be removed. As a result, the inflammatory reaction is more intense.

2. **Much larger amounts of granulation tissue are formed.** Larger defects accumulate a greater volume of granulation tissue to fill in the gap, and provide an underlying framework for the re-growth of tissue epithelium. A greater volume of granulation tissue usually results in **a greater mass of scar tissue (cicatrization).**

3. The feature that most clearly differentiates primary from secondary healing is the phenomenon of **wound contraction.** For example, within 6 weeks large skin defects may be reduced to 5% - 10% of their original size, largely due to **contraction.** Contraction is due to the presence of **myofibroblasts.** These are **modified fibroblasts** that have many of the ultrastructural and functional features of **contractile smooth muscle cells.**

193

Wound strength: How long does it take for a skin wound to achieve its maximal strength? When sutures are removed, usually after first week, wound strength is about 10% of the strength of unwounded skin. It then increases rapidly over the next 4 weeks. The recovery of tensile strength occurs from increased collagen synthesis which exceeds collagen degradation during the first two months, and also from structural modifications of collagen (cross-linking, increased fibre size) when collagen synthesis stops at later times. Wound strength reaches approximately 70% - 80% of normal by the third month. It usually does not improve beyond this point and this strength may persist for life.

Factors Affecting Wound Healing

Both **systemic and local factors** influence wound healing. These are:

Systemic Factors

1. Nutrition plays a very important role in healing, especially proteins. Low protein levels in the diet have an adverse effect on healing. Of special importance are the **two sulphur-containing amino acids methionine and cystine.** In the absence of these amino acids, connective tissue of weak tensile strength is formed. In protein deficiency, few fibroblasts form, and synthesis of collagen is inhibited and healing retarded.

2. Vitamin C (ascorbic acid): Its deficiency is an important cause of poor and delayed wound healing. **Vitamin C increases the conversion of proline to hydroxyproline, and lysine to hydroxylysine.** Thus, deficiency of vitamin C results in impaired synthesis of normal collagen. Absence of hydroxyproline will result in failure to achieve fibril formation (fibrillogenesis). **As a result, fibroblasts produce little collagen and what is produced is of poor quality.**

3. Zinc: Many enzymes, such as the metalloenzymes and DNA and RNA polymerases, **are zinc dependent.** Wound healing is delayed in patients with zinc deficiency, and is restored to normal by zinc administration.

4. Age: It is generally believed that with advancing age, the rate of healing may be considerably impaired, an important factor being the inadequate blood supply in the old age due to generalized vascular disease (arteriosclerosis), particularly in humans.

5. Glucocorticoids: Glucocorticoids have well-documented anti-inflammatory effects, and influence various components of inflammation and fibroplasia. These agents also inhibit collagen synthesis.

Local Factors

1. Local irritants: These, such as bacterial infection, presence of necrotic debris, pus, or foreign bodies in a wound markedly interfere with healing. Of these, **infection is the most important local cause of delayed healing.**

2. Inadequate blood supply (ischaemia): Ischaemia is a local anaemia, a cutting off, of the blood supply to a part. Under such conditions normal healing cannot occur. Arterial disease that limits blood flow (usually arteriosclerosis), and venous abnormalities that delay drainage also interfere with healing.

3. Foreign bodies, such as unnecessary sutures or fragments of wood, steel, glass, and even bone, interfere with healing.

4. Mechanical factors, such as early motion of wounds, can delay healing.

Pathological Aspects of Wound Repair

Complications in wound healing can occur from abnormalities in any of the basic repair processes. These reduce the quality of repair. These factors can be placed into **three groups** (1) Inadequate formation of granulation tissue, (2) excessive formation of granulation tissue, and (3) formation of contractures.

1. Inadequate formation of granulation tissue or assembly of a scar can lead to two types of complications: (i) **wound dehiscence,** and (ii) **ulceration. Dehiscence** or rupture of a wound is most common after abdominal surgery, and is due to increased abdominal pressure. Wounds can **ulcerate** because of inadequate vascularization during healing.

2. Excessive formation of granulation tissue can also complicate wound healing. Abnormalities of growth may occur even in what may begin as normal wound healing. The accumulation of excessive amounts of granulation tissue may protrude above the level of the surrounding skin and block re-epithelialization. It has been called **'exuberant granulation'**, or **'proud flesh'**. The accumulation of excessive amounts of **collagen** may give rise to a raised tumourous scar known as a **keloid.** Keloids are not true tumours, though they may recur after incision. Keloid formation appears to be an individual predisposition, and for reasons unknown, in humans, they are more common in blacks. The mechanisms of keloid formation are still unknown.

3. Contraction in the size of wound is a part of the normal healing process. An excess of this process is called a **contracture**, and results in deformation of the wound and the surrounding tissues. **Contractures** are commonly seen after serious burns and can interfere with the movement of joints.

Healing of Some Special Tissues

Epithelium can in general regenerate easily. Like fibrous tissue, epithelium of the skin, alimentary, respiratory, and urinogenital tracts, has retained its regenerative properties. When the epithelium is lost, repair occurs by proliferation of epithelium from the margin of the wounds. Secretory epithelium of glands, however, is usually not replaced; examples being mammary gland, gastric glands, seminiferous tubules, etc. In the **liver**, epithelial cells regenerate to a limited extent. In the **kidney**, no new nephrons can be formed. The cells can undergo only hypertrophy.

Mesothelium of the serous surfaces is quickly regenerated.

Connective tissue: Fibroblasts proliferate rapidly, replacing their own kind and also others that are not able to regenerate. **When the formed connective tissue is young, it is more cellular and rich in young capillaries. With age, it becomes denser and less vascular.**

Cartilage and bone: Due to avascularity, repair in cartilage is very slow and imperfect. It is usually replaced by fibrous tissue. Repair is very good and complete in the bone, osteoblasts playing the key role.

Tendons and ligaments regenerate slowly but completely.

Elastic tissue is also replaced rather slowly but completely.

Blood vessels are easily replaced by newly formed capillaries. However, the muscular coat (characteristic of arteries and veins) is rarely added.

Muscle: Lost muscles are reunited by fibrous tissue. Skeletal and cardiac muscle never regenerate. A certain amount of regeneration sometimes occurs in smooth muscle.

Nerve cell cannot be replaced. Once destroyed it is lost for ever.

Neuroglia proliferate readily.

Nerves: If the nerve cell is intact, repair of the peripheral nerves can occur. When a peripheral nerve is cut the distal portion first dies but is slowly regenerated by new growth from the proximal end, and although rarely, union can occur between proximal and the original distal end. If, on the other end, a nerve cell dies, then the whole neuron dies and is not replaced. The peripheral nerve then undergoes a series of retrogressive changes known as 'Wallerian degeneration'. The axis cylinder becomes fibrillated and disintegrates. The myelin sheath breaks up into droplets and is removed by the macrophages and the sheath cells, the latter being converted into phagocytes.

Mechanisms of Wound Healing

As stated earlier, **wound healing is a complex but orderly phenomenon**. It involves a number of processes, which include initiation of an acute inflammatory process by the injury, migration and proliferation of both epithelial and connective tissue cells, synthesis of extracellular matrix (ECM) proteins, remodelling of connective tissue and parenchymal components, and collagenization and acquisition of wound strength. The mechanisms underlying these events will now be discussed. As the molecular events involved are very complex, we shall proceed step by step, and begin with a consideration of the size of cell population in a given tissue.

Cell Population

In general, the number of cells in a given tissue **(cell population)** is determined by the rates at which new cells enter and existing cells leave the tissue. Entry of new cells into a tissue depends on their proliferation rates, while cells leave the population either by death (apoptosis) or differentiation into another cell type (Fig. 34). Increased cell number in a given tissue may therefore result from either increased proliferation, or decreased cell death or differentiation.

Control of normal cell growth: Cell proliferation is stimulated by **growth factors,** injury, cell death, or even mechanical deformation of tissues. Particularly, the biochemical mediators and mechanical stressors (stimuli that cause stress) present in the local environment can either stimulate or inhibit cell growth. Thus, an excess of **stimulators** or a deficiency of **inhibitors** results in net cell growth,

197

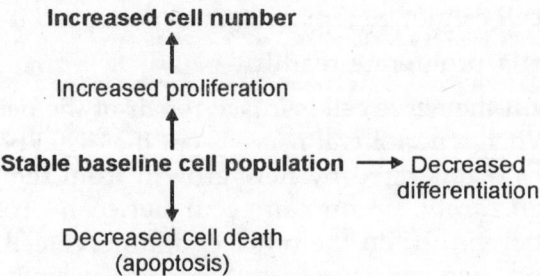

Fig. 34. Mechanisms regulating cell populations. Increased cell number in a given tissue can result from either increased proliferation, or decreased cell death (apoptosis) or differentiation.

and in the case of cancer, uncontrolled growth. Although growth can be achieved by shortening the cell cycle or decreasing the rate of cell loss, **the most important factors are those that recruit resting or quiescent cells (in Go) to enter the cell cycle** (see Fig. 32), as described later. Moreover, the various signals from the local environment may not only change the proliferative rate of cells, but can also alter their differentiation and synthetic capacity.

Normal cell proliferation: The cell cycle: Proliferating cells pass through a series of checkpoints and distinct phases, called the **cell cycle** (Fig. 32). As already stated, the cell cycle consists of: (1) the **pre-synthetic growth phase 1, or G1**, (2) a DNA-**synthetic phase, or S**, (3) the pre-mitotic **growth phase 2, or G2**, and (4) the **mitotic phase, or M**. Quiescent cells are in a physiological state called Go. G1 (pre-synthetic), and S (synthetic) stages take majority of the cell cycle time. **The M (mitotic) phase is very brief.**

With this background, we can now discuss the molecular events involved in cell growth.

Molecular Events in Cell Growth

Molecular events in cell growth are complex and involve a large number of intercellular pathways and molecules. But their understanding is important **because errors in such pathways may underlie the uncontrolled growth in cancer**. This section first discusses different **signalling pathways** and **cell surface receptors**, and then examines the various **intracellular transduction systems**.

Explosion of knowledge in the understanding of molecular events has come from the discovery that **growth factors** cause cell proliferation by affecting the expression of genes involved in **normal**

growth pathways, the so-called **'proto-oncogenes'**. The expression of these genes is tightly controlled during normal growth, regeneration, and repair. **Changes in the structure or expression of proto-oncogenes can convert them into oncogenes, which cause the uncontrolled cell growth characteristic of cancer. Thus, normal and abnormal cell proliferations follow similar pathways** (see Chapter 8).

First, let us examine the various **signalling pathways.**

Signalling pathways: Signalling means communication through signals. There are **three pathways of signalling: autocrine, paracrine,** and **endocrine.** This is based on the distance over which the signals act.

1. Autocrine signalling: In this, a **signalling substance acts on the same cell that secretes it.** Several **growth factors** and **cytokines** act in this manner. When the same cell produces a growth factor and its receptor, an **autocrine loop** is formed. Autocrine signalling also plays a role in compensatory epithelial hyperplasia (e.g., liver regeneration), and particularly, in **tumours.** Tumour cells usually overproduce growth factors that can stimulate their own growth and proliferation.

2. Paracrine signalling: In this, a cell produces signalling substances that **affect only the nearby target cells.** This pathway is important in the connective tissue repair of healing wounds, in which a factor produced by one cell type (a **macrophage**) has its growth effect on nearby cells usually of a different type (e.g., a **fibroblast**).

3. Endocrine signalling: In this, signalling substances (e.g., hormones) are synthesized by cells of endocrine organs and act on **target cells away from their site of synthesis** being carried by the blood.

Next, let us examine the various **cell surface receptors.**

Cell Surface Receptors

Cell growth is initiated by the binding of a signalling molecule (**ligand**), usually a **growth factor**, to a specific receptor. **Most signalling molecules are present at extremely low concentrations.** Therefore, binding to the target cell receptor is a high-affinity and extremely specific interaction. **Receptor proteins** may be **on the cell surface** of the target cell, or found in either the **cytoplasm** or the **nucleus.** A receptor protein specifically binds to particular ligands.

(A **ligand** is a molecule that binds to its specific receptor). The resulting **receptor-ligand complex** initiates a specific cell response (discussed later).

For cell growth, three major classes of cell surface receptors are important (Fig. 35). After ligand binding, they deliver signals to the nucleus by using a variety of **signal transduction pathways** (discussed next). Some pathways are specific to one family of receptors, whereas others are shared. Let us first examine the **various receptors** and their connection to **signalling molecules** (i.e., ligands). **The three major types are** (Fig. 35):

1. Receptors with intrinsic kinase activity: These receptors consist of two molecules. That is, they contain **two regions for receptor binding.** These receptors exist across the cell membrane with an **extracellular ligand-binding domain** and an **intracellular cytosolic domain**. Ligand binding to both receptors makes the two molecules stable (**dimerization**). For example, epidermal growth factor (EGF), fibroblast growth factor (FGF), and platelet-derived growth factor (PDGF) use these receptors because they are dimeric proteins and contain two regions for receptor binding. Ligand binding is followed by **mutual phosphorylation** of the receptor subunits. That is, one receptor molecule phosphorylates the other (**autophosphorylation**). Phosphorylation creates binding sites on the cytosolic domain of the receptor for a series of proteins. They then bind to these intracellular proteins, which include (Fig. 35):   (i) components of the PI3-kinase pathway (phosphatidyl-inositol-3 kinase), (ii) a series of adapter proteins which link the receptor to *ras* signalling pathway, (iii) components of the MAP (mitogen-activated protein) kinase signalling pathway, (iv) phospholipase C-gamma in the **protein kinase C pathway,** and (v) members of the *src* family of tyrosine kinases. **Receptor binding to these intracellular proteins stimulates a chain of events that lead the cell to enter into S phase,** or induce other transcriptional programmes. A very important pathway stimulated by *RAS* activation is the **MAP kinase pathway, which is involved in the intracellular signalling of the growth factors mentioned above** (Fig. 35).

2. G-protein-linked receptors: The receptors of this category contain seven loops that spread across the cell membrane. These receptors are not associated with the regulation of cell growth, but include those for **chemokines** (Chapter 4) as well as the hormones epinephrine (adrenaline) and glucagon. Ligand binding activates intracellular GTP-hydrolyzing proteins, i.e., transducing **G-protein complex** (hence the name **G-protein-linked receptors;** GTP = guanosine triphosphate). After activation, G-proteins dissociate and, in turn, activate an effector system that generates second messengers.

3. Receptors without intrinsic kinase activity: These are usually single molecules spreading across the cell membranes. They have an **extracellular domain** for ligand binding and a cytosolic domain. Ligand binding induces a structural change in the **cytosolic domain**, which then allows this domain to combine with, and also activate, **intracellular protein kinases.** These, in turn, phosphorylate the receptor complex, and stimulate a down-stream activation sequence involving **Janus kinases (JAKs)** and **signal transducers and activators of transcription (STATS).** Receptors of many **cytokines,** involved in the immune system, fall in this category.

Signal Transduction Systems

Signal transduction is the process by which extracellular signals are detected and converted into intracellular signals, that in turn, generate specific cellular responses. Signal transduction systems are composed of **networks of protein kinases.** (A **kinase** is an enzyme that catalyzes the transfer of phosphate groups from a high-energy phosphate-containing molecule, such as ATP, to an acceptor. **That is, it brings about phosphorylation**). The most important kinases in the regulation of cell growth are: (1) PI3-kinase, (2) mitogen-activated protein kinase (MAP-kinase), (3) inositol triphosphate (IP3), (4) cyclic adenosine monophosphate (cAMP), and (5) the JAK/STAT signalling system (Fig. 35).

1. Mitogen-activated protein (MAP) kinase pathway: The **MAP-kinase pathway** is particularly important in respect of **growth factors**. As we have seen, ligand binding by a receptor with tyrosine kinase activity results in **autophosphorylation** of the receptor and binding of adapter proteins. These proteins ultimately lead to activation of the **RAS protein.** RAS belongs to the guanosine triphosphatase (GTPase) superfamily of proteins. **Ras,** in turn, stimulates **MAP-kinases.** The **distal MAP kinase** enters into the **nucleus,** where it **activates nuclear transcription factors,** which, in turn, **activate gene expression. The net result of this pathway is that it stimulates quiescent cells to enter into the cell cycle, initiates DNA synthesis, and ultimately ends in cell division.**

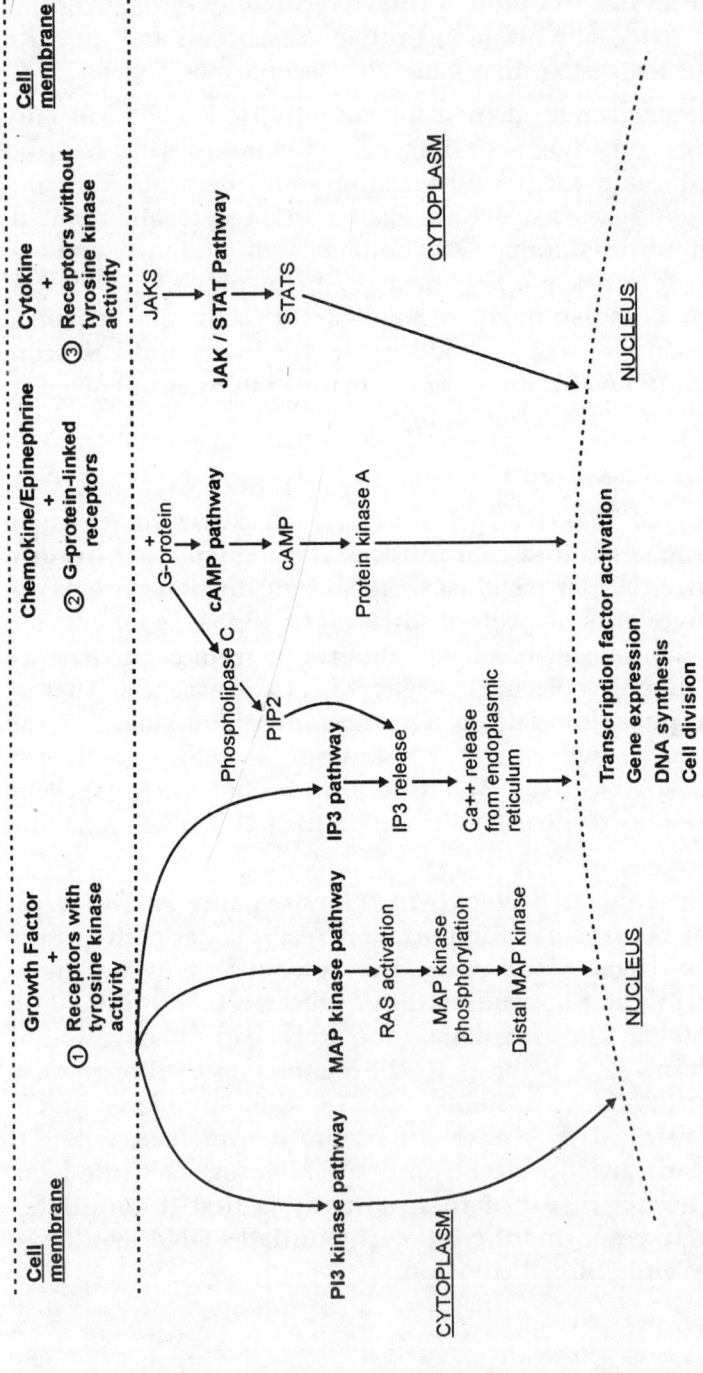

Fig. 35. The major types of cell surface receptors and their principal signal transduction pathways leading to transcription factor activation and translocation into the nucleus (see text). PI3-kinase = phosphatidyl-inositol-3-kinase; MAP-kinase = mitogen-activated protein kinase; cAMP = cyclic adenosine monophosphate; IP3 = inositol triphosphate; JAK = Janus kinase

2. Phosphatidyl inositol 3-kinase (PI3-kinase) pathway: Although many growth factors act by binding to a receptor with kinase activity, **they do not all convey the same signals.** For example, growth factors can differ in their ability to generate signals for cell proliferation and cell survival. This is because these growth factors differ in their ability to activate the PI3-kinase pathway. This kinase generates second messengers, which activate a series of intracellular kinases. The activity of these kinases ultimately leads to cellular responses that are connected with **cell survival**, such as phosphorylation of glycogen synthase kinase 3 and increased glycogen synthesis.

3. Inositol triphosphate pathway (IP3): The IP3 signalling system can be associated with either tyrosine kinase, or G-protein-linked receptors. Binding of a ligand causes activation of a G-protein, which in turn activates **phospholipase C**. Phospholipase C splits PIP2 (phosphatidyl inositol bisphosphate) into inositol triphosphate (IP3) and diacylglycerol (DAG). The IP3 diffuses through the cytoplasm and interacts with IP3-sensitive calcium channels in the endoplasmic reticulum, causing release of calcium ions (Ca^{++}) and **cellular responses**.

4. Cyclic adenosine monophosphate (cAMP) pathway: Binding of hormones, such as epinephrine (adrenaline) and glucagon or chemokines to G-protein-linked receptors, is linked through G protein to activation of adenylate cyclase and generation of second messenger cAMP. Increased cAMP levels activate **protein kinase A** which, through a series of steps, stimulates expression of target genes.

5. JAK/STAT pathway: As discussed earlier, after ligand binding to receptors without tyrosine kinase activity, these receptors associate with and activate one or more protein kinases present in the cytosol, known as **Janus kinases (JAKs)**. The JAKs phosphorylate the receptors as well as down-stream proteins known as **signal transducers and activators of transcription (STATs)**. In general, JAK/STAT system mediates functional and not proliferative responses.

Transcription Factors

The signal transduction systems just described transfer information to the nucleus, where specific changes occur in the regulation of gene expression (Fig. 35). This regulation is achieved at the level of **transcription of genes**. Transcription of genes is controlled by regulatory factors known as **transcription factors**, which play a vital role in controlling cell growth. The end-result is the

transfer of activated transcription factors into the nucleus. These transcription factors are **proteins** that can bind to certain DNA sequences called **promoters** and **enhancers** that lie up-stream of particular genes. Binding of the transcription factors causes DNA conformational (structural) changes that modify the down-stream transcription of these genes. **Depending on the nature of the transcription factor, binding may activate or inactivate gene transcription.**

Regulation of Cell Cycle/Cell Division

So far, we have examined the molecular pathways stimulated by the growth factors. But what are the mechanisms that control the journey of cells through certain specific phases of the cell cycle and also organize the events leading to cell division?

Two types of molecular controls regulate such events: (1) a group of proteins called **cyclins**, and (2) a set of **checkpoints** that monitor (check) whether the molecular events have been successfully completed and, if required, delay progress of the cycle to the next phase.

1. Cyclins: Entry and progress of cells through the cell cycle, are controlled by a family of proteins called **cyclins** (Fig. 36). Cyclins (termed A, B, and E) are synthesized only at certain specific phases of the cell cycle, after which they are rapidly destroyed as the cell enters into the next phase. Because of the cyclic nature of their production and degradation, these proteins are called 'cyclins'. Cyclins perform their functions by forming complexes with a group of newly synthesized enzymes called **cyclin-dependent kinases (CDKs).** These enzymes are activated only when complexed with cyclins. When the cyclins are destroyed, the relevant CDK becomes inactive (Fig. 36). Different combinations of cyclins and CDKs are associated with each of the important transitions in the cell cycle, and they exert their effects through **phosphorylation.** (CDK is a kinase. As stated earlier, a **kinase** is an enzyme that transfers phosphate groups from a high-energy phosphate-containing molecule, such as ATP, to an acceptor. **Phosphorylation** is the process of combining with phosphate groups.) **Cyclin-CDKs complexes** phosphorylate a selected group of protein substrates (Fig. 36). Depending on the protein, phosphorylation can lead to **conformational (structural) changes** that can (i) activate or inactivate an enzymatic activity, (ii) induce or interfere with protein-protein interactions, (iii) induce or inhibit binding of a protein to

DNA, and (iv) induce or prevent the breakdown of a protein.

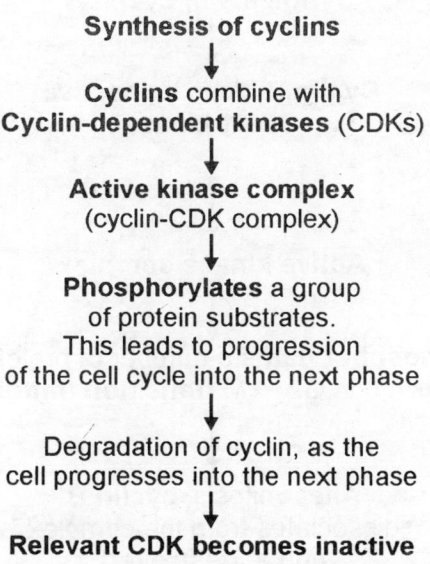

Synthesis of cyclins
↓
Cyclins combine with
Cyclin-dependent kinases (CDKs)
↓
Active kinase complex
(cyclin-CDK complex)
↓
Phosphorylates a group
of protein substrates.
This leads to progression
of the cell cycle into the next phase
↓
Degradation of cyclin, as the
cell progresses into the next phase
↓
Relevant CDK becomes inactive

Fig. 36. Control of cell cycle progress.

Let us take a specific example. Enzyme CDK1 controls the important transition from **G2 to M.** As the cell moves into G2, **cyclin B is synthesized,** and it binds to **inactive CDK1 kinase** (Fig. 37, 38). This **cyclin B-CDK1 complex,** whose activity is necessary for cells to enter into M phase, is activated by **phosphorylation.** The **active kinase complex** then phosphorylates a variety of proteins involved in regulating **G2** to **M transition,** that is, **mitosis.** These include those involved in DNA replication, depolymerization of nuclear lamina, and mitotic spindle formation. After cell division, cyclin B (i.e., the relevant cyclin) dissociates from the complex and is destroyed by a specific pathway (**ubiquitin-proteasomal pathway**). This leaves behind the **inactive CDK1 kinase,** which can re-enter the cycle at the next G2 stage. Until there is a new growth stimulus and synthesis of new cyclins, the cells do not undergo further mitosis.

2. Checkpoints

A checkpoint is a place, where travellers are stopped and their vehicles and documents are inspected. A similar system operates in the cell cycle.

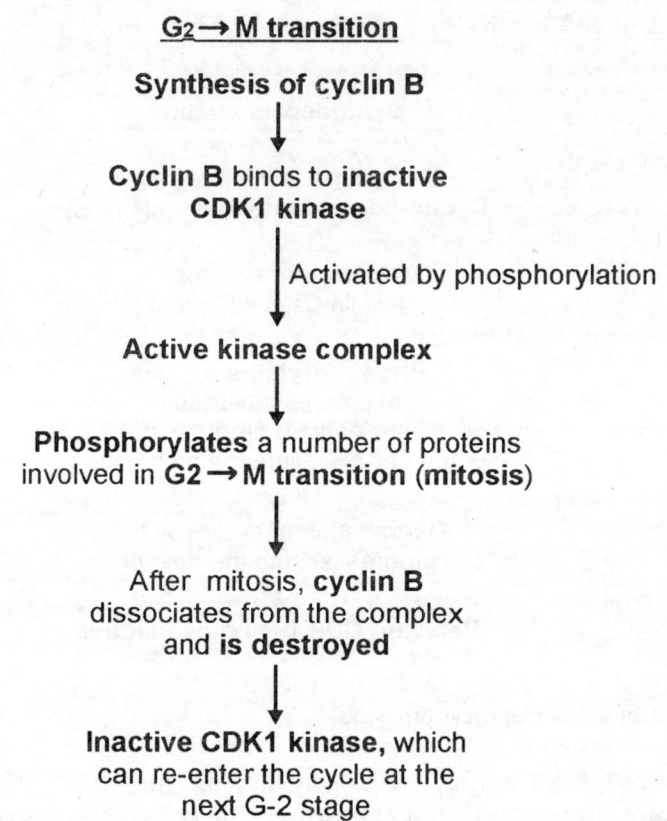

G$_2$ → M transition

Synthesis of cyclin B

↓

Cyclin B binds to **inactive CDK1 kinase**

Activated by phosphorylation

↓

Active kinase complex

↓

Phosphorylates a number of proteins involved in **G2 → M transition (mitosis)**

↓

After mitosis, **cyclin B** dissociates from the complex and **is destroyed**

↓

Inactive CDK1 kinase, which can re-enter the cycle at the next G-2 stage

Fig. 37. Regulation of **CDK1 kinase** activity by **Cyclin B** in the **G2** to **M transition.**

The **cyclin-CDK complexes** are also regulated by the binding of **CDK inhibitors. These inhibitors control the cell cycle** by balancing activity of the cell cycle. The interaction of these opposing signals determines whether a cell progresses or not through the cell cycle. These inhibitors are particularly important in regulating **two cell cycle checkpoints (G1** to **S** and **G2** to **M).** These are the points at which the cell examines whether its DNA has been properly replicated **and all the mistakes got corrected, before progressing any further.** Failure to properly check the accuracy of DNA replication leads to **accumulation of mutations and possible malignant transformation.** For example, when DNA is damaged by ultraviolet irradiation, **tumour suppressor protein TP53** (previously **P53,** a phosphorylated protein, see Chapter 8) is stabilized and induces the transcription of **CDKNIA** (previously **P21), a CDK inhibitor. This arrests the cells**

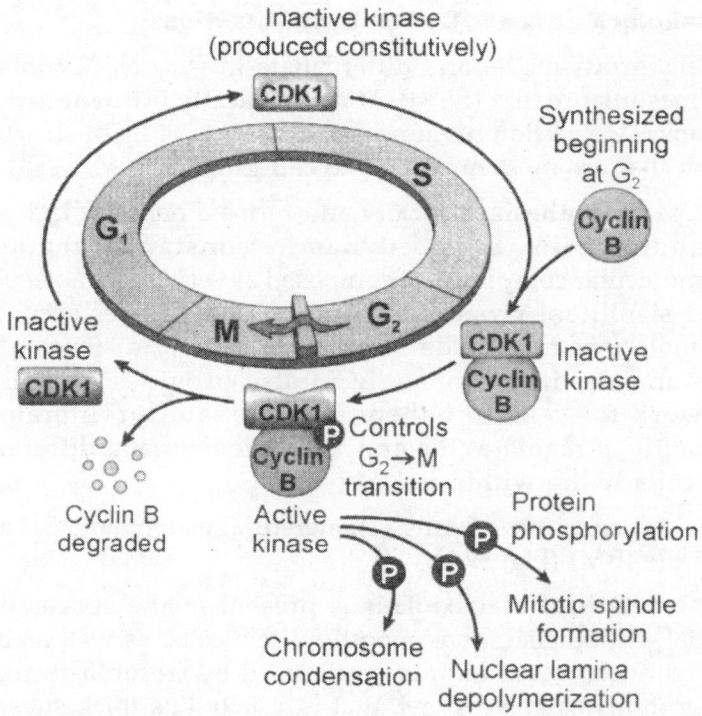

Inactive kinase
(produced constitutively)

CDK1

S

G_1

Synthesized
beginning
at G_2

Cyclin B

Inactive
kinase
CDK1

M

G_2

CDK1 Cyclin B Inactive
kinase

Cyclin B
degraded

CDK1 Cyclin B P Controls $G_2 \rightarrow M$ transition

Active
kinase

Protein
P phosphorylation

P P

Mitotic spindle
formation

Chromosome
condensation

Nuclear lamina
depolymerization

Fig. 38. This is same as Figure 37, but is presented in an illustrated form.

in G1 or G2 until the DNA is repaired. At this point, the TP53 levels fall, CDKNIA decreases, **and the cells can proceed through the checkpoint.** If the DNA damage is too extensive, TP53 initiates a chain of events **to convince the cell to commit suicide (apoptosis)** (see Chapter 3 and 8).

To summarize the molecular events, growth factors bind to their receptors and activate them. Many of these receptors possess kinase activity. Activated receptors then phosphorylate a number of substrates involved in signal transduction and the generation of second messengers. The resulting kinase sequence leads to the activation of nuclear transcription factors, initiates DNA synthesis, **and ultimately ends in cell division.** The process of cell proliferation is controlled by a family of proteins called **cyclins**. Cyclins, when complexed with **CDKs,** control the phosphorylation of proteins involved in cell cycle progression.

Extracellular Matrix and Cell-Matrix Interactions

Cells grow, move, and differentiate in very close contact with the extracellular matrix (ECM). **Matrix critically influences these cell functions**. This section discusses those aspects of ECM structure and function that are most important to **cell growth.**

ECM is synthesized locally and forms a network in the spaces surrounding cells. **It is a dynamic, constantly remodelling macromolecular complex** (i.e., composed of very large molecules) and forms a significant proportion of any tissue. Besides accumulating water molecules to provide turgidity (a state of distension) to soft tissues and rigidity to bone, ECM also provides an underlying framework for cells to adhere, migrate, and proliferate. **More importantly, it regulates the growth, movement and differentiation of the cells living within it.**

ECM occurs in two forms: (1) **interstitial matrix,** and (2) **basement membrane (BM)** (Fig. 39A).

1. Interstitial matrix: This is present in the spaces between epithelial, endothelial, and smooth muscle cells, as well as between cells in connective tissue. It is synthesized by **fibroblasts** and forms an amorphous (shapeless) gel, that is, a jelly-like thick substance. It consists of **fibrillar** (type I, III, V) and **non-fibrillar collagens,** as well as the **proteoglycan** and **glycoprotein elements** described later.

2. Basement membrane (BM): BM is a highly organized interstitial matrix around epithelial cells, endothelial cells, and smooth muscle cells. BM sits under epithelium and is synthesized by overlying epithelium and underlying fibroblasts. It tends to form a flat thin sheet-like mesh (net). BM consists of a network of amorphous **non-fibrillar collagen** (mostly type IV), and **adhesive glycoproteins** discussed later.

Functions of Extracellular Matrix

1. To provide mechanical support for cell attachment. In the absence of adhesion, **most cell types die.**

2. To control cell growth. Growth and differentiation are regulated by cell **adhesion.** Generally, the more adherent a cell is, the more proliferative (and less synthetic) it will be.

3. To maintain cell differentiation. The type of ECM also affects the degree of differentiation. The same ECM may have different effects depending on the **mechanical context** in which it is presented,

208

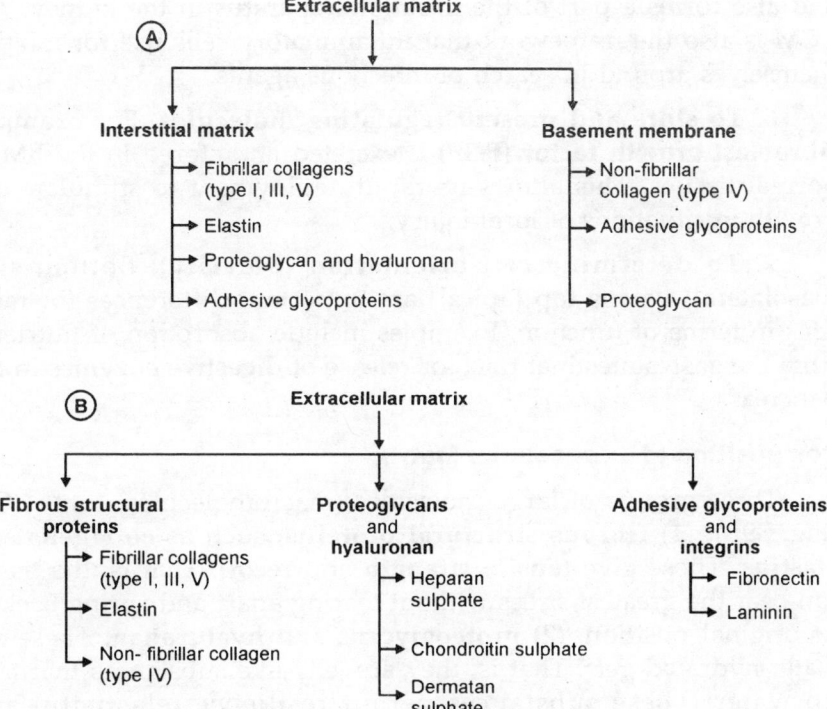

Fig. 39. A. Structural, and **B**. biochemical composition of extracellular matrix.

that is, **flexible or rigid.**

4. To provide scaffolding (a supporting framework) for tissue renewal (regeneration). All tissues renew themselves, and maintenance of normal structure requires support of a basement membrane. It is important that although labile and stable cells are capable of regeneration, injury to these tissues does not always result in restoration of the normal structure. The integrity of the underlying stroma (framework) of the parenchymal cells, **and in particular the basement membrane,** is most important for the organized regeneration of the tissues. **When basement membrane is disrupted cells proliferate in haphazard ways**. This results in disorganized and non-functional tissues. Extensive injury to labile or stable cells ends mainly in scar formation due to the expansion of fibroblast populations.

5. To establish microenvironments. Basement membrane acts as a boundry between epithelium and underlying connective tissue, and also forms a part of the filtration apparatus in the kidney. The ECM is also the framework that inflammatory cells use for moving themselves around in search of infectious agents.

6. To store and present regulating molecules. For example, **fibroblast growth factor (FGF)** is excreted and stored in the BM in normal tissues. This allows its rapid deployment to stimulate cell growth in situations of local injury.

7. To determine cell orientation (polarity). Bottom side (basolateral) versus top (apical) are important differences for most cells in terms of function. Examples include absorption of nutrients from the gastrointestinal tract, or release of digestive enzymes in the pancreas.

Composition of Extracellular Matrix

Three groups of large molecules (macromolecules) form ECM (Fig. 39B). (1) **fibrous structural proteins**, such as **collagens** and **elastins**. These give **tensile strength** and **recoil**. That is, the tissue can bear the greatest stress without tearing apart and spring back to its original position. (2) **proteoglycans and hyaluronan**. These are water-hydrated gels. That is, they are jelly-like substances that take up water. These substances permit resilience (elasticity) and lubrication. (3) **adhesive glycoproteins**, including **fibronectin** and **laminin**. These connect one matrix element with another and to cells.

1. Collagen: Collagen is the most common protein in the body, and provides the extracellular framework. Without collagen, an animal would be reduced to a group of cells, inter-connected by a few neurons. Collagens are **fibrous structural proteins** that give tensile strength. **They are synthesized by fibroblasts**. Collagens are composed of three separate polypeptide alpha chains woven together into **a rope-like triple helix.** The individual chains are able to tightly intertwine (twist together) because the polypeptide chains have **glycines present at every third position.** Mutations changing the glycines to other amino acids result in defective ECM synthesis, with damaging effects on bone, skin, aorta, and other tissues. **More than 30 distinct peptide chains form about 18 different types of collagen.** Some collagen types (type I, III, and V) form **fibrils (fibrillar or interstitial collagen)** by virtue of **lateral cross-linking** of the triple helix. **These are the most abundant.** Other collagens (type IV) are **non-fibrillar** and are components of **basement membranes.** The **tensile strength** of the fibrillar collagen is due to their **cross-linking, a process**

dependent on vitamin C. The fibrillar collagens form a major proportion of the connective tissue in healing wounds, particularly in scars, and are discussed further later.

Briefly, synthesis of collagen is initiated by DNA transcription from specific genes coding for the polypeptide chains on ribosomes. The alpha chain then comes off the ribosome into the cisternae of the rough endoplasmic reticulum (RER). Here, they undergo a series of biochemical modifications; one important change being **hydroxylation of the amino acid proline.** This provides collagen with its characteristic high content of **hydroxyproilne. This hydroxylation is dependent on the availability of vitamin C (ascorbic acid), and is important because it is necessary to hold the three alpha chains inside the RER.**

The **triple helix** is assembled in the RER. It is then transported through the Golgi apparatus and larger vacuoles to the cell surface. Shortly after excretion from the cell, peptidases clip the terminal peptide chains of procollagen (i.e., the basic unit of collagen - a long rod). This results in the formation of fibrils in the extracellular space. These fibrils give strength to connective tissue.

Another important biochemical modification is **lysine oxidation.** This results in **cross-linkages** between alpha chains of neighbouring molecules, **and is the basis of the structural stability of collagen.** Inhibition of lysine oxidation results in malformation of the skeleton, skin, and blood vessels. Thus, cross-linking plays a major role in the tensile strength of collagen.

2. **Elastin**

Tissues require elasticity for their function. That is, ability to get stretched, but returning to their original size or shape after being released. **Although tensile strength is provided by the fibrillar collagen, ability of the tissues to recoil (spring back) and return to their position after physical stress, is provided by the elastic fibres. Elastic fibres can stretch to several times their length and then return to their original size after release of the tension.** Fibroblasts also synthesize elastic fibres.

Elastic fibres consist of a central core of **elastin protein**, surrounded by a network of **fibrillin glycoprotein**. Large amounts of elastin are present in the walls of large blood vessels, such as the aorta, and in the uterus, skin, lungs, and ligaments. Like collagen, elastin requires a **glycine** in every third position, but it differs from

211

collagen by having little hydroxyproline and no hydroxylysine residues. Also elastin has fewer cross-links than collagen. The **fibrillin network** serves as a scaffold (platform) for the **deposition of elastin** and **assembly of elastic fibres.**

3. Proteoglycans and hyaluronan: These molecules form highly hydrated gels (i.e., thick jelly-like substances that bind water) and give resilience (elasticity) and lubrication, such as in the cartilage in joints. **Proteoglycans** consist of large polysaccharides called **glycosaminoglycans** attached to **a protein backbone,** like bristles on a test-tube brush. Some of the most common glycosaminoglycans are **heparan sulphate, chondroitin sulphate**, and **dermatan sulphate.**

Hyaluronan is a **huge** molecule that consists of **many repeats of a simple disaccharide without a protein core.** It is also an important component of the ECM, mainly because of its **ability to bind a large amount of water** into a viscous (thick and sticky), gelatin-like matrix.

Besides providing compressibility to a tissue, **proteoglycans in the extracellular matrix also act as reservoirs of growth factors.** For example, **heparan sulphate** binds basic fibroblast growth factor (bFGF) secreted into the ECM. Any injury to the ECM then releases the bound growth factor, **which can initiate the healing process.** That is, the released bFGF stimulates recruitment of inflammatory cells, fibroblast activation, and new blood vessel formation. **Proteoglycans** can also be essential cell membrane proteins and in that capacity control cell growth and differentiation. For example, a proteoglycan spreading across the cell membrane called **syndecan** has attached extracellular glycosaminoglycan side chains that can bind matrix growth factors like bFGF. This binding facilitates the interactions of bFGF with appropriate cell surface receptors. **Syndecan** also attaches to the intracellular actin cytoskeleton and thus helps in maintaining the normal epithelial sheet morphology.

4. **Adhesive Glycoproteins and Integrins**

Structurally, these proteins are of different kinds. **Their main property is to bind ECM components with one another, and also to link ECM to cells through cell surface integrins.** The important adhesive glycoproteins include **fibronectin** (major component of the interstitial ECM and **laminin** (major component of the basement membrane). These two adhesive glycoproteins, and the integrin family of cell surface receptors will now be discussed.

1. Fibronectin: It is a large multi-functional adhesive

glycoprotein, consisting of two chains held together by disulphide bonds (Fig. 40). It is synthesized by a variety of cells that include **fibroblasts, monocytes,** and **endothelium**. Fibronectin is associated with cell surfaces, basement membranes, and pericellular matrix. It binds to a wide range of ECM components (collagen, fibrin, heparin, and proteoglycans) through **specific domains**, and can also attach to cells through cell receptors (**integrins**) that recognize the specific amino acid sequence of the **tripeptide arginine-glycine-aspartic acid (RGD)** present on fibronectin. This RGD recognition sequence plays a key role in cell-ECM adhesion. Fibronectin is believed to be directly involved in attachment, spreading, and migration of cells. In addition, it increases the sensitivity of certain cells, such as capillary endothelial cells, to the proliferative effects of growth factors.

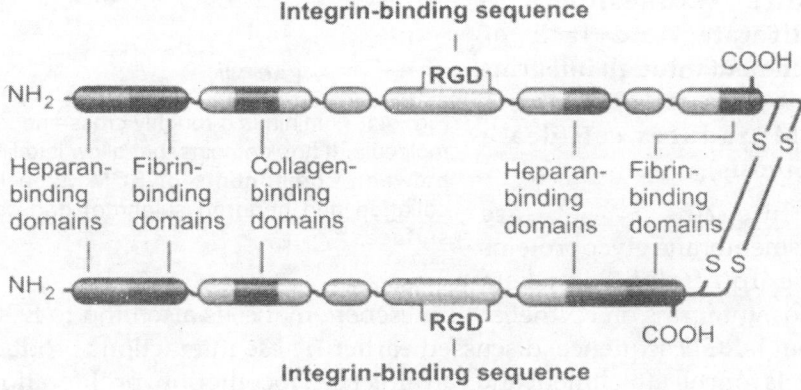

FIBRONECTIN

Fig. 40. The fibronectin molecule consists of two chains held together by disulphide bonds (S-S bonds). It has various domains (regions) that bind to ECM components (heparin, fibrin, collagen). Note that the cell-binding domain (i.e., integrin-binding domain) contains the **arginine-glycine-aspartic aid (RGD) sequence.**

2. **Laminin:** Laminin is the most abundant glycoprotein in the basement membrane. It binds cells to underlying ECM components, such as type IV collagen and heparan sulphate (Fig. 41). Besides binding to basement membrane, laminin also regulates survival, proliferation, differentiation, and motility of various cells.

213

3. Integrins: Integrins are the main cell surface receptors that mediate attachment of cells to the ECM. Remember that in Chapter 4 we discussed some of the integrins present on the surface of leukocytes that mediate important cell-cell interactions involved in leukocyte adhesion and emigration across endothelium at sites of inflammation. **Some cells require adhesion to proliferate, and lack of attachment through integrins to an extracellular matrix (ECM) induces cell death (apoptosis).**

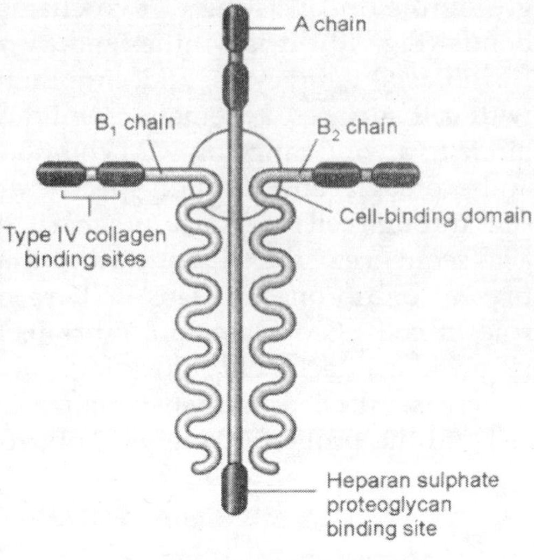

Integrins are transmembrane glycoproteins made up of alpha and beta chains. Integrins on epithelial or mesenchymal cells also bind to ECM through RGD sequence, discussed earlier. These interactions produce signals for cell attachment and can affect cell locomotion, proliferation, or differentiation. **Integrin-ECM interactions utilize the same intracellular signalling pathways used by growth factor receptors. In this manner, extracellular mechanical forces can be linked to intracellular synthetic and transcriptional pathways** (Fig. 42).

Fig. 41. Laminin is a roughly cross-shaped molecule. It has domains that allow it to link between components of ECM (type IV collagen and heparan sulphate) and cell surfaces

Thus, adhesive matrix proteins, such as **fibronectin** and **laminin**, can directly mediate the attachment, spread, and migration of cells. By activating intracellular signalling pathways, **fibronectin** also increases the sensitivity of certain cells (e.g., endothelium) to the proliferative effects of **growth factors**. In the early stages of healing (e.g., skin wounds), large quantities of plasma-derived **fibronectin** accumulate in the extracellular matrix and provide a temporary framework for the ingrowth (inward growth) of endothelium and fibroblasts. After 2 or 3 days, **fibronectin** in the healing wound is **actively synthesized by the proliferating endothelial cells.**

214

To summarize, cell growth and differentiation involve at least two types of signals, acting together. One comes from **soluble mediators** (growth factors, growth inhibitors), the other involves **insoluble elements of ECM** (fibronectin, laminin) interacting with cellular integrins (see Fig. 42).

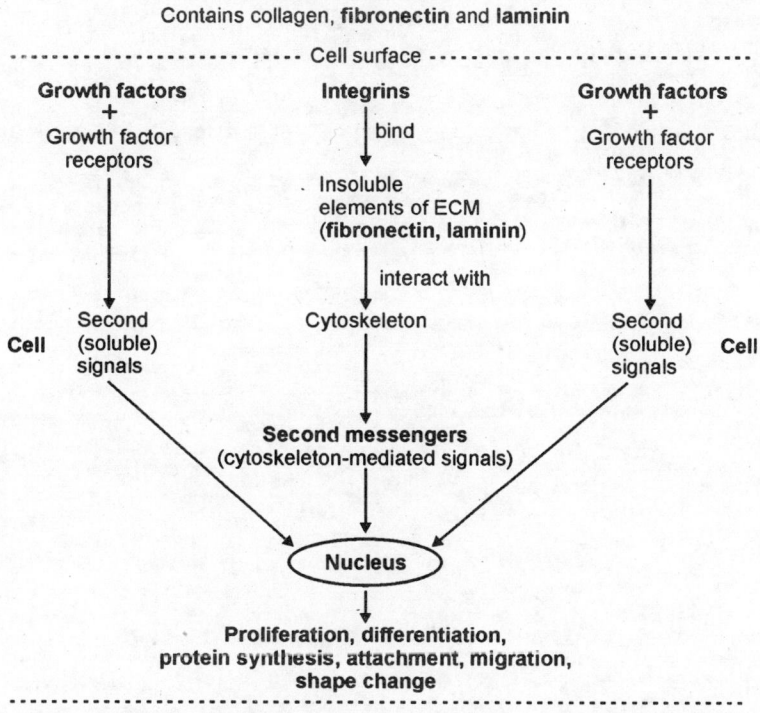

Fig. 42. Mechanisms by which ECM components (fibronectin, laminin) and growth factors can influence cell growth, motility, differentiation, and protein synthesis. Integrins bind ECM components (fibronectin, laminin) and interact with the cytoskeleton. This initiates the production of intracellular second messengers (cytoskeleton-mediated signals). Cell surface receptors for growth factors also initiate second signals. Together, these are integrated by the cell to yield various responses, including changes in cell growth, locomotion, and differentiation.

Chapter 6

Haemodynamic Disorders

T he health of cells and tissues depends on an **intact circulation** that delivers oxygen and removes wastes. However, what is less realized is that **their health also depends on normal fluid homeostasis (fluid balance).** Depending on the species, approximately 60% of lean body weight is water. This is divided between the **intracellular compartment** (40%) and the **extracellular compartment** (interstitial fluid 15%; plasma water 5%). Derangements of either blood supply or fluid balance cause some of the most commonly encountered disorders in veterinary medicine: hyperaemia and congestion; haemorrhage; three inter-related conditions - thrombosis, embolism, and infarction; oedema; and shock. We shall begin our discussion with hyperaemia since it is the most basic of these alterations.

HYPERAEMIA AND CONGESTION

Both terms **hyperaemia** and **congestion** indicate an increased volume of blood in the vessels of a particular tissue. **Hyperaemia** is an **active process** resulting from increased blood flow due to arteriolar dilation, whereas **congestion** is a **passive process** resulting from defective venous return from a tissue. In other words, an increased volume of blood in a given area can occur in **two ways:** too much blood being brought in by the arteries with dilation of arteries and arterioles, or too little blood being drained out by the veins. Thus, **hyperaemia** is of **two types: active hyperaemia** indicates that the increased volume of blood is of **arterial origin,** whereas **passive hyperaemia** (or **passive congestion,** or simply **congestion**), results from **interference with venous drainage.** When used alone, the term **hyperaemia** means **active hyperaemia** and the term **congestion** means **passive hyperaemia.** For a further classification of hyperaemia and its better understanding, refer to Table 10.

Active Hyperaemia

Active hyperaemia is an increased amount of blood in the arterial side of the vascular system. Usually it is associated with inflammation. **All active hyperaemias are acute. Chronic active hyperaemia does**

217

not occur. Active hyperaemia is the method employed by the body to supply additional nutrients and oxygen to the tissues, when an increased rate of metabolism is required. The additional nutrient and oxygen as well as the removal of waste materials are beneficial. **Active hyperaemia** may be **general** or **local**. Both general and local active hyperaemias are **acute, as chronic active hyperaemia does not occur**. Thus, in all, we have **only two types of active hyperaemia:** (1) acute general active hyperaemia (Acute GAH), and (2) acute local active hyperaemia (Acute LAH) (see Table 10).

Table 10. Classification of hyperaemia

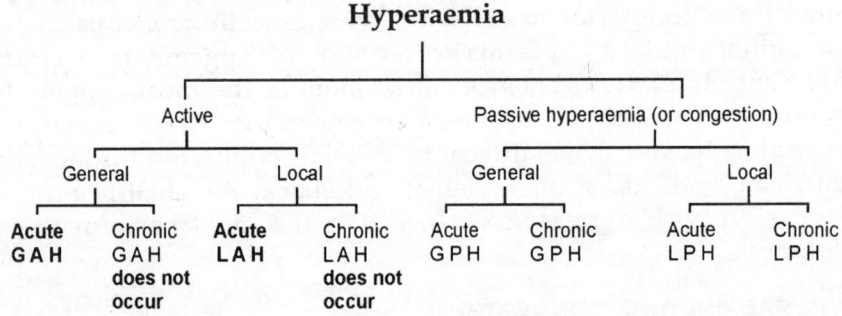

(i) Acute General Active Hyperaemia

This is an increased amount of blood in the arterial system throughout the entire individual. This type of hyperaemia is observed in **various systemic diseases, such as pasteurellosis and erysipelas**, as a result of the rapidly beating heart engorging the arterial system with blood. It can also occur in individuals with retention of body fluids due to renal disease. **Macroscopically,** the **arteries throughout the body are distended** with blood, and the organs and tissues have **a bright red colour of arterial blood. Microscopically,** the **arteries and capillaries are dilated** and filled with blood. **Significance and result:** It disappears as soon as the causative factor is removed.

(ii) Acute Local Active Hyperaemia

This is an increased amount of blood in the arterial system within a local area (leg, stomach, or lung) of an individual. It is the most common type of hyperaemia. **Usually, when the term hyperaemia is used unqualified, it refers to this type of hyperaemia.**

Aetiology: The causes are either physiological or pathological. **Physiological acute local active hyperaemia** occurs in: (1) the stomach and intestine following a meal (2) the lactating mammary gland, (3) the genital tract during oestrus, (4) the organs of locomotion such as muscles during exercise, and (5) blushing, in humans. Here, the hyperaemia is induced by neurogenic mechanisms. **Pathological acute active hyperaemia** is the **first stage of inflammation**. **Macroscopically**, the part is enlarged, swollen, and is heavier than normal due to the increased amount of blood. The colour is bright red. Blood vessels are larger and distended with blood. If the hyperaemia involves skin, the area has an increased temperature because warm blood from interior is brought to the exterior more rapidly than heat dissipation can occur.

Microscopically, when viewed in the living tissues with a magnifying lens, arteries, arterioles, and capillaries are distended with blood. Active hyperaemia is difficult to detect in the dead animal, because when the heart ceases to beat, arterial walls contract and force the blood out into the veins. Thus, very little blood is found in the arterial system. Active hyperaemia is therefore best detected during life by the cardinal sign of inflammation - redness.

Significance and result: Acute local active hyperaemia is beneficial in an area of inflammation, because the increased amount of blood brings additional oxygen, nutrient, leukocytes, and antibodies, which are needed in combating the irritant. Also, the irritant is diluted and rendered less harmful. In addition, the waste products of the increased rate of metabolism are quickly removed. The hyperaemia disappears as soon as the causative factor is removed.

Passive Hyperaemia (or Congestion)

This is **an increased amount of blood in the venous side of the vascular system** due to some form of hindrance to the flow of blood from an organ or region. As already stated, the word **congestion** is sometimes used to indicate passive hyperaemia. It is **general** if the interference is central, i.e., in the heart or lung, and **local** if in the vein of an organ or part of the body. Both general and local passive hyperaemia can be **acute** or **chronic** (see Table 10), but chronic is more common.

(i) Acute General Passive Hyperaemia

This is an increase in the amount of blood in the venous side of the circulatory system due to a **sudden obstruction** to the flow of blood **in the heart or lungs**. The hyperaemia involves the entire venous side of the circulatory system.

219

Aetiology: The aetiological factor is present **for only a short period of time,** and **involves the heart or lungs.** The principal causes are: (1) degeneration and necrosis of the myocardium. The cardiac muscles are unable to overcome the elasticity of the arteries. The arteries control and force the blood through the capillaries into the venous system where it accumulates. This commonly occurs just before death, and causes terminal acute general passive hyperaemia and oedema of lungs. (2) sudden myocardial accidents, such as myocardial infarction resulting from a thrombus or an embolus in a coronary artery. Again, the injured myocardium is unable to contract. (3) pneumonia. The capillaries in the lungs are compressed by the pulmonary exudate, and the passage of blood through the organ is retarded. (4) pulmonary thrombosis and embolism. This prevents the flow of blood through the lung causing it to accumulate in the venous system. (5) hydropericardium, haemopericardium, or pyopericardium. Transudate, blood, or exudate in the pericardial sac presses on the heart and prevents a normal diastole. This causes low blood pressure and passive hyperaemia. (6) hydrothorax, haemothorax, and pyothorax. Transudate, blood, or exudate pressing on the lungs and heart prevents the free flow of blood through these organs and causes it to accumulate in the venous system.

Macroscopically, organs throughout the body have **an intense bluish red (cyanotic) colour** due to the large amount of deoxygenated haemoglobin in the blood **(cyanosis)**, which they contain. The veins are distended with blood. The organs are enlarged and heavier than normal due to increased amount of blood. When organs are incised, blood oozes freely. **Microscopically, veins and capillaries are distended with blood. Significance and result:** If the alteration in the heart or lungs is slight and can be corrected, acute passive hyperaemia **quickly disappears.** When the cardiac or pulmonary change is severe and cannot be corrected, it may result in the **death of the animal.** If the vascular change is not severe enough to cause death, permanent changes of chronic general passive hyperaemia may occur.

(ii) Chronic General Passive Hyperaemia

This is an increase in the amount of blood in the venous side of the circulatory system **that persists for a long period of time and results in permanent alterations (atrophy and fibrosis)** in various tissues and organs throughout the body.

Aetiology: The lesions have a **central location in the heart or lungs**. Lesions involving heart are: (1) **stenosis of a valvular opening.** Stenosis is a **narrowing** of the total size of the valvular opening. It is a common cause of chronic general passive hyperaemia, and usually involves the **atrio-ventricular valves.** Septic thrombi on the valves are the common causes. These are the result of inflammation, mainly **valvular endocarditis** caused by infections. Stenosis results in a decrease in the amount of blood that can pass the valve in a given time. Unlike humans, **in animals, tricuspid (right atrio-ventricular) valvular disease is more common than mitral (left atrio-ventricular) disease.** When mitral valve is involved, there is a hindrance to the flow of blood on the left side of the heart, that is, interference to the free and prompt movement of blood from lungs into the systemic circulation. This leads to **chronic passive hyperaemia (or congestion) of the lungs**. When the right atrio-ventricular valve is involved, the blood is thrown back into the vena cava and its tributaries, and in this case, it leads to **chronic passive hyperaemia (congestion) of the liver.** (2) **valvular insufficiency**. Insufficiency results because of failure of the **cusps of the valve** to close properly, which is usually the result of irregular thickening of their surfaces with inflammatory granulation tissue, or because of thrombi on the valve. Part of the blood then **regurgitates** into the preceding chamber. In other words, when the ventricle contracts some of the blood is forced backward through the leaky valve that obstructs the incoming flow. Insufficiency may also result when cusps become retracted due to shrinking of fibrous scars, so that they do not completely close the lumen. (3) **myocardial failure** from degenerating or necrotic cardiac muscle and injury to the myoneural conducting system. In such cases, the myocardial contraction is strong enough to maintain arterial blood pressure. As a result, the arteries contract and blood accumulates in the venous system. (4) **anomalies of the heart**, such as **persistent foramen ovale,** inter-ventricular defects, or dextro-position of the aorta. These defects allow blood to be shunted from one chamber to another causing abnormal intracardial blood pressure. Normal arterial blood pressure is then not maintained, arteries contract, and blood accumulates in the venous system. (5) **constrictive lesions of the pericardium** and **epicardium,** such as **traumatic pericarditis in cattle.** These lesions compress the heart and prevent its normal expansion and contraction, arterial pressure is not maintained, and blood accumulates in the venous system. The most common lung lesions are: (1) **obliteration of the capillary bed**. This alteration prevents the free flow of blood

221

through the lung, with retardation of the flow through the right side of the heart, and backing up into the liver. It occurs in **chronic alveolar pulmonary emphysema in horses, in pneumonia, and pneumoconiosis.** These lesions compress the capillaries in the alveolar walls, thus hindering the flow of blood through the lungs. **Hydrothorax, haemothorax,** and **pyothorax** cause pressure atelectasis of the lung, compression of the capillaries, and prevent the free flow of blood through the lungs. (2) **compression of major pulmonary vessels by tumours, cysts, or abscesses.** The flow of blood through the lung is impeded by the vascular obstruction and blood accumulates in the venous side of the circulating system.

Morphology: Veins throughout the body are engorged with blood. The blood has a **bluish-red (cyanotic) colour** due to large amount of poorly oxygenated blood. Oedema of the tissue is a prominent lesion, especially in the ventral portion of organs, the under-surface of the body, and in the legs. In long-standing cases, there is atrophy of the parenchyma of organs such as liver, and hyperplasia of connective tissue, and fibrosis. The stasis of poorly oxygenated blood causes chronic hypoxia, which may lead to degeneration or even death of parenchymal cells. **The lungs, liver, and spleen develop the most noticeable changes.**

Lungs: Lungs are affected in the **left-sided heart failure**, that is, due to lesions in the **mitral valve.** The alveolar capillaries are engorged with blood and often become tortuous, with small aneurysmal dilatations. Rupture of distended capillaries may cause **minute intra-alveolar haemorrhages.** The haemosiderin released from the disintegrating red cells is phagocytosed by **alveolar macrophages.** Since chronic passive hyperaemia of the lung is usually due to **valvular heart diseases**, as just explained, the haemosiderin-laden macrophages in the alveolar spaces are called **'heart-failure cells'.** In severe forms of chronic passive hyperaemia, the alveolar septa are widened due to dilatation of alveolar capillaries and collection of oedema fluid in the alveolar septa. In time, the oedematous septa become **fibrotic**, and produce the condition known as **'brown induration of the lung'.** The lung is indurated (hardened) because of fibrous thickening of the alveolar septa. **The brown colour is due to haemosiderin.**

Liver: Liver is affected in **right-sided heart failure**, that is, due to lesions in the **right atrio-ventricular valve, or** in the **lungs.** The liver is slightly increased in size and weight. On sectioning, it shows a prominent **'nutmeg pattern'.** That is, the central veins are prominent, and the area surrounding it **(centrilobular region) is red-blue (congested).** This congested area is surrounded by **paler hypoxic peripheral regions.** This pattern is referred to as **'nutmeg liver'**, because it resembles the surface of a cut nutmeg. **Microscopically, the central vein and the sinusoids of the centrilobular regions are distended with blood.** This is because the hepatocytes in this area undergo **atrophy due to chronic hypoxia**, whereas the peripheral hepatocytes, suffering less severe hypoxia, develop **fatty change**. In some cases, the severe central hypoxia produces **centrilobular necrosis** along with sinusoidal congestion. If the patient does not die, the central areas in time become fibrotic, causing so-called **'cardiac cirrhosis'** or **'cardiac sclerosis'.**

Spleen: Spleen is slightly enlarged and slightly cyanotic. **Microscopically,** sinusoids are markedly distended. **Significance and result: Atrophy of the parenchyma and hyperplasia of the interstitial connective tissue are permanent changes.** If the cause is removed, the remaining parenchymatous tissue tries to compensate for the loss.

(iii) **Acute Local Passive Hyperaemia**

This is an increase in the amount of blood in the veins of an area (foot, tail, kidney, spleen) as the result of a **sudden obstruction** to the flow of blood from an organ or region.

Aetiology: Any factor which causes compression of the veins of a portion, such as: (1) malposition of the viscera (intussusception, volvulus, and torsion) in which veins are compressed. (2) external pressure from ligatures, tourniquets, bandages, and rubber bands cause compression of veins and obstruction of blood flow.

Macroscopically, the veins are engorged with blood. If the obstruction persists, the endothelial cells of the blood vessels undergo necrosis, and haemorrhages may occur. The surrounding tissues soon undergo degenerative changes. In intestinal tract, putrefactive organisms may invade the dead tissue and cause gangrene. **Microscopically, veins and capillaries are distended with blood.** Necrosis and suppurative inflammation may be present. **Significance and result:** If the obstruction is only partial and persists for only a short period, no permanent changes occur. If the obstruction persists, and adequate nutrient and oxygen cannot be supplied, death of the tissue occurs. If the obstruction is partial, or when some collateral circulation is present, necrosis does not occur, but hyperaemia persists and permanent changes of atrophy and fibrosis occur.

(iv) Chronic Local Passive Hyperaemia

This is an increase in the amount of blood that persists **for a long time** in the veins of a portion, and causes permanent tissue changes (**atrophy and fibrosis**) in the area. **Aetiology:** Any factor which brings about a gradual or partial obstruction of the venous circulation in the area. Two types of changes produce this form of hyperaemia: (1) **external pressure** upon a vein, such as from **enlarging neoplasms, lymph nodes,** and **abscesses.** These press upon veins and cause **gradual stenosis (narrowing)** of the vessel. Bandages and harnesses are the other examples. (2) obstruction within a vein, such as caused by **a thrombus**.

Macroscopically, the affected organ in the beginning is larger than normal. Later, when scarring (fibrosis) takes place, it becomes smaller. The veins are engorged with blood, and blood has a bluish-red colour being un-oxygenated. The involved tissues are oedematous due to increased permeability of capillaries. Later, because of inadequate circulation, cells undergo atrophy and organs become smaller than normal. When fibrosis occurs, tissues become firmer than normal. **Microscopically, veins and capillaries are distended with blood** and cells in the involved tissue are separated by a transudate, which stains faintly pink with eosin. Atrophy and fibrosis are present in varying degrees depending on the severity of passive hyperaemia and the length of time it has been present. **Significance and result:** Atrophy and fibrosis are permanent alterations. Other alterations associated with chronic passive hyperaemia interfere with the function of tissues and organs.

HYPOSTATIC CONGESTION

This is an accumulation of blood in the ventral portions of the body **due to the influence of gravity. Aetiology:** It occurs whenever heart is unable to maintain sufficient blood pressure to overcome the force of gravity. For example, it is observed in cardiac injury; and **in recumbent, restrained, or inactive animals** in which the circulation becomes so sluggish that blood accumulates in the ventral portions of the body. Especially in large animals, there is a strong tendency for blood to gravitate to the lower side of the body. **It is particularly common in organs such as the lungs that have poorly supported capillaries.** The congestion occurs in the **lung that is ventral.** Hypostatic congestion that occurs at the time of death, when the failing heart is no longer able to maintain blood pressure, is called **agonal** congestion. When it is observed after death, it is known as **postmortem congestion.**

Macroscopically, the veins in the ventral portion of an organ are distended with blood. For example, the ventral portion of the lung is engorged with blood, while the dorsal contains very little blood. The same vascular change is observed in the kidneys and intestine. Complications of the hypostatic congestion are **pneumonia in** the case of **lungs,** and **gangrene of the intestine** from bacterial invasion. **Microscopically,** the veins and capillaries are distended with blood. Oedema, haemorrhage, inflammation, and necrosis are the complicating changes. In tissue sections, the affected veins will contain erythrocytes, on it will be a layer of leukocytes, and above this a zone of plasma. **Significance and result: Hypostatic congestion indicates the side of the animal that was ventral at the time of death.** It is an indication that heart was not able to maintain adequate blood pressure. Its location is used **in medico-legal cases** to indicate the position of the body at the time of death, and whether or not, the carcass was removed after death.

HAEMORRHAGE

Haemorrhage is the escape of blood from a vessel. It is of two types: (1) **haemorrhage by rhexis,** when there is rupture or break of a blood vessel, and (2) **haemorrhage by diapedesis,** when blood leaves through an apparently intact vascular wall. It is a microscopic haemorrhage, but just how the erythrocytes escape is still not completely understood. It is believed that the cells escape one by one through minute or imperceptible imperfections in the vessel walls. It is likely that certain injurious influences damage the walls of the capillaries and venules, make them more permeable, and bring about diapedesis.

Aetiology: There are a number of factors that cause haemorrhage. (1) **physiological causes:** Physiological haemorrhage occurs during **parturition,** menstruation in women, rupture of the graffian follicles and rupture of the umbilical vessels. (2) **trauma:** mechanical injuries like laceration, incisions, contusions, and ruptures all cause breaks in the continuity of vessels that allow escape of blood. (3) **bacterial and viral diseases:** Toxins of various bacteria (**Salmonella, Clostridium, Streptococcus,** and **Pasteurella**) may injure the endothelium of blood vessels, especially capillaries, and cause haemorrhages. Haemorrhages are characteristic lesions of enterotoxaemia of sheep, caused by the toxin of *Clostridium perfringens*. Swine fever (hog cholera) virus invades the endothelial cells and causes degenerative changes. The cells in the injured vessel wall rupture and haemorrhage occurs. The toxins produced by the septicaemic infections are chiefly responsible for petechiae and ecchymoses seen on serous and mucous membranes. (4) **parasites** cause erosion of intestinal mucosa (e.g., coccidia), induce aneurysms (e.g., strongyles), and inject anticoagulants (e.g., hookworms and tapeworms). (5) **necrosis and destruction of vessel wall:** Arteriosclerotic changes weaken walls of blood vessels, and then blood pressure causes rupture of the vessels. Prior to rupture, the vessel wall may dilate greatly forming an aneurysm. An aneurysm is a local dilatation of an artery or vein. The walls of aneurysm are very thin and rupture easily. (6) **neoplasms**: Vessel walls may be attacked and destroyed by an extending erosive cancer, thus causing haemorrhage. (7) **toxic chemical agents**: Many chemical substances, such as phosphorus, chloroform, cyanide, arsenic, and certain plant poisonings, such as **Crotalaria** poisoning, injure endothelial cells and cause haemorrhage. (8) **haemorrhagic diatheses** (bleeding disorders): These are a group of clinical disorders characterized by increased bleeding tendency. The cause can be divided into four categories. (i) **increased vascular fragility,** such as in vitamin C deficiency or scurvy. Most animals synthesize adequate vitamin C and are not subject to deficiency. However, scurvy is seen in guinea pigs and nonhuman primates (monkeys and apes). (ii) **reduced platelet number (thrombocytopaenia).** Example: purpura haemorrhagica in horses, in which haemorrhage is prominent characteristic of the disease. (iii) **defective platelet function.** (iv) **abnormalities in clotting factors.** Examples: (i) haemophilia A (or classical haemophilia) due to factor VIII deficiency. Haemophilia is important in humans, but also occurs in **dogs, cats,** and **horses,** (ii) von Willebrand's disease, due to deficiency of factor VIII-von Willebrand factor complex. It is observed in **dogs, cats, horses,** and **pigs,** (iii) combination of the above factors. Example: disseminated intravascular coagulation (DIC). This occurs in a variety of diseases. (9) **passive hyperaemia**: In passive hyperaemia, the endothelial cells undergo degenerative changes because of inadequate amounts of oxygen and nutrient. The damaged vascular wall ruptures and causes haemorrhage.

Classification of haemorrhages: Haemorrhages are classified according to the **source** of the blood, **size** of the extravasated blood, and **location** of the bleeding. (i) **source:** The words cardiac, arterial, venous, and capillary haemorrhages indicate the source of blood. (ii)

size and shape: Petechial haemorrhages or **petechiae** (singular, petechia), are tiny and punctate (minute, **pinpoint size**), having a diameter not larger than 1-2 mm. **Purpura** are haemorrhages up to approximately 3-5 mm in size. **Ecchymotic haemorrhages** or **ecchymoses** (singular, 'ecchymosis') are large and blotchy, about 1 to 2 cm in diameter. When blood is enclosed within a tissue, the accumulation is referred to as a **haematoma or haematocyst**. Diffuse, flat, often irregular areas of bleeding are termed **suffusions**. When haemorrhages in the tissues spread over considerable areas, they are called **extravasations**. Haemorrhages that appear as lines on the crests of folds in the mucous membrane of the intestine are called **linear haemorrhages**. Petechiae or ecchymoses arising in association with the death struggle are called **agonal haemorrhages**. (iii) **location:** Haemorrhages may be perivascular, perirenal, subserous, subcutaneous, parenchymatous, subcapsular, **haemothorax, haemopericardium, haemoperitoneum, haemometra** (in uterus), and **haemarthrosis** (in joints). Bleeding from various body openings may be **epistaxis** (bleeding from nose), **haemoptysis** (blood in sputum), **haematemesis** (blood in vomit), **enterorrhagia** (intestinal haemorrhage), **metrorrhagia** (uterine bleeding), **haematuria** (blood in urine), **melena** (blood in stools/faeces), **haematocele** (bleeding in tunica vaginalis - serous lining of the testicle), **haemosalpinx** (bleeding in oviducts), and **apoplexy** (brain haemorrhage).

Microscopically, haemorrhage is recognized by the presence of erythrocytes outside blood vessels. If haemorrhage is recent, the erythrocytes are intact and stain sharply. Soon they begin to disintegrate due to the action of tissue enzymes and are also degraded and phagocytosed by macrophages. The released **haemoglobin** (red-blue colour) is then enzymatically converted into **bilirubin** (blue-green colour) and eventually into **haemosiderin**. Haemosiderin appears as **golden-brown granules** that are irregular in both size and shape. They are insoluble and remain in the area of haemorrhage, where eventually they are phagocytosed and retained in macrophages. Haemosiderin contains iron and gives a **Prussian blue reaction** when potassium ferrocyanide and hydrochloric acid are applied.

Significance and result: The significance of haemorrhage depends on the volume and rate of blood loss, and the site of haemorrhage. Sudden losses of up to 20% of the total volume, or slow losses of even large amounts, may have little clinical significance. Larger or more accurate losses may induce **haemorrhagic**

227

(hypovolaemic) shock. The size and location of the haemorrhage are of great importance. For example, a small haemorrhage in the brain may prove fatal to the animal, while a haemorrhage of similar size in skeletal muscle or subcutaneous tissues may be hardly noticed. Haemorrhage in the pericardial sac is always serious because the mass of blood presses on the heart, preventing diastole. Rupture of the aorta with haemorrhage into the pericardial sac is commonly observed in the horse. Haemorrhage in the respiratory tract results in death. This is usually observed in canine distemper. Repeated haemorrhages such as from the skin, gastrointestinal tract, or female genital tract, cause not only loss of blood but also of valuable iron. The chronic loss of iron may lead to iron deficiency anaemia.

THROMBOSIS

Thrombosis is the formation of a clotted mass of blood within the cardiovascular system. The mass is called thrombus (plural, thrombi). A thrombus must be differentiated from a blood clot. The thrombus is formed by a complex process involving the interaction of: (1) blood vessel walls, (ii) formed elements of the blood, and (iii) coagulation system. In contrast, formation of a blood clot involves only the blood clotting system. As we know, clotting occurs when the blood is drawn into a test tube, or when a blood vessel is cut. Clotting also occurs after death, which is known as postmortem clotting of the blood. The composition of a thrombus also differs from that of a blood clot. Thrombi in the rapidly moving arterial or cardiac circulation are composed largely of platelets and fibrin, whereas blood clot is composed primarily of fibrin. However, with very sluggish venous flow thrombi may closely resemble blood clots.

Obviously, the development of a blood clot is life-saving when a vessel ruptures or is cut. However, when the thrombus develops in the cardiovascular system, it may be life-threatening. Thrombi may diminish or obstruct venous flow, causing ischaemic injury, or become dislodged or break into fragments to create emboli. An embolus is an intravascular solid, liquid, or gaseous mass carried in the bloodstream. Most emboli are derived from thrombi. Indeed, thrombosis and embolism are so closely inter-related as to give rise to the term thromboembolism. Thromboembolic occlusion of an artery may lead to infarction. Infarcts are localized areas of ischaemic necrosis.

Tremendous advances have taken place recently in our

understanding of the pathogenesis of thrombosis. However, to understand the pathophysiology of thrombosis, it would be helpful first to review **normal haemostasis** (i.e., **arrest of bleeding**).

Normal Haemostasis

Nature has devised complex but masterly system to ensure that the blood remains fluid in the vascular system, and yet it can form rapidly a solid plug to close holes made by ruptures, or other forms of injury to blood vessels. Thrombosis is, basically, a pathological extension of the normal haemostatic mechanism, and depends on three components: (i) the vascular wall, (ii) platelets, and (iii) the blood clotting system.

1. Endothelium: It is remarkable that, despite its relatively simple structure, the vascular endothelial cell is functionally and metabolically very active, and secretes a variety of biologically important substances (Fig. 43). **Normal endothelium is thromboresistant**, but when injured, **it promotes thrombosis**. These effects are on account of two mechanisms: (i) passive, and (ii) active. The **passive mechanism** involves **endothelium**, which is not only **thromboresistant** but it also insulates the circulating blood elements **from the highly thrombogenic subendothelium**. The **active mechanisms** involve a number of both **antithrombotic** and **prothrombotic factors** (Fig. 43). The endothelial cells possess these factors on their surface, or can actively produce them. **Under normal conditions, these opposing factors are in balance, and a non-thrombogenic endothelial surface is maintained.** Disturbances by a variety of stimuli, as we shall see, may favour the prothrombotic side, causing thrombosis, or the antithrombotic side, predisposing to excessive bleeding.

Antithrombotic Properties

These properties are present in the **endothelial cells** and inhibit thrombosis.

1. Antiplatelet effect: An intact endothelium prevents platelets from coming in contact with the highly thrombogenic subendothelial extracellular matrix (ECM). Non-activated platelets do not adhere to the endothelium, a property intrinsic to the plasma membrane of endothelium. Moreover, if platelets are activated after endothelial injury, they are inhibited from adhering to the surrounding uninjured endothelium by endothelial **prostacyclin (PGI₂)** and **nitric oxide (NO)** (see Chapter 4; also Fig. 43). **Both are powerful inhibitors of platelet**

Antithrombotic	**Prothrombotic**

(1) Inhibition of platelet aggregation

- Prostacyclin (PGI$_2$)
- Nitric oxide (NO)

(2) Binding and inhibition of thrombin

- **Heparin-like molecules**
  These allow antithrombin III to inactivate thrombin, factor Xa, and other coagulation factors

- **Thrombomodulin.** It binds to
  ↓
  Thrombin. Thrombin is then converted from
  ↓
  Procoagulant to ⟶ **Anticoagulant form**
  ↓
  Anticoagulant thrombin activates **Protein C**
  |← Requires cofactor **S**
  ↓
  Activated protein C inhibits clotting by cleaving factors Va and VIIIa

(3) Fibrinolysis
- Tissue plasminogen activator (t-PA)

(1) Favour platelet adhesion and aggregation

- von Willebrand factor

(2) Favour coagulation

- Tissue factor (Thromboplastin)
- **Inhibition of fibrinolysis**

  Inhibitors of plasminogen activators (PAIs)

Fig. 43. Antithrombotic (inhibiting thrombosis) **and prothrombotic** (favouring thrombosis) **properties of the endothelial cells.**

aggregation. PGI$_2$ is an arachidonic acid derivative, whereas nitric oxide is formed enzymatically in the endothelial cells from the amino acid arginine. Their synthesis by endothelial cells is stimulated by a number of factors, such as **thrombin** and **cytokines**, produced during coagulation. Endothelial cells also produce enzyme **adenosine diphosphatase** that degrades **adenosine diphosphate (ADP)** and further inhibits platelet aggregation (see later).

2. Anticoagulant properties: Two factors protect against the unchecked action of **thrombin**. Thrombin is the terminal enzyme of coagulation system that converts fibrinogen to fibrin (see Fig. 45). These two factors are **heparin-like molecules** and **thrombomodulin**. The **heparin-like molecules** act indirectly. They are cofactors that allow antithrombin III to inactivate thrombin, factor Xa, and several other coagulation factors (see later). **Thrombomodulin**, a surface protein, is a specific thrombin receptor. It also acts indirectly. It binds to **thrombin** and converts it from **procoagulant to anticoagulant**. As an anticoagulant, thrombin activates **anticoagulant protein C**. **Activated protein C, in turn, inhibits clotting** by proteolytic cleavage (i.e., enzymatic splitting) of factors Va and VIIIa. Protein C requires **protein S**, synthesized by endothelial cells, as a cofactor (Fig. 43).

3. Fibrinolytic properties: Endothelial cells react against blood clots by synthesizing **tissue plasminogen activator (t-PA)**. t-PA promotes fibrinolytic activity in the blood to clear fibrin deposits from endothelial surfaces, and also participates in the dissolution (dissolving) of intravascular thrombi.

Prothrombotic Properties

The **endothelial cell** is very strange. On the one hand, it inhibits thrombus formation, but on the other, it favours thrombosis by affecting platelets, coagulation proteins, and the fibrinolytic system. For example, endothelial injury leads to **adhesion of platelets** to subendothelial collagen. This is facilitated by **von Willebrand factor (vWF)** (Fig. 43), which is an essential cofactor for binding platelets to collagen and other surfaces. It should be noted that **vWF is a product of normal endothelium and is found in the plasma.** It is not specifically synthesized after endothelial injury. In addition, endothelial cells are triggered by cytokines, such as tumour necrosis factor (TNF) and interleukin-1 (IL-1), or bacterial endotoxin to secrete **tissue factor (thromboplastin),** which as we shall see, activates the **extrinsic clotting pathway.** By binding to activated coagulation factors IXa and Xa (see later), endothelial cells further increase the catalytic activities of these proteins. **Finally**, endothelial cells also secrete **inhibitors of plasminogen activator (PAIs).** These decrease fibrinolysis and therefore favour persistence of thrombi.

In summary, intact endothelial cells inhibit platelet adherence and blood clotting. Injury or activation of endothelial cells, however, results in a procoagulant activity that increases local clot formation.

2. Platelets: Platelets play a central role in thrombosis. After vascular injury, platelets come in contact with the extracellular matrix (ECM) components, present under an intact endothelium. These include **collagen (most important)**, proteoglycans, fibronectin, and other adhesive glycoproteins. **On contact with ECM, platelets undergo three reactions** (1) adhesion and shape change, (2) secretion (release reaction), and (3) aggregation (Fig. 44). These changes are collectively referred to as **platelet activation.**

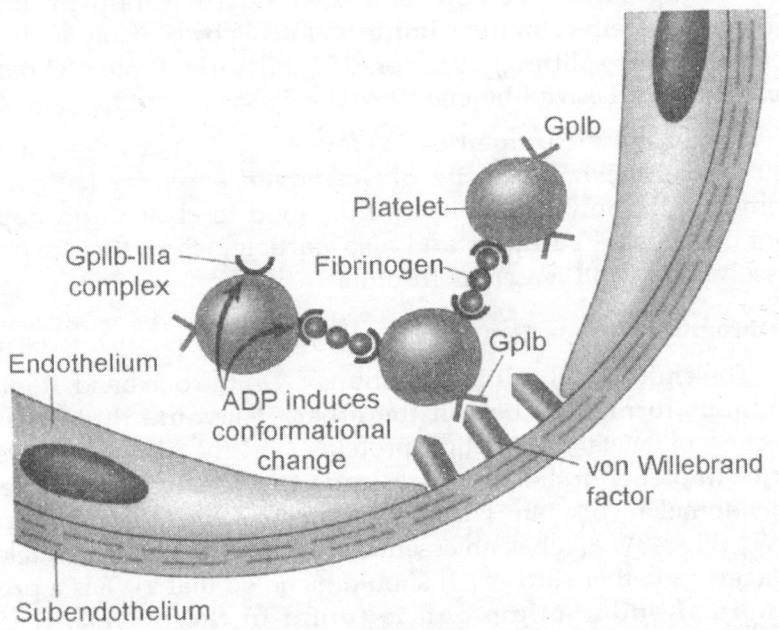

Fig. 44. Platelet adhesion and aggregation. von Willebrand factor functions as an adhesion bridge between subendothelial collagen and the glycoprotein Ib (GpIb) platelet receptor. Aggregation is achieved by fibrinogen's binding to platelet GpIIb-IIIa receptors and bridging many platelets together. ADP = adenosine diphosphate.

(i) Platelet adhesion to ECM is mediated through **vWF**. vWF acts as a bridge between platelet surface receptors (mostly glycoprotein Ib (GPIb) and exposed collagen (Fig. 44). Although platelets can adhere directly to ECM, **vWF-glycoprotein Ib association** is the only interaction sufficiently strong to overcome the high sheer forces (i.e., internal forces) of flowing blood. Genetic deficiencies of vWF (**von Willebrand disease**), or its receptors, result in serious bleeding disorders, highlighting the importance of these interactions.

(ii) **Secretion (release reaction):** Secretion of the contents of two specific types of platelet granules occurs soon after adhesion: (1) **alpha-granules**, and (2) **dense bodies. Alpha granules contain fibrinogen**, fibronectin, platelet factor 4 (an antiheparin), factor V and VIII, platelet-derived growth factor (PDGF), transforming growth factor-alpha (TGF-alpha), and express the adhesion molecule P-selectin on their surface. **Dense bodies contain** adenine nucleotides (**ADP** and **ATP**), **ionized calcium** (Ca^{++} ions), histamine, 5-hydroxytryptamine (serotonin), and epinephrine (adrenaline). Of these, release of the dense body contents is especially important because **calcium** is required in the coagulation process, and **ADP is a powerful mediator of platelet aggregation**, that is, platelets adhering to other platelets (see later). ADP also increases further ADP release from other platelets, leading to amplification of the aggregation. **Finally**, with platelet activation, a **phospholipid complex** gets exposed on the platelet surface. It provides the surface an important binding site for calcium and coagulation factors in the **intrinsic clotting pathway** (see later). Thus, platelet activation contributes to the intrinsic pathway of blood clotting and the formation of **thrombin**.

(iii) **Platelet aggregation** follows adhesion and secretion. **Besides ADP, thromboxane A2 (TXA2)** (see Chapter 4), secreted by platelets, is also an important stimulus for platelet aggregation.

3. **Coagulation system:** The coagulation system is **the third main contributor to thrombosis. To sum up**, the pathways are presented in Fig. 45. **Briefly,** the coagulation sequence is a series of enzymatic changes, converting inactive proenzymes into activated enzymes and ending in the formation of **thrombin**. Thrombin then converts the **soluble** plasma protein **fibrinogen** into the **insoluble** fibrous protein **fibrin**. The blood coagulation system is divided into **an intrinsic and an extrinsic pathway.** Both converge at the point where factor X is activated (see Fig. 45).

The **intrinsic pathway** is activated following endothelial injury (Fig. 45). **First, factor XII (Hageman factor) is activated** by its surface contact with collagen, or other negatively charged substances, and in the reactions that follow, factors XI and IX are activated. Then factor X is activated to factor Xa, as follows. On the phospholipid surface of platelets, factor IXa (the enzyme), factor X (the substrate), and factor

233

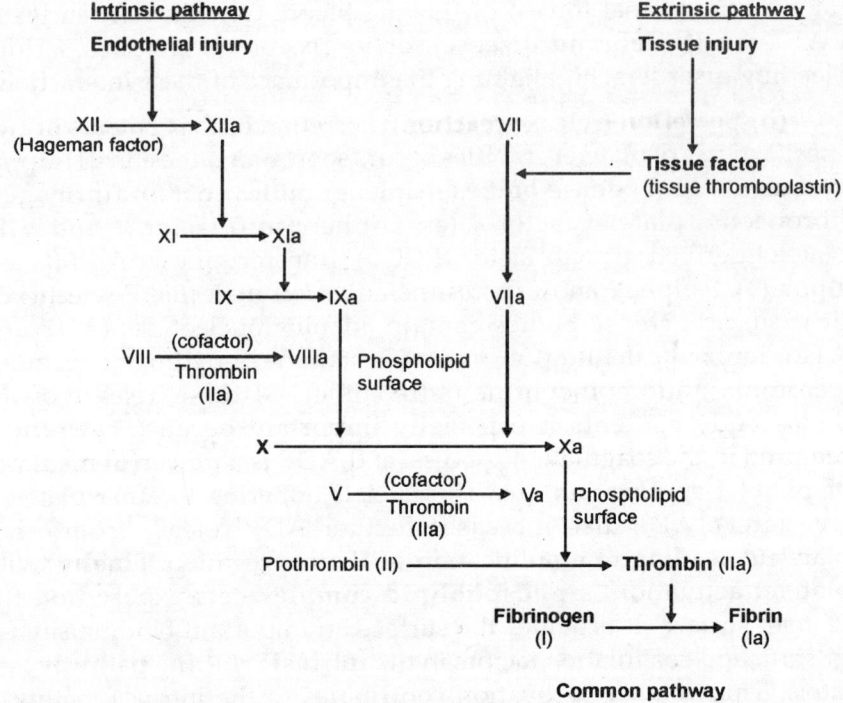

Fig. 45. The coagulation system. Note the common link between the intrinsic and extrinsic pathways at **factor X.** Activated factor is indicated by adding suffix 'a'.

VIIIa (the reaction accelerator) are assembled (Fig. 45). Calcium ions hold the assembled components together and in the reaction that occurs, factor X is converted to factor Xa. **The extrinsic pathway** is activated by **tissue factor (tissue thromboplastin)** released at sites of injury. Tissue factor activates factor VII, which in turn activates factor X. Then, in the **common pathway,** on the platelet surface (phospholipid complex), factors Xa and Va interact with calcium ions and convert **prothrombin to thrombin.** Thrombin converts fibrinogen to fibrin. **Thrombin is a powerful platelet aggregator and,** as we shall see, **plays an important role in thrombosis.**

Anticoagulant Mechanisms

Once activated, the coagulation sequence must be restricted to the site of endothelial injury to prevent clotting of the entire vascular system. Enough thrombin is produced by the clotting of only 1 ml of blood to coagulate all the fibrinogen in 3 litres of blood. The mechanisms to control clotting are: (1) **Antithrombins**, for example, **antithrombin III**. Antithrombins inhibit the activity of thrombin and other clotting factors such as IXa, XIa, and XIIa. **Antithrombin III** is activated by binding to **heparin-like molecules** on endothelial cells. This explains the usefulness of administering heparin in clinical situations to minimize thrombosis. (2) **Proteins C and S:** These are two vitamin K-dependent proteins that inactivate the factors Va and VIIIa. (3) **Fibrinolytic system:** This system by dissolving fibrin limits size of the final clot. This is achieved mainly by the activation of **plasmin**. Plasmin is derived from enzymatic breakdown of its inactive precursor **plasminogen**, present in blood, either by a factor XII-dependent pathway (Chapter 4) or by **plasminogen activators (PAs)**. The most important among plasminogen activators is the **tissue-type PA (t-PA)**. **Tissue-type plasminogen activator** is synthesized mainly by endothelial cells and is most active when attached to fibrin. The affinity for fibrin makes t-PA a useful therapeutic agent. **Plasmin breaks down fibrin**. The resulting **fibrin split products (FSPs)**, also called **fibrin degradation products** (see Chapter 4) can also act as weak anticoagulants. (4) Endothelial cells further regulate the coagulation/anti-coagulation balance by secreting **plasminogen activator inhibitors (PAIs)** (see Fig. 43). These block fibrinolysis and give an overall pro-coagulation effect. The PAIs are increased by certain cytokines, and play a role in the intravascular thrombosis.

But, before taking up the **pathogenesis of thrombus formation**, let us first consider its **aetiology**.

Aetiology

Three major influences predispose to thrombus formation, the so-called **'Virchow triad'** (1) endothelial injury, (2) alterations in normal blood flow, and (3) blood hypercoagulability. **(1) Endothelial injury** is the **single most important factor** and by itself can lead to thrombosis. It is particularly important in thrombus formation in the heart and arteries. Many factors can injure the endothelium. The most common are the **mechanical forces** that cause contusions, abrasions, lacerations, ruptures and crushing injuries. **Parasites** may also injure endothelium. For example, this occurs in the anterior mesenteric artery of the horse when it is invaded with strongyle larvae. **Bacteria** are common causes of thrombosis. **Clumps of bacteria** can lodge in capillaries, injure the endothelium, and cause thrombosis. The passage of bacteria and their toxins through chambers of the heart over a considerable period of time predisposes to thrombosis by injuring the lining endothelium,

235

especially in heart valves. This explains the formation of valvular thrombi in association with **Erysipelothrix, Streptococcus,** and **Corynebacterium** infections. Some viral agents, especially swine fever, injure the endothelium of blood vessels and induce thrombosis. **Arteriosclerotic lesions** can also provide the endothelial injury needed for thrombus formation. This is a common cause of thrombosis in humans, especially in aorta and coronary arteries. Tumours frequently invade the walls of blood vessels, injure endothelium, and cause thrombosis.

However, it is important to note that endothelium does not have to be injured to develop thrombosis. Any disturbance in the dynamic balance of prothrombotic and antithrombotic effects can influence blood clotting events. Regardless of the cause, physical loss of endothelium leads to exposure of subendothelial collagen, adherence of platelets, release of tissue factor, and local depletion of PGI_2 and PA.

2. Alterations in normal blood flow: The rate of flow is extremely important in the formation of a thrombus. In normal blood flow, the larger particles, such as white cells and red cells, occupy the central, the most rapidly moving **axial stream**. The smaller platelets are carried in the more slowly moving **plasmatic or laminar stream** outside the central column. The periphery of the bloodstream, in contact with the endothelium, moves more slowly and is free of all blood elements. **Turbulence** contributes to arterial and cardiac thrombosis by causing endothelial injury, as well as by forming counter-currents and local pockets of stasis. **Stasis** (stoppage of the normal flow) is a major factor in the development of venous thrombi. **Together, stasis and turbulence therefore** (1) disrupt laminar flow and bring platelets into contact with the endothelium, (2) prevent fresh-flowing blood from diluting activated clotting factors, (3) prevent inflow of clotting factor inhibitors and thus prevent build-up of thrombi, and (4) promote endothelial cell activation, thus predisposing to local thrombosis, leukocyte adhesion, and a variety of other endothelial cell effects.

3. Hypercoagulability: Hypercoagulability usually plays a less significant role in thrombosis, but all the same it is an important factor. An increased tendency to thrombosis is associated with a variety of conditions, such as following severe trauma (including fractures) or burns, disseminated cancer, suppurative processes, especially suppurative pneumonia, during late pregnancy and following delivery, and several others. Whereas an **increased amount of fibrinogen** and a **more rapid clotting time** are associated with suppurative processes, the basis for the hypercoagulability is not the same in all these settings. In fact, it is not always understood. It may involve: (1) increased levels of fibrinogen, prothrombin and factors VIIa, VIIIa, and Xa. (2) Increased numbers (or stickiness) of platelets, or (3) decreased levels of inhibitors such as antithrombin III, protein C, and fibrinolysins. Hepatic diseases result in a decrease in the formation of prothrombin. A deficiency of bile in the intestine results in diminished absorption of vitamin K from the intestine. Vitamin K deficiency prolongs clotting time and decreases the amount of fibrin in thrombi.

After having discussed the normal haemostasis and aetiology, we can now consider the **pathogenesis of thrombosis.**

Pathogenesis

Endothelial injury exposes highly thrombogenic subendothelial extracellular matrix (ECM), the most important component being **collagen**. Endothelial injury also releases tissue factor and causes local depletion of prostacyclin (PGI_2) and plasminogen activator (PA). Thus, **endothelial injury allows platelets to adhere to collagen and become activated.** That is, platelets undergo a shape change and release secretory granules (**release reaction**). The activated platelets release **ADP**, a powerful mediator of **platelet aggregation**. The released ADP, in turn, releases more ADP from other platelets, amplifying aggregation. Platelet activation also results in surface expression of a **phospholipid complex** that provides a binding site for calcium and coagulation factors in the **intrinsic clotting pathway**. Besides ADP, **thromboxane A_2 (TXA_2)** synthesized and secreted by platelets, is also an important stimulus for platelet aggregation. **Together ADP and TXA_2 set up an autocatalytic reaction**, and within minutes lead to the formation of an enlarging platelet aggregate, the **primary haemostatic plug. This primary aggregation is reversible.**

However, with activation of the coagulation system, **thrombin** is generated. Thrombin binds to platelet surface receptor, and **along with ADP and TXA_2 cause further aggregation of platelets.** This is followed by **platelet contraction**. Contraction, mediated by the intraplatelet actomyosin (complex of actin and myosin), creates a fused mass of platelets known as **'viscous metamorphosis'**. This mass of platelet forms the **'secondary haemostatic plug'. This secondary aggregation is irreversible.** At the same time, **thrombin converts fibrinogen to fibrin** within and around the platelet plug. The **fibrin** acts like **cement for the 'platelet bricks'. This further stabilizes the plug and through fibronectin attaches it firmly to its site of origin.**

Fibrinogen is also important in platelet aggregation. Activation of platelets by ADP causes a change in the shape of their surface receptors (GpIIb-IIIa) so that they can bind fibrinogen. Fibrinogen then connects many platelets together to form large aggregates (see Fig. 44).

It is worth noting that **prostacyclin PGI$_2$** (synthesized by endothelium) is a vasodilator and **inhibits platelet aggregation**, whereas TXA$_2$ a platelet-derived prostaglandin is a vasoconstrictor and **promotes platelet aggregation.** The interplay between PGI$_2$ and TXA$_2$ constitutes a finely balanced mechanism of regulating platelet function. **In the normal state, it prevents intravascular platelet aggregation, but after endothelial injury, it favours formation of haemostatic plugs.** The clinical use of aspirin (a cyclooxygenase inhibitor) in human patients at risk of coronary thrombosis is due to its ability to inhibit synthesis of TXA$_2$. Like PGI$_2$, nitric oxide also acts as a vasodilator and inhibits platelet aggregation.

The complex events of pathogenesis can be summarized as follows: (1) platelets recognize the sites of endothelial injury and adhere to the exposed **subendothelial collagen, (2)** following activation, platelets secrete granule products (e.g., **ADP**) and synthesize **thromboxane A$_2$, (3)** platelets also expose phospholipids complexes important in the activation of **intrinsic coagulation pathway, (4)** at the same time, the tissue factor released from injured or activated endothelial cells activates **extrinsic coagulation pathway, (5) ADP** released from platelets stimulates formation of a **reversible primary haemostatic plug** of aggregated platelets, **(6)** soon the primary plug is converted into a larger **irreversible secondary plug by ADP, thrombin, and TXA$_2$,** and **(7) deposition of fibrin** (derived from platelets and plasma fibrinogen) within and around the aggregated platelets **stabilizes the mass (thrombus) and attaches it firmly to its site of origin.**

Platelets accumulating on the endothelial surface produce a white or pale coloured mass at the site of injury, known as a **white or pale thrombus.** They soon fuse into a homogeneous mass. **Fibrin is seldom observed in rapid blood flow**, since the process of fibrin formation requires at least four minutes. In this length of time, both tissue factor (thromboplastin) and fibrinogen are swept away. As a result, in the heart and major arteries, where the current is swift, only **white**

thrombus is formed. In slowly moving streams of blood, as in veins, strands of fibrin become attached to platelets. Erythrocytes and leukocytes then get trapped in the fibrin network. Sometimes the thrombi in veins resemble closely coagulated blood, but close examination reveals aggregated platelets and fibrin. The erythrocytes impart a red colour to the thrombus and it is then called a **red thrombus**.

The thrombus gradually increases in size, and may even completely obstruct the blood vessel. With slowing of the blood flow, formation of fibrin is facilitated. The platelets come in contact with the vessel wall, and this in turn, enlarges the thrombus rapidly. If the vessel is occluded, the flow of blood ceases. When this occurs, there is a stagnant column of blood on either side of the thrombus. Presence of thromboplastin leads to clotting of the stagnant columns. When this mass of clotted blood protrudes into the bifurcation of a vessel where flowing blood is present, platelets are deposited on it. **In this manner, a thrombus can extend for long distances through the vascular system.**

Location of thrombi: Thrombi may develop anywhere in the cardiovascular system: within the cardiac chambers, on valve cusps, arteries, veins, or capillaries. They are of variable size and shape. The main component of a thrombus is the platelet, while that of blood clot - fibrin. **In rapid blood flow**, such as in the aorta and major arteries, the platelets are held more or less in the centre, and only plasma touches the endothelial surface. However, if there is a sudden change in the direction of blood flow which may produce **turbulence** (**counter-currents**, previously known as **'rolling'** or **'eddying currents'**), such as in arch of the aorta, then platelets come into contact at the greater curvature, and if there is endothelial injury, a thrombus will occur. Due to the anatomical characteristics of the species, this occurs in **human beings** and **monkeys. A second common site** is the bifurcation of a vessel where the sudden change in the direction of blood flow produces turbulence and platelets are forced against the vessel wall. In the more slowly moving venous circulation, stasis (sluggish blood flow) contributes to thrombosis by bringing platelets in contact with the endothelium. Within the heart, the surging of blood through valvular openings, together with sudden changes in directional flow produce turbulence, and platelets have no difficulty in coming in contact with the endothelium, especially that covering the valves. The valvular thrombi thus produced are referred to as

239

vegetations. The most common cause of vegetations is a blood-borne bacterial infection that seeds the heart valves (e.g., swine erysipelas) and thus provides a site of injury on which a thrombotic mass of fibrin and platelets builds up to produce **infective vegetative endocarditis**. Capillaries are so small that platelets have no difficulty in coming in contact with the endothelium.

Classification of thrombi: Thrombi vary in colour, location, and composition. They may therefore be classified as follows:

I. Classification According to Location within the Blood Vascular System

1. Cardiac thrombi: These are located in the heart, and may be attached to valves (**valvular thrombi**) or walls (**mural thrombi**). Valvular thrombi are most commonly observed in the **pig** when the valve is invaded with *Streptococcus pyogenes* or *Erysipelothrix rhusiopathiae*. *Corynebacterium pyogenes* **in cattle** and *Streptococcus equi* **in horses** also cause valvular thrombi. Mural thrombi, particularly on the wall of left auricle, are observed in *Clostridium chauvoei* infection **in cattle**. An acute fibrinous endocarditis with mural thrombosis is pathognomonic of blackquarter.

2. Arterial thrombi: These are located within the arteries, and are usually firmly attached to the damaged arterial wall. **In domestic animals** these are more common than cardiac or venous thrombi. **In horses**, *Strongylus vulgaris* larvae in the anterior mesenteric artery produce thrombi.

3. Venous thrombi: These are found in the veins. These are also known as **phlebothromboses**, and sometimes incorrectly as **thrombophlebitis** in the mistaken impression that inflammation of the veins caused the thrombi. **They are not as important in animals as in humans**, because diseases of veins that produce thrombosis are relatively uncommon in animals. In addition, all animals, even when ill, move about, thus preventing slowing of circulation in the injured veins. In contrast, when the human being is ill, he goes to bed. The circulation then becomes sluggish, and this favours thrombosis. Also, a contributing factor in human is his erect position. In the presence of general passive hyperaemia, this causes an unusual distension of veins affected with phlebitis. The slowing of the bloodstream favours thrombosis. Venous thrombi in humans are particularly common in the femoral, popliteal, and iliac veins of elderly bedridden individuals. These are also serious because they may embolize. **In animals,** venous thrombi are observed in the nasal vascular sinuses of the **cow** and

horse, the veins of the broad ligament of the **cow**, and in the scrotal plexus of the **horse**. They are often attached to the underlying vessel wall.

4. Capillary thrombi: These are located within the capillaries. They are mostly associated with inflammation because the aetiological agents easily injure the vascular endothelium.

5. Lymphatic thrombi: These are found in blood vessels and sinuses of lymph nodes, and are composed of fibrin. They are usually observed in lymphatics draining an area of inflammation in which bacteria are present. The lymphatic thrombi are useful in that they prevent spread of infectious agents by the lymphatic system.

II. **Classification According to Location within the Heart or Blood Vessels**

1. Mural thrombi are attached to the wall of the heart or blood vessel. They generally occur within the cardiac chambers and aorta.

2. Valvular thrombi are attached to the heart valves.

3. Lateral thrombi are attached to one side of a vessel wall.

4. Occluding thrombi are attached to the entire circumference of the vessel.

5. Saddle thrombi sit on the bifurcation of blood vessels just as saddle straddles the back of a horse.

6. Canalized thrombi are those thrombi in which new blood channels have been formed through the clot. These channels allow a partial restoration of the blood circulation. The channels are lined with endothelium.

III. **Classification According to the Infectious Agent**

1. Septic thrombi are those, which contain bacteria.

2. Parasitic thrombi are those, which contain parasites, for example, *Strongylus vulgaris* larvae in the **horse** and *Dirofilaria immitis* in the **dog**.

3. Aseptic thrombi are those, which do not contain bacteria or parasites.

IV. **Classification According to Colour**

1. A pale or white thrombus is white in colour and is composed almost entirely of platelets. It is observed in heart and blood vessels (aorta, carotid, and femoral arteries).

2. A red thrombus is red in colour, and is composed of platelets, fibrin, erythrocytes, and leukocytes. The red colour is due to erythrocytes trapped in the fibrin meshwork. A red thrombus is usually observed in veins. **It should not be confused with a postmortem clot.**

3. A **mixed thrombus** is composed of both white and red thrombi, and is the most common type. The white portions form when the blood flow is rapid and the red portions form when slow.

4. A **laminated thrombus** is a type of mixed thrombus composed of alternating layers of paler platelets mixed with some fibrin, separated by darker layers containing more red cells. It is the result of variations in the rapidity of the flow of blood through the vessel. For example, during exercise, the rapidity of blood flow through the leg is increased and a white thrombus is formed. When the animal is at rest, the blood flow is slow, and a red thrombus is formed.

Fate of the Thrombus

1. Propagation: The thrombus may accumulate more platelets and fibrin (propagate), and by its enlargement eventually cause obstruction of a vessel.

2. Emboli formation: The thrombus may give rise to emboli that are carried away from their sites of origin. These emboli are dangerous because they lodge in smaller vessels and cause infarction. If emboli contain bacteria, new foci of suppurative inflammation are established at the sites of obstruction.

3. Abscessation: Abscesses appear in thrombi when pyogenic bacteria are present.

4. Dissolution: Thrombi may be removed by fibrinolytic activity. A thrombus activates the plasminogen-plasmin system. If the thrombus is small and fresh, it may undergo complete digestion through fibrinolysis. The freshly formed fibrin is more susceptible to lysis, than older fibrin.

5. Organization and re-canalization: Thrombi may cause inflammation and fibrosis (organization), and may eventually become re-canalized (re-establish vascular flow). Enzymes derived from leukocytes and platelets begin to digest the thrombus. At the same time, fibroblasts and capillaries proliferate and invade the base of the thrombus. In time, the entire intravascular mass is organized and converted into a **vascularized connective tissue**. The capillaries anastomose to provide new channels that cross the thrombus, and through which blood flow may partly be re-established. The process is known as **re-canalization of the thrombus**. When fibrous tissue contracts, the thrombus is incorporated into the thickened vessel wall or cardiac chamber, as a fibrous lump or thickening

6. Calcification: Since a thrombus contains degenerating and necrotic tissue, it may undergo dystrophic calcification. This is usually seen in venous thrombi.

Significance: The significance of thrombosis depends upon its effects, which are:

1. Negligible effects: No effects are noticed when thrombi occur in vessels which are not required. Experimentally, both jugular veins and both carotid arteries can be ligated in the **dog** with no adverse effects if the animals are not forced to move about.

2. Beneficial effects: The primary haemostatic plug assists in the control of haemorrhage, and is life-saving.

3. Harmful effects: The harmful effects depend on which vessel is thrombosed, and on collateral circulation in the area. Thrombosis in **'end-arteries'** results in infarction. This is commonly observed in coronary arteries in humans. Portions of the thrombi may break, float in the bloodstream as **emboli**, get lodged in smaller arteries and cause **infarction**. Thrombi in veins cause local passive hyperaemia. When lymphatics are thrombosed, **oedema** of the area drained by the lymph vessel occurs. Thrombosis weakens the vessel wall and this may cause its local dilatation known as **aneurysm**. This is observed in the anterior mesenteric artery of the **horse** following an invasion with strongyle larvae.

Differentiation of Postmortem Clots from Venous Thrombi

A thrombus must not be confused with the postmortem clot. **Table 11** presents differences between the two. **Postmortem clots** are of **two types: (1) Red or currant jelly clots** are those in which components of the blood are evenly distributed. This occurs when there is rapid clotting of blood and its composition is normal. **(2) Yellow or chicken-fat clots** are those in which components of the blood are not evenly distributed. The ventral portion of the clot is red and contains erythrocytes, while the dorsal portion is yellow and is composed of fibrin and plasma. These clots occur when erythrocytes do not remain in suspension and settle out. Example: In

243

prolonged clotting time of the blood and increased erythrocyte sedimentation rate (ESR).

Table 11. Comparison of a thrombus and a postmortem clot

Thrombus	Postmortem clot
1. Granular, dry and rough	1. A rubbery, gelatinous coagulum
2. White or pale in colour	2. Intense red or yellow in colour
3. Attached to the vessel wall	3. Not attached to the vessel wall
4. Stratified in structure	4. Uniform in structure
5. Composed mainly of platelets	5. Composed mainly of fibrin
6. Vascular endothelium below the thrombus is damaged and rough	6. Vascular endothelium below the clot is undamaged, smooth, and glistening
7. Forms in a flowing stream of blood	7. Forms in a stagnant column of blood
8. Forms in the living animal	8. Forms in the dead animal
9. May be partially organized	9. No indication of organization
10. Caused by endothelial injury	10. Initiated by thromboplastin (tissue factor)

Disseminated Intravascular Coagulation

Disseminated intravascular coagulation (DIC) is characterized by the appearance of an extremely large number of **fibrin thrombi** within the small blood vessels, including capillaries and sinusoids. While these thrombi are not visible grossly, they are readily seen microscopically. DIC is not a primary disease, but it can be a complication of any condition associated with **widespread activation of thrombi. In humans,** most cases are associated with sepsis, obstetric complications, malignancy, and major trauma. **In animals,** it is seen in severe systemic infections, septic (endotoxic) shock, neoplastic diseases, extensive trauma or burns, and following extensive surgery. Viral diseases associated with DIC include swine fever, infectious canine hepatitis, and bluetongue. DIC has also been seen in cattle with acute sarcocystosis, resulting from endothelial damage by schizonts.

Pathogenesis: DIC is due to the release of **tissue factor (tissue thromboplastin),** factors from damaged endothelium, or the direct activation of clotting factors by substances released into the circulation

244

in the various disorders mentioned. These factors activate the coagulation system and lead to the generation of **thrombin. Thrombin**, in turn, converts **fibrinogen** into **fibrin**. The thrombi may be seen in any organ or tissue, but are usually seen in the lungs, kidneys, liver, spleen, adrenal gland, heart, and brain where they lead to **infarction**. The generation of extensive thrombosis depletes the circulation of platelets and the various clotting factors, hence the other name **'consumption coagulopathy'**. At the same time, **fibrinolytic mechanisms** are activated (e.g., plasminogen), which digest fibrin, fibrinogen, and factors V and VIII. The net effect of this loss of platelets and clotting factors leads to failure of further coagulation, and **severe bleeding** becomes one of the main clinical findings.

EMBOLISM

An **embolus** (plural **emboli**) **is any foreign body floating in the blood**. In other words, an embolus is an intravascular solid, liquid, or gaseous mass that is carried by the blood to a site away from its point of origin. The **process** of a foreign body moving through the circulatory system and becoming lodged in a vessel causing obstruction is known as **embolism**.

Location of emboli: Emboli may occur within either the arterial, or the venous system. However, the embolus **almost always lodges in an artery or a capillary** since the diameter of these vessels progressively decreases. An embolus does not ordinarily lodge in a vein because the flow of blood is always into a vessel of increasing diameter, and so the passage of foreign body is not prevented. **In domestic animals, embolism almost always occurs in arteries and not in veins. In humans**, on the other hand, venous embolism is very common. This is because within the veins of the legs, thrombosis is common in humans (see 'thrombosis'). In more than 95% of cases in humans, venous emboli originate from thrombi within the deep veins of the leg. These emboli, then circulate through progressively larger channels, pass through right side of the heart, and become lodged in the pulmonary circulation. That is, either in the pulmonary artery itself or within its branches. This is know as **pulmonary embolism**, and is the most serious form of thromboembolic disease in humans. **In humans**, it is also an extremely important and common clinical problem. The consequences of pulmonary embolism depend on the size of the embolus and on the size of the occluded pulmonary artery. **Pulmonary embolism is rare in animals, because thrombosis within the veins of the legs is uncommon in animals** (see 'thrombosis'). Both in humans and animals, rarely, an embolus originating from venous thrombi, instead of getting caught in the lungs, may pass through a congenital inter-auricular or inter-ventricular defect and gain access to the systemic circulation. This is known as **paradoxical embolism**. Embolism may also occur in lymphatics. The emboli then get lodged in the sinuses of the lymph nodes.

Aetiology: Many objects can become emboli, but the most common group of substances found in the arterial circulation are:

1. Thrombi: A great majority of arterial emboli arise in thrombi, hence the commonly used term **thromboembolism**. Thrombi usually disintegrate and fragments are carried away as emboli. Most arterial emboli arise from thrombi within the heart from fragmentation of a vegetation on a heart valve. Less common sources of arterial emboli include thrombi developing in relation to aortic aneurysms and ulcerated atherosclerotic plaques in the aorta, or some other large artery. Emboli are especially dangerous if they contain bacteria. A disintegrating thrombus having a central location (heart or aorta) is much more dangerous than one located in a peripheral artery, because emboli in that case are scattered throughout the body.

2. Bacteria: Bacterial emboli are frequently observed in many diseases, and occur as single cells or clumps of bacteria. Single organisms do not produce a vascular obstruction, but when several agglutinate, or become enclosed within a phagocyte, the mass gets covered with platelets and fibrin. Then due to an increase in size they are stopped in capillaries, to which they are carried after leaving the heart. Interference with the circulation is not significant, but such groups of bacteria usually multiply at the places where they lodge and set up a new focus of infection, than scattered single organisms would do. Such a transfer of infection is known as **metastasis**. Two factors determine the frequency of metastasis in an organ: (1) the amount of blood flowing through it, and (ii) the extent of the fine capillary network. **This means that lungs, liver, and kidneys are the most frequent organs of metastatic infections.**

3. Parasites: Parasites are a common type of emboli. Examples: Canine heartworm *Dirofilaria immitis* in the pulmonary artery of the **dog; schistosomes** in the portal, mesenteric, and nasal blood vessels in **cattle, sheep, goats**, and **horses**; agglutinated trypanosomes; and the larvae of many parasites (**ascarids** in **pigs, hookworms** in **dogs,** and **strongyles** in **horses**) exist as emboli in the bloodstream, but usually due to their small size, do not cause obstruction.

4. Neoplasms: These are a common source of emboli, because it is by clumps of tumour cells carried in the blood that malignant neoplasms are able to colonize in new locations. The growing tumour cells invade arteries or lymphatics and are carried away as tumour emboli. Wherever they lodge, they may produce new tumour growth at the site of obstruction.

5. Fibrin: Fibrin emboli may occur during blood transfusions. This is likely when blood is improperly defibrinated, or when inadequate amounts of anticoagulants are used.

6. Fat emboli: Minute fat globules may be found in the lungs when fractures of long bones occur, which have fatty marrows. The fat globules enter the ruptured blood vessels in the bone marrow and are then transported to lungs. **Firm fat** of the **cattle** and **sheep** is less likely to form emboli than the **soft fat** of **humans, guinea pigs,** and **chickens.** Extensive fat embolism is fatal through interference with the pulmonary circulation. It may cause unexpected death soon after accidents. The condition is more important in **humans,** and is manifested clinically as **'fat embolism syndrome'.** The syndrome is characterized by acute respiratory distress, neurological symptoms and tachycardia; and is fatal in about 10% of cases.

7. Clumps of normal body cells: These appear in circulation when tissues and organs have been **injured.** For example, hepatic cells are transported to lungs by the bloodstream in crushing injuries to liver. **In humans, amniotic fluid embolism,** is a rare but extremely grave complication of labour, characterized by infusion of amniotic fluid and its contents into the maternal circulation, through a tear in the placental membranes and rupture of uterine veins. It is an important cause of maternal mortality in women. The clinical signs include profound respiratory difficulty with cyanosis, cardiovascular shock, seizures, coma, and death. **Amniotic fluid embolism is rare in domestic animals because of the differences in placental and uterine structures.**

8. Air or gas emboli: Bubbles of air or gas within the circulation obstruct vascular flow and damage tissues. Air or gas may gain access to the circulation following injuries to neck region when negative air pressure sucks air into the jugular veins. Small amounts of air that may enter the circulation during intravenous injection are of no significance because they are quickly absorbed. Large amounts of air, more than 100 ml, are required to produce clinical effects. **Caisson disease** or **decompression sickness** occurs **in human beings and animals** exposed to sudden changes in atmospheric pressure. **The disease is important in humans.** Those at particular risk are underwater construction workers, deep sea and **scuba** (self-contained underwater breathing apparatus) divers, and in individuals in unpressurized aircrafts that ascend rapidly to high altitudes. As underwater construction workers move down to greater depths in their underwater compartments, air pressure is increased within the compartment to compensate for the water pressure. When air is breathed under high pressure, increased amounts of gas (particularly nitrogen) dissolve in the blood and tissue fluid. If the worker comes out of the underwater compartment suddenly, that is, if he decompresses too rapidly, **the dissolved oxygen, carbon dioxide, and nitrogen** may come out of the solution in the form of minute bubbles. **Oxygen and carbon dioxide are readily soluble, but the nitrogen is of low solubility and persists to form gaseous emboli within the blood vessels.** These watertight chambers used in construction work under water are known by the French name **caisson**, and the disorder is therefore called **caisson disease**. It is also known as the **bends**, because of the severe cramping pain that occurs when the individual is released from pressure. The emboli may induce foci of necrosis in the brain, heart, or other tissues or organs; stop the flow of capillaries; and the condition is sometimes fatal. **The remedy is to release the pressure slowly.**

9. Other types of emboli include red bone marrow, or even fragments of bone following **fractures, foreign bodies such as broken needles, hair** introduced in venipuncture, and atheromatous debris from ruptured atherosclerotic plaques.

Significance and result: Importance of embolism depends on several factors: **(i) character of the emboli (a) size**: The larger the emboli, the larger will be the vessels that will be blocked. It will then be difficult for the collateral circulation to supply the vascular needs. **(b) septic or aseptic:** Septic emboli are more serious. Since they contain bacteria, new foci of infection may be established wherever emboli lodge. **(c) neoplastic or normal cells:** Neoplastic cells may grow wherever they lodge and produce new tumour growths. Normal cells do not grow in new location. **(ii) number of emboli:** The more emboli in circulation, the greater will be the number of vascular obstructions. The collateral circulation may then fail and infarction of the organ may result. **(iii) organ involved:** If the embolus lodges in an organ or tissue (liver, lung, or muscle) where there is an abundant blood supply from an anastomosing network of blood vessels, very little injury will occur. However, if the embolus enters organs (heart, kidney or spleen) in which an abundant network of blood vessels (collateral circulation) is not present, death of the area (infarction) occurs.

INFARCTION

An infarct is an area of ischaemic necrosis caused by occlusion of either the arterial supply, or rarely the venous drainage in a particular tissue. Occlusion of the arterial blood supply produces ischaemic necrosis more certainly than does obstruction to venous drainage. This will be discussed later. The area involved is that supplied by a single **'end artery'** whose flow has been arrested. However, even arterial occlusion does not always produce an area of **ischaemic necrosis (infarction)**, as will soon be seen. It may cause only atrophy, or focal cell death, or may even be without effect. The word infarction is derived from the Latin word **'infarcire'**, meaning 'to stuff or to fill fully'. In most infarctions, there is at some time an actual stuffing with blood.

Aetiology: The aetiological agents that obstruct the flow of blood through an artery and cause infarction are usually located within the lumen of the vessel, in the wall of the artery, or in the periarterial tissue. **Thrombi and emboli are common causes of infarction.** Emboli arising in the heart, or major arteries, impact in arteries. Similarly, venous emboli lodge in the pulmonary arterial system. Rarely, narrowing of an artery and infarction may be caused by other forms of vascular disease, such as large atherosclerotic plaque, or by compression of arteries by **expanding tumours, abscesses, cysts, or by inflammatory fibrous adhesions.** Even ligatures and tourniquets may do this. Vascular narrowing, or occlusion may also be caused by poisonous compounds or drugs, such as ergot by inducing contraction of the musculature of arterial walls. This leads to infarction most commonly in the extremities (legs, tail, ear, wattle, and comb) where limited collateral circulation of blood exists.

Although venous occlusion of an organ or tissue, such as from venous thrombosis, may cause infarction due to obstruction of its drainage, usually bypass channels develop which provide some outflow from the area. This in turn improves the arterial outflow. However, infarcts caused by venous obstruction may occur in the case of a strangulated intestine (torsion). This is because veins are more readily compressed than arteries. Also, in organs **having a single outflow without bypass channels,** occlusion of venous outflow may induce infarction, such as in testis and ovary.

Types of Infarcts

Infarcts are classified on the basis of their **colour** as **pale, white or anaemic,** and **red or haemorrhagic**. This distinction is quite arbitrary and is based on the **amount of haemorrhage that occurs** in the area. The haemorrhage in turn depends on two factors: (1) the **solidity of the organ** involved, and (ii) the **type of vascular occlusion,** whether arterial or venous. Whenever infarcts occur in **solid organs** and are caused by arterial occlusion, they are **pale or white**. In fact, most infarcts in **solid organs** result from arterial occlusion and are pale or white. The solidity of the organ limits the amount of haemorrhage into the area of ischaemic necrosis. **The kidneys, heart, and spleen are examples of solid compact organs that develop pale or white infarcts.** In contrast, **loose spongy organs,** such as the **lung** usually suffers **red or haemorrhagic infarction**. The loose spongy organ permits blood to collect in the infarct from the anastomotic capillary circulation in the margins of the necrotic area. Infarcts are also classified as either **septic** or **bland,** depending on the presence or absence of **bacterial infection** in the area of necrosis.

Pathogenesis: The first alteration that must occur in infarction is **obstruction of the arterial blood supply** to portions of organs. Whether red or pale, all infarcts tend to be **wedge-shaped,** with the occluded vessel at the apex and the periphery of the organ forming the base. Sometimes the margins are quite irregular. This depends on the pattern of vascular supply from adjacent vessels. **At the outset, all infarcts are slightly haemorrhagic and poorly defined**. To understand the pathogenesis of events, let us take the example of an infarct that involves kidney.

Immediately after obstruction of the artery, the area supplied by that vessel first undergoes **transient ischaemia**. The capillaries then **begin to dilate** in an attempt to increase the blood supply. Blood is forced from the neighbouring arterial systems by blood pressure through the abundant network of anastomosing capillaries into the ischaemic area. **The capillaries dilate to their maximum and become engorged with blood.** As a result, the area that earlier showed **ischaemia** now becomes much redder and is then known as a **red**

infarct. Due to hypoxia, changes occur in the endothelium of capillary walls. This results in haemorrhage by diapedesis. The area is now called **haemorrhagic infarct**. After two hours, the erythrocytes stuffed into the area begin to fuse into a homogeneous mass. Cells in the area show degenerative changes. Within 24 hours, the cells in the centre of infarction undergo **coagulation necrosis**. Necrosis then progresses toward the periphery of the infarct. The entire area of infarction usually becomes necrotic and more sharply defined **within 72 hours**. In **solid organs**, like **kidney**, in which the lesions have relatively less haemorrhage, the red cells are lysed and the released haemoglobin either diffuses out or is transformed to haemosiderin. When this occurs, the area loses its intense red colour and is then known as a **pale** or **anaemic infarct**. In **spongy organs**, such as the **lungs**, too many red cells are present, and therefore the **infarct does not become pale**.

Dead tissue is irritating. In response to this irritation, **an inflammatory reaction (zone of inflammation)** appears between the living and dead tissue. Macrophages accumulate in this area, and fibroblasts and new blood vessels proliferate. When all necrotic tissue has been removed, most infarcts are ultimately **replaced by scar tissue**. The scar usually has a yellow or brown colour due to the **haemosiderin** it contains. Scar tissue deposited in the area begins to contract and may lead to considerable distortion of the organ. When an infarct is produced by an **infected embolus (septic embolus)**, as may occur with a fragment of a bacterial vegetation from a heart valve, the infarct is virtually converted to an **abscess**.

Factors that Influence Development of an Infarct

Occlusion of an artery, or venous drainage, may have little or no effect on the involved tissue, or it may cause death of the tissue and also of the individual. **The major determinants include**: (1) nature of the vascular supply, (2) rate of development of occlusion, (3) vulnerability of the tissue to hypoxia, and (4) oxygen content of blood.

1. The nature of blood supply: The availability of an alternative blood supply (**collateral circulation**) is the **most important factor** in determining whether occlusion of a vessel will cause damage. For example, **lungs** have a **double blood supply** from pulmonary and bronchial artery. The same applies to **liver**, with its double blood supply of hepatic artery and portal vein. In these organs, blockage of pulmonary arterial tree or hepatic artery may be without effect. On

251

the other hand, some organs like **kidney** and **spleen** have a **'single'** **arterial supply** with few anastomoses insufficient to provide adequate bypass channels, so-called **end-arteries**. Occlusion of one of the major branches, or of the main renal artery, is followed by ischaemic necrosis (infarction). The **heart** is an example of an organ that has an **intermediate pattern** of fairly rich inter-arterial anastomoses and may compensate for occlusion of one of the trunks of the coronary arterial system. There are fine inter-arterial anastomoses joining each of the major coronary trunks to the others. When one major trunk is blocked, the collateral supply from an unaffected trunk may suffice to prevent ischaemic injury. Thus, the anatomic pattern of the vascular supply of an organ modifies the result of a vascular occlusion.

2. Rate of development of occlusion: Slowly developing occlusions are less likely to cause infarction. This is because they provide time for the development of alternative pathways of flow and anastomotic bypass channels to develop.

3. Vulnerability to hypoxaemia (ischaemia): Tissues of the body differ widely in their susceptibility to ischaemic hypoxia, and this influences the possibility of infarction. Neurons undergo irreversible damage within only 3-4 minutes. Myocardial cells, although hardier than neurons, are also quite sensitive and die after 20-30 minutes of ischaemia. In contrast, the fibroblasts within the myocardium remain viable (alive) after many hours of ischaemia.

4. Oxygen content of blood: The anaemic patient tolerates arterial insufficiency less well than does the normal patient. Occlusion of a small vessel might lead to an infarction in anaemic patients, whereas it would be without effect at normal level of oxygen transport.

Macroscopically, in general, infarcts have **a cone-shaped (wedge-shaped) appearance** with the apex of the cone at the point of arterial obstruction and the base of the cone at the periphery of the organ. They are most frequently observed in those organs, which have **end-artery circulation** (kidney and spleen). **Red and haemorrhagic infarcts bulge** because they are **stuffed with blood**, whereas **pale or anaemic infarcts usually have a slightly depressed surface** because haemosiderin and other substances have diffused out of the area. When an infarct gets organized, **contraction of connective tissue causes a depressed surface and puckering of the organ.**

The **important characteristics of infarcts in various organs** are as follows:

Infarcts in the kidneys are usually **pale** or **anaemic**. The infarct is usually **cone-shaped** with its apex in the vicinity of the arcuate arteries, and its base at the capsule. The capsule, since it has different blood supply, does not become necrotic and remains intact. Renal infarcts are usually the result of emboli from cardiac thrombi. **Infarcts in the spleen**, because of large amount of blood and the many vascular sinuses, are usually of the **red type in animals.** Even when haemoglobin diffuses, they are not as anaemic as in kidney. Splenic infarcts are usually observed along the border of the spleen where the arterial circulation is poorest and end arteries are most numerous. They are mostly the result of emboli from cardiac thrombi, or as the result of endothelial injury caused by swine fever virus. In contrast to animals, splenic thrombi in humans are white to pale. **Infarcts in the heart**, unlike in humans, are **rare in animals** because coronary thrombosis as the result of atherosclerosis is not common in animals. They have an irregular border, and depending on the length of time and its size, it may be **red** or **pale**. In humans, they are usually pale. If the area of infarction is large, death occurs before necrosis takes place. Smaller areas undergo coagulative necrosis.

True infarcts of the liver are almost non-existent. Since liver has a double blood supply from hepatic artery and portal vein, both sources must be obstructed before infarction can occur. This may occur in hepatitis produced by bacteria in which invasion of the liver can cause thrombosis of all vessels in the area. This is observed in *Clostridium haemolyticum* infection in **cattle**. Infarcts in the intestinal tract usually involve the entire circumference. Two adjacent arteries must be obstructed at the same time, or the obstruction must occur in one of the major branches of the anterior mesenteric artery before infarction will occur. **In horses**, this occurs due to thrombi and emboli produced as the result of vascular injury caused by migrating strongyle larvae. Infarcts are always in the **red** or **haemorrhagic stage** because the animal dies early. Moist gangrene may be an early complication due to the presence of saprophytic bacteria in the intestine and may cause death. **In animals, infarction of the lungs is not** common. The lungs have a double blood supply from pulmonary and brachial artery, and before infarction can occur, obstruction must be present in both. This may occur from pulmonary emboli or thrombi in branches of the pulmonary artery, accompanied by impaired arterial or pulmonary venous circulation in bronchi, due to pneumonia, passive hyperaemia or hypostatic congestion. The emboli usually originate from the broad ligaments of the uterus of the cow and the scrotal

253

venous plexuses of the **horse**. Infarcts in the lungs are also observed in **pigs** when swine fever virus injures the endothelium of pulmonary vessels; and in **cattle, sheep**, and **pigs** affected with *Pasteurella multocida*. The areas of infarction are of the **red** or **haemorrhagic type. Infarcts in the brain are mostly seen in dogs.** They are usually anaemic and quickly reach a state of liquefactive necrosis. Mechanical injury to the brain from automobile accidents is the common cause in **dogs. In animals, infarction in the brain is not common as in human** because they have relatively little arteriosclerosis of the central nervous system.

Significance and Results

The outcome of infarction depends on **location of the infarct and its size**, which is as follows: (1) **death of tissue** supplied by the obstructed artery. If the area is small, no clinical manifestations are observed. (2) **organization** of the infarct and production of a scar occurs in infarcts which do not kill the host. (3) **shock** may occur from absorption of the toxic products when areas of infarction are large, for example, infarction from obstruction of anterior mesenteric artery. (4) **bacterial** invasion of the necrotic tissue from saprophytes, as in the intestinal tract, may result in gangrene. If pyogenic bacteria are present, an abscess occurs. (5) **death of the individual** occurs when infarct involves a vital organ such as heart, brain, or intestine. The animal may die from shock, or when bacteria invade the necrotic tissue from septicaemia.

OEDEMA

Oedema is a condition characterized by an excessive accumulation of fluid in the interstitial tissue spaces or body cavities. Cells may also accumulate an abnormal amount of fluid, but this phenomenon is referred to as **cellular swelling** or **cellular odema** (see Chapter 3). Oedema may occur as a **generalized** or **localized disorder.** When oedema is severe and generalized and causes swelling of the subcutaneous tissues, it is called **anasarca**. Collection of oedema fluid in the peritoneal cavity is known as **hydroperitoneum** (commonly called **ascites**), in the pleural cavity as **hydrothorax**, in the pericardial sac as **hydropericardium** or **pericardial effusion**, and in the ventricles of the brain as **hydrocephalus. Hydrocele** refers to a local accumulation of fluid in the tunica vaginalis of the testicles.

The oedema fluid is non-inflammatory and is referred to as a **transudate**. It is **low in protein** and other colloids, with a specific gravity below **1.012.** In contrast, inflammatory oedema, due to increased vascular permeability is **protein-rich** and therefore has a high specific gravity, usually over **1.020.** The inflammatory fluid is called **exudate**. The differences between a transudate and an exudate have been given in Chapter 4 (see Table 6).

Pathogenesis: Oedema is the result of **an increase in the forces that tend to move fluids from the intravascular compartment into the interstitial tissue spaces.** The volume of each compartment is maintained within narrow limits in health, but there is a constant interchange between them. The exchange between intravascular and interstitial compartment is governed **by Starling's forces.** According to Starling's hypothesis, the normal fluid balance is maintained by two opposing sets of forces, namely, **vascular hydrostatic pressure and plasma osmotic pressure**. Fluid moves from intravascular to the interstitial compartment at the arteriolar end of the microcirculation largely under the influence of the **hydrostatic pressure**. It returns to the intravascular compartment at the venular end mainly because of the **osmotic pressure**. The balance of these factors is such that there is only a small excess of fluid in the interstitial tissue spaces but this fluid is normally drained off through lymphatics, **and no oedema occurs.** Thus, the volume of interstitial fluid depends on the hydrostatic pressure of the blood at the arterial end of the capillary, the level of plasma proteins, and the adequacy of the lymphatic drainage. The following illustration will show the relationship of hydrostatic pressure and osmotic pressure in the exchange of fluids through vessel walls in a **normal resting leg.**

Hydrostatic pressure at the arterial end of the capillary	=	45 mm Hg (mercury)
Osmotic pressure at the arterial end of the capillary	=	30 mm Hg
		15 mm rate of fluid flow into the tissues
Osmotic pressure at the venular end of the capillary	=	30 mm Hg
Hydrostatic pressure at the venular end of the capillary	=	15 mm Hg
		15 mm rate of fluid flow into the vein

Thus, fluid leaves at the arterial end of the capillary bed because 45 mm of hydrostatic pressure is overcoming the 30 mm osmotic pressure of the blood plasma, and fluid is being forced into the tissues at the rate of 15 mm Hg. At the venular end of the capillary, hydrostatic pressure of 15 mm Hg cannot overcome 30 mm osmotic pressure of blood, and fluid flows from the interstitial tissue spaces into the venular end of the capillary at the rate of 15 mm Hg. Since it is entering the tissues at the rate of 15 mm Hg and leaving at the same rate, **there is a continuous circulation and no accumulation of fluid occurs in the interstitial spaces**. However, not all of the fluid in the interstitial spaces returns to the venules, **some is drained off through the lymphatics.**

From this brief review of the formation and drainage of interstitial fluid, it is obvious that **oedema will occur when there is**: (1) an increase in intravascular hydrostatic pressure, (2) a fall in colloid osmotic pressure of the plasma, and (3) impairment in the flow of blood. These are the important primary causes of oedema. To this list must be added retention of sodium and water, which may be a primary disturbance when there is kidney disease.

Causes of Oedema

1. Increased hydrostatic pressure: This may result from an impaired venous return. **In animals, this is a less important cause of oedema, than in humans.** Increased hydrostatic pressure occurs **in general or local passive hyperaemia**, and is due to increased venous hydrostatic pressure caused by a central obstruction in the heart or lungs, or local obstruction in a vein (see 'passive hyperaemia'). The accumulation of fluid in the interstitial spaces is explained as follows:

Hydrostatic pressure at the arterial end	=	45 mm Hg
Osmotic pressure at the arterial end	=	30 mm Hg
		15 mm Hg rate of fluid flow into the tissues
Osmotic pressure at the venular end	=	30 mm Hg
Hydrostatic pressure at the venular end	=	20 mm Hg
		10 mm Hg rate of fluid flow into the vein

Net result: 15 mm Hg minus 10 mm Hg = 5 mm Hg. **Therefore, at the rate of 5 mm Hg fluid accumulates in the tissues.**

256

This type of oedema is mild. Since the usual cause of venous stasis is impaired cardiac function (a weakened heart), oedema caused in this way is known as **cardiac oedema**.

2. **Reduced plasma osmotic pressure:** This results from **excessive loss or reduced synthesis of serum albumin.** As is known, serum proteins, **mainly albumin**, determine the osmotic pressure of plasma. Although this is the most common cause of general oedema both in humans and animals, **in domestic animals this cause is more common than increased hydrostatic pressure.** Continued removal of blood protein can produce **hypoproteinaemia.** In **cattle** and **sheep**, this occurs as a result of heavy infestation **with trichostrongyles (stomach worms), and some other intestinal parasites.** The blood sucking bites of these parasites, and possibly an anticoagulant toxin, result in repeated minute haemorrhages in large numbers. This daily loss of blood, with inadequate replacement, account for **parasitic oedema.** Loss of blood protein may also occur when slowly bleeding gastric ulcers, especially in **dogs** and **pigs**, are present.

Blood protein can be lost when renal injury is present. This is a common cause of oedema in humans, but is **of little importance in domestic animals.** This is because **nephrotic syndrome**, which is the most important cause of increased loss of albumin from kidney, does not occur in animals. Also, glomerular nephritis, which permits protein to escape from kidneys, is uncommon in animals. Oedema on account of kidney diseases is known as **renal oedema**. In animals, renal amyloidosis can be a rare cause of renal oedema.

Advanced liver disease, usually in the form of **cirrhosis**, can also lead to **hypoproteinaemia** due to decreased synthesis of plasma proteins. **During starvation/malnutrition** also, liver is unable to produce adequate amounts of these essential proteins. In either case, there is a decrease in the osmotic pressure of the plasma and then oedema occurs. Protein deficiency and **cachexia** also cause serious deficiency of blood protein. This situation is the cause of **nutritional oedema** or **cachectic oedema**. The accumulation of fluid into the interstitial spaces, or body cavities, is explained as follows:

Hydrostatic pressure at the arterial end   =   45 mm Hg
Osmotic pressure at the arterial end   =   20 mm Hg

-----

25 mm Hg rate of fluid
flow into the tissues

Osmotic pressure at the venular end   =   20 mm Hg
Hydrostatic pressure at the venular end   =   15 mm Hg

---

5 mm Hg rate of fluid
flow into the vein

Net result: 25 mm Hg minus 5 mm Hg = 20 mm Hg. **Therefore, at the rate of 20 mm Hg fluid accumulates in the tissues. This type of oedema is severe.**

3. Lymphatic obstruction: Interference with **lymphatic drainage** will cause accumulation of the interstitial fluid. This usually leads to **local oedema**, and may result from inflammatory or neoplastic obstruction. This occurs when **tumours, cysts, abscesses, bandages, rubber bands,** or **harnesses press on lymph vessels.** It is also observed when tumours or thrombi are found within lymphatics or lymph nodes. **Parasites (filaria** or *Demodex canis* **mites)** can obstruct lymph vessels. **In humans, filariasis,** a parasitic infection often causes massive fibrosis of the lymph nodes and lymph channels in the inguinal region. The resulting oedema of the lower limbs is so extreme it is called **elephantiasis.**

Although the endothelial lining is relatively impermeable to the passage of proteins, a small amount of albumin normally leaks into the interstitial space along with the normal interchange of fluid between vascular and interstitial compartments. Thus, with lymphatic obstruction, neither the small amount of fluid lost from the blood vessels nor the protein within the interstitial fluid can be drained off, **thus reducing the net effective osmotic pressure of the blood. This leads to local oedema,** sometimes called **lymphoedema**. The local accumulation of fluid into the interstitial spaces is explained as follows:

Hydrostatic pressure at the arterial end   =   45 mm Hg
Osmotic pressure at the arterial end   =   25 mm Hg

---

20 mm Hg rate of fluid
flow into the tissues

Osmotic pressure at the venular end   =   25 mm Hg
Hydrostatic pressure at the venular end   =   15 mm Hg

---

10 mm Hg rate of fluid
flow into the vein

Net result: 20 mm Hg minus 10 mm Hg = 10 mm Hg. **Therefore, at the rate of 10 mm Hg fluid accumulates in the tissues.**

4. Sodium and water retention: The osmotic activity of sodium largely determines volume of fluid in the interstitial spaces. Excess consumption of either salt or water by a normal individual does not cause oedema. **However, failure to excrete sodium in the urine resulting in water retention does lead to generalized oedema.** Reduced urinary excretion of sodium can occur in congestive heart failure, in nephrosis and nephritis, or in acute renal failure. Sodium retention causes expansion of the intravascular fluid volume, a decrease in the vascular colloid osmotic pressure, and secondarily, an increase in the interstitial fluid volume.

The **changes of oedema** are much **more visible grossly than microscopically. Grossly,** the oedematous part is **swollen, increased in weight, and if external, cold.** Temperature of extremities is lower than normal because of the suppressed rate of flow of blood through the area, greater heat dissipation because of the increase in size, and a lower rate of metabolism because of inadequate blood circulation. **Colour is less intense than normal and pain is absent.** However, a **sense of fullness and turgidity exists** due to distension of the tissues with fluid. **Incision** results in the flow of oedematous **fluid** from the cut surface. The swollen tissue has a firm and doughy consistency. It **'pits on pressure',** meaning that if finger is pressed into the oedematous tissue, the fluid is dispersed into the nearby tissue spaces. When the finger is removed, the pit remains for a moment, since a certain interval of time is required for the fluid to filter back through the network of tissue cells and fibrils. **Fibrosis** occurs when oedematous fluid has been present in the area for a considerable period of time. **Microscopically,** the spaces between adjacent cells, fibrils, or other structures, are enlarged. **During life, they were filled with fluid.** In the **microscopic section,** they may contain a finely granular material that **stains faintly pink with eosin.** The intensity of eosin staining depends on the amount of protein (mainly albumin) in the transudate. **Atrophy** of the parenchymatous cells and fibrosis occur in the area, if the oedematous fluid persists for a long period of time.

Significance and result: Oedema disappears if the cause is removed. **In the brain and the lungs, oedema may be fatal,** but subcutaneous oedema and oedema of other viscera are usually of little functional significance. Oedema of the subcutaneous tissues may impair healing of wounds.

259

SHOCK

Shock is a haemodynamic disorder characterized by inadequate systemic blood circulation (hypoperfusion) due to a reduction either in the cardiac output, or in the effective circulatory blood volume. This results in abnormally low pressure (hypotension), which in turn leads to poor blood flow to tissues, resulting in cellular hypoxia. That is, in a deficiency of oxygen reaching to cells of the body. Although these changes at the beginning cause only reversible cellular injury, persistence of the shock eventually leads to irreversible injury and can end up in the death of the patient.

Aetiology: Shock, also called 'cardiovascular collapse' may develop following any serious attack on the body's homeostasis. Shock may be precipitated by any massive insult to the body, such as profuse haemorrhage, extensive trauma or burns, and uncontrolled bacterial sepsis. In humans, extensive myocardial infarction and massive pulmonary embolism are also important causes of shock. Shock associated with crushing injuries, especially those that invade the chest and abdomen, are frequently observed in dogs injured by automobiles. Profuse haemorrhage and burns are common causes of shock in domestic animals. Cold, exhaustion, depression, and general anaesthesia predispose the animals to shock.

Classification: Based on cause, shock is at times classified as haemorrhagic shock (blood loss), traumatic or surgical shock (probably neurogenic), burn shock (fluid loss), septic or endotoxic shock, and neurogenic shock (trauma, pain, psychic). However, this haemodynamic disorder in the clinical conditions is best divided into four pathophysiological types: (1) hypovolaemic shock, (2) cardiogenic or cardiac shock, (3) septic or endotoxic shock, and (4) neurogenic shock. The mechanisms underlying hypovolaemic and cardiogenic shock are simple and involve low cardiac output. In contrast, mechanism of septic shock is complicated. Less commonly, anaphylactic shock, caused by a generalized immunoglobulin E-mediated hypersensitivity response, is seen in systemic vasodilation and increased vascular permeability. In anaphylactic shock, widespread vasodilation causes a sudden increase in the capacity of the vascular bed, which cannot be filled adequately by the normal circulatory blood volume. Thus, tissue hypoperfusion and cellular anoxia may result.

1. Hypovolaemic shock: Hypovolaemia means abnormally decreased volume of circulating blood in the body. Hypovolaemic

shock results from loss of blood or plasma volume. This may be caused by haemorrhage, fluid loss from extensive skin burns, exudation from large traumatic wounds, diarrhoea, and vomiting.

Pathogenesis: On account of reduced perfusion (blood flow), there is insufficient delivery of oxygen and nutrients to cells and tissues, and inadequate clearance of metabolites. With persistent oxygen deficiency (**cellular hypoxia**) there is defective intracellular aerobic respiration, followed by anaerobic glycolysis, and excessive production of lactate, which often induces metabolic lactic acidosis (see 'cell injury', Chapter 3). The lowering of pH in the tissues reduces the vasomotor response: arterioles dilate and blood begins to pool in the microcirculation.

Under normal conditions, in most, if not all parts of the body, more than half of the capillaries remain closed, especially if the organ or part is resting. But when capillaries throughout the body dilate, so much space becomes available in the general capillary bed (microcirculation) that all blood in the body can be contained within the capillaries. When capillaries dilate their walls become permeable, and fluid leaves the vessels and enters the tissues. With loss of fluid, the blood becomes concentrated (**haemoconcentration**), becomes more viscous, and the total blood volume is decreased. Deficiency of blood in the heart and major blood vessels results in decreased cardiac output, which finally reaches the point where adequate circulation can no longer be maintained. Thus, **peripheral pooling of blood** not only worsens the cardiac output, it also favours anoxic injury to endothelial cells. Persistence or worsening of the shock leads to widespread tissue hypoxia and irreversible injury, which in turn, lead to death of cells, and sometimes, the patient.

2. Cardiac shock: Cardiac shock results from **myocardial pump failure.** The **causes** include myocardial damage (infarction), external compression from haemopericardium (cardiac tamponade), or outflow obstruction (pulmonary embolism). The basic mechanisms of cardiogenic shock are the same as in hypovolaemic shock, that is, inadequate cardiac output, hypotension, impaired tissue perfusion, and cellular hypoxia.

3. Septic or endotoxic shock: Pathogenesis of septic shock is much more complex. It is caused by **systemic microbial infections** usually caused by Gram-negative bacteria, but it can also occur with Gram-positive bacteria and fungi. Septic shock results from spread and expansion of an initially localized infection, such as abscess,

261

peritonitis, or pneumonia, into the bloodstream.

Septic shock is mostly caused by **endotoxin-producing Gram-negative bacilli**, such as *Escherichia coli* and *Pseudomonas aeruginosa*, hence the name 'endotoxic shock'. Endotoxins are bacterial cell wall lipopolysaccharides (LPSs) released when the cell walls are destroyed, for example, in an inflammatory response. LPS consists of (1) a toxic fatty acid core common to all Gram-negative bacteria (**lipid A**), and (2) a complex polysaccharide coat that is unique for each species (**O antigens**). Similar molecules in the walls of Gram-positive bacteria (e.g., peptidoglycans in streptococci) and fungi can also cause septic shock.

Pathogenesis: All the cellular and haemodynamic effects of septic shock are caused by LPS (Fig. 46). Free LPS attaches to a circulating LPS-binding protein and the complex then binds to a specific receptor called **CD14** on monocytes, macrophages, and neutrophils. Engagement of CD14, even at extremely minute doses such as 10 picogram/ml (a picogram is one trillionth of a gram), results in intracellular signalling through a specific receptor, and this leads to profound activation of mononuclear cells with production of powerful cytokines, such as **interleukin-1 (IL-1)** and **tumour necrosis factor (TNF)** (Fig. 46).

At low doses, LPS mainly activates monocytes, macrophages, and neutrophils (Fig. 46) to increase their ability to eliminate invading bacteria. LPS also directly activates complement, which contributes to local bacterial removal. The mononuclear phagocytes respond to LPS by producing TNF, which in turn induces IL-1 synthesis. Both TNF and IL-1 act on endothelial and other cells to produce further cytokines, such as IL-6 and IL-8, and produce adhesion molecules. The initial release of LPS results in a cytokine sequence that increases the **local acute inflammatory response** and improves clearance of the infection (Fig. 46).

With moderately severe infections, **higher levels of LPS** are involved and therefore there is a greater production of cytokines. As a result, cytokine-induced secondary effectors, such as nitric oxide (NO) and platelet-activating factor (PAF) (see Chapter 4), become important (Fig. 46). In addition, systemic effects of TNF and IL-1 begin to be seen, including fever, increased production of acute-phase reactants, and increased production of circulating neutrophils (Fig. 46). **Finally, at still higher levels of LPS, the syndrome of septic shock appears (**Fig. 46). The same cytokines and secondary mediators

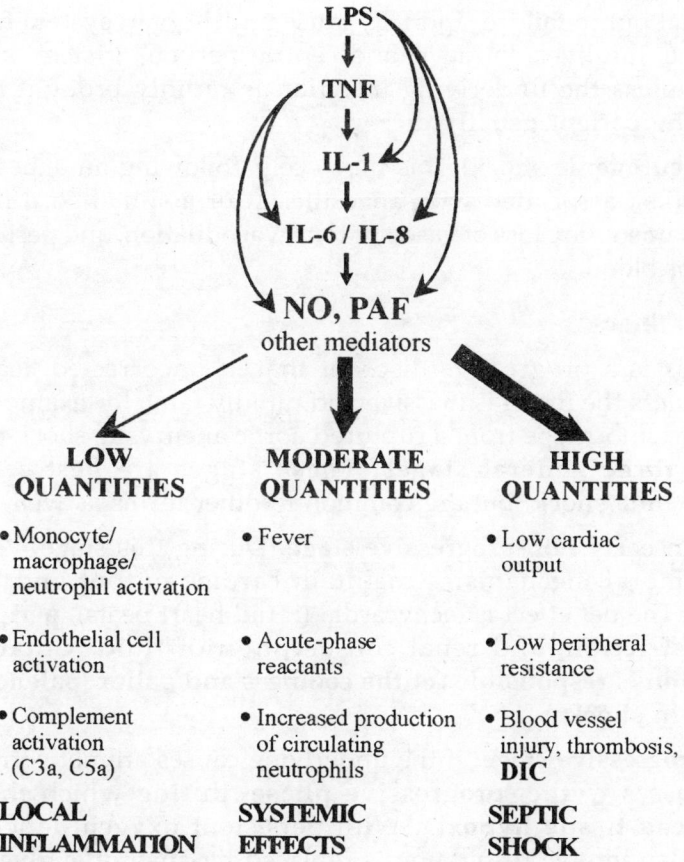

Fig. 46. Effects of lipopolysaccharide (LPS) and pathogenesis of septic or endotoxic shock.

now at a higher levels result in:

1. Systemic vasodilation (**hypotension)**

2. Diminished myocardial contractility

3. **Widespread endothelial injury and activation.** These cause systemic leukocyte adhesion and diffuse alveolar capillary damage in the lung.

4. Activation of the coagulation system, resulting in **disseminated intravascular coagulation (DIC).**

The **hypoperfusion** (inadequate systemic blood circulation), which results from the combined effects of widespread vasodilation, myocardial pump failure, and DIC cause **multi-organ system failure** that affects the liver, kidneys, and central nervous system, among others. Unless the underlying infection is rapidly brought under control, **the patient usually dies.**

4. Neurogenic shock: This may occur following an anaesthetic accident (i.e., associated with anaesthesia) or a spinal cord injury. The mechanisms are loss of vascular tone, vasodilation, and peripheral pooling of blood.

Stages of Shock

- Shock is a progressive disorder that, if uncorrected, leads to death. Unless the insult is massive and rapidly fatal, for example in a massive haemorrhage from a ruptured aortic aneurysm, shock passes through **three general stages. These stages are best seen in hypovolaemic shock,** but are common to other forms as well.

1. An early non-progressive stage. During this stage, various neurohumoral mechanisms maintain cardiac output and blood pressure. The net effect is tachycardia (rapid heart beats), **peripheral vasoconstriction,** and renal conservation of fluid. **Cutaneous constriction is responsible for the coolness and pallor (paleness) of the skin in shock.**

2. Progressive stage: If the underlying causes are not corrected, shock passes to the **'progressive phase'** during which there is **widespread tissue hypoxia.** With persistent oxygen deficiency, intracellular aerobic respiration is replaced by **anaerobic glycolysis** with excessive production of **lactic acid.** The resultant metabolic **lactic acidosis lowers the tissue pH and blunts the vasomotor response.** As a result, arterioles dilate, and blood begins to pool in the microcirculation. Peripheral pooling not only worsens the cardiac output, but also puts endothelial cells at risk of developing anoxic injury with subsequent DIC. **With widespread tissue hypoxia, vital organs are affected and they may begin to fail.** Clinically, the stage is characterized by abnormally rapid respirations (**tachypnoea**) and marked reduction in urinary output (**oliguria**) owing to reduced renal blood flow. Obviously, **this stage registers a marked deterioration in the condition of the patient.**

`3. Irreversible stage:** The process eventually enters an **'irreversible stage'** in which even the treatment does not stop the deteriorating condition of the patient. This phase is then a transition from the reversible to irreversible stage. There is a progressive reduction in the cardiac output and a progressive fall in the blood pressure. The reduced blood flow to the brain, heart, and kidneys leads to **ischaemic (hypoxic) cell death in these organs. This may lead to coma, renal failure, uraemia, and death.**

Morphology: The cellular and tissue changes induced by shock are essentially those of hypoxia (Chapter 3). They are particularly seen in brain, heart, lungs, kidneys, adrenals, and gastrointestinal tract. In the brain, the cells most vulnerable to ischaemia are neurons, and they suffer first reversible and then irreversible damage (called **ischaemic encephalopathy**). The heart may reveal subepicardial and subendocardial haemorrhages and necrosis. The kidneys show acute tubular necrosis. Since lungs are somewhat resistant to hypoxic injury they are seldom affected in pure hypovolaemic shock. But changes may appear in endotoxic and neurogenic shock. The adrenal changes comprise the common stress response. The gastrointestinal tract may suffer patchy mucosal haemorrhages and necrosis referred to as **'haemorrhagic enteropathy'.** The liver may develop fatty change and even central haemorrhagic necrosis.

Macroscopically, there is an acute general passive hyperaemia. The organs have a diffuse cyanotic colour due to the partially oxygenated blood that they contain. Petechial haemorrhages are numerous throughout the carcass. The body cavities (peritoneal, pleural, or pericardial) contain oedematous fluid. **Microscopically,** the capillaries and small veins are distended with blood. Focal haemorrhages are present. Cells and tissue fibres are separated by the transudate.

Symptoms: The animal feels cold and without strength. The animal is depressed, lethargic, and expression is anxious and worried. The body temperature is subnormal and skin cold. **The fundamental change is a tremendous fall in blood pressure.** Respirations are shallow and irregular. Blood pressure is low, pulse is rapid, and heart rate is very rapid. The animal becomes unconscious, **and finally dies from circulatory failure.**

Significance and results: The animal recovers with timely and appropriate therapeutic measures that are directed towards restoring blood volume, increasing cardiac output, and improving blood pressure. Death occurs if the blood volume cannot be restored and adequate circulation is not maintained.

Chapter 7

Cellular Adaptations of Growth and Differentiation

As discussed earlier, cells must constantly adapt (adjust themselves) to changes in their environment, even under normal conditions. These **physiological adaptations** (adjustments) usually represent responses of cells to normal stimulation by hormones or endogenous chemical substances, for example, enlargement of the mammary gland (breast in humans) and induction of lactation by pregnancy. **Pathological adaptations** share the same underlying mechanisms but they allow the cells to modulate (change) their internal environment, and thus escape injury. **Cellular adaptation, then, is a state that lies between the normal (unstressed) cell and the injured (over-stressed) cell.**

Cellular adaptation can occur by a number of mechanisms. Some adaptive responses are associated with the stimulation of new protein synthesis by the target cell. These proteins, for example, **heat shock proteins**, may protect cells from certain forms of injury (see 'heat shock proteins'). Still other adaptations involve a **switch** from producing one type of protein to another, or marked over-production of a specific protein. For example, this occurs in the cells synthesizing various collagens and extracellular matrix proteins in **chronic inflammation** and **fibrosis** (Chapter 4). Cellular adaptive responses can thus involve a number of mechanisms, including receptor binding; signal transduction; or protein transcription, translation, or export.

In this section, the adaptive changes in cell growth and differentiation that we shall consider include **atrophy** (decrease in cell size), **hypertrophy** (increase in cell size), **hyperplasia** (increase in cell number), and **metaplasia** (change in cell type).

However, first let us consider the two important disturbances of growth, namely, **aplasia** (failure of an organ to develop) and **hypoplasia** (incomplete development of an organ). These present themselves as congenital malformations (see Chapter 14).

Normal adult cells do not differ significantly in size in different species of animals. The cells of the same tissues in a cat are

267

approximately of the same size as those in a horse. **The difference in the size of the two animals depends on the total number of cells in their bodies.** Alterations in nutrition, however, can cause some change in the size of the cells. With reduced nutrition, they shrink, and with good nutrition, accompanied by some other factors, they enlarge.

Aplasia

Aplasia is the failure of an organ or tissue to develop. This disturbance occurs in the embryo or foetus during intrauterine development. **Causes** include (1) hereditary defects in germplasm, (2) death of a cell at some critical point in the development of the individual. For example, if the cell that forms the arm or leg bud dies in foetal life, then that limb will not develop. Diseases, particularly viral, of the dam during gestation, may invade the foetus and cause cellular damage. **Macroscopically**, there is an absence of that organ or tissue. In place of the aplastic organ, a fatty or fibrous mass may be present. Aplasia of a vital organ, such as heart, brain, or pituitary is incompatible with life. The foetus dies immediately after birth if it is born alive. Aplasia of a kidney, an adrenal, or a testicle (paired organs) is not serious because the remaining organ undergoes hypertrophy and hyperplasia and assumes the function of the organ that failed to develop.

Hypoplasia

Hypoplasia is a failure of cells, tissues, or organs to attain their mature size. In other words, it is incomplete development or underdevelopment of an organ, with decreased number of cells. It differs from atrophy in that atrophic cells already attain their adult size before reverting to small form. **Causes** include (1) congenital anomalies. Examples: hypoplasia of kidney in all animals; hypoplasia of one or both eyes in pups, baby pigs and Jersey calves; hypoplasia of the cerebellum in kittens, lambs, and calves, (2) inadequate blood supply, (3) inadequate innervation. Example: faulty innervation of limb or organ following infantile paralysis in humans. The part does not develop properly and the individual then has a short or distorted leg, and (4) malnutrition.

Macroscopically, some of the tissue or organ is present but it never attains its normal adult size. This variation in size can be determined by weight, volume, or measurement when compared with normal tissue or organs. **Microscopically**, cells in the hypoplastic tissue are not as large as normal cells and are fewer in number. Usually there is an excessive amount of connective tissue and fat. **Significance and results**: Hypoplasia may involve one or many organs in the body. However, it does not necessarily result in death of the individual. But the damage is permanent since the disturbance of growth cannot be corrected.

Atrophy

Atrophy is shrinkage in size of the cell from loss of cell substance. When a sufficient number of cells is involved, the entire tissue or organ diminishes in size, and becomes atrophic. It is emphasized that **although atrophic cells may have diminished function, they are not dead. Also, atrophy is not to be confused with hypoplasia, which is failure of cells to attain their adult size, whereas atrophy occurs in cells that have reached their full development.**

Causes of atrophy include: (1) physiological (physiological atrophy). **Examples**: (i) disappearance of the thymus as an organism reaches sexual maturity, (ii) involution of the uterus after pregnancy, (iii) involution of mammary gland after lactation, and (iv) atrophy of the endometrium during anoestrus. **(2) aging (senile atrophy)**: The aging process is associated with **cell loss**. Senile atrophy is a general atrophy involving all cells of the body, but certain cells show it earlier and to a greater extent than others. The organs of reproduction (testes and ovaries) are among the first to show senile changes. **(3) inadequate nutrition (starvation atrophy)**: During starvation, glycogen and fat are the first to disappear, then the protein of the body musculature, and finally the protein of the vital organs. This results in **marked muscle wasting. (4) decreased workload (disuse atrophy)**. In this, there is a reduction in the size of cells as a result of decreased workload or inactivity. When a broken limb is immobilized in a plaster cast, atrophy of skeletal muscle occurs. The race horse kept inactive in the stable experiences a decrease in the size of his body musculature. **(5) loss of innervation (denervation or neurotropic atrophy)**. Normal function of skeletal muscle depends on its nerve supply. Damage to the nerves leads to rapid atrophy of the muscle fibres supplied by them. Examples: (i) when the nerve supply to a limb is cut muscles of that limb atrophy. (ii) horses which have nerves cut in the treatment of lameness often show marked atrophy of muscles, tendons, and ligaments of their affected limb. (iii) the muscles of the shoulder of the horse undergo atrophy (sweeny), when the suprascapular nerve is injured. (iv) injury to the recurrent laryngeal nerve in horses results in the atrophy of muscles of the larynx. **(6) diminished blood supply (angiotrophic atrophy)** may result from anaemia, ischaemia, or chronic passive congestion. In horse, atrophy in the hind limbs occurs when a parasite (strongylus larvae) occludes the femoral artery. Chronic passive congestion prevents adequate oxygen and nutrients from reaching cells. This type of atrophy is seen in the central lobular region of the liver. **(7) pressure (pressure atrophy)**. Presssure atrophy occurs when a mild mechanical force is applied continuously to cells over a long period of time. Basically it is due to malnutrition associated with ischaemia. It is commonly observed in tissues adjacent to tumours, abscesses, and haematocysts, as well as in the necks, shoulders, and backs of horses when collars and saddles are pressed. **(8) loss of endocrine stimulation (endocrine atrophy)**. Endocrine atrophy occurs either from loss of endocrine stimulation, or from excessive endocrine secretion. Examples: (i) hypersecretion of the thyroid results in extreme emaciation and atrophy as a result of greatly increased rate of metabolism. (ii) oestrogen produced by testicular tumours causes atrophy of the seminiferous cells of testicle and epithelium of the accessory sex glands. (iii) atrophy of the prostate gland following castration. (iv) atrophy of the uterus after ovariectomy (removal of ovaries).

As an Adaptive Response

Some of the causes mentioned are **physiological** (e.g., involution of the uterus after pregnancy) and others **pathological** (e.g., denervation), but the basic cellular changes are similar. **They represent a retreat (withdrawal) by the cell to a smaller size at which survival is still possible.** Thus, a new equilibrium is achieved between cell size and diminished blood supply, nutrition, or trophic stimulation. **Although atrophic cells may have diminished function, they are not dead.** However, atrophy may progress to the point at which cells are injured and die. If the blood is inadequate even to maintain life of shrunken cells, injury and cell death may supervene. The atrophic cells are then replaced by connective and adipose tissue. The part, however, returns to near normal if the cause is removed before the atrophic cells entirely disappear.

Biochemical Mechanisms

In atrophy, there is a reduction in the structural components of the cell. The **biochemical mechanisms** underlying this process ultimately affect the balance between synthesis and degradation

270

(destruction). **Decreased synthesis, increased catabolism, or both may cause atrophy.** In normal cells, synthesis and degradation of cellular components are influenced by a number of hormones, including insulin, thyroid-stimulating hormone, and glucocorticoids.

The regulation of protein degradation plays a key role in atrophy. Cells contain **two proteolytic systems: (i) lysosomes** contain proteases and other enzymes that degrade **molecules endocytosed** from outside, as well as senescent (old) cytoplasmic organelles (mitochondria, lysosome, ribosome), and **(ii) ubiquitin-proteasome pathway**. This pathway degrades many **cytosolic and nuclear proteins**. Proteins to be destroyed by this pathway are conjugated (joined) to **ubiquitin**, a 76-amino acid cytosolic peptide. The protein is then destroyed within a large cytoplasmic proteolytic complex called 'proteasome'. **This pathway is thought to be responsible for increased proteolysis in atrophy.**

Macroscopically, there is a decrease in the size of the organ or the tissue involved. The part is flabby, soft, and lacks its normal tissue tone. Also, it loses its normal tissue colour and appears anaemic. **Microscopically**, cells undergoing atrophy are smaller than normal, and fewer in number, or may have entirely disappeared. In many situations, atrophy is also accompanied by marked increase in the number of **'autophagic vacuoles'**. These are membrane-bound vacuoles within the cell that contain fragments of cell components (mitochondria, endoplasmic reticulum), which are to be destroyed. This is achieved by fusion with lysosomes and discharge of their enzymes. The cellular components are then digested. Some of the cell debris within the autophagic vacuole may resist digestion and persist as membrane-bound residual bodies (e.g., **lipofuscin granules**) in the cytoplasm. When present in sufficient amounts, they impart a brown discoloration to the tissue (**brown atrophy**).

Hypertrophy

Hypertrophy is an increase in the size of cells and, as a result, an increase in the size of the organ. Thus, the hypertrophied organ has no new cells, just bigger cells. The increase in size of cells is not due to cellular swelling, but because of the increased synthesis of structural proteins and organelles. In contrast, **hyperplasia** (discussed next) is characterized by an increase in cell number.

Causes: Hypertrophy of an organ can be **physiological or pathological** and is **caused by increased functional demand or by**

271

specific hormonal stimulation. Hypertrophy and hyperplasia can also occur together. Both result in an enlarged (hypertrophic) organ. Pure hypertrophy (without hyperplasia) occurs only in those organs in which cells have lost the ability to divide; for example, skeletal and cardiac muscle. **(1) Physiological hypertrophy:** the massive physiological growth of the uterus during pregnancy involves both hypertrophy and hyperplasia, and occurs from oestrogen stimulation. In contrast, development of muscles in a race or draft horse, or a weight lifter, occurs only from hypertrophy of individual muscle cells induced by increased workload. **(2) Adaptive response:** hypertrophy as an adaptive response occurs as muscular enlargement in **two settings**. The **striated muscle cells** in both **heart** and the **skeletal muscles** can undergo only hypertrophy in response to increased demand, because in the adult they cannot divide to produce more cells to share the increased workload. Therefore, synthesis of more proteins and myofilaments occurs for each cell. This achieves a balance between the demand and the cell's functional capacity. The greater number of myofilaments permits an increased workload with a level of metabolic activity per unit volume of cell not different from that carried out by the normal cell. Thus, the draft horse readily pulls the load. Whatever the exact mechanism of hypertrophy, eventually a limit is reached beyond which enlargement of mass can no longer compensate for the increased burden. In the case of heart, cardiac failure occurs. **(3) compensatory hypertrophy.** This form of hypertrophy may be a physiological or pathological response. It is usually the result of impaired function of an organ system. For example, compensatory hypertrophy occurs when one of a pair of organs is destroyed. When one kidney is damaged, the other gradually enlarges and compensates for the loss. In horse, hypertrophy of the muscular coats of the distal end of oesophagus occurs following spasms of the cardiac sphincter of the stomach. Other examples include hypertrophy of the myocardium following stenosis (narrowing) of a valvular lumen; hypertrophy of the terminal portion of the ileum in horse and pig in case of a defective ileo-caecal valve; and hypertrophy of the musculature in lung in asthma. This also occurs in pulmonary adenomatosis in cattle.

Macroscopically, the organ or tissue is larger and heavier than normal, as can be appreciated by large muscles of the race or draft horse. **Microscopically**, there is an increase in the size of cells, and therefore there are fewer cells in each microscopic field. **Significance and results:** Compensatory hypertrophy results in an increased

272

function of an organ or tissue. Thus, the hypertrophied muscles of a race horse enable him to run rapidly, and the draft horse readily pulls the heavy load that would break the back of a pony. When one tissue of an organ enlarges out of proportion to other tissues, the resulting distortion may cause obstruction of hollow organs, e.g., in the oesophagus of horse and the ileum of horse and pig.

Hyperplasia

Hyperplasia is an increase in the number of cells in an organ or tissue. Just as enlargement of cells (hypertrophy) represents a response to increased functional demand, **cells capable of mitotic division may divide when stressed or stimulated by increased activity, and thus constitute hyperplasia.** Hypertrophy and hyperplasia are closely related. They often develop together so that both may contribute to an overall increase in organ size. They are usually found together in **prostate** and are difficult to differentiate. **Pregnant uterus** is another example of hypertrophy and hyperplasia. **Goitre** is a hypertrophy and hyperplasia of the thyroid gland. Cardiac and skeletal muscle cells have no capacity for hyperplastic growth, and thus undergo only hypertrophy. On the other hand, even potentially dividing cells, such as **renal epithelial cells**, undergo hypertrophy but not hyperplasia. Hyperplasia can be **physiological** or **pathological**.

Physiological hyperplasia is divided into: **(1) hormonal hyperplasia**, for example, proliferation of the glandular epithelium of the mammary gland at puberty and during pregnancy. **(ii) compensatory hyperplasia**: That is, hyperplasia which occurs when a portion of the tissue is removed (e.g. in partial hepatectomy). The mitotic activity in the remaining cells begins within 12 hours, eventually restoring the liver to its normal weight. The stimuli for proliferation are polypeptide growth factors, produced by remaining hepatocytes (see 'growth factors').

Pathological hyperplasia: Causes include **(1) repeated and prolonged irritation** by mechanical, chemical, and thermal agents. **Examples**: Calluses on the elbows and stifles of dogs, and the hands of workmen. Excessive heat or cold, toxic chemical substances, and highly chlorinated naphthalenes cause hyperplasia. **(2) endocrine disturbances:** Hyperplasia of the prostate occurs in old dogs but can be prevented if the animal is castrated, or if oestrogen is administered. Also in dogs hyperplasia of epithelium and connective tissue of the mammary gland occurs, and can be produced experimentally by the administration of excessive amounts of oestrogen. **(3) nutritional disturbances**: Iodine deficiency results in hyperplasia of the thyroid (goitre). Vitamin A deficiency results in hyperplasia and hyperkeratinization of epithelium in oesophagus of the chicken. **(4) infectious causes**: The pox viruses (cowpox, fowl pox, and pigeon pox) cause hyperplasia of epithelium. Hyperplasia of the epithelium of the lips occurs in sheep infected with contagious ecthyma virus. Wart viruses cause hyperplasia of epithelium in cattle. The hyperplasia may be due to increased sensitivity of cells to normal levels of growth factors. Thus, the common skin wart is caused by an increased expression of various transcription factors by the infecting **papillomavirus. Any minor stimulation of the cell by growth factors results in an excessive mitotic activity**, and **(5) wound healing**: Hyperplasia is also an important response of connective tissue cells in wound healing, in which growth factor-stimulated fibroblasts and blood vessels proliferate to facilitate repair (Chapter 5).

Significance and results: Hyperplastic epithelial tissue usually disappears if the cause is removed. However, connective tissue hyperplasia is a permanent change and persists for the life of the individual. The great danger associated with hyperplasia is that the cells have changed their normal pattern and rate of growth. **Pathological hyperplasia, thus, constitutes a fertile soil in which cancerous proliferation may eventually arise.** For example, human patients with hyperplasia of the endometrium are at increased risk of developing endometrial cancer. In the domestic animals, this is usually observed in the mammary glands of dogs.

Metaplasia

Metaplasia is a reversible change in which one adult cell type (epithelial or mesenchymal) is replaced by another cell type. It is **an adaptive response** in which cells sensitive to a particular stress are replaced by other cell types better able to withstand the adverse environment. **The transformation is an alteration from a less specialized cell type to a more specialized cell type** (cuboidal to columnar epithelium, columnar to stratified squamous epithelium, fibrous connective tissue to bone, cartilage to bone).

Causes include: **(1) Repeated and prolonged irritation:** Adaptive metaplasia is best seen in the **squamous metaplasia** that occurs in the respiratory tract in response to chronic irritation. Bronchial epithelium changes from pseudostratified columnar ciliated epithelium to stratified squamous epithelium as the result of injury from lungworms.

274

Similar change occurs in the trachea and bronchi of habitual cigarette smokers. Gallstones injure the gallbladder mucous membrane and change the epithelium from columnar to stratified squamous. A persisting eversion of the uterus results in an epithelial change from columnar to stratified squamous. Continued irritation of a serosal surface (peritoneum) may also result in a change from simple squamous epithelium to cuboidal, columnar, or even stratified squamous epithelium. In all these cases, the more tough stratified squamous epithelium is able to survive under circumstances in which the more fragile specialized epithelium would have succumbed. **(2) Nutritional disturbances:** A deficiency of vitamin A causes cuboidal or columnar epithelium to change to stratified squamous epithelium in a variety of locations, including the lachrymal ducts and renal pelves. It is easily seen in the mucous glands of the oesophagus of the chicken. **(3) Endocrine disturbances:** The mammary gland tumour in dogs is caused by endocrine disturbances. In this neoplasm, the epithelial and connective tissue elements of the glands undergo metaplasia and produce stratified squamous epithelium, cartilage, bone, and muscle. The columnar epithelium of the prostate gland of dogs may change to stratified squamous epithelium when Sertoli-cell tumours of the testicle are present. Rarely, the scars of abdominal wounds develop metastatic bone.

Thus, metaplasia may also occur in mesenchymal cells (**connective tissue metaplasia**), **but less clearly as an adaptive response**. Fibroblasts may get transformed to chondroblasts or osteoblasts to produce cartilage or bone, where it is normally not found. For example, bone formation in muscle (**myositis ossificans**), or occasional formation of bone in soft tissues, particularly in foci of injury.

Significance and results: Being a reversible change, metaplastic epithelium returns to its original type when the cause is removed. However, formation of cartilage and bone are permanent alterations. Squamous metaplasia may function as a protective mechanism. **However, the influences that cause such metaplasia, if persistent, may induce malignant transformation in metaplastic epithelium.**

Dysplasia

Dysplasia (L. dys = disordered; plasein = to form) is a term used to describe **disorderly, but non-neoplastic proliferation**. It is seen mainly in the epithelial cells. **Dysplasia is a loss in the uniformity of individual cells and a loss in their architectural orientation.** Dysplastic cells exhibit considerable variation in size and shape, and usually have deeply stained (hyperchromatic) nuclei that are abnormally large for the size of the cell. Mitotic figures are more abundant than usual, and appear in abnormal locations. In dysplastic stratified squamous epithelium mitoses are not confined to the basal layers, **but appear at all levels and even in surface cells.** When dysplastic changes are marked, and involve the entire thickness of the epithelium, the lesion is referred to as **carcinoma** *in situ* - a pre-invasive stage of cancer.

Dysplasia is not an adaptive response, but is considered here because it is closely related to hyperplasia, and is sometimes called **'atypical hyperplasia'.** Dysplastic change is important mainly in human pathology, and is mostly encountered in the cervix and in the respiratory tract of habitual cigarette smokers. In both cervix and the respiratory tract, dysplasia is strongly implicated **as a precursor of cancer. However, dysplasia does not necessarily progress to cancer.** Mild-to-moderate changes that do not involve the entire thickness of epithelium may be reversible, and with removal of the inciting causes, the epithelium may revert to normal.

Chapter 8

Neoplasia

Neoplasia means 'new growth'. A neoplasm (Greek neo = new + plasma = a thing formed) **is a growth of new cells that proliferates without control, serves no useful function, and has no orderly arrangement. Neoplastic cells are transformed cells.** They continue to replicate (grow), completely ignoring the regulatory influences that control normal cell growth. **Thus, fundamental to the origin of all neoplasms is loss of responsiveness, that is, insensitivity to normal growth controls.** Neoplasms therefore behave as parasites and compete with normal cells and tissues for their metabolic needs. Thus, neoplasms flourish, whereas the patients undergo wasting. They also enjoy autonomy (self-government) and steadily increase in size regardless of the nutritional status of the host. All neoplasms depend on the host for their nutrition and blood supply.

Generally, a neoplasm is referred to as a **tumour**. Strictly speaking, a tumour is simply a swelling (Latin tumour = a swelling), but it does not mean that all swellings are tumours. Many swellings may be tumour-like, for example, cold abscesses, haematocysts (haematomas), chronic inflammation, parasitic nodules, and masses of intra-abdominal fat necrosis. Most of these processes develop for a time and then subside. Today, the term tumour is applied to **neoplastic masses** that may cause swelling on the body surface. **Its use for non-neoplastic lesions has been dropped.**

The study of tumours (neoplasms) is called **oncology** (G. oncos = tumour + logos = study of). In oncology, division of neoplasms into benign and malignant category is most important. A tumour is said to be **benign** (Latin = mild) when it remains localized, does not spread to other sites, can be removed surgically, and does not cause death, unless its location interferes with an important body function. **Malignant** (Latin = evil in nature) neoplasms, on the other hand, can invade and destroy adjacent structure, spread to distant sites (metastasize), and cause death. **Malignant tumours are commonly called cancers.** The word **cancer** is derived from Latin and means a **crab**, because cancers adhere to any part that they seize very firmly like a crab.

Nomenclature

Neoplasms are divided into **two major groups: (1) benign,** and **(2) malignant**. As stated, a **benign tumour** usually does not kill the patient, grows slowly, and does not spread to distant organs. A **malignant tumour**, on the other hand, kills the patient by progressive local invasion and also by spread to distant organs (metastasis).

All tumours, both benign and malignant, have two basic components: **(1) the parenchyma.** This is made up of transformed or neoplastic cells and **(2) the supporting**, host-derived non-neoplastic **stroma**, made up of connective tissue and blood vessels. The **parenchyma** determines the biological behaviour of the neoplasm. The **stroma** carries the blood supply and provides support for the growth of parenchymal cells. **It is very important for the growth of neoplasm.**

In general, benign tumours are designated by attaching the suffix '**- oma'** to the cell type from which the tumour arises. For example, a benign tumour of fibrous tissue is a **fibroma**, and a benign tumour of cartilage is a **chondroma**. The nomenclature of benign epithelial tumours is more complex. The nomenclature of malignant tumours is basically similar to that of benign tumours, with certain additions and exceptions. The following simple classification will make things clear.

Tumour Classification

(A) Epithelial: Tumours derived from epithelial surfaces, either squamous or glandular.

(1) **Benign**

(a) Papilloma: involves an epithelial surface.

(b) Adenoma: involves glandular epithelium.

(2) **Malignant**

(a) Carcinoma: involves either squamous or glandular epithelium.

(B) Non-epithelial: Tumours derived from connective tissue in general (fibrous tissue, cartilage, bone, muscle).

(i) Benign: The name of the tissue plus 'oma' (fibroma, chondroma, osteoma).

(ii) Malignant: Indicated by the term sarcoma (fibrosarcoma, chondrosarcoma, osteosarcoma).

(C) Dermal cyst tumour: This tumour arises from an embryonic defect in growth and is composed of one germ layer only, the ectoderm, and contains teeth, hair, and other dermal structures.

(D)Teratoma: This tumour also arises from an embryonic defect in growth and is composed of two or more germ layers.

Thus, the term **papilloma** refers to a benign epithelial tumour growing on any epithelial surface that produces microscopic or macroscopic finger-like projections. The term **adenoma** is applied to a benign tumour of the glandular epithelium. **Malignant neoplasm** originating from mesenchymal tissue is called a **sarcoma**. A cancer of fibrous tissue is a **fibrosarcoma**, and that composed of chondrocytes is a **chondrosarcoma**. Thus, sarcomas are designated by their histogenesis, that is, the cell type of which they are composed. Malignant tumour of epithelial origin is called a **carcinoma**. It must be remembered that epithelium of the body is derived from all three germ-cell layers: ectoderm, mesoderm, and endoderm. Therefore, a malignant neoplasm of the skin (ectoderm), renal tubular epithelium (mesoderm), and lining epitheiium of the intestine (endoderm) are all **carcinoma**. Thus, it is interesting that **mesoderm** can give rise to both **carcinomas** (epithelial) and **sarcomas** (mesenchymal). Carcinomas are further classified as **squamous-cell carcinoma** and **adenocarcinoma**. The former originates from stratified squamous epithelium and the latter from glandular epithelium. **Cystadenomas** are hollow cystic masses, typically seen in the ovary. A **teratoma** contains cells derived from more than one germ-cell layer, and sometimes all three. Teratomas take origin from totipotential cells (i.e., capable of differentiating into all the three germ layers). Such cells are normally present in the ovary and testis. These cells have the capacity to differentiate into any type of cell found in the adult body. Therefore, they can give rise to neoplasms that have bits of bone, epithelium, muscle, fat, nerve, and other tissues. When all the components are well differentiated, it is a **benign teratoma**; when less well differentiated, a **malignant teratoma**.

Frequently tumour cells are composed of more that one type of tissue. This is particularly true of the neoplasms of the mammary gland of the dog. In such a case, the tumour is **a mixed tumour**, for example, a mixed mammary gland tumour. The term is then followed by a list of the types of neoplastic tissues present, for example, mixed mammary gland tumour composed of fibrous connective tissue, cartilage, and bone. The other alternative is to list the components of the tumour in compound words; the least important, or the least malignant tissue is placed last, e.g., fibro-chondrosarcoma, osteo-fibro-chondrosarcoma.

The pathologist classifies tumour on a histogenetic basis, that is, according to the origin of cells (Table 12). However, this is often difficult because it is not always possible to identify the type of cell present. The more undifferentiated (anaplastic) the cells are, the more difficult it is to classify the tumour.

Table 12. Histogenetic classification of neoplasms

Tissue of origin	Benign	Malignant
(A) Tumours of mesenchymal origin		
1. Connective tissue and derivatives		
Fibrous connective tissue cell	Fibroma	Fibrosarcoma
Embryonal connective tissue that produces mucin	Myxoma	Myxosarcoma
Adipose tissue cell	Lipoma	Liposarcoma
Chondrocyte	Chondroma	Chondrosarcoma
2. Endothelial and related tissues		
Blood vessels	Haemangioma	Haemangiosarcoma
Lymph vessels	Lymphangioma	Lymphangiosarcoma
Mesothelium	—	Mesothelioma
Meninges	Meningioma	Invasive meningioma
3. Tumours of haematopoietic cells		
Lymphoid cells	—	Lymphoid leukaemia
	Lymphoma	Lymphosarcoma
Myeloid cell	—	Myeloid leukaemia
Plasma cells	—	Multiple myeloma
4. Tumours of muscle		
Smooth	Leiomyoma	Leiomyosarcoma
Striated	Rhabdomyoma	Rhabdomyosarcoma
(B) Tumours of nervous tissue		
Glia		Glioma Gliosarcoma
Neuron	Neuroma	Neuroblastoma
(C) Tumours of epithelial origin		
1. Stratified squamous	Papilloma	Squamous-cell (or epidermoid) carcinoma

2. **Basal cells of the skin** or adnexa	—	Basal cell carcinoma
3. **Glandular epithelium**	Adenoma	Adenocarcinoma
4. **Neuroectoderm** (melanocytes)	Melanoma	Melanocarcinoma
5. **Urinary tract epithelium** (transitional)	Transitional cell papilloma	Transitional cell carcinoma
6. **Testicular epithelium** (germ cells)	—	Seminoma

Macroscopic Appearance

Neoplasms have no definite size, shape, colour, or consistency. Several factors such as location, the type of tumour, blood supply, rate of growth, and the length of time the tumour has been present, influence the macroscopic appearance of the neoplasm.

In **size**, neoplasms measure from one to two millimetres to several centimetres in diameter. In **weight**, they vary from a few milligrams to as much as 60 kilograms, or even more. The tumours may be larger than the host in the smaller animals, such as mice. The **shape** is quite variable. It may be round, elliptical, or multi-lobulated. A slowly growing tumour tends to be spherical or pedunculated. A rapidly growing neoplasm is usually irregular in shape, or is multi-lobulated.

The **colour** of a neoplasm is usually greyish white, but may be yellow, red, brown, or black. Areas of necrosis often appear as white or yellow. Fat pigmented with lipochromes, if present, imparts neoplasm a yellow colour. Haemorrhage or hyperaemia gives the tumour a pink or red colour. The presence of melanin results in black colour. The **consistency** varies with the type of tissue. Tumours of bone are very hard. If tumours of connective tissue contain considerable amounts of collagen, they are dense and firm. They are said to be **sclerotic** or **fibrotic** in consistency. Certain tumours induce a dense, abundant, fibrous stroma (**desmoplasia**) making them hard, so called **scirrhous** tumours. Some tumours are very soft and friable and are called **encephaloid** in consistency, because they resemble brain tissue. Tumours may be soft and liquefied, if degeneration, suppuration, and necrosis are present. Some tumours are watery in consistency because of oedema. If tumours contain mucin, they are slimy in consistency.

Microscopic Appearance

The appearance of neoplastic cells varies with the degree of malignancy of the tumour. The more benign the tumour, the more

281

the cells resemble the adult cell type. The more malignant the tumour, the more the cells resemble the immature or the embryonal cell type. When a tumour cell becomes malignant, it reverts to the more embryonal type, and this reversion is called **anaplasia** (discussed next). The more anaplasia a tumour shows, the more malignant is the neoplasm. **Anaplasia is characterized by:**

1. Hyperchromasia and enlargement of the nucleus: The nuclei are extremely hyperchromatic and large. The nuclear-cytoplasmic ratio may be 1:1, instead of the normal 1:4 or 1:6. Nuclei also vary in their size and shape, and reveal odd or unusual forms.

2. Enlargement of the nucleolus: The nucleoli are also extremely large, and may become two or three times their normal size.

3. Increased number of mitotic figures: The more rapidly the cells are multiplying, the greater the number of mitotic figures. Mitotic figures are distinctly atypical.

4. Giant cells: These cells are much larger than the neighbouring cells, and possess either one very big nucleus, or several nuclei. The nucleus is dividing more rapidly than cytoplasm and, as a result, multiple nuclei are found within the cell. Such cells are called tumour giant cells.

5. Hyperchromasia of the cell: The more anaplastic the cell, the more intensely the cell stains with haematoxylin, especially the nucleus. The intensity of the haematoxylin staining gives an indication as to the lack of differentiation, or maturity of the cell.

6. Embryonal type cells: The cell loses its resemblance to the cells from which it originated, and approaches the undifferentiated embryonal cell type. **This indicates that cell growth is no longer under the control of growth regulating mechanism of the body.**

Characteristics of Benign and Malignant Neoplasms

Benign tumours are harmless unless their location interferes with the function of an important organ. They grow slowly, usually become encapsulated, are often pedunculated if located on a surface, do not metastasize, and do not recur when removed. Malignant tumours are harmful because they spread locally, grow rapidly, are not encapsulated, spread to other parts of the body by metastasis, and recur after excision or irradiation. These differences between benign and malignant neoplasms are discussed under four headings: (1) differentiation and anaplasia, (2) rate of growth, (3) local invasion, and (4) metastasis.

1. Differentiation and Anaplasia

Differentiation and anaplasia refer only to the **parenchymal cells,** because these are the cells that form the transformed elements of neoplasms. Although the stroma carrying the blood supply is very important for the growth of tumours, it does not help in differentiating benign from malignant tumours. The amount of stromal connective tissue, however, does determine the consistency of a neoplasm. Certain cancers induce a dense, abundant fibrous stroma (**desmoplasia**), making them hard, so-called **scirrhous tumours**. The differentiation of parenchymal cells means the extent to which they resemble the normal cells, both morphologically and functionally.

Benign neoplasms are composed of well-differentiated cells that closely resemble normal cells. A **lipoma** is made up of **mature fat cells** and a **chondroma** of **mature cartilage cells.** In well-differentiated benign tumours, mitoses are extremely small in number and are of normal configuration.

Malignant neoplasms exhibit a wide range of parenchymal cell differentiation, from well- differentiated to completely undifferentiated cells. Malignant neoplasms composed of undifferentiated cells are said to be **anaplastic. Lack of differentiation, or anaplasia, is the characteristic feature of malignancy.** The word **anaplasia** is of Greek origin (Greek ana = backward + plasma = a thing formed) and means 'to form backward'. **Anaplasia therefore means reversion of cells to a more primitive or undifferentiated form.** It indicates de-differentiation, or loss of the structural and functional differentiation of normal cells. (De-differentiation means reversion of cells to a primitive form). However, as most cancers arise from stem cells in tissues, **it is now believed that failure of differentiation, rather than de-differentiation of specialized cells, accounts for undifferentiated tumours** (i.e., anaplasia).

Anaplastic cells show marked **pleomorphism**, that is, marked variation is size and shape (see 'microscopic appearance'). The **nuclei** are **extremely hyperchromic** and **large**. The **nuclear-cytoplasmic ratio** may be 1:1, instead of the normal 1:4 or 1:6. **Giant cells** may be formed. They are much larger than the neighbouring cells, and possess either one very big nucleus, or several nuclei. **Anaplastic nuclei vary in size and shape and show odd or abnormal (bizarre) forms.** The chromatin is coarse and clumped, and **nucleoli** may be **extremely large**. More important, **mitoses are numerous and atypical**. Multiple abnormal spindles may be seen. Sometimes spindles are seen as tripolar (three) or quadripolar (four) forms in which one spindle is usually large and others very small.

Regarding functional differentiation of neoplastic cell, if differentiation is better, the cell completely retains its functions like normal cells. For example, benign neoplasms, and even well-differentiated cancers of endocrine glands, elaborate hormones. Well-differentiated squamous-cell carcinomas form keratin, and well-differentiated liver cancers secrete bile. In fact, there are few differences in the enzyme profiles of well-differentiated tumours and their normal counterparts. On the other hand, higly anaplastic undifferentiated cells of malignant neoplasms differ markedly from the normal cells from which they have originated. They may even elaborate foetal proteins not produced by normal cells (see 'biochemical assays'). Also, **cancers of non-endocrine origin** may produce hormones, called **'ectopic hormones'**. Thus, the more rapidly growing and the more anaplastic a tumour, the less likely it will have specialized functional activity. **To summarize**, the cells in benign tumours are well differentiated and resemble their normal cells of origin, whereas cells in malignant tumours are usually undifferentiated.

The term **dysplasia** means disorderly but non-neoplastic proliferation of cells. It is seen mainly in the epithelium. It is a loss in the uniformity of individual cells and also in their architectural orientation. Dysplastic cells exhibit considerable pleomorphism (variation in size and shape) and usually possess deeply stained (hyperchromatic) nuclei that are abnormally large for the size of the cell. Mitotic figures are more than usual, but conform to normal patterns. However, often mitoses appear in abnormal locations. For example, in dysplastic stratified squamous epithelim, mitoses are not confined to the basal layers, where they normally occur, but may appear at all levels and **even in surface cells**. Also, there is disordered architectural arrangement. For example, the normal pattern of maturation of basal cells to flattened surface cells is lost, and replaced by a disordered scrambling of dark basal-appearing cells. When dysplasia is marked, and involves the entire thickness of the epithelium, the lesion is referred to as **carcinoma *in situ***, a pre-invasive stage of cancer. **However, dysplasia does not necessarily progress to cancer**. Mild and moderate changes are reversible, and with removal of the inciting causes, the epithelium may revert to normal.

2. Rate of Growth

Benign tumours grow slowly over a period of months to years. Malignant tumours, on the other hand, grow much faster, spread locally and to distant sites (metastasis), and eventually cause death. However, there are several exceptions to these generalizations. The rate of growth of malignant tumours correlates with their level of differentiation. Thus, there are wide variations. Some grow slowly, others rapidly. Most cancers take years, and in humans, even decades to become a clinically detectable lesion. Rapidly growing malignant tumours often contain **central mass of ischaemic necrosis**. This is because the blood supply fails to keep pace with the oxygen requirements of the expanding mass of cells.

3. Local Invasion

A benign tumour remains localized at its site of origin. It does not have the capacity to infiltrate, invade, or metastasize to distant sites, as do cancers. As benign tumours (fibromas, adenomas) slowly expand, **most develop an enclosing fibrous capsule** that separates them from the host tissue. This capsule is derived from the stroma (supporting framework) of the native tissue, following atrophy of the parenchymal cells under the pressure of the expanding tumour. **However, not all benign tumours are encapsulated.** Thus, whereas, presence of capsule means that the tumour is benign, its absence does not imply that a tumour is malignant.

Malignant tumours (cancers) grow by progressive infiltration, invasion, destruction, and penetration of the surrounding tissue. They do not develop capsules. Sometimes a slowly growing malignant tumour appears to be enclosed by the stroma of the surrounding tissue, but microscopic examination shows **tiny, crab-like feet penetrating the margin** and infiltrating the neighbouring structures. This **invasion** occurs along anatomical planes of cleavage, that is, the path of least resistance. **Next to metastasis, local invasiveness is the most important feature that distinguishes malignant from benign tumours.**

Although all tissues in the body can be involved by malignant tumours, there are differences in their susceptibility. The connective tissue stroma of the organ is the common path. Within the connective tissue, elastic fibres are much more resistant than collagen fibres. **This is due to a greater content of collagenase than elastase in malignant tumours.** However, dense collagen present in membranes, tendons, and joint capsules resists invasion. Muscle is not a suitable medium

285

for the growth of most tumour cells. Cartilage is the most resistant of all tissues to invasion.

4. Metastasis

Metastasis means development of **secondary growths (metastases)**. These are not continuous with the primary tumour, but develop in the remote tissues. The spread of malignant cells from one part of the body to another, through the blood vessels or lymphatics (as an embolus), is called **metastasis**. The secondary growths so formed in distant organs or tissues are called **metastases**. The term **metastasize** is verb, and the term **metastatic** adjective. **The property of metastasis is the most characteristic feature of malignant tumours, than any other attribute.** However, not all cancers have the same ability to metastasize. For example, basal cell carcinomas of the skin and most primary tumours of the central nervous system are highly invasive in their sites of origin, **but rarely metastasize.** On the other hand, osteogenic (bone) sarcomas have usually metastasized to lungs, at the time of their first detection.

In general, the more anaplastic and larger the primary tumour, the more likely is the metastatic spread. However, there are exceptions. Extremely small cancers have been known to metastasize, whereas some large lesions may not spread.

Pathways of Spread

Malignant tumours spread by one of the three pathways: (1) haematogenous spread, (2) lymphatic spread, and (3) seeding within body cavities. **(1) Haematogenous spread:** This is the **favoured pathway for sarcomas**, but is also used by carcinomas. **Arteries are more resistant to invasion than veins and lymphatics.** This is not only due to thickness of the arterial walls, but also due to **elastin** content of the arterial walls and their secretion of **protease inhibitors**. Once in veins, the tumour cells follow the venous flow draining the site of the neoplasm. Most tumour cells lodge in the **capillaries. The lungs and liver are the most commonly involved secondary sites in such haematogenous spread.** All caval blood flows to the lungs, and all portal area drainage flows to the liver. **(2) Lymphatic spread:** This is the **favoured pathway for carcinomas**, just as haematogenous route is for sarcomas. However, as there are numerous inter-connections between the lymphatic and vascular systems, all forms of cancer may spread through either or both systems. Lymphatic spread invariably involves the regional lymph nodes. Here, the reduced diameter of the sinuses serves as a filter, and retains the metastatic cells. However, enlargement of regional lymph nodes may not always mean cancerous involvement. The necrotic products of neoplasm and tumour antigens (see 'tumour antigens'), usually produce reactive changes in the lymph nodes, such as enlargement and hyperplasia of the follicles (lymphadenitis) and proliferation of macrophages in the subcapsular sinuses (sinus histiocytosis). **3. Seeding within body cavities:** Seeding of malignant tumours (**transplantation, implantation**), is the transfer of tumour cells from one serous or mucous surface to another **by direct contact**. Seeding of malignant tumour occurs when they invade a body cavity. Peritoneum is the most commonly involved, but any other cavity, namely, pleural, pericardial, subarachnoid, and joint spaces may be affected. This method of spread is particularly characteristic of **cancers of ovary** (adenocarcinoma), which often cover the peritoneal surfaces widely. Another example of seeding is the **venereal granuloma in the dog**, where tumour cells are spread by coitus. **Neoplasms of the central nervous system** such as **ependymoma**, may penetrate the cerebral ventricles and are carried by the cerebrospinal fluid to re-implant on the meningeal surfaces either in the brain or spinal cord.

Table 13 summarizes the differences between benign and malignant neoplasms.

Table 13. Comparison of benign and malignant neoplasms

Benign	Malignant
Macroscopic comparison	
1. They occur singly. Since benign tumours do not spread, only a single original tumour is found.	1. These may appear as single or multiple tumours. This is on account of metastases.
2. The shape is round, elliptical, wart-like, or pedunculated. Since the tumour grows slowly, pressure is equal in all directions. Therefore, tumour tends to be round or elliptical. On epithelial or mucous surface, it grows as a pedunculated, or wart-like mass.	2. The shape is irregular. This is because the tumour grows rapidly, and extends in all directions.
3. Encapsulation is present.	3. Encapsulation is not present.
4. The rate of growth is slow.	4. The rate of growth is rapid.

287

5. Degenerative and necrotic changes within the tumour are slight. Since the tumour grows slowly, the blood vessels within the tumour are able to meet the requirements.

5. Degenerative and necrotic changes within the tumour are extensive. Because the tumour grows rapidly, the blood vessels are not able to meet the requirements. As a result, portions of the tumour undergo degeneration and necrosis. In addition, the infiltrating tumour may invade its own vessels, whose thrombosis and occlusion further result in necrosis.

6. Removal is not difficult. This is due to encapsulation, and lack of local invasion.

6. Removal of the tumour is difficult. This is on account of local invasion and metastasis, and also lack of encapsulation.

7. The tumour is not toxic to the patient. This is because the degenerative and necrotic changes that liberate toxic materials do not occur.

7. The tumour is toxic to the patient. This is due to extensive degeneration and necrosis. The toxic products absorbed are extremely harmful.

8. Metastases are lacking.

8. Infiltration, metastasis, and transplantation are present.

9. There is no recurrence of the tumour.

9. The tumour tends to recur after apparent removal.

10. Death of the individual does not occur.

10. Death of the individual occurs. This is on account of local invasion, metastasis, and tissue destruction.

Microscopic comparison

1. The morphology of the tumour is approximately normal in relation to adjacent tissues.

1. The morphology of the tumour is abnormal in relation to adjacent tissues.

2. The tumour shows minimal evidence of anaplasia, and generally appears mature. Mitotic figures are few in number, and may not be seen.

2. The tumour shows marked evidence of anaplasia and lack of maturity of cells. Mitotic figures are present and may be abundant.

3.	The tumour is confined by adjacent tissues. It does not extend beyond the basement membrane, or the basal layer of cells.	3.	The tumour is not confined by adjacent tissues. The tumour extends beyond the basement membrane, or the basal layer of cells.
4.	The tumour does not penetrate, or infiltrate connective tissue capsule.	4.	The neoplasm penetrates or infiltrates through any connective tissue capsule.
5.	The tumour does not grow beyond the blood supply.	5.	The tumour grows beyond the blood supply.
6.	Degenerative and necrotic changes within the tumour are slight.	6.	Degenerative and necrotic changes within the tumour are extensive.
7.	There is no invasion of blood vessels or lymphatics.	7.	Invasion of the blood vessels and lymphatics occurs.

Aetiology of Cancer

The factors associated with the aetiology (causation) of neoplasms can be divided into two main groups: (1) **the intrinsic factors**, and (2) **the extrinsic factors**.

Intrinsic (Predisposing) Factors

1. Heredity: A tremendous amount of work has been done in the field of genetics in relation to neoplasia. Strains of mice unusually susceptible or resistant to tumours have been produced. All these investigations have clearly established that, at least in some species of animals, heredity plays an important role in the appearance of a neoplasm. In the chicken, strains of birds have been produced that have considerable resistance to the lymphoid leukosis virus, and the incidence of leukosis has been greatly reduced. However, it is difficult to apply the results of mice and chicken experiments to the larger domestic animals. Moreover, the fundamental basis for decreased and increased susceptibility is not known.

The **human studies** have revealed that hereditary predisposition undoubtedly exists, an example being breast cancer. The first-degree relatives of breast cancer patients are at markedly increased risk. The evidence is strong that carcinogenesis (production of cancer) involves mutations in the genome. One or more such mutations may be inherited in this germ line. Such individuals are then more predisposed to cancers than, others. Thus, familial predisposition has been noted with common neoplasms such as carcinoma of the breast, colon, ovary, prostate, and uterus, and with melanocarcinomas. **In mice,** high cancer strains can be produced by genetic inbreeding. However, there is no understanding how the factors operate in the induction of neoplasm. Again, in humans, a great predisposition to lung cancer has been suggested. Other examples include childhood retinoblastoma and familial adenomatous polyposis syndrome. However, attempts at defining markers of genetic susceptibility have been unsuccessful. Information on these aspects in domestic animals is, at present, lacking.

2. Age: In general, the frequency of cancer increases with age. The rising incidence with age may be due to the accumulation of somatic mutations over a period of time that are needed for the development of cancer. The decline in immune competence that accompanies aging may also be a factor. The type of tumour varies somewhat with the age of the individual. **Sarcomas** (malignant tumours of connective tissue) are more frequently observed in younger individuals, while **carcinomas** (malignant tumours of epithelial tissue) are found in older animals.

3. Pigmentation: Colour is a factor in white-skinned animals. Examples: In white and grey horses, melanosarcomas are more common; in Hereford cattle squamous-cell carcinoma of the eye is more common.

4. Sex: Tumours occur in both males and females. However, there is a difference between the male and the female in the incidence of tumours in genital organs.

5. Tumour immunity: Both cell-mediated and humoral immunity have anti-tumour activity. This topic is discussed later under 'Host defence against tumours: tumour immunity'.

Extrinsic Factors

Genetic damage lies at the centre of carcinogenesis, that is, production of cancer. But what agents cause such damage? A large number of external agents have been shown to induce neoplastic transformation of cells *in vitro*, and cancers in experimental animals. These are known as **carcinogenic agents**, and fall into six categories: (1) chemicals, (2) radiant energy, (3) chronic irritation, (4) hormones, (5) parasites, and (6) oncogenic viruses. It is important to note that several agents may act together, or sequentially, to produce many genetic abnormalities characteristic of neoplastic cells.

Chemical Carcinogens

The London surgeon **Sir Percival Pott** was the first to point out that chemical agents could be carcinogenic. More than 200 years ago (1775), he correctly attributed scrotal skin cancer in the chimney sweeps (persons who clean chimneys) to chronic exposure of soot. In 1915, **Yamagiwa** and **Ichikawa** induced cancer in a rabbit's ear with repeated application of **coal tar**. Subsequently, **Kennaway and Cook** extracted 50 grams of chemically pure carcinogen 3, 4- benzapyrene, from **two tons of crude tar**. These pioneering observations demonstrated the carcinogenicity of chemicals (polycyclic aromatic hydrocarbons). **Since then hundreds of chemicals have been shown to be carcinogenic in animals**.

It is clear that the industrial age has increased the hazards in our environment. Those individuals employed in gas-production, tar, and pitch plants; in industries in which coal by-products are in abundance; men working with petroleum products; in operations associated with the production and fractionation of tar; and road workers using tars, all these workers show a high incidence of tumours. Paraffins (wax) with impurities; oils sprayed for the control of mosquitoes; creosote; anthracene, a product obtained from tar and used in the production of grease and diesel engine fuel; chlorinated naphthalene; the aniline dyes such as butter yellow; colouring matter used in pastries, candies, fruit juices, fruit preservatives, butter, dyes, cosmetics and deodorants; dyes used in the clothing industry; chronic irritation from smoking tobacco, large amounts of alcohol consumption; chewing of betel nuts, lime, and tobacco; plastics such as cellophane, Dacron, nylon, polystyrene, polyethene and others - all have been, in some way or the other, implicated with tumours.

Chemical carcinogens are of different kinds, and include both natural and synthetic products (Table 14). They **fall into two categories: (1) direct-acting agents**. They do not require chemical transformation for producing cancer, and (2) **indirect-acting agents**. These become active only after metabolic conversion. Such agents are referred to as **'procarcinogens'**, and their active end products are called **'ultimate carcinogens'**. **Majority of the chemical carcinogens are indirect-acting**.

291

Table 14. Major chemical carcinogens

1. **Direct-acting carcinogens**

   Alkylating agents

   Anti-cancer drugs (cyclophosphamide, chlorambucil, nitrosoureas)

2. **Indirect-acting carcinogens** (procarcinogens that require metabolic activation)

   (i) **Polycyclic and heterocyclic aromatic hydrocarbons**

   Benzanthracene

   Benzapyrene

   Dibenzanthracene

   3-Methylcholanthrene

   7, 12-Dimethylbenzanthracene

   (ii) **Aromatic amines, amides, azo dyes**

   Benzidine

   2-Naphthylamine (beta-naphthylamine)

   2-Acetylaminofluorene

   Butter yellow

   (iii) **Natural plant and microbial products**

   Aflatoxin B1

   Griseofulvin

   Betel nuts

   (iv) **Miscellaneous agents**

   Asbestos

   Arsenic

   Chromium, nickel, vinyl chloride

   Insecticides, fungicides

   Nitrosamines and amides

1. Direct-Acting Agents

These substances **require no metabolic conversion to become carcinogenic. They are**, in general, **weak carcinogens**. All the same, they are important because some of them are cancer chemotherapeutic drugs (cyclophosphamide, chlorambucil, nitrosoureas) that have successfully cured, controlled, or delayed recurrence of certain types of cancers. But, unfortunately, later on they produce a second form of cancer, usually leukaemia.

2. Indirect-Acting Agents

Polycyclic aromatic hydrocarbons: These chemicals require metabolic conversion before they are active. They represent some of the most potent carcinogens, such as benzanthacene, benzapyrene, methylcholanthrene and others (Table 14). When painted on the skin, benzanthracene causes skin cancers; when injected subcutaneously, it induces fibrosarcomas. Brain tumours can easily be produced in experimental animals by injecting dibenzanthracene and methylcholanthrene. The polycyclic hydrocarbons are of particular interest because benzapyrene and other carcinogens are produced in the combustion of tobacco in cigarette smoking, and are involved in the causation of lung cancer in cigarette smokers. They are also produced from animal fats in the process of broiling meats, and are present in smoked meats and fish. Over 1200 substances have been counted in cigarette smoke. They include both **initiators** (polycyclic aromatic hydrocarbons, such as benzapyrene) and **promoters** (such as phenol derivatives).

Aromatic amines and azo dyes: These are important in humans. Before it became known that **beta-naphthylamine** was carcinogenic, in the past, it caused 50-fold increased incidence of bladder cancers in workers heavily exposed to the aniline dye and rubber industries. Some of the **azo dyes** were developed to colour food, for example, butter-yellow to colour margarine and scarlet-red for cherries.

Natural plant and microbial products (naturally occurring carcinogens): Among the several known chemical carcinogens produced by plants and microorganisms, **aflatoxin B1**, the **hepatic carcinogen**, is the most important. It is produced by some strains of *Aspergillus flavus*, a mould that grows on improperly stored grains and groundnuts. There is a strong correlation between the dietary level of **aflatoxin B1** and the incidence of liver cancer (hepatocellular carcinoma) in humans. It is believed that aflatoxin and hepatitis B virus may act together to produce hepatic cancers, in humans.

Miscellaneous agents: A large number of other chemicals have been implicated as carcinogens. Exposure to **asbestos** has been associated with an increased incidence of lung (bronchogenic carcinoma) and gastrointestinal cancers, in both humans and animals. Skin cancer associated with **arsenic**, in both animals and humans, is also well established. **Chromium, nickel**, and other metals, when inhaled have caused cancer of the lung. Many **insecticides**, such as aldrin, dieldrin, and chlordane and **fungicides** are carcinogenic in animals. **Nitrosamines** and **nitrosamides** are important because they can be formed in the acidic environment of the stomach in humans, and have been implicated in gastric carcinoma. **Saccharin** and **cyclamates** have been found carcinogenic in experimental animals. However, their role in human carcinogenesis remains in doubt.

Steps Involved in Chemical Carcinogenesis

Carcinogenesis, that is, production of cancer, is a multi-step process. From the work carried out in experimental animals (mainly mouse), **chemical carcinogenesis** can be divided into two stages: (1) **initiation**, and (2) **promotion**. The following concepts have emerged from these experiments:

1. **Initiation** results from exposure of cells to a carcinogen (polycyclic hydrocarbons - initiator) (Fig. 47). An initiated cell is an altered cell and can give rise to a tumour. **However, initiation alone is not enough for tumour formation.**

2. **Initiation causes permanent DNA damage (mutations).** It is therefore rapid and irreversible and has **'memory'**.

3. **Promoters can induce tumours in initiated cells, but they are not tumour-producing by themselves.** Moreover, tumours do not occur when the promoting agent (e.g., croton oil) is applied before, rather than after, the initiating agent. This indicated that **in contrast to initiators, the cellular changes resulting from the application of promoters do not affect DNA directly and are reversible.**

Mechanisms of Chemical Carcinogenesis

Initiation of carcinogenesis: As already stated, **direct-acting chemical carcinogens** do not require chemical transformation for cancer production. On the other hand, **indirect-acting agents (pro-carcinogens)** require metabolic conversion to produce 'ultimate carcinogens' capable of transforming cells. **All direct-acting and ultimate carcinogens are highly reactive electrophiles, that is, they have electron-deficient atoms that can react with nucleophilic (electron-rich) sites in the cell.** These reactions result in the formation of 'addition products' between chemical carcinogen and a nucleotide in DNA (Fig. 47). The electrophilic reactions may attack several electron-rich sites in the target cells, including DNA, RNA, and proteins. Sometimes they produce lethal damage (Fig. 47). In initiated cells, the interaction is non-lethal and DNA is the primary target.

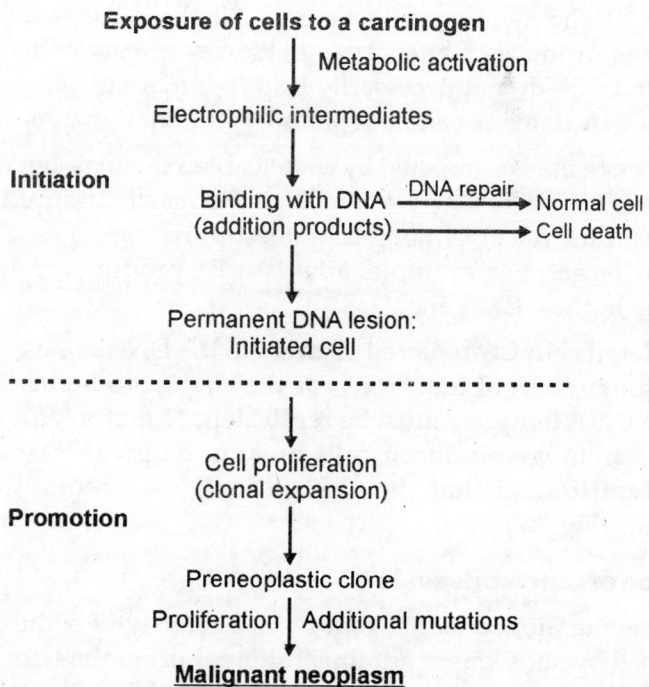

Exposure of cells to a carcinogen

⬇ Metabolic activation

Electrophilic intermediates

Initiation

Binding with DNA ──DNA repair──▶ Normal cell
(addition products) ──────────▶ Cell death

Permanent DNA lesion:
Initiated cell

Cell proliferation
(clonal expansion)

Promotion

Preneoplastic clone

Proliferation │ Additional mutations

Malignant neoplasm

Fig. 47. Events in chemical carcinogenesis.

Metabolic activation of carcinogens: Most of the known chemical carcinogens are metabolized by **cytochrome P-450-dependent monooxygenases.** The genes that encode these enzymes are polymorphic (occur in many forms). Because these enzymes are essential for the activation of pro-carcinogens, the susceptibility to carcinogenesis is regulated in part by **polymorphism** in the genes that encode these enzymes.

Molecular targets of chemical carcinogens: Malignant transformation results from **mutations** that affect oncogenes, cancer-suppressor genes, and genes that regulate apoptosis. Therefore, majority of the initiating chemicals are mutagenic (i.e., induce mutations). Their mutagenic potential is investigated by **Ames test**. This test uses the ability of a chemical to induce mutations in the bacterium *Salmonella typhimurium*. Up to 90% of known chemical carcinogens score positive in the Ames test.

That DNA is the primary target for chemical carcinogens is now well established. But there is no single change that is associated with initiation of chemical carcinogenesis. All the same, each class of carcinogens produces DNA damage. However, carcinogen-induced changes in DNA do not necessarily lead to initiation, because several forms of DNA damage can be repaired by cellular enzymes (Fig. 47).

Any gene may be targeted by chemical carcinogens, but mutations in *ras* genes are particularly common in chemically induced tumours in rodents (rats, mice). Among tumour-suppressor genes, *TP53* is an important target. For example, aflatoxin B1 produces characteristic mutations in the *TP53* gene.

Initiated cell: Un-repaired changes in the DNA are essential first steps in the process of initiation. **For the change to be heritable, the damaged DNA template must be replicated. Therefore, for initiation to occur, carcinogen-induced cells must undergo at least one cycle of proliferation, so that the change in DNA becomes fixed, or permanent** (Fig. 47).

Promotion of Carcinogenesis

It was mentioned earlier that carcinogenicity of some chemicals is increased by subsequent administration of **promoters**, for example, phorbol esters, hormones, phenols, and drugs. **These by themselves are not carcinogenic (tumourigenic).** They are not electrophilic (electron-deficient) compounds, and they do not damage the DNA. To be effective these promoters must be applied **after** application of the carcinogenic chemical, which acts as an **'initiator'.** That is, their repeated or sustained exposure must **follow** the application of initiator. **This initiation-promotion sequence is important in chemical carcinogenesis** (Fig. 47). Some chemicals possess the capability of both initiation and promotion. They induce tumours without any added factors. They are called **'complete carcinogens'**, to differentiate them from **'incomplete carcinogens'**, which are capable of only initiation.

Since promoters are not themselves mutagenic, how do they contribute to cancer production (tumourigenesis)? Studies with TPA, a phorbol ester and the best-studied tumour promoter, have revealed that it activates **protein kinase C (PKC)** (see 'chemotaxis'). PKC is an enzyme of several signal transduction pathways, including those initiated by growth factors (see Chapter 5).

No single genetic damage is enough for neoplastic transformation. While the application of initiator may cause mutational activation of an oncogene, (such as *ras*), it can only give rise to a preneoplastic or hyperplastic lesion. Subsequent application of promoters causes proliferation and clonal expansion of initiated (mutated) cells (Fig. 47). **Initiated cells respond differently to promoters than normal cells**, and therefore expand selectively. Such cells require less amount of growth factor and are also less responsive to growth initiator signals. Thus, forced to proliferate, the initiated clone (group) of cells suffers more mutations, **developing ultimately into a malignant neoplasm** (Fig. 47).

It is emphasized that carcinogen-induced damage to DNA does not necessarily lead to initiation of cancer. Several forms of DNA damage are repaired by cellular enzymes. Defects of DNA repair lead to increased risk of cancers. Examples include a greatly increased risk of cancers caused by ultraviolet light and certain chemicals.

Radiation Carcinogenesis

Radiation, whatever its source, ultraviolet (UV) rays of sunlight, x-rays, nuclear fission, radionuclides (i.e., radioactive nuclides. A nuclide is a species of atom.), **is an established carcinogen**. Examples: certain parts of USA, Africa and Australia have an extremely high incidence of skin cancer in **cattle** due to the effect of solar (sun) radiation. In particular, it causes ocular and periocular squamous-cell carcinoma in white-faced Hereford cattle, due to lack of protective pigmentation in the eyelid. Likewise, carcinoma of the skin, following solar radiation, is observed in light-coloured Australian cattle that have developed photosensitization after eating certain plants. **In humans**, x-ray (roentgen ray) workers may develop skin cancers; exposure to sunlight (UV rays) in persons with fair skin can lead to skin cancer; correlation between nuclear fission and leukaemia; and, even therapeutic irradiation has been found to be carcinogenic. **Thus, it is clear that radiation is strongly oncogenic.**

The oncogenic effect of ultraviolet (UV) rays highlights the importance of DNA repair in carcinogenesis. Natural UV radiation derived from the sun can cause skin cancers. UV light has several biological effects on cells. Of particular importance in carcinogenesis is the **ability of UV light to damage DNA by forming pyrimidine dimers. In normal persons, the altered DNA is repaired by a series of repair enzymes**. But in a small group of disorders, one or more of the DNA repair enzymes are defective or deficient. Patients with such diseases have greatly increased predisposition to skin cancers, predominantly in the sun-exposed areas of the skin. **UV light causes mutation in the *TP53* gene.**

Mechanisms of Radiation Carcinogenesis

Electromagnetic (x-rays, gamma rays) and particulate (alpha particles, beta particles, protons, neutrons) radiations are all carcinogenic. However, the precise event responsible for neoplastic transformation is still unknown. Radiant energy causes chromosomal breakage, translocations, and point mutations. It also alters proteins, inactivates enzymes, and injures membranes. **Two theories** dominate the mechanism of action: (1) **Direct theory**: The radiation directly ionizes critical cellular components, and (2) **Indirect theory**: It first reacts with water or molecular oxygen to produce free radicals (see 'free radicals') that mediate the damage. Through either pathway, the DNA is damaged inducing a somatic mutation. The mutagenic effect of ionizing radiation is well established.

Like chemical carcinogens, ionizing radiation is known to activate *ras* genes and inactivate tumour suppressor genes. **Thus, the mutagenesis-carcinogenesis sequence takes place.** Since the latent period of irradiation-induced cancer is very long, it is thought that cancer appears only after the progeny of initially damaged cells acquire **additional mutations**, induced by other environmental factors.

Chronic Irritation

It was long observed that the incidence of squamous-cell carcinoma was higher in scars resulting from severe burns, branding of cattle, and other injuries, than in normal skin. **Burns often resulted in skin tumours.** It was observed that among the people of Kashmir, carcinoma of the skin of abdomen was frequent, but almost unknown in other races and nationalities. These people had a habit of carrying a pot filled with hot coals under their clothes during the winter to keep them warm. These warming pans rested on the anterior belly wall. Frequent burning of the abdominal wall occurred, and after a period of years a skin tumour developed at the site. Similarly, the incidence of cutaneous neoplasms on the feet and legs appears to be much higher among bare-foot people than those whose feet are clad. Carcinomas of the mouth are very common in the natives of the Orient, particularly India and the Philippines, who chew the betel nut obtained from the betel palm.

Although the concept of chronic irritation in the past came to occupy a prominent place for many years, **the present view is to discount ordinary physical injury as a cause of neoplasm.**

Hormones

Administration of massive doses of the **oestrogenic hormones in the mice** induces neoplastic growth of the interstitial cells in the **testes. High oestrogen levels** associated with retention of milk in the mammary gland produce **mammary tumours in mice.** The **dog** has a very high incidence of **mammary tumours** associated with disturbances of hormone balance. Drugs such as stilbestrol (synthetic oestrogen) are established carcinogenic agents in animals.

There is a similarity in the structural formulas of the carcinogenic hydrocarbons, such as benzanthracene and cholanthrene, to those of certain hormones produced in the body, particularly oestrogens, progesterone, testosterone, and corticosteroids. This led to the belief that disordered metabolism of these hormones may result in their transformation into carcinogenic compounds. **However, there is no real evidence that this happens.**

In humans, endogenous oestrogen excess, or more accurately, hormonal imbalance, clearly plays a significant role in the production of breast cancer (carcinoma). Functioning ovarian tumours that secrete oestrogen are associated with breast cancer in post-menopausal women. Also prolonged post-menopausal oestrogen therapy in women moderately increases the risk of breast cancer. In one Swedish study a two-fold increase in breast cancer was observed in those who took synthetic oestrogen oestradiol. The effect of adding progesterone to oestrogen on the risk of breast cancer was also recorded. Recent studies have revealed that the normal breast epithelium possesses oestrogen and progesterone receptors. These are also often present in breast cancer cells. A variety of growth factors, namely, TGF-alpha, PDGF, and FGF (see 'growth factors', Chapter 5) are secreted by human breast cancer cells. Moreover, oestrogen stimulates the production of growth factors in both normal breast epithelial cells and cancer cells. It is therefore thought that the oestrogen and progesterone receptors normally present in breast epithelium, and often present in breast cancer cells, may interact with growth factors (that act as growth promoters), to create an autocrine mechanism of tumour development. (In an autocrine mechanism cells respond to the signalling substances that they themselves secrete).

Again, in human, uterine leiomyomas (fibroids) are thought to be caused by excessive oestrogenic stimulation. Similarly, carcinoma of the endometrium is also influenced by increased or prolonged oestrogen stimulation. Any such information to explain mammary tumours in domestic animals is, at present, lacking.

Parasites

Parasites, by causing chronic irritation, may lead to neoplasia. Examples: A small nematode *Gongylonema neoplasticum* may cause carcinoma of the gastric mucosa in the rat; *Cysticercus fasciolaris*, the larval stage of the cat tapeworm *Taenia taeniaeformis* developing in the rat liver, may cause sarcomas; in the dog, a nematode *Spirocerca lupi* invades the wall of the lower oesophagus and may produce fibrosarcomas or osteosarcomas. Following its migration, it may also produce fibrosarcomas in the wall of the aorta. A number of them have also been reported as metastasizing to the lungs. Gastric adenomas are found in horses and mules when nematode *Habronema megastoma* (stomach worm) is present. *Eimeria stiedae* invasion of the liver of the rabbit results in multiple adenomas of the bile ducts. In humans, a nematode *Schistosoma haematobium* has been considered a cause of carcinoma of the human bladder. Thus, the occurrence of neoplasia in animals from parasites appears to be established. However, it is not known whether the carcinogenic effect is physical or chemical.

Viral Oncogenesis (Oncogenic Viruses)

Since the subject of viral oncogenesis is complex, only the basic principles are presented, giving special emphasis to the mechanism of action of oncogenic (tumour-causing) viruses in animals.

As early as 1876, Novinsky successfully transplanted venereal granuloma (transmissible histiosarcoma) from one dog to another dog. Since 1908, it has been shown that extracts of animal tumours, free of cells and bacteria, were capable of inducing new tumours upon injection into a susceptible host. Ellerman and Bang were the first (1908) to give a demonstration of an oncogenic virus in avian leukosis. In 1910, Rous produced similar results with fowl sarcoma, commonly known as Rous sarcoma. In 1933, Shope discovered that viruses were the aetiological agents of papillomas in rabbits. These demonstrations of viral-associated neoplasms have been followed over the years by many others (Table 15). The role of viruses in the causation of human

papilloma (benign warts) has also been established. Today, a large number of viruses have proved to be oncogenic in a wide variety of animals, ranging from birds and amphibian (frogs) to primates (monkeys and apes), indicating that some viruses can cause tumours in birds, invertebrates, and mammals. Further, the evidence is growing even stronger that certain viruses (e.g., human T-cell leukaemia virus type 1, Epstein-Barr virus, hepatitis B virus) are responsible for some forms of human cancer.

Table 15. Some virus-induced neoplasms

Year	Species	Neoplasm	Investigator
1908	Chicken	Fowl leukosis	Ellermann and Bang
1910	Chicken	Fowl sarcoma	Rous
1920	Cow	Bovine papilloma	Magalhaes
1932	Dog	Oral papilloma	DeMonbreun and Goodpasture
1932	Rabbit	Fibroma	Shope
1933	Rabbit	Cutaneous papilloma	Shope
1933	Chicken	Lymphomatosis, myelomatosis	Furth
1936	Mouse	Mammary adenocarcinoma	Bittner
1938	Frog	Renal adenocarcinoma	Lucke
1943	Rabbit	Oral papilloma	Parsons and Kidd
1951	Mouse	Malignant lymphoma	Gross
1953	Mouse	Tumour of parotid gland	Gross
1953	Squirrel	Fibroma	Kilham, Herman, and Fisher
1954	Goat	Cutaneous papilloma	Moulton
1955	Deer	Fibroma	Shope *et al.*
1957	Mouse, hamster	Polyoma	Stewart and Eddy
1964	Cat	Malignant lymphoma	Jarrett *et al.*
1964	Rodents	Sarcoma	Harvey
1966	Mouse	Osteosarcoma	Finkel, Biskis, and Jinkins
1967	Guinea pig	Malignant lymphoma	Opler
1967	Mouse	Leukaemia	Friend
1969	Simian primates	Malignant lymphoma	Melendez *et al.*
1969	Cat	Sarcoma	Snyder and Theilen
1971	Simian primates	Sarcoma	Theilen *et al.*

Oncogenic viruses fall into two classes: RNA viruses and DNA viruses (Table 16). **RNA oncogenic viruses** come under a single group called **Oncornaviruses**, also known as **Oncoviruses**, or more commonly as **Retroviruses**, whereas **DNA oncogenic viruses** include members of the genera **Papovavirus, Herpesvirus, Hepadnavirus,** and **Adenovirus** (Table 16).

Table 16. Some Important Oncogenic Viruses

Group/Genus	Virus	Host	Tumour formed
RNA Viruses (Retroviruses)			
1. Rapidly (or Acutely) Transforming Viruses			
Type B Oncovirus Group	Mouse mammary tumour virus	Mouse	Mammary adenocarcinoma
Type C Oncovirus Group	Feline sarcoma virus	Cat	Sarcoma
	Murine sarcoma virus	Mouse	Various sarcomas
	Rous sarcoma virus	Chicken	Sarcoma
Alpha-retroviruses (previously 'Avian type C oncornaviruses')	Avian sarcoma chicken virus	Chicken	Various sarcomas
	Reticuloendotheliosis virus	Chicken	Reticuloendotheliosis
2. Slowly (or Slow) Transforming Viruses			
Alpha-retroviruses (Previously 'Avian type C oncornaviruses')	Lymphoid leukosis and many of the avian leukosis viruses	Chicken	Various carcinomas, lymphomas, and leukaemias
Type C Oncovirus Group	Feline leukaemia virus	Cat	Leukaemias and lymphomas
	Bovine leukaemia virus	Cattle	Leukaemias and lymphomas
	Murine leukaemia virus	Mouse	Leukaemias
	Primate leukaemia virus	Monkey	Leukaemia in apes
Type D Oncovirus Group	Human T-cell leukaemia virus type 1	Human	T-cell leukaemia/ lymphoma

<u>DNA Viruses</u>

1. Papovaviruses

A. Polyomaviruses	**Polyomavirus muris**	Young mice, rats, guinea, pigs, rabbits, hamsters	Sarcomas and carcinomas
	Polyomavirus maccacae (**SV40**)	Young mice, hamsters	Sarcomas and lymphomas
B. Papillomaviruses	Bovine and other papilloma viruses (BPV)	Cattle; other mammals (horse, sheep, dog, rabbit)	Genital, alimentary and skin warts, oesophageal cancer
	Human papillomaviruses (HPV)	Human	Genital, laryngeal, and skin warts. *In situ* and invasive cancers of the vulva and uterine cervix
2. Herpesviruses	Marek's disease virus	Chicken	Neural lymphoma
	Epstein-Barr virus	Human	Burkitt (B- cell) lymphoma; nasopharyngeal carcinoma
3. Hepadnavirus	Hepatitis B virus	Human	Liver cancer
4. Adenoviruses	Certain serotypes	Experi- mentally in newborn mice, rats, hamsters	Sarcomas

RNA Oncogenic Viruses

All RNA oncogenic viruses are **retroviruses. That is, they contain the enzyme reverse transcriptase which allows reverse (L. retro = reverse) transcription of viral RNA into DNA**, the reverse of what occurs in most biological systems. To understand how retroviruses induce tumour formation, it would be better if we first examine the genomic structure of a retrovirus and review the steps involved in its replication.

The **genome of animal retroviruses** contains three sets of genes: *gag*, *pol*, and *env* (**Fig. 48**). The *gag* gene encodes **structural core proteins** and **protease**; the *pol* gene **reverse transcriptase** and **integrase**; and the *env* gene **envelope glycoproteins**. **All the three genes (*gag*, *pol* and *env*) are required for viral replication.** As shown in Fig. 48, these genes are flanked on the 5' and 3' ends of the genome by sequences of nucleotides referred to as **'long terminal repeats'** or **'LTRs'**. These LTRs contain the same sequences, but the left 5' LTR enhances and promotes transcription of the viral genome, whereas the right 3' LTR specifies the site of polyadenylation of the mRNA transcript, which prevents it from being rapidly destroyed in the cytoplasm. The **gag** (core protein) transcript contains a **protease**, whereas the **gag-pol** polyprotein is eventually split and processed to form **reverse transcriptase** and **integrase** required for integration of proviral DNA into host-cell DNA. These final processing events involving **gag** and **gag-pol** proteins are mediated by the virally encoded **protease** after the virions have been assembled.

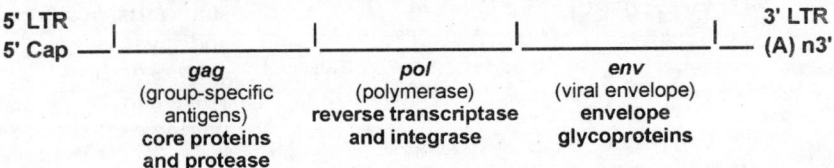

Fig. 48. Gene sequence of the proviral DNA of a standard replicatively competent retrovirus.

Replication of a retrovirus: The retrovirus genome consists of two identical strands of single-stranded, positive RNA. Briefly, replication of a retrovirus is as follows: Virus enters the cell through a receptor present on the cell membrane. Viral RNA is released in the cytoplasm and under the influence of **reverse transcriptase** a strand of **negative viral DNA** is synthesized on the template of viral RNA. Reverse transcription then synthesizes a complementary strand of **positive viral DNA**. Both the strands get covalently linked to produce **linear** double-stranded viral DNA called a **'provirus'** or **'proviral DNA'**. Proviral DNA then migrates to nucleus, and becomes integrated into the host-cell DNA under the influence of an enzyme **'integrase'** encoded by *pol* gene of the virus. The proviral genes (proviral DNA) are integrated in the same order as their RNA copies in the virion (*gag, pol, env*) and are flanked on either side by exactly similar sequences of nucleotides called **'long terminal repeats (LTR)'** (see **Fig. 49**) (discussed next).

Formation of new virions (virus particles) is the result of transcription and translation of proviral DNA. After integration, the proviral DNA is transcribed by the cell's own machinery to form viral messenger RNA (mRNA) and genomic RNA. The genomic RNA is incorporated into new virions. The mRNAs are translated to produce the protein and enzyme products of the *gag, pol,* and *env* genes that form the **'virion'.** The virion (virus) then comes out of the cell by budding, and thus the viral life cycle is completed. The **envelope** is acquired while budding through the cell membrane.

Mechanism of Action of RNA Oncogenic Viruses

Studies on oncogenic retroviruses in animals have provided remarkable insights in recent years into the genetic basis of cancer. **Animal retroviruses transform cells by two mechanisms.** Some, called **rapidly or acutely transforming viruses** contain a transforming **viral oncogene (v-*onc*).** Others, called **slowly transforming viruses, do not contain a viral oncogene,** but the proviral DNA is **always** inserted near a cellular oncogene. Under the influence of a strong retroviral promoter, the adjacent normal or mutated cellular oncogene is over-expressed. This mechanism of transformation is called **'insertional mutagenesis'.** But before we discuss these two mechanisms, in some detail, let us first understand the **differences between a proto-oncogene, an oncogene, and a viral oncogene.**

Those genes involved in **normal cell division,** that is, in the normal growth control pathways, are called **proto-oncogene.** As discussed under tissue repair (Chapter 5), expression of these genes is tightly regulated during normal regeneration and repair. Alteration in the structure and expression of proto-oncogene can convert them into **oncogenes,** which cause uncontrolled cell growth characteristic of cancer. In other words, when a mutated proto-oncogene results in neoplastic transformation, the affected gene is referred as an **'oncogene'.** The name **'proto-oncogene'** derives from the fact that they represent the cellular precursors of **'viral oncogenes'. Let us understand this.**

DNA hybridization studies have revealed that the **viral oncogene** sequences are the same found in the normal DNA of all cells in all species. These normal genes, as stated, are referred to as **proto-oncogenes** because they were the **first** to evolve in nature (Greek proto = first) and have the potential to induce tumour when they are converted to **oncogene** (Greek **onco** = tumour, thus **oncogene** = tumour-producing gene), hence the name **proto-oncogene.** It is now believed that **viral oncogenes** (v-*oncs*) are not viral genes at all. **They** are, in fact, copies of the proto-oncogenes that got incorporated (transduced) into the viral genome during the process of viral replication in a normal cell, at some earlier time in evolution of the virus. Thus, v-*oncs* are mere travellers in the viral genome, imparting virus the ability to transform cells, **at the expense of the ability to replicate. That is, such retroviruses are unable to replicate (replication-defective).** The conservation of proto-oncogenes throughout evolution in all species in the biological kingdom suggests that they play essential roles in cell differentiation. **Proto-oncogenes** are cellular genes, which **are not oncogenic** in the physiological state, but as stated, on alteration in their structure or expression can give rise to cancer-causing **oncogenes.** This occurs when proto-oncogenes are incorporated into rapidly (acutely) transforming retroviruses, giving rise to **viral oncogenes,** as described above.

With this background, we can now discuss the mechanisms involved in retroviral oncogenesis. **Oncogenic retroviruses** can be divided into **two distinct types, based on the efficiency and rapidity with which they transform cells.** These are: **(1) rapidly or acutely transforming retroviruses,** and **(2) slowly transforming retroviruses.** Each category represents a different mechanism. **However, both the mechanisms are involved in tumour transformation by avian retroviruses.**

Rapidly or Acutely Transforming Viruses

These viruses produce tumours rapidly within a few days or weeks. They are responsible for naturally occurring tumours of animals (see Table 16). Each virus in this group carries a **viral oncogene (v-oncogene)** in its genome, which was acquired originally from a host-cell proto-oncogene by recombinant events at some earlier time in evolution of the virus. There are about 30 known retrovirus oncogenes that have genetic similarity with avian and mammalian proto-oncogenes. **All oncogene-containing retroviruses, except that of Rous sarcoma, are 'defective' in replication** (Fig. 49A). This is because they have acquired the oncogene **at the expense of all, or a portion of one of the three genes (*gag, pol, env*),** essential for viral replication (Fig. 49B). **Therefore, these defective viruses require a helper virus to replicate.** The helper retrovirus, when it infects a cell containing a defective retroviral gene, provides the missing gene product needed for the defective oncogenic retrovirus to replicate. **Rous sarcoma virus is the only rapidly transforming retrovirus that is not defective. It contains all the three genes (*gag, pol, env*)**

306

required for replication of the virus, plus a viral oncogene known as v-*onc* (sarcoma) (Fig. 49A).

The transforming capacity of the rapidly transforming retroviruses does not depend on the proviral DNA integrating at a specific site within the host-cell DNA, **as occurs in the case of slowly transforming retroviruses** (Fig. 49C). **In fact, every cell that is infected with a rapidly transforming virus becomes transformed.** This is because transcription of the integrated proviral DNA is under the control of left LTR of the provirus, **and not the host-cell regulatory genes.** As a result, transcription of the viral genome occurs **more or less continuously** in the infected cell with the accumulation of large quantities of viral oncogene product within the cell. For example, the *v-src* gene of Rous sarcoma virus encodes a transformation-specific phosphoprotein, **p60**, in the infected cell with protein kinase activity. Morphological change associated with high levels of p60 is believed

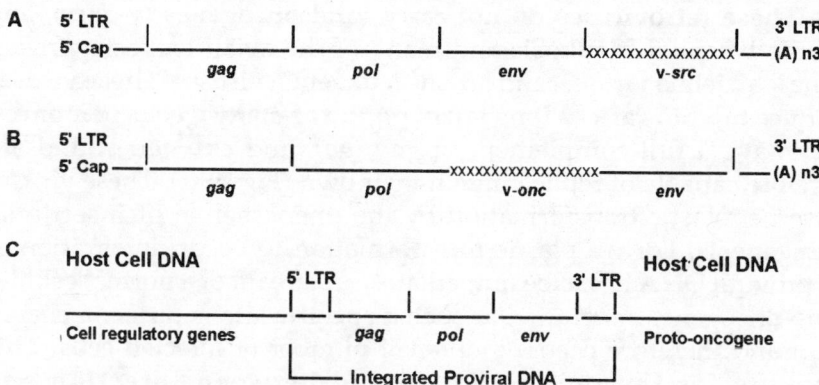

Fig. 49. Diagram showing proviral genome of rapidly transforming and slowly transforming retroviruses. **A.** Genomic organization of **Rous sarcoma virus**. This is the only replicatively competent rapidly transforming retrovirus (i.e., non-defective). Note that **the virus has all the three genes** (*gag, pol, env*), but in addition it has acquired the **oncogene v-src**, derived from the proto-oncogene *src*. **B.** Genomic organization of **a typical 'defective' rapidly transforming retrovirus**. These viruses have acquired a v-oncogene from proto-oncogene, but in doing so **they have lost a portion of *pol*** and ***env* genes** which are required for viral replication. **C.** The diagram shows **integration of the proviral DNA of a slowly transforming retrovirus into the host cell DNA**. Note that the proviral DNA is inserted at a site between a normal cell proto-oncogene and its regulatory sequences. This results in the proto-oncogene coming under the control of the promoting and enhancing sequences of the 3'LTR of the virus. **This results in unregulated production of the proto-oncogene product and malignant transformation.**

to be responsible for the transformed state. The **v-*onc*** genes associated with other rapidly transforming viruses encode other transformation-associated proteins.

There are no negative feedback mechanisms that control v-oncogene expression, as they are in the case of proto-oncogene expression in normal cells. The uncontrolled synthesis of viral oncoprotein causes infected cells **to divide continuously and become immortalized.** Because many cells in a host animal are transformed soon after infection, the tumours caused by this group of viruses are **polyclonal in origin** (i.e., derived from many cells). This means that the proviral DNA is integrated **at random sites** within the host-cell DNA in the population of cells making up the neoplasm. **This is in marked contrast to what is found in cells transformed by slowly transforming retroviruses.**

Slowly Transforming Retroviruses

These retroviruses do not carry viral oncogenes (**v-*oncs***), and include **lymphoid leukosis** and many of the avian leukosis viruses, feline leukaemia viruses, and bovine leukaemia viruses. **These viruses produce tumours after a long latent period of many weeks or months.** They have a full complement of *gag*, *pol*, and *env* genes, and are therefore capable of replicating on their own (Fig. 49C). These viruses cause neoplastic transformation by the phenomenon of **insertional mutagenesis.** For neoplastic transformation to occur, integration of the proviral DNA has to be immediately upstream of a normal cellular proto-oncogene. Integration at such a **specific site** is purely a chance event and therefore occurs in a small number of infected cells. **This accounts for the long latent period between infection and development of a neoplasm.**

Two events occur when a proviral DNA molecule integrates upstream from a cellular proto-oncogene. **Firstly,** the insertion (integration) of the proviral DNA immediately adjacent to a proto-oncogene **effectively removes the proto-oncogene from control by its normal host-cell regulatory genes. Secondly,** the promoting and enhancing sequences of the 3' LTR of the proviral DNA cause continuous and uncontrolled expression of the neighbouring proto-oncogene, leading to increased synthesis of gene product. **This results in uncontrolled proliferation and malignant transformation (Fig. 49C).**

Tumours caused by slowly transforming retrovirus, because they result from the progeny of a single transformed cell, are

monoclonal in origin. This means that all cells making the neoplasm have the proviral DNA integrated at exactly the same site within the tumour-cell DNA.

To conclude, slowly transforming viruses, since they do not contain viral oncogenes, transform cells indirectly by activation of a proto-oncogene.

Human T-Cell Leukaemia Virus Type 1

This is **the only known slowly transforming retrovirus that is associated with cancer in humans.** It appears to cause a form of T-cell leukaemia/lymphoma which is endemic in certain parts of Japan and the West Indies. It is interesting that HTLV-1 causes cancer by **yet another mechanism**. In contrast to rapidly transforming viruses, **HTLV-1 does not contain a viral oncogene**, and in contrast to slowly transforming retroviruses, **no consistent integration next to a cellular proto-oncogene** has been discovered. Like the AIDS virus, HTLV-1 has **tropism for CD4+ T-cells** (see 'AIDS', Chapter 9), and therefore these cells are the major target for neoplastic transformation.

In addition to the usual retroviral genes, the genome of HTLV-1 contains a unique region called *pX*. This region encodes several proteins, including one called **TAX**. The **TAX protein** can activate the transcription of host genes encoding the cytokine IL-2 (interleukin-2) and its receptors (IL-2R) and the gene for GM-CSF (myeloid growth factor). In addition, TAX can prevent the function of several tumour suppressor genes that control the cell cycle. These include the **CDKIs** and *TP53*.

To conclude, IL-2, a T-cell growth factor, in turn, reacts with its receptor on the same cell, **setting up an autocrine system of proliferation** (see 'growth factors'). Simultaneously, the GM-CSF produced acts on the neighbouring macrophages (**a paracrine pathway**), and induces increased secretion of other T-cell mitogens, such as IL-1. Along with these growth-promoting activities, inhibition of growth suppressive pathways also occurs. Initially, the T-cell proliferation is **polyclonal** (involving many cells), because the virus infects many cells. The proliferating T-cells may later undergo mutations, which ultimately lead to **a neoplasm of monoclonal T-cell population** (i.e., derived from a single cell).

DNA Oncogenic Viruses

As indicated in Table 16, several DNA viruses have been associated with the causation of cancer in animals. Some, such as adenoviruses, cause tumours **only in laboratory animals**, whereas others such as the **bovine papilloma viruses** cause benign as well as malignant neoplasms in their natural hosts. Established viral oncogenicity in animals has led to great interest in the possible role of viruses in **human cancers**, and the mechanisms involved in neoplastic transformation. Of the various DNA viruses, **three**, namely, human papillomavirus (HPV), Epstein-Barr virus (EBV), and hepatitis B virus (HBV) have been implicated in the causation of **human cancer.**

Mechanism of Action of DNA Viruses

The mechanisms by which DNA viruses cause neoplastic transformation are as different as the viruses themselves, **and are extremely complex.** Therefore, only the basic principles are discussed, genus-wise, as per Table 16. But, first, let us review certain features shared by oncogenic DNA viruses.

1. **To be transformed by a virus, the cell must survive the infection and should not die.** Cells in which virus replication can be completed are called **permissive.** Such cells **cannot be transformed because they die** with the release of newly formed virus. On the other hand, **non-permissive cells**, which do not allow the virus to complete its life cycle, **can be transformed into neoplastic cells.**

2. With most oncogenic viruses, **only those portions of the genome that are transcribed <u>early</u> in the viral life cycle are essential for transformation.** The protein products of **'early genes'** have been identified and the molecular basis of their action examined (see 'polyomaviruses' and 'adenoviruses').

3. In **non-permissive cells**, oncogenic DNA viruses form stable association with the host genome. This usually occurs by **integration** of viral DNA into chromosomes. However, **only those integration events that interrupt late viral genes can produce transformed cells** (see 'polyomaviruses').

Polyomaviruses

These viruses usually cause latent infections, and have revealed their oncogenic potential **only under experimental conditions.** Two such agents have been studied extensively, namely: (1) **polyomavirus of mice**, and (2) **simian (monkey) virus 40.**

1. **Murine** (mouse) **polyomavirus** occurs as a latent infection of **wild mice**, but is rare in commercially raised mice. It can cause **a wide variety of neoplasms** (hence the name **polyoma**) in **newborn** or **suckling mice, rats, guinea pigs, rabbits**, and **hamsters**. The tumours

include sarcomas and carcinomas. (i) **In permissive cells,** as mentioned earlier, virus replication is completed and such cells die (**lytic infection**). Thus, permissive cells do not get transformed. (ii) **Polyomavirus,** like certain papillomavirus and adenovirus, can also become integrated into the host-cell DNA and cause **non-permissive, permanently transforming infections**. Thus, when polyomavirus DNA gets integrated into the host-cell DNA, **only the early proteins are expressed** through the action of the viruses' own promoter sequences. In such cases, the complete viral genome and late structural genes of the virus are integrated upstream from the viral promoter sequences, and therefore are not transcribed. **When this occurs, viral replication cannot take place and only the early genes of the virus are expressed.**

Polyomavirus encodes for **three early proteins (oncoproteins): large, middle,** and **small 'T-proteins' (transforming proteins)**. The presence of both large and middle-sized T-proteins of polyomavirus is necessary to acquire the malignant transformation. **The large T-protein** is a nuclear DNA-binding protein. It enhances both viral and DNA transcription during a lytic cycle. Integration of the viral DNA into the host-cell genome does not allow viral replication, but only cellular DNA replication. **This forces the cell to continue to divide.** The **middle T-protein** is a membrane-bound protein. It interacts with *src*, a normal cellular **proto-oncogene** product with tyrosine kinase activity. The integration causes a fifty-fold increase in the enzyme activity of this oncoprotein, **thus providing the second step required for transformation.**

2. **Simian (monkey) virus 40 (SV40)** occurs as a **latent infection** of **rhesus monkeys**. It causes disease in monkeys (nephritis, pneumonia, **but no tumours**) only when they become immunocompromized. However, SV40 is highly oncogenic when inoculated into **newborn mice** and **hamsters**. It causes a variety of **sarcomas**, including **lymphosarcoma**. Similar to murine polyomavirus, SV40 infection can be **permissive and lytic,** or **non-permissive and transforming,** depending on whether the viral DNA is present in the nucleus in episomal or integrated form. The permissive cells die as a result of viral replication, whereas the non-permissive cells get transformed as a result of integration of the viral genome. The transforming capacity of SV40 is similar to murine polyomavirus, **except that** SV40 encodes two, rather than three, early proteins. These are called large T and small T. The **large T-protein** is a nuclear protein, and functions the same way as protein of murine polyomavirus. **It**

311

binds to and inactivates TP53 (previously p53) and RB, both of which are products of tumour-suppressor genes (see 'RB gene' and 'TP53 gene'). However, it also has a component that binds to plasma membrane and it functions like the middle T protein of murine polyomavirus.

Papillomaviruses

Papillomaviruses cause benign neoplasms known as **papilloma** or **warts** on the skin and oral and genital mucous membranes of **animals** and **humans**. **In humans**, specific virus types (16 and 18) also have been implicated in the production of squamous-cell carcinoma of the cervix, and anal, perianal, vulva, and penile (of penis) cancers. There are numerous types of papillomaviruses in both animals and humans. In humans alone, more than 50 different types have been identified. Papillomaviruses are relatively host-specific.

Human papillomaviruses encode two early proteins, E6 and E7. These are the products of two early viral genes, *E6* and *E7*, and are responsible for the oncogenic potential of the virus. **E7 protein** binds to and inactivates the **retinoblastoma protein (RB protein)**, a product of tumour-suppressor *RB* gene (see '*RB* gene and cell cycle'). It also inactivates the cyclin-dependent kinase inhibitors (CDKIs) (see 'cyclins' and 'cyclin-dependent kinases'). **E6 protein binds and inactivates the TP53 protein** (see '*TP53* gene').In addition E6 mediates degradation of **BAX**, a pro-apoptotic member of the BCL2 family (see 'apoptosis'), and it activates **telomerase** (see 'limitless replication potential').

To summarize, papillomaviruses cause loss of tumour suppressor genes (*RB* and *TP53*), activate cyclins, and inhibit apoptosis. Inactivation of both the above tumour-suppressor genes results in pronounced proliferation of squamous cells. The viral genome is integrated in a manner that allows only the **early (transforming) genes** of the virus (*E6* and *E7*) to be transcribed. Therefore, no viral replication or cytolytic effect occurs. This results in malignant transformation and carcinoma, in contrast to the benign, self-limiting nature of the virally permissive papillomas.

Herpesviruses

Herpesviruses replicate in the nucleus of infected cells. The viral genome remains in the nucleus as non-integrated molecule of circular DNA. **Different herpesviruses cause malignant transformation by different mechanisms.**

Epstein-Barr virus (EBV), a typical example of lymphotropic herpesvirus, is the cause of several human tumours. Of these, an important tumour is **Burkitt lymphoma**, a B-cell tumour endemic in certain parts of Africa **and infects many B-cells, causing them to proliferate.**

The molecular basis of B-cell proliferations induced by EBV is complex. One of the EBV-encoded genes, called *LMP-1*, acts as an oncogene and its expression induces **B-cell lymphomas**. *LMP-1* promotes B-cell proliferation by activating signalling pathways that resemble B-cell activation through the B-cell surface molecule CD40. At the same time, *LMP-1* prevents apoptosis by activating *BCL2* (see 'apoptosis').

In immunologically normal individuals, EBV-caused polyclonal B-cell proliferation is readily controlled. Malaria or other infections, if present may impair immune competence, allowing sustained B-cell proliferation. In addition, the B-cells do not express cell surface antigens. Such B-cells are at increased risk of acquiring mutations, such as the translocation between chromosomes 8 and 14 [t (8:14)]. This translocation causes mutation in the normal *MYC* proto-oncogene (see 'nuclear transcription factors'). *MYC* is one of those genes that regulate transcription of DNA. The **mutated *MYC* gene** induces persistent and over-production of **Myc protein** (an oncoprotein), which causes sustained proliferation of B-cells and development of Burkitt lymphoma.

Hepadnaviruses

The term **'hepadnavirus'** is an acronym derived from **hepa**-titis **DNA virus**. There are no viruses under this genus that cause cancers in animals, but **in humans, hepatitis B virus (HBV)** of this genus is linked with cancer (hepatocellular carcinoma) of the liver. The oncogenic effect of the virus seems to involve many factors. (1) by causing chronic cell injury and repair, HBV predisposes the cells to **mutations. Aflatoxin B1**, a toxin produced by the mould **Aspergillus** may also induce mutations. Thus, HBV and aflatoxin may act together to produce liver cancers. (2) HBV encodes a regulatory protein called **'HBX protein'.** This protein disrupts normal growth control by activation of host-cell proto-oncogenes and disruption of cell cycle control. (3) cytosolic signal transduction pathways (e.g., RAS-MAP kinase) are turned on by HBV (see 'signal transduction pathways' under Chapter 5, and 'TAX proteins' of HTLV-1 under 'RNA oncogenic viruses'). (4) As with human papillomaviruses, certain HBV proteins bind to and inactivate the tumour-suppressor gene *TP53* (see '*TP53* gene').

Adenoviruses

These DNA viruses occur commonly in infections of the respiratory and alimentary tracts of **animals** and **humans, but they do not produce neoplasm in any species**. However, experimentally some serotypes of adenoviruses are highly oncogenic if injected into newborn **mice, rats**, and **hamsters**. Neoplasms caused by adenovirus contain copies of the viral DNA integrated into their genome **so that only early genes of the virus are transcribed and not the late genes** required for complete virus replication. Some of these early genes encode intranuclear proteins, called '**T proteins**' ('T' for tumour).These early adenovirus proteins (**E1A** and **E1B**) bind to a normal cellular protein known as **TP53**, which is a product of the tumour-suppressor gene *TP53*. In normal cells, TP53 protein arrests cells in G1 phase of the cell cycle (see '*TP53* gene'). **Inactivation of p53 protein** by virus-encoded T proteins **results in uncontrolled expression of cellular proto-oncogenes and neoplastic transformation**. As already pointed out, a similar mechanism underlies the neoplastic transformation caused by the **papovaviruses**. The family of 'papovaviruses' is divided into two genera 'polyomavirus' and 'papillomavirus' (see 'polyomaviruses' and 'papillomaviruses').

Molecular Basis of Cancer

Since this topic is so vast and complex, only the basic principles will be discussed. We may begin by considering certain fundamental principles, before going into the minor details of the genetic basis of cancer.

1. For carcinogenesis (cancer production), the genetic damage (or mutations) must be non-lethal. That is, it must not kill the cell. Such genetic damage may be from the action of environmental agents, such as chemicals, radiation, or viruses, or it may be inherited in the germ line. The genetic hypothesis of cancer indicated that a tumour results from the clonal expansion (growth) of **a single cell** that has suffered the genetic damage. **That is, tumours are monoclonal** (derived from a single cell).

2. Three classes of normal regulatory genes, namely: (1) growth-promoting proto-oncogenes, (2) growth-inhibiting cancer-suppressor genes (anti-oncogenes), and (3) genes that regulate programmed cell death (apoptosis) are the main targets of genetic damage. Mutant

forms (alleles) of proto-oncogenes are called 'oncogenes'. **Mutant alleles** of **proto-oncogenes** are considered **dominant** because they transform cells despite the presence of their normal counterpart. Since an allele is an alternative form of that gene on the same site (locus), this means that **proto-oncogene** being dominant, it can transform the cell even if, of the two, only one proto-oncogene is damaged and the other is normal. In contrast, both normal alleles (forms) of the **tumour-suppressor genes** must be damaged for transformation to occur. Therefore, this family of genes is often referred to as 'recessive oncogenes'. Genes that regulate **apoptosis** may be dominant like proto-oncogenes, or they may behave as cancer-suppressor genes.

3. In addition to the above three classes of genes, **a fourth category of genes**, which **regulate repair of damaged DNA**, are also important. **DNA repair genes** affect cell proliferation or survival **indirectly**. They influence the ability of the organism to repair non-lethal damage in proto-oncogenes, tumour-suppressor genes, and genes that regulate apoptosis. **A disability in the DNA repair genes can predispose to widespread mutations in the genome and hence to neoplastic transformation.**

4. **Carcinogenesis is a multi-step process** at both phenotypic (visible) and genetic levels. For example, a malignant tumour has several **phenotypic features**, such as excessive growth, local invasiveness, and the ability to form distant metastases. These characteristics are acquired in a step-wise fashion, a phenomenon called **tumour progression**. **At the molecular level**, progression results from accumulation of genetic lesions that in some cases are favoured by defects in DNA repair. Recently it has been revealed that genetic changes that increase tumour progression, involve not only growth regulatory genes, **but also genes that regulate angiogenesis, invasion, and metastases.**

With this background (see Fig. 50), we can now discuss the **molecular pathogenesis of cancer**. In the 1980s and 1990s, hundreds of cancer-associated genes were discovered. Each of the cancer genes has a specific function, and its dysregulation contributes to the origin or progression of cancer. These **cancer-related genes** will now be discussed in relation to **six basic changes** in cell physiology, which together produce cancer.

1. Self-sufficiency in growth signals
2. Insensitivity to growth-inhibitory signals
3. Evasion of apoptosis

4. Limitless replicative potential

5. Sustained angiogenesis, and

6. Ability to invade and metastasize

Mutations in genes that regulate these cellular events are seen in every cancer. The occurrence of mutations depends on the strength and efficiency of the **DNA repair machinery of the cell.** When genes that normally detect and repair DNA damage are impaired or lost, the resulting genomic instability favours **mutations** in genes that regulate the above-mentioned six acquired features of cancer cells. This group of genes (**enabler genes**) is discussed last. This is because it affects genes in all other pathways. In the discussion that follows, it should be noted that **genes are in italics, but their protein products are not.** Example: *RB* gene and **RB** protein.

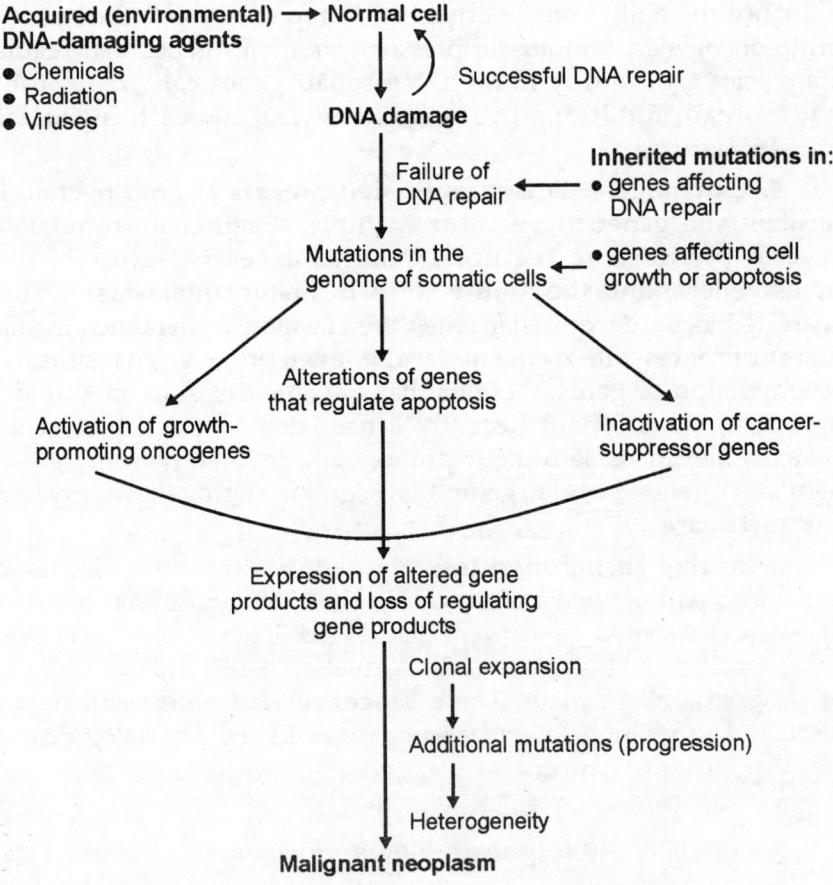

Fig. 50. A simplified scheme of the molecular basis of cancer.

316

1. Self-Sufficiency in Growth Signals

Oncogenes are cancer-causing genes. They are derived by mutations in **proto-oncogenes**, cellular genes that promote normal growth and differentiation. **Oncogenes** are characterized by their ability to **promote cell growth in the absence of normal growth-promoting signals.** The discovery of proto-oncogenes was not straightforward. These cellular genes were first discovered as 'travellers' within the genome of **acutely-transforming retroviruses** by J. Michael Bishop and Harold Varmus. For this pioneering contribution, they received the Nobel Prize in 1989. Protein products of oncogenes are called **oncoproteins**. **Oncoproteins** resemble the normal products of proto-oncogenes except that oncoproteins are **devoid of important regulatory elements**, and their production in the transformed cells does not depend on growth factors or other external signals. To understand the nature and functions of oncoproteins, it is necessary to review briefly the sequence of events that occur in normal cell proliferation (see Fig. 35, and Chapter 5 for details). These include:

a. Binding of a growth factor to its specific receptor on the cell membrane.

b. Activation of the growth factor receptor. This, in turn, activates several signal-transducing proteins on the inside of the plasma membrane.

c. Transmission of the transduced signal across the cytosol to the nucleus, through second messenger.

d. Induction and activation of the nuclear regulatory factors that initiate DNA transcription.

e. Entry and progression of the cell into the cell cycle, resulting in cell division.

With this background, we can now discuss the ways and means by which cancer cells acquire **self-sufficiency in growth signals.**

(a) Growth Factors

All normal cells require stimulation by growth factors to undergo proliferation. Most growth factors are made by one type of cell and act on a neighbouring cell to stimulate proliferation (**paracrine**

action). However, many cancer cells acquire self-sufficiency in growth by acquiring the ability to synthesize the same growth factors to which they respond (**autocrine action**). Such is the case with **platelet-derived growth factor (PDGF)** and **transforming growth factor-alpha (TGF-alpha).** Many glioblastomas secrete PDGF and sarcomas make TGF-alpha. Similar **autocrine loops** are quite common in many types of cancer. In many cases, the growth factor gene itself is not altered or mutated, but the **products of other oncogenes** (e.g., *RAS*) **cause over-expression of growth factor genes**. As a result, the cell may be forced to secrete large amounts of growth factors, such as **TGF-alpha.**

(b) Growth Factor Receptors

The next group in the sequence of signal transduction (transmission) involves **growth factor receptors. Several oncogenes that encode growth factor receptors have been found.** Mutations of such genes and pathological over-expression of normal forms of growth factor receptors have been found in many tumours. **Mutant receptor proteins** deliver continuous mitogenic (cell dividing) signals to cells, **even in the absence of growth factor**. More common than mutations is the **over-expression of growth factor receptors. This over-expression** can make cancer cells **hyper-responsive** to normal levels of the growth factor, **a level that would not normally trigger proliferation**. Best examples of over-expression involve epidermal growth factor (EGF) receptor family. EGF receptor (*ERBB1*) is over-expressed in 80% of squamous-cell carcinomas of the lung. A related receptor (*ERBB2*) is amplified in breast cancers and cancers of the lung, ovary, and salivary glands. **These tumours are extremely sensitive to the mitogenic effects of even small amounts of growth factors.**

(c) Signal-Transducing Proteins

A common mechanism by which cancer cells acquire **growth autonomy (self-sufficiency)** is by **mutations in genes that encode various components of the signalling pathways**. These **signalling molecules** connect growth factor receptors to their nuclear targets. Many such **signalling proteins** are present on the inside of the plasma membrane, where they receive signals from activated growth factor receptors **and transmit them to the nucleus.** Two important members of this category are *RAS* and *ABL*. Of these, only the *RAS* **gene** will be discussed, being most important.

RAS gene: About 30% of all human tumours contain mutated forms of the *RAS* gene. In some tumours, the incidence of *RAS* mutations is even higher. **Mutation of *RAS* gene is the most common oncogene abnormality in human tumours.** Normal RAS proteins, products of normal *RAS* genes, move back and forth between inactive and active state (Fig. 51A). In the **inactive state**, RAS proteins bind GDP (guanosine diphosphate). When cells are stimulated by growth factors, inactive RAS becomes **activated** by exchanging GDP for GTP (guanosine triphosphate) (Fig. 51A). The **activated** RAS, in turn, activates **regulators of proliferation**, including *RAF-MAP* kinase mitogenic pathway (Fig. 51A, see also Fig. 35, Chapter 5), **which**

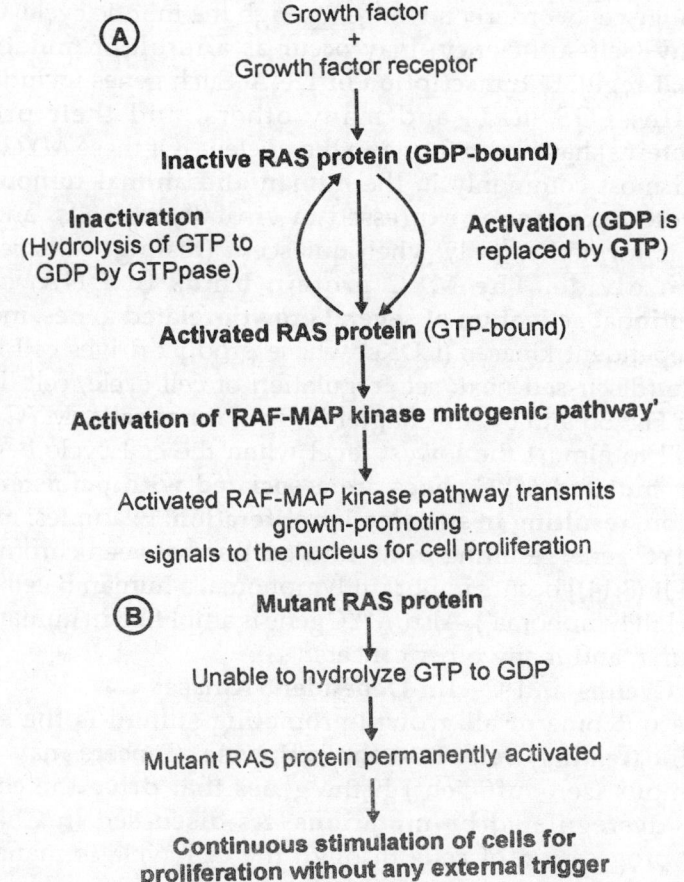

Fig. 51. A flow chart showing the action of *RAS* genes. A. Result of normal *RAS* gene. B Result of mutant *RAS* gene.

floods the nucleus with signals for cell proliferation. The **active state of RAS** is **short-lived**, because its intrinsic GTPase (guanosine triphosphatase) hydrolyzes GTP to GDP (Fig. 51A). This returns **active RAS** to its **inactive state. The mutant RAS protein is unable to hydrolyze GTP. Therefore, mutant RAS protein is trapped in its activated GTP-bound form, and the cell remains under the impression that it must continue to proliferate** (Fig. 51B). The *RAS* gene is commonly activated by **'point mutations'** (see 'point mutations').

(d) Nuclear Transcription Factors

Ultimately, all signal transduction pathways enter the nucleus and affect the large numbers of responder genes (genes that respond) that arrange cell's orderly advance through the mitotic cycle. Growth autonomy (self-sufficiency) may occur as a result of **mutations in genes that regulate transcription of DNA.** Such genes include *MYC, MYB, JUN, FOS, REL,* and many others, and their products (**oncoproteins**) have been found in the nucleus. Of these *MYC* **gene** is involved most commonly in the **human and animal tumours.** The *MYC* **proto-oncogene** is expressed in virtually all cells, and **MYC protein** is formed rapidly when quiescent (resting) cells receive a signal to divide. **The MYC protein binds to DNA,** causing **transcriptional activation of several growth-related genes,** including cyclin-dependent kinases (CDKs) whose product drives cell into the cell cycle (discussed next; see 'regulation of cell cycle/cell division, and also Fig. 36 and 37, in Chapter 5). **In normal cells,** MYC protein levels fall to almost the lowest level when the cell cycle begins. **In contrast, mutated *MYC* genes are associated with persistent over-expression, resulting in sustained proliferation.** Examples: mutation in the *MYC* gene, resulting from translocation between chromosomes 8 and 14 [t (8:14)] occurs in Burkitt lymphoma, a human B-cell tumour (see 'Burkitt lymphoma'). Also, *MYC* gene is amplified in human breast, colon, lung, and many other cancers.

(e) Cyclins and Cyclin-Dependent Kinases

The outcome of all growth-promoting stimuli is the **entry of quiescent (resting) cells into the cell cycle.** Cancers may become autonomous (self-sufficient) if the genes that drive the cell cycle become dysregulated by **mutations.** As discussed in Chapter 5, orderly progression of cells through the cell cycle is managed by **cyclin-dependent kinases (CDKs)** after they are **activated** by binding with another family of proteins called **'cyclins'** (Fig. 52A, 53; see also 'regulation of cell cycle/cell division' and Fig. 36 and 37 in Chapter 5). CDKs are expressed during the cell cycle in an **inactive form**. **Cyclins** are synthesized during specific phases of the cell cycle, and their function is to **activate CDKs** by binding them. After completing their job, cyclin levels fall rapidly (Fig. 52A). The cell cycle can be seen as a relay race, in which each lap (segment) is regulated by a separate set of cyclins, and as one set of cyclin leaves the track, the next set takes over (Fig. 52A). For example, cyclin D/CDK4, cyclin D/CDK6 and cyclin E/CDK2 regulate the **G1 to S transition**, whereas cyclin A/CDK2 and cyclin A/CDK1 are active in the **S phase**. Cyclin B/CDK1 is essential for the **G2 to M transition** (Fig. 52A). While cyclins activate CDKs, their **inhibitors** inhibit the CDKs and stop the cell cycle.

Although each phase of the cell cycle is monitored carefully, the transition from **G1 to S** is an **extremely important checkpoint** in the cell cycle (see 'checkpoints'). When a cell comes in contact with growth-promoting signals, levels of the **D family of cyclins** go up, and **CDK4 and CDK6 are activated** (Fig. 52B, 53). The checkpoint is guarded by a protein called **'retinoblastoma protein'** (RB protein). Phosphorylation of RB (pRB), carried out by D cyclins and CDKs (D/CDK4, D/CDK6), overcomes the G1 to S hurdle (Fig. 52B) and allows entry of cells into the DNA synthetic (S) phase. Further progress from S phase to G2 phase is brought about by cyclin A and CDKs (A/CDK2, A/CDK1). Early in the G2 phase, **B cyclin** takes over. By forming complexes with **CDK1**, B cyclin moves the cell from **G2 to M** (Fig. 52B).

The activity of CDKs is regulated by **two families of CDK inhibitors** (CDKIs) (Fig. 52C, 53). **One family** of CDKIs is composed of three proteins, called CDKNIA (p21), p27, and p57, and inhibits all CDKs, whereas the **other family** of CDKIs acts on cyclin D/CDK4 and cyclin D/CDK6. The four members of this family include p15, CDKN2A (p16), p18, and p19 (Fig. 52C, 53).

With this background, it is easy to understand that **mutations** which dysregulate the activity of **cyclins** and **CDKs would favour cell proliferation** (Fig. 52D). Mishaps affecting the expression of cyclin D or CDK4 genes are common events in neoplastic transformation. **The cyclin D genes are over-expressed in many cancers** (Fig. 52D), including those affecting the breast, oesophagus, and liver. **Amplification** of the CDK4 gene occurs in melanomas, sarcomas, and glioblastomas. **Mutations** affecting **cyclin B** and **cyclin E** and other **CDKs** also occur in certain malignant neoplasms, but they are much less common than those affecting **D/CDK4** (Fig. 52D).

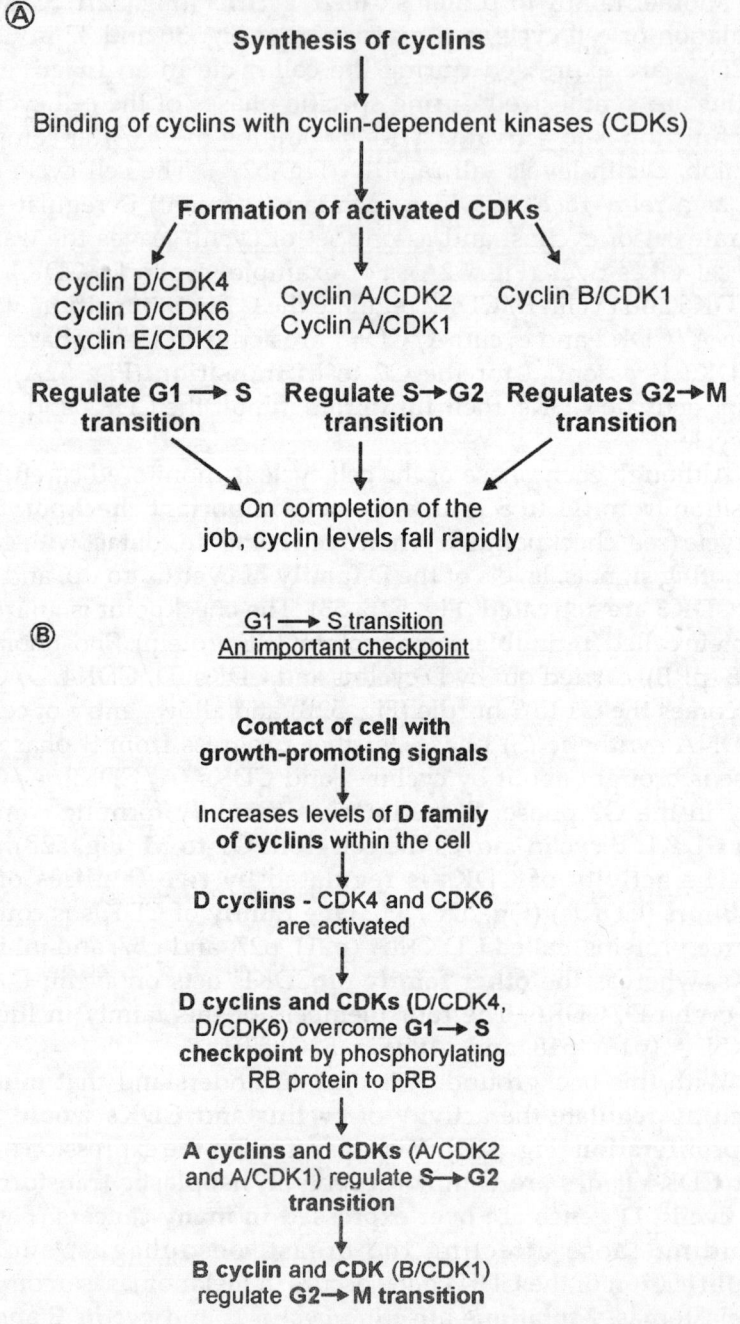

Ⓐ **Synthesis of cyclins**

Binding of cyclins with cyclin-dependent kinases (CDKs)

Formation of activated CDKs

Cyclin D/CDK4
Cyclin D/CDK6   Cyclin A/CDK2   Cyclin B/CDK1
Cyclin E/CDK2   Cyclin A/CDK1

Regulate G1 → S   **Regulate S→G2**   **Regulates G2→M**
transition   **transition**   **transition**

On completion of the
job, cyclin levels fall rapidly

Ⓑ   G1 ──→ S transition
             An important checkpoint

**Contact of cell with
growth-promoting signals**

Increases levels of **D family
of cyclins** within the cell

D cyclins - CDK4 and CDK6
are activated

**D cyclins and CDKs (D/CDK4,
D/CDK6)** overcome **G1→ S**
checkpoint by phosphorylating
RB protein to pRB

A cyclins and **CDKs (A/CDK2
and A/CDK1)** regulate **S→G2
transition**

B cyclin and **CDK (B/CDK1)**
regulate **G2→ M transition**

Fig. 52. Flow chart showing the role of cyclins, cyclin-dependent kinases (CDKs), and cyclin-dependent kinase inhibitors (CDKIs) in regulating the cell cycle. (**A**) Synthesis of cyclins, (**B**) G1 to S transition,

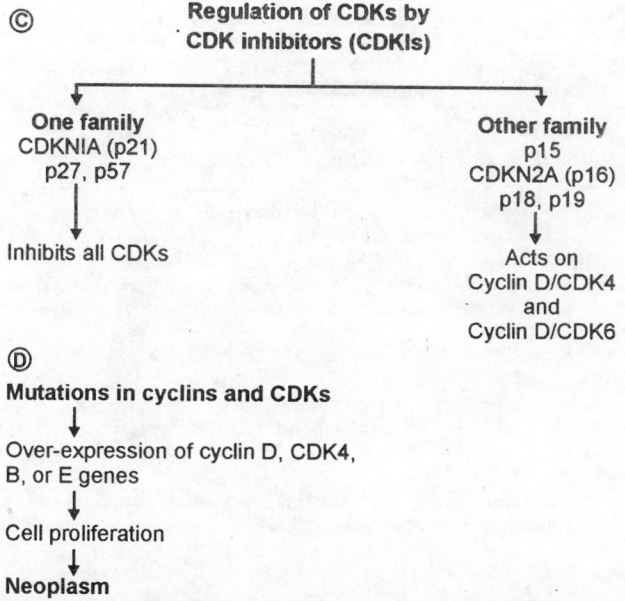

(C) Regulation of CDKs by CDK inhibitors (CDKIs), and (D) Mutations in cyclins and CDKs.

Activation of Oncogenes

We have discussed how **mutant forms of proto-oncogenes** provide unnecessary and uncalled-for growth-stimulating signals. We shall now discuss the **mechanisms by which proto-oncogenes are transformed into oncogenes.** This is brought about in **two ways.**

(i) From **changes in the structure of the gene.** This results in the synthesis of an abnormal gene product (oncoprotein), which has an abnormal function.

(ii) From **changes in the regulation of gene expression.** This results in increased or inappropriate production of the structurally normal growth-promoting proteins.

Let us now examine the **specific lesions (mutations)** that cause structural and regulatory changes in the proto-oncogenes.

Mutations

A mutation is a permanent change in the DNA. Mutations that affect the **germ cells** are transmitted to the progeny and may give rise to inherited diseases. Mutations that arise in the somatic cells do not cause hereditary diseases, **but are important in the production of cancer. Mutations** can be of **three types:**

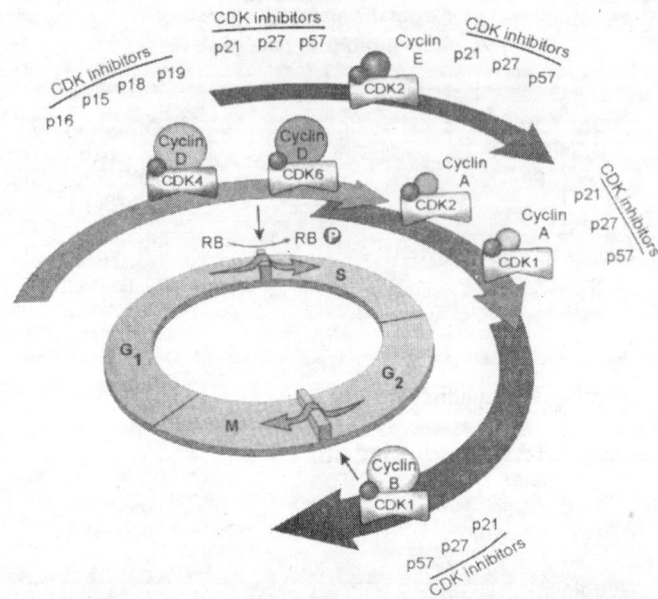

Fig. 53. Schematic illustration of the role of cyclins, cyclin-dependent kinases (CDKs), and cyclin-dependent kinase inhibitors (CDKIs) in regulating the cell cycle. Cyclin D/CDK4, cyclin D/CDK6, and cyclin E/CDK2 regulate the G1 to S transition by phosphorylation of the RB protein (pRB). Cyclin A/CDK2 and cyclin A/ CDK1 are active in the S phase. Cyclin B/CDK1 is essential for the G2 to M transition. Two families of CDK inhibitors, so-called INK4 inhibitors composed of p16, p15, p18, and p19, act on cyclin D/CDK4 and cyclin D/CDK6. The other family of three inhibitors p21, p27, and p57, can inhibit all CDKs.

(i) **Genome mutations** involve loss or gain of whole chromosomes. **These are rare.**

(ii) **Chromosome mutations** result from rearrangement of genetic material. **Two** types of **chromosomal rearrangements** can activate **proto-oncogenes - translocations** and **inversions**. Of these, chromosomal translocations are much more common. **Translocations result in over-expression of proto-oncogenes.** The best example of translocation-induced over-expression of a proto-oncogene is that of Burkitt lymphoma in humans (see Burkitt lymphoma). The Philadelphia chromosome, characteristic of chronic myeloid leukaemia in humans, is another example of genetic damage brought about by translocation.

(iii) **Gene mutations** may result in partial or complete deletion of a gene or, more often, **affect a single base**. For example, a single nucleotide base may be **substituted** by a different base, resulting in a

point mutation. The *ras* oncogene represents the best example of activation by point mutations. Less commonly, one or two base pairs may be **inserted** into or **deleted** from the DNA, leading to alterations in the reading frame of the DNA strand. Therefore, these are referred to as **'frameshift mutations'**.

A **point mutation (single base substitution) within coding sequences** may alter the code in a triplet of bases, and lead to the replacement of one amino acid by another in the gene product. These mutations alter the meaning of the genetic code. **Mutations within non-coding sequences** may also result in harmful effects. As is known, transcription of DNA is initiated and regulated by promoter and enhancer sequences that are found down-stream or up-stream of the gene. Point mutations or deletions involving these regulatory sequences may interfere with binding of transcription factors and thus lead to a marked reduction in, or total lack of transcription.

Mutations also occur **spontaneously** during the process of DNA replication. Certain environmental influences, such as chemicals, radiation, and viruses, increase the rate of **'spontaneous mutations'**.

(iv) Reduplication and manifold amplification of the DNA sequences in **proto-oncogene** may result in their activation. This leads to **over-expression of their products.** Such amplification may produce several hundred copies of the proto-oncogenes in the tumour cell. This occurs in human neuroblastoma and in breast cancers.

2. Insensitivity to Growth-Inhibitory Signals

Whereas oncogenes encode proteins that promote cell growth, **products of tumour-suppressor genes apply brakes to cell proliferation**. **Loss of tumour-suppressor genes** makes cells insensitive to growth inhibition, and this situation resembles the growth-promoting effects of oncogenes. In this section, we shall discuss briefly **cancer-suppressor genes, their products, and** possible **mechanisms** by which loss of their function results in **unregulated cell growth.**

Let us begin with the **retinoblastoma (*RB*) gene, the first cancer-suppressor gene** to be discovered.

The *RB* gene was discovered in a rare tumour of children known as **retinoblastoma**. It was found that **two mutations** in the normal *RB* gene were required to produce the tumour. That is, **both** the normal *RB* alleles (both forms of the normal *RB* gene on the same locus in a chromosome) must be lost (mutated). Afterwards, it was found that, apart from retinoblastoma, homozygous loss of this gene

325

(i.e., loss of **both** normal *RB* alleles) was fairly common in several human tumours, including breast cancer.

At this point, let us understand a few facts. A cell **heterozygous** at *RB* locus is not malignant. That is, when it has **only one** mutated *RB* gene, the other being normal. **Cancer develops only when the cell becomes homozygous.** That is, when there is loss (mutations) of both the normal forms (alleles) of the *RB* gene. Because loss of both normal alleles of the *RB* gene is required for neoplastic transformation, this and other cancer-suppressor genes are often called **'recessive cancer genes'** (see point '2' of the 'molecular basis of cancer', discussed earlier).

However, how anti-growth signals prevent cell proliferation is less well understood than those for growth promotion. In principle, anti-growth signals can prevent cell proliferation by **two mechanisms:** (1) The anti-growth signals may cause dividing cells to go into the quiescent (resting) phase (Go), or (2) the cells may enter a post-mitotic, differentiated pool and loose replicative (growth) potential. **It is now clear that at the molecular level anti-growth signals exert their effects on the G1 to S checkpoint of the cell cycle** (see 'cell cycle', Chapter 5). **This transition is controlled by the RB protein,** a product of *RB* gene.

With this background, let us examine how cancers dodge (avoid) the growth inhibitory mechanisms. That is, how they become insensitive (resistant, unresponsive) to growth-inhibitory signals **and continue to grow.** Let us again focus on the *RB* gene, since it controls G1 to S checkpoint.

RB Gene and Cell Cycle

Since *RB* gene was the first tumour-suppressor gene discovered, much more is known about it. The *RB* gene product (**RB protein**) is a DNA-binding protein and is expressed in every cell type examined. It exists in an **active (hypophosphorylated)** and an **inactive (hyperphosphorylated)** state (Fig. 54A). In its **active state**, RB protein acts as a **brake** in the progress of cell from **G1 to S phase** of the cell cycle. When cells are stimulated by growth factors, the RB protein is inactivated by phosphorylation, **the brake is released, and the cells travel through the G1 to S checkpoint** (Fig. 54B). When cells enter the **S phase**, they divide without additional growth factor stimulation. In the **M phase**, the phosphate groups are removed from RB protein by cellular phosphatases, regenerating the **dephosphorylated form of RB.**

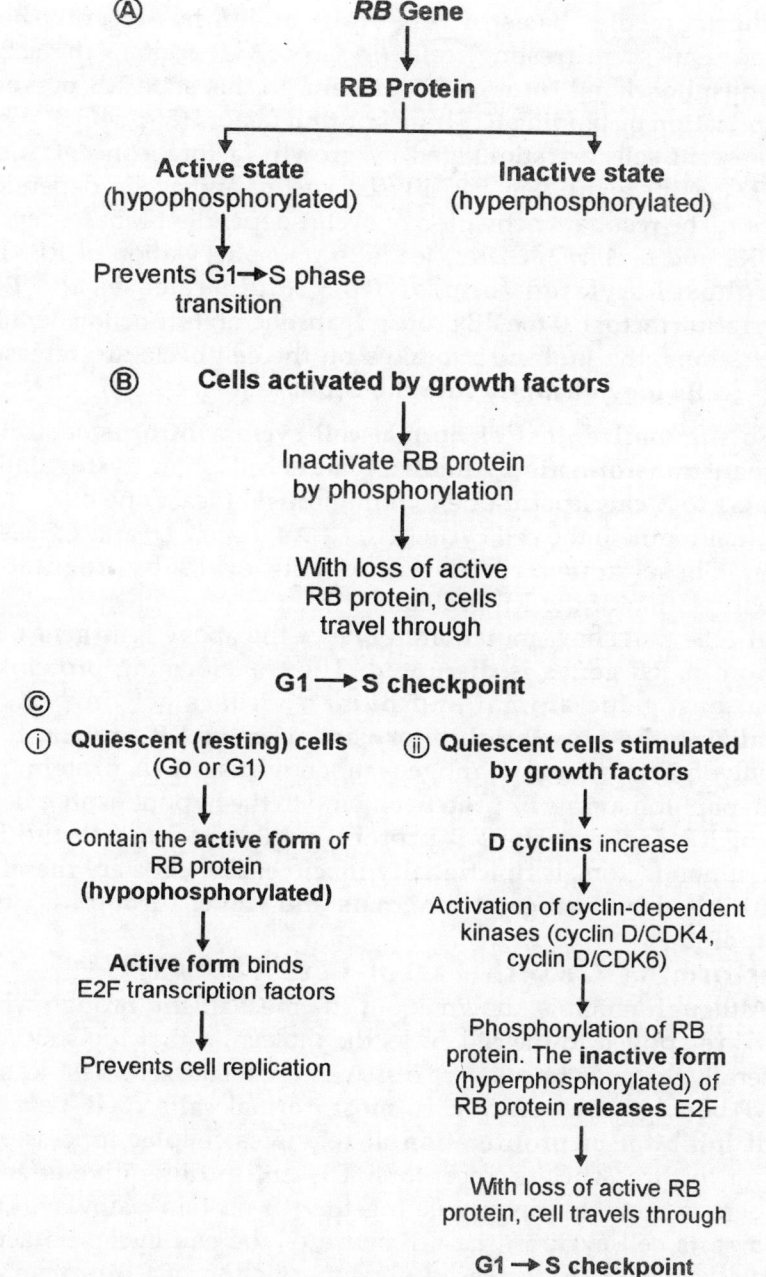

Fig. 54. The role of RB protein in regulating the G1 to S checkpoint of the cell cycle. **(A)** Two forms of RB protein. **(B)** Role of RB protein on activation of the cell by growth factors. **(C)** Different role of RB protein in a resting cell and in a cell stimulated by growth factors.

327

The molecular basis of this brake action has recently been revealed. Quiescent (resting) cells (in Go or G1) contain the active **hypophosphorylated form of RB protein**. In this state **RB prevents cell replication** by binding **E2F transcription factors** (Fig. 54C-i). When the quiescent cells are stimulated by growth factors, concentrations of the **D cyclins** go up (Fig. 54C-ii) (see 'cyclins and cyclin-dependent kinases'). The resultant activation of cyclin-dependent kinases (cyclin D/CDK4 and cyclin D/CDK6) leads to phosphorylation of RB. The **hyperphosphorylated form of RB protein** releases the ERF transcription factors. If the RB protein is **absent**, or its function derailed by **mutations**, the **molecular brakes** on the cell cycle are **released**, and the **cells move happily into the S phase** (Fig. 54C-ii).

To summarize, **loss of normal cell cycle control is central to malignant transformation.** Almost all cancer cells show **dysregulation of the G1 to S checkpoint** due to mutation in at least one of the four genes that regulate the cell cycle (*RB*, *CDK4*, *cyclin D*, and *CDKN2A* (p16)). These genes regulate the cell cycle by regulating phosphorylation of the RB protein.

In cells that show mutation in one of the above four genes, **the function of *RB* genes is disrupted.** The transforming proteins of several oncogenic **animal and human viruses** act, in part, **by neutralizing the growth-inhibitory activities of RB protein.** SV40 and polyomavirus large T antigens, adenoviruses **EIA protein**, and human papillomavirus **E7 protein** all bind to the hypophosphorylated form of RB protein. The **RB protein**, unable to bind to the E2F transcription factors, is **functionally inactive. The cells are therefore not inhibited by anti-growth signals and travel through G1 to S checkpoint.**

Transforming Growth Factor-Beta Pathway

Although much is known about the mechanism through which brakes are applied to the cell cycle, the molecules that transmit anti-proliferative signals to cells are less well characterized. **Best known is TGF-beta, a growth factor. In most normal cells, TGF-beta is a potent inhibitor of proliferation.** It regulates cellular processes by binding to three specific receptors. The anti-proliferative effect of TGF-beta is mediated by regulating the RB protein pathway. TGF-beta arrests cell cycle in the G1 phase of the cell cycle. Its action eventually results in decreased phosphorylation of RB protein and cell cycle arrest. **In many forms of cancer**, the growth-inhibiting effects of TGF-beta pathway are lost by mutations in the TGF-beta signalling pathway.

TP53 Gene: Guardian (protector) of the Genome

The *TP53* tumour-suppressor gene (previously *p53*) is one of the most commonly mutated genes in **human** and **animal cancers**. It has many functions. **TP53**, a protein product of *TP53* **gene**, has not only **anti-proliferative effect but it also regulates apoptosis. Basically *TP53* gene is a monitor of stress**. Under stress, it directs the cell towards an appropriate response, whether it is **cell arrest or apoptosis**. A variety of stresses can trigger the *TP53* gene response pathway, one of the important being damage to the integrity of DNA. By managing the DNA damage, *TP53* **gene plays a key role in maintaining integrity of the genome**.

Normal TP53 protein in non-stressed cells has a short half-life (20 minutes). This short life is due to its association with a protein called **MDM2**, which leads to its destruction. **When the cell is stressed**, as in DNA damage, TP53 protein is released from **MDM2** and its half-life is increased. By this process, **TP53** protein gets activated as a transcription factor. It then triggers transcription of many genes. These genes can be grouped into **two** categories: (1) those that cause **cell cycle arrest**, and (2) those that cause **apoptosis**.

Arrest of cell cycle by TP53 protein is the primary response to DNA damage. It occurs **late in the G1 phase** and is caused by *TP53* gene-dependent transcription of the cyclin-dependent kinase inhibitor [CDKNIA (p21)] (Fig. 55). The *CDKNIA (p21)* **gene**, as described earlier, prevents phosphorylation of RB protein essential for cells to enter G1 phase. **This leads to the cell arrest in G1 phase.** Such a pause in cell cycle is welcome, because it gives the cell time to repair its DNA. *TP53* gene also does one more thing to repair the damage. It stimulates formation of certain proteins, such as GADD45 (Growth Arrest and DNA Damage), involved in DNA repair. If DNA damage is repaired successfully, *TP53* gene up-regulates transcription of MDM2, which then down-regulates *TP53* genes, removing cell cycle block (obstruction). **If during the pause DNA damage cannot be successfully repaired, normal Tp53 protein directs the cell to death by triggering apoptosis** (Fig. 55). It does so by stimulating apoptosis-inducing genes, such as *BAX*. How *TP53* gene comes to know about DNA damage and how it determines the adequateness of DNA repair are not completely understood.

329

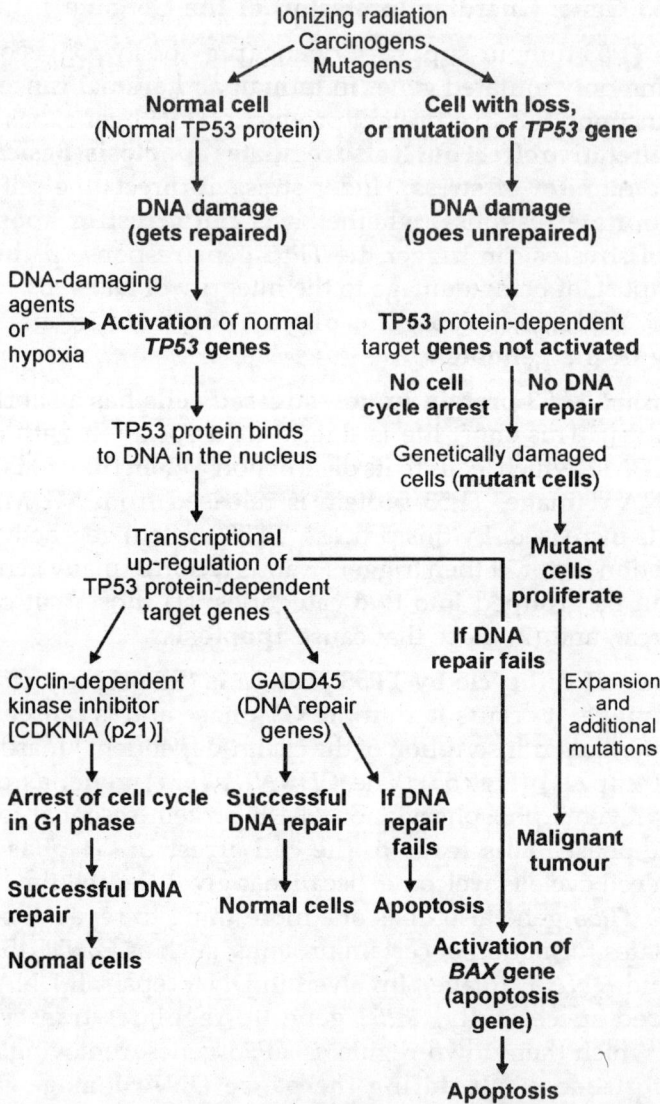

Fig. 55. Role of *TP53* gene in maintaining integrity of the gene (see text).

To summarize, TP53 protein somehow comes to know about DNA damage. It then tries to repair DNA by causing arrest of cell in G1 stage and by stimulating DNA repair genes. A cell with damaged DNA that cannot be repaired is directed by TP53 protein to undergo apoptosis (Fig. 55). Thus, *TP53* gene acts as a **'molecular policeman'**

that prevents the progression of genetically damaged cells. In view of these activities, *TP53 gene* has been called as **'Guardian (protector) of the genome'**. With homozygous loss of the *TP53* (i.e., loss of both the alleles), DNA damage goes un-repaired, mutations become fixed in dividing cells, and the cell enters into a one-way street that leads to **malignant transformation.**

The importance of *TP53* gene can be realized from the fact that more than 70% of human cancers (and possibly also of animals) have a defect in this gene, and the remaining have defects in genes up-stream or down-stream of *TP53*. Homozygous loss of the *TP53 gene* is found in almost every type of human cancer, including carcinomas of the lung, colon, and breast.

As with RB protein (see **'RB gene'**), normal **TP53 protein** can also be made non-functional by certain **DNA viruses**. Proteins encoded by oncogenic human papillomaviruses (HPVs), hepatitis B virus (HBV), and possibly Epstein-Barr virus (EBV) **can bind to normal TP53 protein and nullify (make ineffective) their protective functions. Thus, DNA viruses can ruin two of the best-understood tumour-suppressor genes,** namely, *RB* and *TP53*.

3. Evasion of Apoptosis

Accumulation of neoplastic cells may result not only from: (1) activation of growth-promoting oncogenes, or (2) inactivation of growth-inhibiting tumour-suppressor genes, but also from (iii) **mutations in the genes that regulate apoptosis.** Just as cell growth is regulated by growth-promoting and growth-inhibiting genes, **cell survival is determined by genes that promote and inhibit apoptosis.**

A large family of genes that regulate apoptosis has been identified. However, to understand how tumour cells avoid apoptosis, it is necessary to review briefly the **biochemical pathways of apoptosis** (see 'apoptosis', Chapter 3). Fig. 56 shows the sequence of events that lead to apoptosis when cell is signalled (triggered) through the **death receptor CD95 (Fas) and by DNA damage.** When **CD95** is bound to its ligand **CD95L**, CD95's death domains in cytoplasm attract adapter (connecting) protein **'FADD'**. FADD, in turn, attracts **procaspase 8** to form a complex called **'death-inducing signalling complex'**. Procaspase 8 is activated by its cleavage (split) into smaller subunits. **Activated caspase 8,** in turn, activates down-stream caspases, an important being **caspase 3. Caspase 3 is a typical executioner (killer) caspase. It cleaves DNA and other substrates to cause cell death (apoptosis).**

331

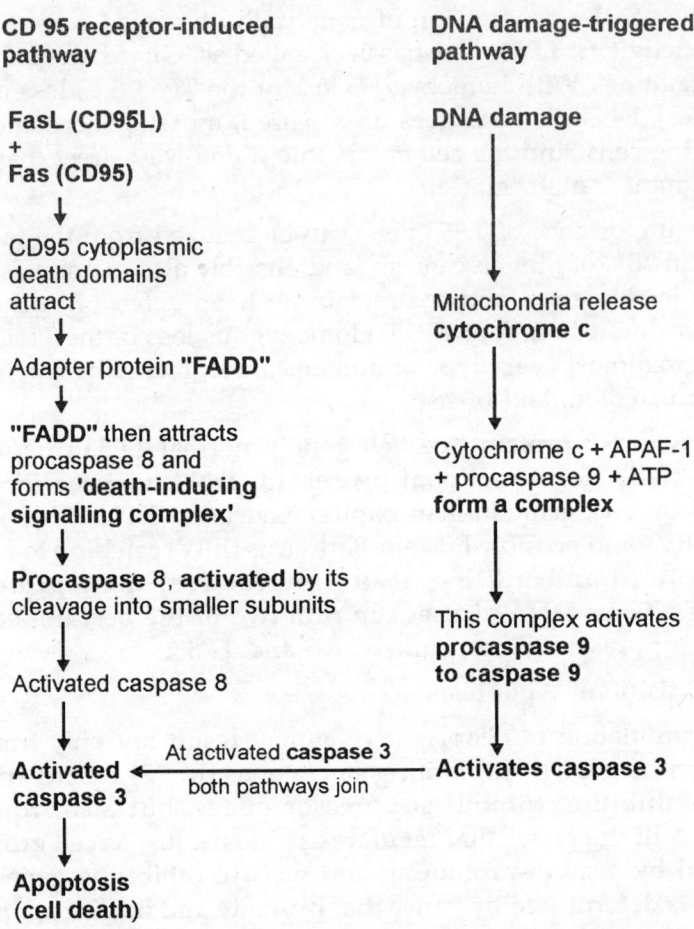

CD 95 receptor-induced pathway

FasL (CD95L)
+
Fas (CD95)
↓
CD95 cytoplasmic death domains attract
↓
Adapter protein **"FADD"**
↓
"FADD" then attracts procaspase 8 and forms **'death-inducing signalling complex'**
↓
Procaspase 8, **activated** by its cleavage into smaller subunits
↓
Activated caspase 8
↓
Activated caspase 3 ← At activated **caspase 3** both pathways join — **Activates caspase 3**
↓
Apoptosis (cell death)

DNA damage-triggered pathway

DNA damage
↓
Mitochondria release **cytochrome c**
↓
Cytochrome c + APAF-1 + procaspase 9 + ATP **form a complex**
↓
This complex activates **procaspase 9 to caspase 9**
↓
Activates caspase 3

Fig. 56. CD95 receptor-induced and DNA damage-triggered pathway of apoptosis (see text).

The other pathway of apoptosis is initiated by DNA damage (stress, radiation, chemicals) and other causes, such as growth factor deprivation (Fig. 56). Mitochondria play a key role in this pathway by releasing **cytochrome c.** Cytochrome c, in turn, forms a complex with **apoptosis-inducing factor-1** (APAF-1), procaspase 9, and ATP. With this complex, **procaspase 9** is activated to **caspase 9**, which then triggers **caspase 3** that ultimately leads to cell death. **Release of cytochrome c is a key event in apoptosis.** It is regulated by genes of the *BCL2* family. Some members of this family (*BCL2, BCL-X$_L$*) **inhibit apoptosis**, whereas others (*BAD, BAX, BID*), **promote**

apoptosis by favouring cytochrome c release (see 'apoptosis'). When triggered by DNA damage, *TP53* gene promotes apoptosis by up-regulation (increased synthesis) of BAX protein. Similarly, **caspase 8** promotes apoptosis by activating synthesis of proapoptotic protein **BID.**

With this background, it would be easy to understand the many sites at which apoptosis is prevented by cancer cells (Fig. 57). (1) Starting from the cell surface, **reduced levels of CD95 (e.g., in liver cancer) make tumour cells less susceptible to apoptosis by FasL. CD95 levels are regulated by TP53 protein**, and loss of TP53 protein may be responsible for reduced CD95 (Fig. 57-1). (2) Some tumours have high levels of a protein called **FLIP (or FLICE)** (Fig. 57-2). This protein can bind death-inducing signal complex and **prevent activation of caspase 8**. (3) Of all the genes, **best established is the role of *BCL2* in protecting tumour cells from apoptosis.** Certain tumours show **over-expression** of the BCL2 protein. Examples: B-cell lymphomas of the follicular type and Burkitt lymphoma, of humans. **Over-expression of BCL2 protein protects lymphocytes from apoptosis** and allows them to survive for long periods (Fig. 57-3). Therefore, there is a gradual accumulation of B-lymphocytes. Because BCL2-overexpressing lymphomas arise mainly from reduced cell death, rather than explosive cell proliferation, they tend to be slow growing compared to most other lymphomas.

As mentioned earlier, ***TP53* is an important apoptotic gene. It causes apoptosis in cells that are unable to repair DNA damage.** The actions of *TP53* are mediated, in part, by activation of *BAX* gene. **Two new mechanisms** by which tumour cells escape apoptosis have recently been discovered: (1) Certain tumour cells (e.g., melanoma) show **loss of APAF-1** (Fig. 57-4). This blocks the mitochondrial-cytochrome c pathway. Such cells are **resistant to apoptosis induced by *TP53* gene** through activation of *BAX* gene. (2) In some tumours, there is **up-regulation (increased synthesis) of inhibitors of apoptosis** (Fig. 57-5) that inactivate caspases (caspase 9). **This prevents apoptosis.**

4. Limitless Replicative (Proliferative) Potential

To follow this topic, let us first understand what happens when cells undergo division. Normal cells grown in culture undergo a limited number of cell divisions **and then die**. Within the body, most normal cells have a capacity of 60-70 doublings. After this, cells lose the

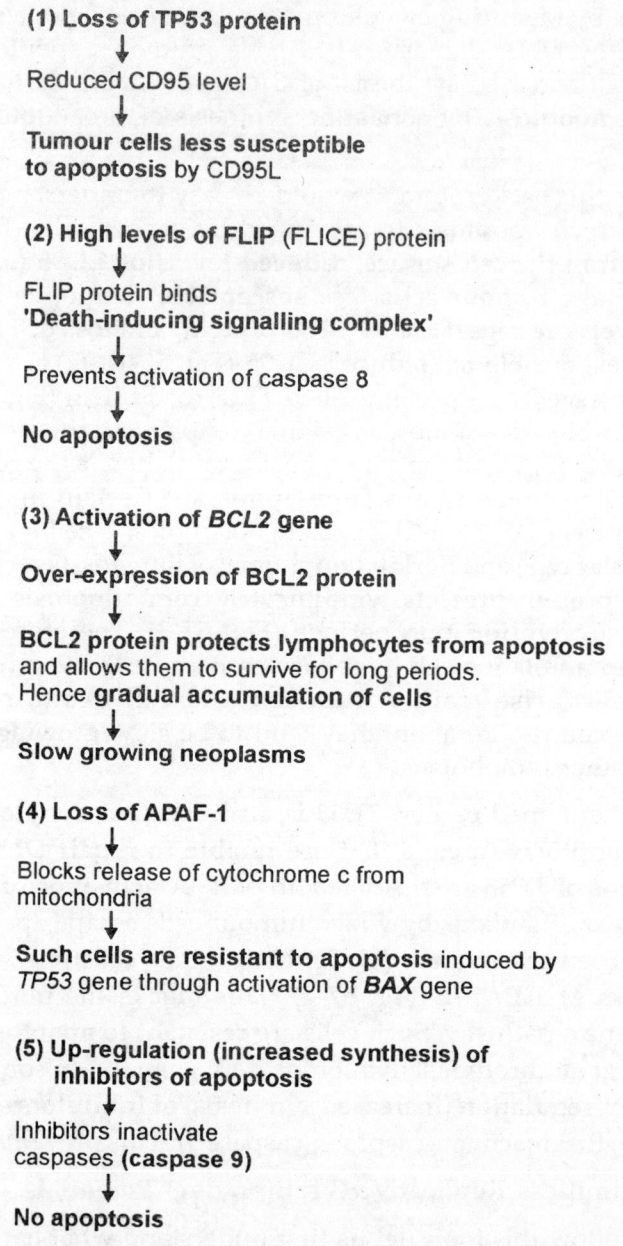

(1) Loss of TP53 protein
↓
Reduced CD95 level
↓
**Tumour cells less susceptible
to apoptosis** by CD95L

(2) High levels of FLIP (FLICE) protein
↓
FLIP protein binds
'Death-inducing signalling complex'
↓
Prevents activation of caspase 8
↓
No apoptosis

(3) Activation of *BCL2* gene
↓
Over-expression of BCL2 protein
↓
BCL2 protein protects lymphocytes from apoptosis
and allows them to survive for long periods.
Hence **gradual accumulation of cells**
↓
Slow growing neoplasms

(4) Loss of APAF-1
↓
Blocks release of cytochrome c from
mitochondria
↓
Such cells are resistant to apoptosis induced by
TP53 gene through activation of ***BAX*** gene

**(5) Up-regulation (increased synthesis) of
inhibitors of apoptosis**
↓
Inhibitors inactivate
caspases **(caspase 9)**
↓
No apoptosis

Fig. 57. Mechanisms used by tumour cells to avoid cell death (apoptosis).

capacity to divide and enter into a non-replicative (non-dividing) state known as **cellular senescence (cellular aging)**. The mechanisms of DNA replication is such that with each cell division each chromosome gets slightly shortened. Shortening of chromosome results from progressive shortening of short, repeated sequences (i.e.,nucleotides) of non-transcribed DNA that sit at the end of chromosomes called 'telomeres'. As a result, with each cell division, telomeres are shortened. Thus, telomeres provide a buffer of non-transcribed DNA that can be repeatedly shortened without affecting the replication of functional genes. Beyond a certain point, however, loss of telomeres leads to massive chromosomal abnormalities and **cell death**. In **germ cells** and **stem cells** (but not in somatic cells), in which unlimited number of cell divisions are required, telomere length is restored after each cell division by a specialized enzyme called 'telomerase'. **Interestingly, telomerase is also activated in immortal cancer cells.** This indicates that **preservation of telomere length is a critical step in the development of cancer.** Let us examine how this occurs.

In contrast to normal cells, transformed cells in the culture can be maintained indefinitely. This is because transformed cells do not undergo the progressive telomeric shortening that occurs in normal cells with each cell division. Transformed cells contain **repair mechanisms that maintain normal telomere length** lost during cell division. One such mechanism involves activation of the enzyme **telomerase**.

It was found that aging of cells in culture (e.g., fibroblasts) could be partially overcome by inactivating their tumour-suppressor *RB* and *TP53* genes. But, ultimately, these cells underwent death. This meant that for tumours to grow indefinitely loss of growth restraint alone is not sufficient. **Tumour cells also must develop ways to avoid cellular aging (senescence).** As mentioned, this is achieved by the enzyme **telomerase**, which can maintain normal telomere length. Telomere maintenance is seen in almost all types of cancers. In 85% to 95% of cancers, this is **due to up-regulation (increased synthesis) of the enzyme telomerase.**

5. Development of Sustained Angiogenesis

Even with all the genetic abnormalities discussed so far, **tumours cannot enlarge beyond 1-2 mm in diameter or thickness, unless they**

are vascularized (become vascular). The 1-2 mm zone is the maximum distance across which oxygen and nutrients can diffuse from blood vessels. Beyond this size, the tumour fails to enlarge without vascularization because hypoxia (deficiency of oxygen) causes apoptosis (cell death) by activation of *TP53* gene (see '*TP53* gene'). **Angiogenesis** (formation of new blood vessels), also called '**neovascularization**' (see Chapter 5), has a double effect on tumour growth: (i) diffusion of blood supplies nutrients and oxygen, and (2) newly formed endothelial cells stimulate the growth of neighbouring tumour cells **by secreting polypeptides**, such as insulin-like growth factors, platelet-derived growth factor (PDGF), granulocyte-macrophage colony-stimulating factor (GM-CSF), and interleukin-1 (IL-1). **Angiogenesis is required not only for continued tumour growth but also for metastasis**. Without the availability of blood vessels, tumour cells cannot metastasize. **Angiogenesis is a necessary biological requirement of malignancy.**

How do then **growing tumours develop a blood supply?** Tumours themselves contain factors that can form new blood vessels. Such **tumour-associated angiogenic factors** may be of two types: (1) those that are produced by tumour cells, and (2) those that are derived from inflammatory cells (e.g., macrophages) that infiltrate tumours. Of the dozen tumour-associated angiogenic factors, the two most important are: (1) **vascular endothelial growth factor (VEGF)**, and (2) **basic fibroblast growth factor (bFGF)**. It is now known that tumour cells not only produce **angiogenic factors**, but also induce **anti-angiogenesis molecules**. The current belief is that **tumour growth is controlled by the balance between angiogenic factors and factors that inhibit angiogenesis. Anti-angiogenesis factors** may be produced by the tumour cells themselves (e.g., thrombospondin-1), or their production may be induced by tumour cells (e.g., angiostatin, endostatin, and vasculostatin).

Early in their growth, most tumours do not produce angiogenesis. They remain small, or *in situ* (in position), for years until the **angiogenic switch** terminates the stage of vascular quietness. The molecular basis of angiogenic switch involves increased production of angiogenic factors, or loss of angiogenesis inhibitors. *TP53* gene inhibits angiogenesis by inducing synthesis of the anti-angiogenic molecules **thrombospondin-1**. With **mutational inactivation of both** *TP53* **alleles** (common in many cancers), the levels of thrombospondin-1 drop suddenly, **tilting the balance in favour of angiogenic factors.**

6. Ability to Invade and Metastasize

Local invasion and distant spread (metastasis) are the most important biological features of malignant tumours. We shall now discuss the **mechanisms** by which tumours spread locally, and are also transported to distant sites.

The spread of tumours is a complex process. For tumour cells to break loose from a primary growth, enter blood vessels or lymphatics, and produce a secondary growth at a distant site, they must go through a series of steps. These are summarized in Figure 58. This sequence of steps can be interrupted at any stage by either host-related or tumour-related factors. Experimental studies in mice have revealed that of the million of cells released into circulation each day from a primary tumour, **only a few metastases are produced.** Why? What is the basis of the inefficiency of this process? As is discussed later (in 'tumour progression and heterogeneity'), cells within a tumour differ in their **metastatic potential.** Only certain groups (subclones) possess the right combination of gene products to complete all the steps outlined in Fig. 58. The spread of tumours can be divided into two phases: (1) invasion of the extracellular matrix, and (2) vascular dissemination and homing (localization) of tumour cells.

I. Invasion of Extracellular Matrix

To understand this topic better, review first the composition of extracellular matrix (ECM) given in Chapter 5 (see also Fig. 39).

Tissues are organized into a series of compartments. The compartments are separated from each other by two types of ECM (1) **basement membranes,** and (2) **interstitial connective tissue.** Both the ECMs are composed of collagens, glycoproteins, and proteoglycans. For a tumour to metastasize, its cells must interact with ECM at several stages (Fig. 58). For example, a carcinoma must first breach (break) the underlying basement membrane, then travel through the interstitial connective tissue, and ultimately enter into the circulation by penetrating the vascular basement membrane. This cycle is repeated when tumour cell emboli come out of the blood vessels at a distant site. **Invasion of the ECM by tumour cells** is an active process that can be divided into **four steps.**

1. Detachment of tumour cells from each other
2. Attachment of tumour cells to matrix components
3. Degradation of extracellular matrix
4. Migration of tumour cells

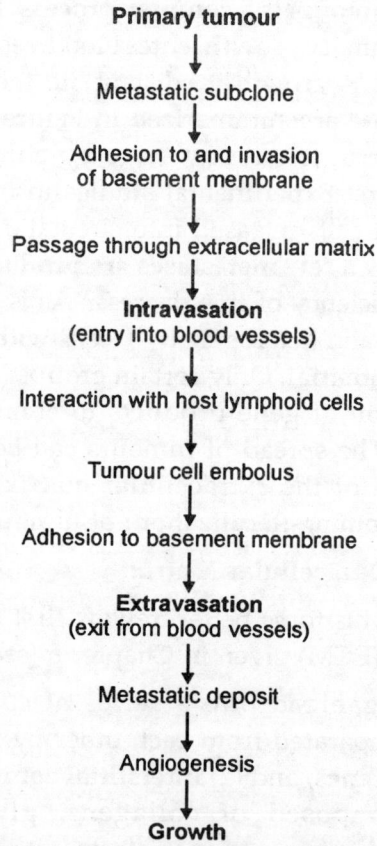

Primary tumour

↓

Metastatic subclone

↓

Adhesion to and invasion
of basement membrane

↓

Passage through extracellular matrix

↓

Intravasation
(entry into blood vessels)

↓

Interaction with host lymphoid cells

↓

Tumour cell embolus

↓

Adhesion to basement membrane

↓

Extravasation
(exit from blood vessels)

↓

Metastatic deposit

↓

Angiogenesis

↓

Growth

Fig. 58. Sequential steps involved in the haematogenous spread of a tumour.

1. Detachment of Tumour Cells from Each Other

The first step in metastasis is a **loosening of tumour cells.** Normal cells are nicely glued together to each other by a variety of **adhesion molecules.** Of these, the **cadherin family** of transmembrane glycoproteins is the most important. **E-cadherins** act as intracellular glues and keep the cells together. Recently it has been found that in almost all epithelial cancers, there is a down-regulation (decreased synthesis) of E-cadherin by mutational inactivation of *E-cadherin* genes. As a result, E-cadherin function is lost. This leads to loosening of intercellular junctions. **The tumour cells then detach from each other because of reduced adhesiveness.**

E-cadherins are attached to the cytoskeleton of cells by a family of proteins called **'catenins'**, which lie under the plasma membrane. The normal function of E-cadherin depends on its attachment to catenins (**beta-catenin**). In some tumours, **E-cadherin is normal, but its expression is reduced** because of mutations in the genes for beta-catenin. This also contributes to detachment of cells.

2. Attachment of Tumour Cells to Matrix Components

To penetrate ECM, the tumour cells must first attach to the matrix components. Attachment of tumour cells to ECM proteins such as **laminin** and **fibronectin** is important for invasion and metastasis. Normal epithelial cells have **receptors** for basement membrane **laminin** that are grouped at their basal (lower) surface. **In contrast**, carcinoma cells have **many more receptors**, and they are **distributed all around the cell membrane**. Moreover, there is a correlation between the density of laminin receptors and their invasiveness. In addition to laminin receptors, tumour cells also express **integrins** that serve as receptors for many components of the extracellular matrix. As with laminin receptors, there is a correlation between the expression of certain integrins on carcinoma cells and their ability to attach.

3. Degradation of Extracellular Matrix

After attachment, the next step in invasion is local degradation (destruction) of the basement membrane and interstitial connective tissue. **Tumour cells secrete proteolytic enzymes themselves**, or induce the host cells (e.g., fibroblasts) to secrete **proteases**. Several matrix-degrading enzymes called **'metallo-proteinases'** are involved. These include collagenases, gelatinases, and stromelysins. Type IV collagenase is a gelatinase that cleaves (splits) type IV collagen of the epithelial and vascular basement membranes. **Benign tumours show little type IV collagenase activity, whereas their malignant counterparts over-express this enzyme.** At the same time, the levels of metallo-proteinase inhibitors are reduced. This tilts the balance greatly towards tissue degradation. Similar correlations have been observed with **other proteases**, including **cathepsin D**. Over-expression of cathepsin D occurs in invasive breast cancers.

4. Migration of Tumour Cells

Locomotion is the final step of invasion. Locomotion pushes the tumour cells forward through the degraded basement membranes and zones of ECM proteolysis (digestion). **Migration** is mediated by tumour cell-derived **cytokines**, such as **autocrine (self-derived) motility factors**. In addition, cleavage (split) products of matrix components (e.g., collagen, laminin) and some growth factors (e.g., insulin-like growth factors I and II) **have chemotactic activity for tumour cells.**

II. Vascular Dissemination and Homing of Tumour Cells

Once in circulation, tumour cells are vulnerable to destruction by the host immune cells (see 'anti-tumour effector mechanism'). However, some tumour cells form emboli by aggregating and adhering to circulating leukocytes, particularly platelets. Aggregated tumour cells are thus somewhat protected from the host immune cells. But, most tumour cells circulate as single cells. For free tumour cells or tumour emboli to come out of the blood vessels (extravasation) (Fig. 58), they must first adhere to the vascular endothelium. This is followed by their exit through the basement membrane by mechanisms similar to those involved in invasion.

The **site of extravasation** and the organ in which tumour is going to metastasize usually can be predicted by the location of the primary tumour and its vascular or lymphatic drainage. However, in many cases, the natural pathways of drainage do not easily explain the distribution of metastases. Some tumours (e.g., lung cancers) regularly involve the adrenals, but never spread to skeletal muscle. That is, they show a clear **'organ tropism'**. Such organ tropism (i.e., a natural liking) **or homing** (going to one's natural site, or home) **may be due to:**

1. **Expression of adhesion molecules by tumour cells.** The ligands (molecules that bind) of adhesion molecules are preferentially expressed on the endothelium of target organs.

2. Another mechanism of site-specific homing involves **chemokines and their receptors.** Chemokines are involved in chemotaxis (directed movement) of leukocytes (Chapter 4). Tumour cells also use similar mechanisms to home in (localize) on specific

tissues. Examples, human breast cancer cells express high levels of the **chemokine receptors**. The **ligands** for these receptors (see 'chemokines') are **highly expressed only in those organs where breast cancer cells metastasize.**

3. In some cases, the target organ may be an unfavourable place for the growth of tumour cells. For example, the organ may secrete **inhibitors of proteases** (proteolytic enzymes). These, in turn, prevent the establishment of a tumour colony.

Defects in DNA Repair (Genomic Instability)

So far we have discussed the six characteristic features of malignancy, and also the genetic alterations (mutations) responsible for the attributes of cancer cells. **How do these mutations arise?** Whereas there are so many mutagenic agents in the environment (e.g., chemicals, radiation, sunlight), cancers are relatively rare. **This is because normal cells have the ability to repair DNA damage, and mutations occur when cells fail to repair this damage. In other words, mutations result from defects in DNA repair (genomic instability).** The importance of DNA repair in maintaining integrity of the genome is highlighted by several inherited disorders. In these disorders genes that encode proteins involved in DNA repair are defective. Individuals born with such inherited mutations of DNA repair proteins are at a greatly increased risk of developing cancer.

For example, certain cancers result from **defects in genes involved in DNA mismatch repair.** When a strand of DNA is being repaired, these genes act as **'spelling checkers'**. For example, if there is a wrong pairing of G with T rather than the normal A with T, **the mismatch repair genes correct the defect.** Without these 'proof-readers', errors slowly accumulate in several genes, including proto-oncogenes and cancer-suppressor genes. Thus, DNA repair genes affect cell growth only **indirectly,** by allowing mutations during the process of normal cell division.

Molecular Basis of Multi-Step Carcinogenesis

Tumours must develop those six fundamental abnormalities we have discussed earlier. This means that **each cancer must result from accumulation of multiple mutations.** Every human and animal cancer analyzed has revealed multiple genetic alterations, involving activation of several oncogenes and loss of two or more cancer-suppressor genes.

Each of these alterations represents crucial steps in the progression from a normal cell to a malignant tumour.

Tumour Progression and Heterogeneity

It is well established that many tumours become more aggressive and more malignant over a period of time. This phenomenon is referred to as 'tumour progression'. It must be differentiated from an increase in tumour size. Increasing malignancy, that is, faster growth, invasiveness, and ability to form distant metastases, is usually acquired in a step-wise manner. This progression phenomenon is due to the development of **subpopulations of cells** in the tumour that differ from each other in many ways, such as invasiveness, rate of growth, metastatic ability, karyotype, hormonal responsiveness, and susceptibility to anti-cancer drugs. **Thus, despite the fact that most malignant tumours are monoclonal in origin, by the time they become clinically visible, their cells are extremely heterogeneous (i.e., of different kinds).**

At the molecular level, this is believed to result from **multiple mutations** that accumulate independently in different cells. **This leads to production of subclones (subgroups) with different characteristics.** Some of these mutations are lethal and kill the cells; others may stimulate cell growth by affecting other proto-oncogenes or cancer-suppressor genes. The subclones so formed are exposed to body's immune responses. For example, cells that are highly antigenic are destroyed by host defences (see 'tumour immunity'), whereas those with reduced growth factor requirements are selected. **A growing tumour therefore comes to have populations of those subclones that are able to survive, grow, invade, and metastasize - the so-called 'metastatic subclone'.**

Karyotypic Changes In Tumours

The genetic damage that activates or inactivates tumour-suppressor genes may be subtle, that is, difficult to detect (e.g., point mutation), or large enough to be detected in a karyotype (i.e., chromosomes). The *RAS* oncogene represents the best example of activation by **point mutation**. In certain tumours, karyotypic abnormalities are common. Specific abnormalities have been identified in most leukaemias and lymphomas. The common types of structural abnormalities in tumour cells include balanced translocations, deletions, and cytogenetic manifestations of gene amplification. In addition, whole chromosomes may be gained or lost.

Balanced translocations are extremely common. In this, there is a balanced and reciprocal translocation (change of location) between chromosomes, for example, between chromosome 8 and 14 in Burkitt lymphoma. **Chromosome deletions** are the second most prevalent structural abnormality in tumour cells.

Biology of Tumour Growth

Development of most malignant tumours can be divided into **four phases:** (1) transformation (malignant change in the target cell), (2) growth of the transformed cells, (3) local invasion, and (4) distant metastasis. The molecular basis of transformation has already been considered. Here we outline the **factors that affect growth of the transformed cells.**

Formation of a tumour from the proliferation of a single transformed cell is a complex process. It is influenced by many factors. Some, such as doubling time of tumour cells, are intrinsic to (i.e., originate within) the tumour cells. Others, such as angiogenesis, represent host responses brought about by tumour cells or their products. The multiple factors that influence tumour growth include: (1) kinetics of tumour growth, (2) tumour angiogenesis, and (3) tumour progression and heterogeneity. Of these, second and third have already been covered earlier. Therefore, here, we discuss only the kinetics of tumour cell growth.

Kinetics of Tumour Cell Growth

We may begin by asking a question. How long does it take to produce a clinically visible tumour? The original transformed cell (about 10µm in diameter) must undergo at least 30 population doublings to produce 10^9 **cells (weighing about 1 gm). This is the smallest clinically detectable mass.** On the other hand, only 10 further doubling cycles are required to produce a tumour containing 10^{12} **cells (weighing about 1 kg).** These are minimal estimates, based on the assumption that all descendants of the transformed cell retain the ability to divide, and that there is no loss of cells from the proliferative pool. All the same, this calculation highlights one extremely important concept about tumour growth. **By the time a solid tumour is clinically detected, it has already completed a major portion of its life cycle.** This means that a malignant tumour must be a mass of rapidly and constantly dividing cells. But, this is not entirely correct. Let us examine the facts.

1. The doubling time of tumour cells: The cycle controls exerted by tumour-suppressor genes *RB* and *TP53* and cyclins (see *'Rb* gene', *'TP53* gene', and 'cyclins') are deranged in most tumours. As a result, **tumour cells can be triggered into cycle more readily and without the usual restraints.** We may think that tumour cells must be completing the cell cycle more rapidly than normal cells. However, this is not true. In reality, the total cell cycle time for many tumours is equal to, or even longer than that of corresponding normal cells. **Thus, growth of tumours is usually not associated with a shortening of cell cycle time.**

2. Growth fraction: Growth fraction is the number of cells within the tumour that are in the proliferative (replicative) pool. During the early, sub-microscopic phase of tumour growth, the vast majority of transformed cells are in the **proliferative pool.** As tumours continue to grow, cells leave the proliferative pool due to shedding or death from lack of nutrients, by differentiating, and by reversion to Go (quiescent state). In fact, most cells within cancers remain in the Go or G1 phase. Thus, by the time a tumour is clinically detectable most cells are not in the proliferative pool. Even in some rapidly growing tumours, the **growth fraction is about 20%.**

3. Excess of cell production over cell loss: Ultimately the growth of tumours and the rate at which they grow are determined by the **excess of cell production over cell loss.** In some tumours, especially those with a high growth fraction, the imbalance is large. That is, there is much more cell production than cell loss. In these tumours, the growth is more rapid than those in which cell production exceeds cell loss by only a small margin.

Host Defence against Tumours: Tumour Immunity

Malignant transformation is associated with complex genetic alterations. Some of these may result in the expression of **proteins** that are treated as **non-self** or **foreign** by the immune system. Thus came the concept of **'immune surveillance'** (Fr. surveiller = to watch over, policing), put forward by Lewis Thomas and McFarlane Burnet. **It meant recognition and destruction of non-self tumour cells on their appearance, by the immune system.** The fact that cancers occur suggests that immune surveillance is imperfect and that some tumours escape such policing. In this section, we shall discuss the nature of tumour antigens, the host systems that recognize tumour cells, and the effectiveness of tumour immunity against spontaneous neoplasms.

Tumour Antigens

Tumour cells may differ antigenically from normal cells. They either gain or lose cell membrane molecules. Antigens that produce an immune response have been demonstrated in many experimentally induced and in **animal** and **human cancers**. They are of **two types**: (1) **tumour specific antigens**. These are present only on tumour cells and **not on any normal cells**, and (ii) **tumour-associated antigens**. These are present on tumour cells **and on some normal cells**. **Recent studies have revealed an important role for CD8+ cytotoxic T-cells in tumour immunity.**

(i) Tumour-specific antigens (TSAs): These were first demonstrated in chemically induced tumours of rodents (rats, mice). Many chemically induced tumours express **'private'** or **'unique'** antigens not shared by other histologically similar tumours induced by the same chemical, even in the same animal.

(ii) Tumour-associated antigens (TAAs): Most tumour antigens are not unique (specific) to the individual tumour, but are shared by similar tumours in other hosts.

Anti-Tumour Effector Mechanisms

Both cell-mediated and humoral immunity can have anti-tumour activity. The cellular effectors, that is, cells that mediate immunity have been described in Chapter 9 (see Fig. 59). Here, we briefly characterize these cells.

1. Cytotoxic T-lymphocytes (CD8+ T-cells): The role of cytotoxic T-cells in experimentally induced tumours is well established. In humans and animals, they seem to play a protective role, mainly against virus-associated neoplasms. **By recognizing the MHC class I antigens expressed on tumour cells, cytotoxic T-cells destroy the tumour cells** (Fig. 59).

2. Natural killer cells (NK cells): NK cells are lymphocytes that are capable of destroying tumour cells **without prior sensitization**. Therefore, they provide the **first line of defence against tumour cells**. After activation, with interleukin-2, NK cells can lyse a wide range of animal and human tumours (Fig. 59). **T-cells and NK cells provide complementary (mutually supportive) anti-tumour mechanisms.**

345

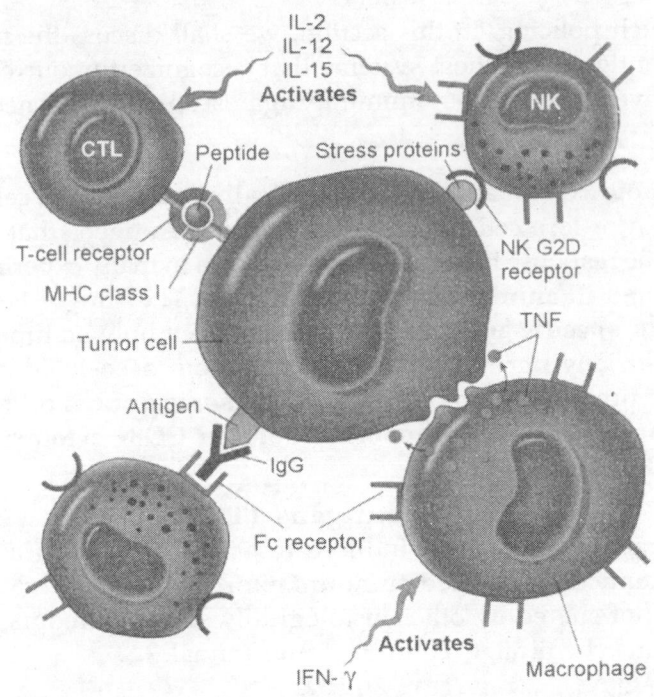

Fig. 59. Cellular effectors of anti-tumour immunity and some cytokines that regulate anti-tumour activities. CTL = cytotoxic T-cell; IFN = interferon; MHC = major histocompatibility complex; NK = natural killer; TNF = tumour necrosis factor.

For example, tumour cells that fail to express MHC class I antigens cannot be recognized by **T-cells**, and therefore T-cells cannot kill them. **However, such tumour cells may be killed by NK cells.** This is because when MHC class I antigens are present on tumour cells, they send **inhibitory signals** to NK cells to stop killing. In the absence of MHC class I antigens, NK cells do not receive any such inhibitory signals from tumour cells, and therefore proceed with killing (see 'natural killer cell' and Fig. 63 in Chapter 9). **Receptors on NK cells** are of different types and belong to several gene families. One such important receptor is **NKG2D** (Fig. 59). These receptors recognize stress-induced antigens. These are expressed mainly on tumour cells. Blocking the NKG2D receptors renders animals more susceptible to cancers. Apart from direct destruction of tumour cells, NK cells participate in **antibody-dependent cellular cytotoxicity (ADCC)**, as described in Chapter 9.

346

3. Macrophage: Activated macrophages show selective cytotoxicity against tumour cells. T-cells, NK cells, and macrophages may work together in their anti-tumour activity. This is because **interferon-gamma**, a cytokine secreted by T-cells and NK cells, **is a potent activator of macrophages** (Fig. 59). Macrophages may kill tumours by mechanisms similar to those used to kill bacteria, for example, production of reactive oxygen metabolites (see 'free radicals', Chapter 3), or by secretion of tumour necrosis factor (TNF) (Chapter 4).

4. Humoral mechanisms may also participate in tumour cell destruction by two mechanisms: (i) by activation of complement (see Chapter 4), and (ii) by induction of antibody-dependent cellular cytotoxicity (ADCC) by NK cells (see Chapter 9).

Immuno-surveillance

We discussed the possible anti-tumour mechanisms. But is there any evidence that they operate in the body to prevent the development of neoplasm? The strongest evidence for the existence of immuno-surveillance is the increased frequency of cancers in immuno-deficient hosts. If immuno-surveillance exists, how do cancers dodge the immune system in immuno-competent hosts? Several **escape mechanisms** have been proposed.

1. During tumour progression, strongly immunogenic subclones may be eliminated.

2. Tumour cells may fail to express normal levels of MHC class I antigen, **thus escaping attack by cytotoxic T-cells.**

3. **Lack of co-stimulation:** Sensitization of T-cells requires two signals, one by foreign peptide antigens presented by MHC and the other by co-stimulatory molecules (see Chapter 9). Although tumour cells may express peptide antigens with MHC class I molecules, **they usually do not express co-stimulatory molecules, such as B7-1.** This not only prevents sensitization, but also may **render T-cells anergic** (see 'anergy'), **or cause them to undergo apoptosis.**

4. **Immunosuppression:** Many oncogenic agents (chemicals, ionizing radiation) suppress host immune responses. **Tumours or tumour products also may be immunosuppressive.** For example, **transforming growth factor-beta (TGF-beta),** secreted in large quantities by many tumours, is a **potent immunosuppressant.** In some cases, the immune response induced by the tumour may inhibit tumour immunity. Another clever mechanism used by tumour is to

347

express **Fas ligand** that binds to **Fas receptor** on the surface of T-cells and sends a death signal to the immune cells (see 'apoptosis').

Clinical Features of Neoplasia

The importance of neoplasms lies in their effects on the host. Any tumour, even a benign one, may cause morbidity and mortality. This section considers: (1) the effects of a tumour on the host, (2) the grading and clinical staging of cancer, and (3) the laboratory diagnosis of neoplasms.

Effect of Tumours on Host

Cancers are far more threatening to the host than benign tumours. Nevertheless, both types of tumours may cause problems because of location and impingement on neighbouring structures, effects on functional activity such as hormone synthesis, and production of bleeding and secondary infections when the lesion ulcerates. Cancer may also be responsible for cachexia (wasting), or paraneoplastic syndromes.

(i) Cancer Cachexia (Wasting)

Many cancer patients suffer progressive loss of body fat and lean body mass, accompanied by profound weakness, anorexia, and anaemia. This wasting syndrome is referred to as **cachexia**. There are many factors responsible for cancer cachexia. Anorexia (reduced food intake) is one. Other important causes are circulating factors, such as tumour necrosis factor (TNF) and interleukin-1 (IL-1), released from activated macrophages. TNF suppresses appetite and inhibits the action of lipoprotein lipase, thereby inhibiting the release of free fatty acids from lipoproteins. A protein-mobilizing factor that causes breakdown of skeletal muscle proteins has been detected in the serum of cancer patients. In healthy animals, injection of this material causes acute weight loss without causing anorexia. Other molecules with lipolytic action also have been found.

(ii) Paraneoplastic Syndromes

Symptoms other than cachexia also appear in patients with cancer. If these symptoms cannot be easily explained either by local or distal spread of the tumour, or by secretion of hormones common to the tissue from where the tumour originated, then they are referred to as **'paraneoplastic syndromes'**. It is important to recognize them for several reasons. They may represent the earliest manifestation of a hidden neoplasm, or may even prove fatal to the patient. The paraneoplastic syndromes are diverse and are associated with many different tumours. **Hypercalcaemia** is one of the most common paraneoplastic syndromes.

Grading and Staging of Cancers

The **grading of a cancer** attempts to form some estimate about its aggressiveness or level of malignancy, based on the cytological differentiation of tumour cells and the number of mitoses within the tumour. The cancer may be classified as grade I, II, III, or IV, in the order of increasing neoplasia.

The staging of a cancer is based on the size of the primary lesion, its extent of spread to regional lymph nodes, and the presence or absence of metastases. This assessment is usually based on clinical and radiological examination, and in some cases surgical explorations. **The TNM system** is the commonly used method of staging (T, primary tumour; N, regional lymph node involvement; M, metastases). In this system, T1, T2, T3, and T4 describe the increasing size of the primary lesion; NO, N1, N2, and N3 indicate progressively advancing lymph node involvement; and MO and M1 reflect the absence or presence of distant metastases. **When compared with grading, staging has proved to be of greater clinical value.**

Laboratory Diagnosis of Cancer

In most cases, the laboratory diagnosis of cancer is not difficult. The clear-cut benign and malignant tumours pose no problems. However, those in the middle are difficult to assess. Here, the clinician (often a surgeon) and the pathologist can collaborate. Clinical data are extremely helpful for correct pathological diagnosis. This is because the laboratory evaluation of a lesion is only as good as the specimen submitted for examination. **The specimen therefore must be adequate, representative, and properly preserved.**

(i) Histological and Cytological Methods

Samples can be biopsy, fine-needle aspiration, and cytological smears. If the specimen is not properly preserved, the centre remains largely necrotic. The pieces should be small and properly immersed in a usual fixative, such as formalin solution. In experienced and competent hands, **frozen-section diagnosis** is accurate and very helpful, particularly during surgical operations. This method, in which a sample is quick-frozen and sectioned, permits histological evaluation within minutes. This helps the surgeon in deciding whether the lesion is malignant and requires wider excision. However, in many cases better histological details provided by the more time-consuming routine histopathological methods are required. In such cases, it is better to wait a few days, than to perform unnecessary surgery.

Fine-needle aspiration of tumours is another method for the detection of cancer. It involves aspiration of cells from a tumour, followed by cytological examination of the smear. It prevents unnecessary surgery and its risks, and in experienced hands, it can be extremely reliable, rapid, and helpful. **Cytological (Papanicolaou) smears** provide another method for the detection of cancer. It is commonly used for many forms of suspected malignancy, such as bladder and prostate tumours and gastric carcinomas in **dogs**; for the identification of tumour cells in abdominal, pleural, joints, and cerebrospinal fluids, and, less commonly, with other forms of neoplasms. **Neoplastic cells are less cohesive (sticking together) than others and so are shed into fluids or secretions. The shed (exfoliated) cells are evaluated for features of anaplasia (exfoliative cytology).** However, cytological interpretation requires a great deal of expertise. A negative report does not exclude the presence of a malignancy. Likewise, all positive findings must be confirmed by biopsy and histopathological examination before deciding the line of treatment. Recent aids in the laboratory diagnosis of cancer include immunocytochemistry (monoclonal antibodies), Southern blot analysis, flow cytometry, and DNA probe analyses. These techniques can be applied to exfoliated cancer cells, tissue aspirations, or biopsy specimens.

(ii) Biochemical Assays

Biochemical assays for tumour-associated enzymes, hormones, and other tumour markers in the blood are also helpful, and in some cases are useful in determining the effectiveness of therapy. A large number of circulating tumour markers have been described and new ones are identified every year. Only a few have stood the test of time and proved to be clinically useful. The two best established in humans are: (1) **carcino-embryonic antigen (CEA)**, and (ii) **alpha-foetoprotein**. However, since these markers are also increased in several other disorders that are not neoplastic, they lack in specificity and sensitivity required for the detection of cancers.

(iii) Molecular Diagnosis

An increasing number of molecular techniques have been recently introduced for the diagnosis of tumours and for predicting their behaviour. The two most important are: (1) **polymerase chain reaction (PCR)** to differentiate between monoclonal (neoplastic) and polyclonal (reactive) proliferations, and (2) **fluorescent *in situ* hybridization (FISH) technique,** useful in detecting translocation characteristic of many tumours.

Molecular Profiling of Tumours

One of the most exciting advances in the molecular analysis of tumours has been made possible by **'DNA-microarray analysis'**. This technique, the so-called **'gene chip technology'** allows simultaneous measurements of the expression levels of several thousand genes.

TUMOURS OF DIFFERENT TISSUES

The description of tumours arising from different tissues is as per the histogenetic classification given earlier in **Table 12.**

Connective Tissue Tumours

As mentioned, the benign form of a tumour is designated by the tissue of origin plus the suffix **'oma'**. The term **sarcoma** indicates the malignant form of the connective tissue tumour. The word sarcoma is derived from the Greek word for flesh (sarkos).

Fibroma and Fibrosarcoma

These tumours originate from **connective tissue cells**, and are common in the **horse** and **dog**. According to the amount of collagen present, fibromas and fibrosarcomas may be either **hard**, or **soft**. **Macroscopically, hard fibromas** and fibrosarcomas are firm and hard. Their cut surface is dry and white or yellowish-white. The tumours are composed of bundles of connective tissue. They may vary in size from tiny nodules to masses weighing more than 45 kilograms. They must be differentiated from chronic inflammatory conditions like tuberculosis, actinobacillosis, actinomycosis and staphylococcosis, in which large amount of connective tissue is deposited. **Soft fibromas** are spongy, more vascular than hard fibromas, and often oedematous. When they involve a mucous membrane, these tumours are often pedunculated and are called **polyps**. Polyps are common in the nasal passages of **horse (nasal polyps)**. The cut surface of soft fibromas may be pink due to their rich blood supply.

Microscopically, the **hard fibromas** are composed of adult type fibrous connective tissue cells. The cells and their nuclei are spindle-shaped. The collagen fibres are seen as compact bundles of wavy

351

fibres, arranged in a concentric manner around blood vessels. The **soft fibromas** contain very little collagen. Intermediate types between the hard and soft fibromas contain moderate amount of collagen. The rapidly growing fibrosarcomas contain numerous blood vessels, and present characters of anaplasia (see 'microscopic appearance').

Regarding **location**, fibromas can occur wherever there is connective tissue. Since connective tissue is abundant in all parts of the body, fibromas occur anywhere. The most common site is the subcutaneous tissue of the head, neck, shoulder, and legs. **Gingival fibromas** are extremely common in the **dog**. They are found along the gum line, and are commonly called as **epuli** (sing. **epulus**). **Neurofibroma** is derived from Schwann cells of the nerve sheath (neurilemma), and occurs in **dogs**, mostly subcutaneously. The **prognosis** of a fibroma is good, if it could be removed surgically. When large, or occur in vital organs, they could be problematic. Fibrosarcomas may metastasize to lungs and other internal organs.

Equine sarcoid: The tumour is believed to be caused by a virus, and arises from fibrous connective tissue. It occurs in **horses**, **mules**, and **donkeys**, and is indistinguishable from fibromas and fibrosarcomas. Even though the tumour recurs after excision, it does not metastasize. It occurs in head, neck, and the forelegs. The growths are irregular in shape and tend to ulcerate. Most tumours have the history suggestive of relationship to trauma. Equine connective tissue is inherently extremely sensitive to injury. **Microscopically**, the neoplastic cells are usually arranged in whorled patterns of spindle-shaped cells. On account of ulceration, it often becomes impossible to separate proliferating tumour from the accompanying inflammatory response of the connective tissue. Areas of necrosis and leukocytic infiltrations are seen throughout.

Spirocerca fibrosarcoma of dogs: This tumour of **dog** is produced by a nematode called *Spirocerca lupi.* Like the mixed mammary tumour of the dog, it has mixed connective tissue components. Briefly, larvae of *S. lupi* penetrate the stomach walls, and then migrate through the adventitia and media of arteries until they reach anterior aorta. They then leave aorta and move to the adjacent caudal portion of the oesophagus, encyst in its submucosa, and periodically discharge eggs into the lumen of the oesophagus. The tumours therefore occur in the wall of the oesophagus, aorta, and stomach.

Macroscopically, invasive fibrosarcomas or osteosarcomas are seen. The tumours are firm, pinkish or greyish, often protruding into the lumen of the oesophagus as polypoid masses. **Microscopically**, there is marked anaplasia characterized by enlarged and hyperchromatic nuclei and mitotic figures in the characteristically spindle-shaped cells.

Transmissible fibropapilloma of cattle: This tumour is produced by the virus of bovine cutaneous papillomatosis, a DNA oncogenic virus (see Table 16). The neoplastic transformation occurs in both squamous epithelium and connective tissue. On non-genital surfaces the epithelial changes are more, whereas in the genitalia the neoplastic proliferation of connective tissue is so extreme that the tumour resembles fibrosarcoma. Growth on the genitalia is benign, does not metastasize, and usually regresses. **Macroscopically**, the tumour usually occurs singly on the penis, or in the vulva, or vagina. They vary in size and have a cauliflower-like appearance. Most of them have an ulcerated surface. **Microscopically**, fibropapillomas consist of connective tissue covered with stratified squamous epithelium of varying thickness. Young tumours appear as fibrosarcomas; fibroblasts being young with many mitotic figures. Older tumours have mature connective tissue with no mitotic figures.

Rous sarcoma of poultry: This is caused by a RNA oncogenic virus (a retrovirus) known as a Rous sarcoma virus (RSV). RSV induces sarcomas (tumours of connective tissue) which include both fibroma and fibrosarcoma; myxoma and myxosarcoma; osteoma and osteosarcoma; and chondrosarcoma.

Shope fibroma of rabbits: Described first by Shope in 1933, Shope fibroma is an example of another **virus-induced tumour**, caused by a DNA oncogenic virus. The tumour occurs as one or more firm subcutaneous masses **in rabbits**. It is composed of spindle-shaped connective tissue cells. The tumour grows slowly, and remains mostly as a localized lesion.

Myxoma and Myxosarcoma

These tumours of **connective tissue are capable of producing mucin**. Normally, it is embryonic connective tissue that produces mucin (e.g., Wharton's jelly of the umbilical cord). Therefore, any mucin-producing tumour cells are anaplastic and hence indicate malignancy. The myxoid change is supposed to be due to metaplasia. **Myxoma and myxosarcomas are not common in animals.**

Macroscopically, the myxomas resemble soft fibromas in appearance and consistency. They are usually not large, rather

353

transparent, and of pale yellow or greenish colour. Their cut surface is moist and slimy because of mucin. **Microscopically**, they consist of spindle-shaped and stellate (star-shaped) connective tissue cells, possessing long, branching fibrils, suspended in an abundance of intercellular mucin. While diagnosing, myxoma should not be confused with soft fibromas.

The tumour **occurs** in the subcutaneous tissue of head and shoulder. Occasionally, they are reported in the heart and uterus in **cows**. The prognosis of a myxoma is good. Myxosarcoma is extremely rare.

Infectious myxomatosis of rabbits: This is caused by a **virus** and occurs as raised nodular growths on the head, face, ears, and abdomen. Large, branching, invasive cells, containing mucin are considered neoplastic and spread rapidly in the subcutaneous tissues. It is a rapidly progressive disease causing death in 10-20 days.

Lipoma and Liposarcoma

These tumours originate from **fat cells**. These are rather common tumours in **most species of domestic animals** in the older age group. **Lipomas are much more common than liposarcomas.**

Macroscopically, they occur mostly singly and vary in size. A lipoma up to 54 kilograms in the abdominal cavity of an aged **mare** has been reported. Others may be so small that they are easily overlooked. They also vary in shape, and may be pedunculated or encapsulated, and mostly either lobulated or nodular. **Lipomas** are soft, cut surface being oily, translucent, white or yellow in colour. Calcification may also occur, and rarely formation of bone from metaplasia. **Liposarcomas** are much more variable in appearance. They may be soft or firm, and have a definite nodular appearance.

Microscopically, lipomas are made up of cells containing either one large fat globule, or several small ones. The nucleus is pushed to the periphery or even obliterated. Interspersed between the fat cells are strands of collagen fibres. In liposarcomas, tumour cells are more difficult to identify as having originated from fat cells. They may be round, stellate, spindle-shaped, or polyhedral. Small globules of fat can be identified only with fat stains. The nuclei are very large. Mitotic figures and giant cells are common.

The tumour **occurs** where fat is abundant such as in the mesentery, peritoneum, subcutis, and submucosa. The most common sites for lipoma and liposarcoma are tissues of the thorax and abdomen, thorax being more common in **dogs**. **Prognosis**: Lipomas are very slow to undergo malignant transformation. They do not recur on excision. Some are so large that they create problem due to their sheer size. Liposarcomas are more infiltrative and more difficult to remove.

Chondroma and Chondrosarcoma

These tumours consist mainly of neoplastic **cartilage cells**. They **occur** in places where cartilage is normally present, e.g., at the epiphyses of long bones of the extremities, the costo-chondral and chondro-sternal junctions, and in the cartilage of the nasal passages, larynx, trachea, and bronchi. These tumours are extremely rare in cattle, pigs, horses, cats and dogs, but have been reported in **sheep** on costo-chondral junctions of the rib, the scapula, humerus, and femur.

Macroscopically, these tumours are hard, lobulated, well-defined and almost always occur singly. They may even attain weight over 9 kilograms in **cattle** and **horses**, and 4.5 kilograms in **sheep** and **dogs**. On section, chondromas are transculent, bluish-white and glistening. Sections of a chondroma show more confluent growth. **Microscopically**, some chondromas are very cellular; others are not. The cells are arranged singly, and not in groups as in normal cartilage. They vary much in size and shape. At the periphery, they are small and at the centre large. Between the cells is a hyaline matrix. As in normal cartilage, there are no vessels. The chondrosarcomas are much more cellular and anaplastic. Nuclei are large and hyperchromatic. Mitotic figures are frequent. Cells vary from spindle to round in shape.

Prognosis: The chondrosarcoma frequently metastasizes to lungs if left untreated. Chondroma seldom recurs after removal.

Osteoma and Osteosarcoma

These are tumours of bone. Their cells have the ability to form osteoid matrix, and even bone. In animals, osteomas are rare except in the **dog**. Osteosarcomas are also relatively more common in the **dogs** and **cats**, and occur rarely in **horses** and **cattle**. An osteoma is at times difficult to differentiate from inflammatory formation of new bone, such as **the exostoses** on the limbs and mandible of **horses**. These are not neoplasms.

355

Macroscopically, osteomas are small, hard, slow growing, sharply defined and encapsulated. They are round or elliptical in shape. The bone near an osteosarcoma usually shows extensive destruction. This is because the bone has a tendency to undergo demineralization whenever active growth is present. **Microscopically**, in benign osteomas the arrangement of lamellae is like that of normal bone. The Haversian canals are not so regular, and run at right angle to the bone axis. In the osteosarcomas, the osteoblasts may be very anaplastic, pleomorphic, and hyperchromatic. They also contain many tumour giant cells.

Most osteomas **occur** in the bone of the head, particularly of the nasal passages and orbital region. They must be differentiated from inflammatory formation of bone (**exostosis**). **Osteosarcomas** in the **dog** may be skeletal or extra-skeletal. This is because in certain connective tissue tumours, the connective tissue has a tendency to undergo metaplasia to **osteosarcoma**, for example, mixed mammary tumour of the dog and **osteosarcoma** associated with *Spirocerca lupi* infection. Skeletal osteosarcomas in dogs occur mostly in the humerus, the middle ribs, and the lower half of the radius, femur, and tibia. They also occur in the jaw and nasal bones of the **horse** and **cow**. **Prognosis**: Like chondrosarcoma, skeletal osteosarcoma usually metastasizes to lungs.

Canine Transmissible Venereal Tumour

Transmissible venereal tumour of the **dog** is of uncertain histogenesis. That is, the cell of origin of this tumour is not known. **The neoplastic cells have 59 chromosomes compared to the normal 78 for dogs.** The tumour is transmitted at coitus by the transfer of intact tumour cells. Both sexes are affected. It occurs in the genital organs, namely, vulva, vagina, penis, or prepuce of dogs. **This is a very common tumour of dogs**. The tumour is also of great historical importance. It was the first neoplasm to be successfully transmitted from one animal to another. M.A. Novinsky, a Russian veterinarian, was the first to demonstrate that it could be transplanted to other dogs. Since the tumour is spread by coitus, it is called **venereal** (resulting from sexual intercourse) **granuloma**.

Grossly, these tumours are single or multiple, small or large, soft or friable, sessile or pedunculated, nodular or papillary masses, grey or red in colour. In the vaginal mucosa, the nodules are often red, ulcerate, and protrude from the vulva. Ulceration, necrosis, and haemorrhage may occur. If metastasis occurs, it usually involves only the regional lymph nodes. **Microscopically**, the cells are large, round, oval, or polyhedral with indistinct outlines and poorly stained cytoplasm. Considerable variation may occur in the size of cells, and mitotic figures are numerous. Other microscopic features include multi-focal necrosis and infiltration of lymphocytes. Lymphocytes may cause **cell-mediated tumour cell lysis**, and this mechanism may be responsible for spontaneous regression of the tumour.

Most of the tumours are confined to genitalia, but occasionally may occur in the skin on other parts of the body, such as face and shoulders. It is a tumour of younger dogs (1-6 years of age), and is **more common in the female**. Care should be taken not to diagnose mast-cell tumour as transmissible venereal tumour. **Prognosis**: Surgical removal of this tumour should be done with great care because the cells can be easily transplanted in the wound of surgery, or other portions of the body. For this reason, recurrence is quite common. Sometimes the tumour spontaneously regresses, and when this occurs, the dog acquires immunity against the tumour.

Mast-cell Tumour (Mastosarcoma, Mastocytoma)

This tumour arises from the **mast cells** of the connective tissue of skin. Since mast cells are produced from undifferentiated mesenchymal cells in the connective tissue, this tumour is grouped here. It is mainly a tumour of the **dog**, and occasionally also of the **cat**. It usually develops on the thighs, and rarely on external genitals. These tumours appear at a later age than venereal granuloma, majority being between 6-15 years. **Macroscopically**, it appears usually as a small, solitary swelling. Most tumours vary in size from 1 cm to 20 cm in diameter, and may ulcerate. Cut surface is grey or white, and has a lobulated appearance. Slowly growing tumours are often soft in consistency, while the rapidly growing are firm. Encapsulation is not present. Metastasis and recurrence are common.

Microscopically, the tumour cells are round, oval, or polyhedral. The nuclei are round or oval. One or more nucleoli may be observed. In H and E stained sections, the metachromatic cytoplasmic granules that characterize this tumour, are not clear. Therefore, it is necessary to use Giemsa or toluidine blue staining methods to demonstrate the granules. Numerous leukocytes such as eosinophils and neutrophils are present. Mitotic figures are few.

357

Tumours of Endothelial and Related Tissues

Tumours may arise from **endothelial cells of capillaries or lymphatics**. Benign tumours are called **haemangiomas** and **lymphangiomas**, and malignant as **haemangiosarcomas** and **lymphangiosarcomas**.

Haemangioma and Haemangiosarcoma

Haemangiosarcomas have been reported in the liver and spleen of **dogs**. They also occur in **horses** and **cattle**. Lymphangiomas and lymphangiosarcomas are extremely rare, and therefore will not be described. Haemangiomas and haemangiosarcomas should not be confused with telangiectasis. **Telangiectasis** is dilatation of pre-existing vessels, most commonly observed in the **liver of cattle**. Telangiectasis usually occurs throughout the liver and there is no invasion of the regional lymph nodes, nor any evidence of metastasis to the lungs. Care should be taken to differentiate these tumours from blood vascular haemartias. **Haemartias** are developmental defects in the blood vascular system. Haemartias are common in the skin (usually shanks) and occasionally internal organs of the White Leghorn chickens, and are detected usually at the postmortem examination. They vary in size from being just visible to round bulging protrusions, measuring up to 3 cm in diameter. Repeated haemorrhage from trauma often leads to the death of the bird. The tendency of birds to pick also favours recurrence of haemorrhage. Histologically, haemartias consist of small capillary nests and large masses of inter-lacing capillaries in the subcutaneous tissue.

Haemangiomas are of **three types**: (i) capillary, (ii) cavernous, and (iii) solid. The **capillary type** consists of capillaries more or less uniform in size. The **cavernous type** is composed of capillaries that are greatly dilated. In contrast, the **solid type** consists of masses of endothelial cells, without any vascular lumen. **Macroscopically**, haemangiomas are dark red in colour and soft in consistency. The more vascular type is red and soft; the more cellular type looks like a sarcoma, and is more firm or solid. They bleed profusely when traumatized. They vary in size, being up to 15 or more cm in diameter. They weigh as much as 2 kilograms. **Microscopically**, the more vascular type of haemangioma consists of newly formed capillaries lined by a single layer of endothelial cells. The capillaries are surrounded by varying amounts of collagen fibres. The more solid type consists of mass of endothelial cells with no vascular lumen. The nuclei of haemangiosarcomas are round or oval with normal or atypical mitotic figures.

These tumours **occur** mostly in the extremities, thorax, perianal region, and in the liver and spleen, particularly in **dogs**. **Prognosis** for haemangiomas is good, as they do not recur after removal. The prognosis for haemangiosarcomas is very unfavourable. Even most haemartias progress to malignancy. Haemangiosarcomas are very prone to metastasize, being a malignant tumour of blood vessels, and cause death.

Haemangiopericytoma

Electron microscopic studies have revealed that these tumours originate from **pericytes**. Pericytes are cells present in the walls of capillaries and venules, external to endothelial cells, and enveloped by basement membrane. Haemangiopericytomas are seen usually in the subcutaneous tissues of older **dogs**, but are extremely rare in other domestic animals.

Macroscopically, they are firm, lobulated masses of several cm in diameter. They occur on the limbs, thorax, abdomen, face, and back. **Microscopically**, the neoplastic cells encircle and closely approach capillaries. These capillaries have distinct endothelium with collagenous sheaths that separate them from neoplastic cells. This forms the basis of their differentiation from endothelial neoplasms. Although some tumours are anaplastic and show mitotic activity, they grow more by expansion and seldom show invasiveness.

Mesothelioma

This tumour originates from mesothelium (lining cells of body cavities) of peritoneum, pleura, and pericardium. **In animals, these tumours are rare**, and have been reported in **cattle** and **horses** only. They should not be confused with inflammatory changes, or tumour metastases. They appear as nodular or papillary growths, covered by proliferating mesothelial cells. **Microscopically**, they show capillary growths of endothelium and supporting stroma.

Meningioma

Tumours involving the meninges are called **meningiomas**. Since they originate from the mesothelial cells of cranial and spinal meninges, they are grouped here. However, for a better understanding, they are described under 'Tumours of nervous tissue'.

Tumours of Haematopoietic Cells

The subject of neoplastic processes involving **haematopoietic cells** in animals is vast and complex, and beyond the scope of this book. It is therefore dealt with only briefly.

Neoplasms involving **haematopoietic cells** are of **two types**: (i) myeloproliferative, and (ii) lymphoproliferative disorders. A **myeloproliferative disorder (MPD)** is a disorder of the haematopoietic stem cells that produce granulocytic, monocytic, and megakaryocytic series. A **lymphoproliferative disorder (LPD)** is restricted to the cells of the lymphoid series (Table 17).

Table 17. A simplified classification of haematopoietic neoplasms

1. **Myeloproliferative disorders**
   i.   Acute myeloid leukaemia
   ii. Chronic myeloid leukaemia
2. **Lymphoproliferative disorders**
   i.   Lymphocytic
        Lymphoma
        Acute lymphocytic leukaemia
        Chronic lymphocytic leukaemia
        Lymphosarcoma
        Hodgkin's disease
   ii. Plasmacytic
        Multiple myeloma

Leukaemias

Leukaemia is a neoplastic disease involving one or more type of cells of the haematopoietic tissues. The total leukocyte count is extremely high (**leukaemoid reaction**) with abnormal or primitive cells in the blood. This permits diagnosis. Leukaemia, however, is not always associated with leukocytosis (**aleukaemic leukaemia**). Also neoplastic blood cells may not be observed in blood films. In fact, in some cases leukopaenia (decrease of white cells) may occur (**subleukaemic leukaemia**) as is common in lymphoma.

The **leukaemias** are further categorized as **acute** or **chronic**, based on cellular maturity, apparent onset, and clinical course. **Acute** leukaemias are characterized by the presence of mostly **immature (blast) cells** in the blood and haematopoietic tissues, and a relatively shorter clinical course. **In humans**, more than 30% blast cells in the bone marrow are sufficient for the diagnosis of acute myeloid leukaemia (AML), and this is true for the **dog** and **cat**. **Chronic leukaemias** are characterized by the predominance of mature leukocytes in the blood and bone marrow, and a relatively longer clinical course. A number of cytomorphological features help in differentiating lymphocytic, granulocytic, and monocytic leukaemias. These include cell size, nuclear shape, type of nuclear chromatin (fine to coarse), number of nucleoli, amount of cytoplasm (nuclear:cytoplasmic ratio), cytoplasmic basophilia, presence of azurophilic and specific granules, and cytological markers (peroxidase, alkaline phosphatase, lipase, non-specific esterase).

The **incidence** of leukaemia in animals varies with the type of leukaemia, the species involved, and the geographic location. Although leukaemia can occur at any age, myeloid leukaemia is common in young animals. The species most commonly affected are **cats** and **dogs**. Leukaemia also occurs in **cattle, horses, sheep, goats,** and **pigs**. A brief description follows.

Feline Leukaemias

Haematopoietic neoplasms represent about one-third of all **cat tumours, and most are lymphoid.** They are caused by **feline leukaemia virus (FeLV).** The FeLV is a C-type oncornavirus (retrovirus), similar to avian and murine leukaemia viruses (see Table 16).

Among the lymphoproliferative disorders, lymphoma and lymphocytic leukaemia are common and may occur singly or in combination. **These two tumours account for 80 to 90% of all feline haematopoietic neoplasms; lymphoma being the most common.** Clinical signs include depression, rapid wasting, fluctuating temperature elevations, vomiting, diarrhoea, and refractory anaemia. Haematological changes in lymphoid malignancies are usually not characteristic of leukaemia. Cats also develop **acute lymphoblastic leukaemia** un-associated with solid tumour masses. **The myeloproliferative disorders (MPD) or myeloid leukaemias** involving the neutrophils, eosinophils, and basophils, are the classical forms of MPD. Monocytic leukaemias are rare in cats.

Canine Leukaemias

Lymphoma is the most common form of lymphoproliferative neoplasia in the **dog**. It occurs in dogs of five years of age and above, with no sex predilection. The cause is still under investigation, and canine leukaemia virus has not been demonstrated to be the cause. **Canine lymphoma** is characterized by a bilateral, painful swelling of the superficial lymph nodes (**bilateral lymphadenopathy**). Oedema of the face, throat or limbs may be present in the late stages of the disease. A definite diagnosis of lymphoma requires finding neoplastic cells in the blood, bone marrow, and cytological aspirates, or in biopsy specimens of the lymph nodes, or other tissues. In addition, **dogs** also suffer from **acute and chronic lymphocytic leukaemias (ALL and CLL).** ALL is a rapidly progressive disease of sudden onset, characterized by high numbers of lymphoblasts in the blood and bone marrow, un-associated with solid tumour masses. Clinical signs include lethargy, anorexia, vomiting, diarrhoea, anaemia, splenomegaly, and hepatomegaly. **CLL** is a disease with long course that manifests over a period of several months or years. It is characterized by the presence of a large number of well-differentiated mature lymphocytes in the blood and bone marrow. **CLL is a disease of B-lymphocytes.**

Myeloproliferative disorders (MPD) include acute and chronic myelogenous leukaemias. Myelogenous leukaemia is more common in **young dogs**, and **lymphoma** is more common in **older dogs**. Clinical signs include progressive weakness and weight loss over a period of several months. In addition, anorexia, vomiting, polydipsia (excessive thirst), polyuria (excessive urination), diarrhoea and anaemia are present in various combinations. The typical blood picture of **myelogenous leukaemia** is a neutrophilia with a left shift to myeloblasts. The neutrophils exhibit variation in shape and size. Monocytic leukaemias also occur in the dog, particularly in young animals.

Bovine Leukaemias

The leukaemias in cattle primarily originate from the neoplastic proliferation of lymphocytes. C-type oncornavirus (retrovirus), known as **bovine leukaemia virus (BLV),** is the cause of abnormal proliferation of lymphocytes. It causes either a **benign persistent lymphocytosis (PL),** or a malignant tumour-forming disease known as **enzootic bovine leukosis,** or the **adult form of lymphoma in cattle.**

Bovine Lymphoma

Lymphoma affects cattle of all breeds and ages, but is **more common in dairy cattle**, after 5 years of age. Lymphoma occurs in two main forms: (i) **enzootic bovine leukosis (EBL),** also known as **adult form of lymphoma.** This is the **most prevalent** form and is caused by BLV, and (ii) **sporadic form.** This is **rare.**

Adult bovine lymphoma is mostly **an afebrile disease,** and is characterized by widespread lymphadenopathy with frequent involvement of the heart, abomasum, and intestine. **Bilateral enlargement of the superficial lymph nodes is the first detectable abnormality.** Rectal palpation of the pelvic and abdominal organs may reveal extensive neoplastic masses. Chronic indigestion, cardiac abnormalities, and partial or complete paralysis may occur because of neoplastic infiltration of the abomasum, myocardium, and nerves of the spinal cord, respectively. The course of illness may vary from a few weeks to several months. The terminal phase is associated with rapid wasting and sudden death. Cardiac failure is the major cause of death. Specific tumour-associated antigens (TAA) appear on the surface of lymphocytes of cattle infected with EBL.

The **diagnosis** of **bovine persistent lymphocytosis** should be based on repeated demonstration of significant lymphocytosis for several weeks. **The lymphocytes are of normal morphology. Lymphoma** is a tumour-forming disease, and is not regularly associated with lymphocytosis, or the occurrence of abnormal lymphocytes in the blood. In suspected cases, such abnormal lymphocytes should be carefully detected, because they are diagnostic. Lymphoblasts, lymphoid cells with multiple asymmetrically lobed nuclei, and mitotic figures are frequently observed in blood during the leukaemic phase.

Equine Leukaemias

Lymphoma is the most important haematopoietic neoplasm in the **horse,** lymphatic leukaemia is infrequent, and myelogenous leukaemia is extremely rare. **The cause is unknown.** Lymphoma, in the **horse,** is not as common as in the **dog, cat,** and **cow.** The clinical picture of equine lymphoma is varied, and the differential diagnosis is difficult. Lymphoma usually occurs in horses of 5 years and above. Clinical signs include peripheral lymphadenopathy, weight loss, ventral oedema, pleural effusion, respiratory distress, and fever. Haematological findings include immature lymphocytes and a moderate leukocytosis. The lymph node biopsy is diagnostic of lymphoma. The usual picture is of an admixture of lymphoblasts, some plasma cells, and a few normal, mature lymphocytes. Mitotic figures are usually present in small numbers. Various types of myeloid leukaemias, that is, myelogenous, eosinophilic, and monocytic have been reported in the **horse**, but are extremely rare.

Leukaemias in Other Species

Leukaemia is rare in other animal species. Sporadic cases have been reported in **sheep, goats, pigs**, and **buffaloes**. Of these, except for **pigs**, MPD has not been described in other animals. **Lymphoma** in **sheep** occurs mostly in adult animals, without sex and breed predilection. The tissues most commonly involved are lymph nodes, spleen, liver, kidney, small intestine, and heart. Ovine lymphoma is caused by a C-type oncornavirus, and the BLV is oncogenic for sheep. **Lymphoma** in **goats** is **rare**, and presents as lymphadenopathy at necropsy. In **pigs**, **lymphoma** occurs mainly as a sporadic disease in young animals, without sex or breed predilection. Clinical signs include ataxia or perhaps paralysis, enlarged superficial lymph nodes, loss of body weight, dyspnoea (laboured or difficult breathing), and sudden death. The **diagnosis** is difficult from the blood examination because the WBC count is often normal, and abnormal lymphocytes may not be present. Single cases of myelogenous (myeloid) leukaemia, eosinophilic leukaemia, and granulocytic sarcoma have been reported in **pigs**.

Lymphosarcoma (Malignant Lymphoma)

The malignant form of lymphoma is called **lymphosarcoma**, or a **malignant lymphoma**. Its parenchyma comprises immature lymphocytes. There is little stroma. It grows rapidly and produces extensive metastases. **Cattle, dogs, pigs**, and **chickens** are most commonly affected. Lymphoma is believed to be **caused by a virus.**

Macroscopically, lymphosarcomas may appear as solitary tumours. They are greyish-white in colour. **In chickens**, they are usually multiple. When the tumour is generalized, all the lymphoid organs become greatly enlarged. As a result, there is splenomegaly, hepatomegaly, and enlargement of the lymph nodes, thymus, and Peyer's patches. The bone marrow is also involved. Extensive involvement of the skin in the **cattle** is occasionally observed. Lymphosarcoma is most common in **aged cats**, and involves internal organs such as intestine and kidney, than the peripheral lymph nodes.

364

Microscopically, the normal architecture of the lymphoid tissue disappears. Besides the normal lymphocytes, there are innumerable anaplastic cells of variable size. The total leukocyte count may show increases up to 5 times the normal number for **horses**, up to 15 for **cattle** and **pigs**, and up to 60 for **dogs**. **The predominating cells are lymphocytes and lymphoblasts**. There is a decrease in the number of erythrocytes, neutrophils and platelets, because the infiltrating leukocytes cause atrophy of the haematopoietic tissue of the bone marrow.

Depending on the maturity of the lymphocytes, **lymphosarcomas in domestic animals are classified into four cytological types**: (1) **lymphocytic type**: The lymphosarcoma is composed of cells resembling mature lymphocytes. (2) **lymphoblastic type**: In this, the cells are more immature and resemble lymphoblasts. (3) **reticulum (or histiocytic) type**: The lymphocytes are still more immature, and (4) **stem cell (or poorly differentiated type),** representing the most anaplastic type of cell. These histological types may not be always separable, and in some cases, two types may occur together. When the neoplastic cells are found circulating in the blood, the term **leukaemia** is used. If the cells are lymphocytic in origin, it is **lymphocytic leukaemia**; if of myeloid origin, **myelocytic leukaemia**. If the cells are not circulating in the blood, the term leukaemia cannot be used, because leukaemia signifies that leukocytes are present in the bloodstream. It is emphasized that **in domestic animals**, the occurrence of immature cells in the blood is much less frequently observed than in humans.

Lymphosarcomas occur in the lymphoid tissues, that is, lymph nodes, spleen, thymus, and other lymphoid organs. On the basis of their distribution, they are classified in **three forms**: multicentric, thymic, or alimentary. (i) **multicentric form**: In this, lymphosarcomas involve most of the lymph nodes as well as other organs. This applies to about **65% of canine cases**. (ii) **thymic form**: in this, the thymus is replaced and greatly enlarged by lymphosarcoma. This is seen in about **20% of feline cases**; and **also** occurs in **cattle, dogs, pigs**, and **sheep**. (iii) **alimentary form**: In this, the tumours appear to arise in Peyer's patches, but invade submucosa and muscularis. Occasionally, a **leukaemic form** occurs. The lymphocytic tumour cells replace the bone marrow, and collect in various organs. **In cattle**, walls of the forestomachs and heart are the frequent locations.

365

Hodgkin's Disease

Hodgkin's disease, **in humans**, is a lymphoid neoplasm recognized by its characteristic histology. The tumour in the lymph nodes begins with lymphocytic hyperplasia. This is followed by a gradual loss of normal architecture with replacement of lymphocytes as the disease progresses. It is characterized by the presence of distinctive binuclear or multinuclear cells called Reed-Sternberg (RS) cells, mixed with inflammatory cells. RS cells are pathognomonic for diagnosis. **Typical Hodgkin's disease has not been found in animals.** However, several cases of possible Hodgkin's disease have been reported in the **dog**. Also, Hodgkin's disease has been diagnosed in a 9-year-old female **cat**. Necropsy revealed splenomegaly. The diagnosis was based on the presence of numerous cells with characteristics of RS cells.

Plasmacytic Lymphoproliferative Disorder: Multiple Myeloma

Multiple myeloma is characterized by proliferation of neoplastic **plasma cells** in bone marrow, often producing multifocal osteolytic (causing softening and destruction of bone) lesions throughout the skeletal system. The malignant plasma cells are **monoclonal** (i.e., derived from a single cell), and therefore secrete a single species of immunoglobulin (**monoclonal gammopathy**) producing M (myeloma) protein. In 80% of the human patients, the M component is IgG and rarely IgM, IgD, or IgE. In the remaining 20% of the human cases, plasma cells produce only kappa and lambda chains. These are of low molecular size and are readily excreted in the urine, where they are termed **Bence Jones proteins**. In such patients, urine contains only Bence Jones proteins (**Bence Jones proteinuria**) and no serum M component, the condition being known as **'light-chain disease'**. However, in 80% of patients the malignant plasma cells synthesize complete immunoglobulin molecules, as well as the light chains. Therefore, both Bence Jones proteins and serum M components are present in the urine.

Whereas **multiple myeloma** is by far the most common of the malignant plasma cell dyscrasias (an abnormal condition) **in humans, this tumour is rare in domestic animals**; and multiple myelomas involving IgG or IgA have been described **only in the dog, cat, and horse**. Moreover, Bence Jones proteinuria was found only in some animals. As in humans, multiple myeloma in animals too usually develops from the neoplastic clonal proliferation of plasma cells in bone marrow, but in **horses** osteolytic lesions apparently do not occur. In rare instances, the tumour may arise at extramedullary sites as **solitary plasmacytoma**, and may later metastasize. Frequent complications in animals include recurrent infections from a diminished immune response and impaired phagocytic activity. Acute or chronic renal failure occurs mainly from the excretion of myeloma proteins. Lameness, bone pain, and fracture from bone marrow infiltration by malignant plasma cells and osteolysis, can occur. Blindness may develop in the **dog** with IgA myeloma from bilateral detachment of retina.

Bence Jones proteins (i.e., light chains) present in the blood are associated with the development of amyloidosis, both in humans and animals (see 'amyloidosis'). **Extramedullary plasmacytoma in a cat was associated with a monoclonal gammopathy, and a systemic amyloid light chain amyloidosis.**

Leukosis/Sarcoma Group

The **leukosis/sarcoma group of diseases of the chicken** comprises lymphoid, erythroid, and myeloid leukoses and a variety of other tumours, such as fibrosarcomas, haemangiomas, and nephroblastomas. These conditions are caused by a group of related retroviruses known as **'avian leukosis/sarcoma viruses (ALSV)'** that belong to **a subgroup of avian type 'C' oncoviruses.** Of the various neoplasms caused by ALSV, only **lymphoid leukosis** is sufficiently prevalent to be of economic importance.

Lymphoid Leukosis (LL)

Lymphoid leukosis is the commonest neoplasm caused by the ALSV. It is characterized by enlargement of the liver by infiltrating **lymphoblasts.** LL appears between the 14th and 30th week of age. Incidence is usually highest at about sexual maturity. External signs of the disease are not specific. **Grossly** visible tumours almost always involve liver, spleen, and bursa of Fabricius. Tumours are soft, smooth, and glistening. Growth may be nodular, granular or diffuse, or a combination of these forms. **Microscopically**, the lesions consist of immature lymphoid cells - **lymphoblasts**. The cytoplasm of most tumour cells contains a large amount of RNA, indicating that the cells are immature and rapidly dividing. **They have B cell markers and carry surface IgM.**

Erythroid Leukosis (Erythroblastosis)

This is a rare and sporadic disease, affecting mainly **adult chickens**. There is always anaemia, which is associated with the presence of a large number of immature red cells in the blood. The disease originates in the bone marrow and a leukaemia is present from the outset. It is a peculiarity of the disease that, the malignant cells remain within the blood vessels throughout the course of the disease. This leads to erythrostasis in sinusoids in organs, such as liver, spleen, and bone marrow, giving them a cherry-red colour that characterizes this condition at postmortem. The liver and spleen are moderately enlarged.

Myeloid Leukosis (Myeloblastosis)

This is also a rare and sporadic disease of adult chickens. It involves proliferation of cells of the granulocytic series. The disease originates in the bone marrow and involves immature cells. The liver and spleen are greatly enlarged.

Other tumours: Solid tumours caused by ALSV include fibrosarcoma, chondroma, endothelioma, haemangioma, nephroblastoma, and hepatocarcinoma. They usually occur sporadically in young or older chickens.

Marek's Disease

Marek's disease (MD) is **a lymphoproliferative disease of chickens caused by a cell-associated herpesvirus**. It is characterized by a mononuclear infiltration of the peripheral nervous system, and to a lesser degree, other tissues and visceral organs. In other words, **the disease is associated with the development of lymphoid tumours - lymphoma**. MD affects chickens from about 6 weeks of age and is mostly seen between 12 and 24 weeks of age. The disease occurs in **two forms**: (1) **classical Marek's disease**, and (2) **acute Marek's disease**. Clinical signs in the **classical form** include paralysis of the wings and legs, torticollis (twisting of the neck), and dyspnoea (difficult breathing). The interval between onset of symptoms and death varies from a few days to several weeks. Rarely, birds may recover. **Acute Marek's disease**: Mortality in this form is much higher than in the classical form. Many birds may die suddenly without preceding symptoms. Others appear depressed before death, and some show paralytic symptoms similar to those seen in the classical form.

The characteristic **gross lesion** in the **classical form** is marked enlargement of one or more peripheral nerves. Nerves commonly affected are the sciatic and brachial plexus, abdominal vagus, and intercostal nerves. Affected nerves are up to 2-3 times the normal thickness. **Acute Marek's disease** is characterized by diffuse lymphomatous involvement and enlargement of the liver, gonads, spleen, kidneys, lungs, proventriculus, and heart. **Microscopically**, the lesion consists of proliferating lymphoid cells, lymphoblasts, and small, medium, and large lymphocytes. The most common lesions in visceral organs are **lymphoid tumours**, showing similar cellular infiltration. **The malignantly transformed cell is a thymus-dependent lymphocyte (T-cell),** and the **lymphoma** consists of a mixture of malignant T-cells and reactive, bursa-dependent lymphocytes (B-cells), T-cells, and macrophages.

Reticuloendotheliosis

Reticuloendotheliosis (RE) includes **three disease conditions** caused by retroviruses of the reticuloendotheliosis virus (REV) group. These viruses are different from those of the leukosis/sarcoma group. In chickens, they produce acute reticulum cell neoplasm and chronic neoplasm of lymphoid and other tissues. **But these are very rare conditions.**

Tumours of Muscle

Leiomyoma and Leiomyosarcoma

These are **tumours of smooth muscle**, found mostly in older animals, particularly in the **dog, cattle**, and **chicken. Macroscopically**, leiomyomas vary in size, are usually spherical or elliptical, and pink in colour. They are firm in consistency, and have areas of degeneration, necrosis, and haemorrhages. On section, they are made up of interlacing fibres and strands of tissue that have a whorled appearance. The surface has a glassy, dry appearance in contrast to the fibroma. The leiomyosarcomas resemble leiomyomas. **Microscopically**, the basic cell is a long spindle-shaped cell containing an elliptical nucleus. At times, the muscle cells are interspersed with connective tissue cells, and it is then difficult to determine whether they are fibroblasts or muscle cells. Connective tissue stains, such as Van Gieson's stain, help in differentiating them; collagen stains red while muscles yellow. The tumour cells are usually arranged in bundles and bands that interlace and form a somewhat whorled pattern. In the more anaplastic leiomyosarcomas, the cells invade the tissues.

These tumours **occur** mostly in the musculature of the tubular and hollow organs such as the digestive, urinary, and genital tract. In **horse**, they occur in the wall of the small intestine; in the **dog**, in walls of the uterus and vagina. Those in vagina are often pedunculated and may protrude through the vulva. Components of leiomyoma and leiomyosarcoma are also seen in the mixed mammary tumour of the dog. Leiomyoma, **in the chicken**, is seen commonly in the nasopharynx as a firm globular mass. **Prognosis**: Leiomyomas can be easily removed surgically. Leiomyosarcomas metastasize and pose a greater problem.

Rhabdomyoma and Rhabdomyosarcoma

These are tumours of **skeletal or cardiac muscle. In animals, rhabdomyomas are rare**, and seldom undergo transformation to rhabdomyosarcomas. **Macroscopically**, rhabdomyomas in the myocardium appear as a globular mass 1-3 cm in diameter. In consistency and colour, they resemble heart muscle. Rhabdomyosarcomas are not so well demarcated from adjacent muscle. It is locally invasive, and reaches a larger size without producing secondary metastases. **Microscopically**, the basic cell is the cardiac muscle cell or the striated muscle cell. They are identified by their cross striations and resemblance to striated muscle.

Rhabdomyomas mostly **occur** in the myocardium, the lateral thoracic wall, or the muscle of the limb, and have been reported in **cattle** and **pigs**. Rhabdomyosarcomas also arise in heart and at other places in the musculature. **Prognosis**: Most rhabdomyomas are found at necropsy, but they do not appear to contribute to the death of the individual. **Rhabdomyosarcomas metastasize and pose as greater problem.**

Tumours of Nervous Tissue

Tumours of the nervous system may be **primary or secondary. Primary tumours** arising in nervous tissue come mainly from neuroglia, i.e., neuro-ectodermal glial cells, and are known as **gliomas**. The **secondary or metastatic tumours** reach the brain by metastasis. Tumours of the nervous system are common in **dog** and **cattle**, but their **incidence is lower in other domestic animals**. The classification of nervous system tumours is presented in Table 18.

Table 18. Classification of nervous system tumours

I.	**Primary tumours**	
	Tumours of neuroglia	
	Astrocytes	Astrocytoma
		Glioblastoma multiforme
	Oliogodendrocytes	Oligodendroglioma
	Ependyma	Ependymoma
	Tumours of neurons	Neuroblastoma
		Ganglioneuroma
	Tumour of primitive undifferentiated cell	Medulloblastoma
	Tumour of pineal cells	Pinealoma
	Tumour of meninges	Meningioma
	Tumour of nerve sheath cells	Schwannoma (neurilemmoma)
II.	**Secondary or metastatic tumours**	

The **primary brain tumours** are usually single and do not metastasize to distant organs, **glioma** being the most common. Malignant tumours are known as **gliosarcoma**. However, no gliosarcoma metastasizes to locations outside the cranial cavity, or spinal cord. The malignant variety infiltrates only in the adjoining areas. Microglia does not form tumours. The **astrocytoma** may be **protoplasmic astrocytoma** or **fibrous astrocytoma**. This tumour occurs in almost any part of the brain, and is of lesser malignancy. Astrocytomas are most common in **dogs**, but are **rare in other species**. The **glioblastoma multiforme** also arises from astrocytes. It is differentiated from other types of astrocytoma by its varied appearance, hence the term 'multiforme'. **In humans**, this tumour is the most frequent of the gliomas, as well the most malignant. **In domestic animals**, they are usually seen in **dogs**. **Oligodendroglioma** also occurs in **dogs**, but is rare. The tumour infiltrates and destroys adjacent tissue. A few cases have also been reported in **cats** and **cattle**. Tumours involving the ependymal cells of the ventricles are called **ependymomas**. Ependymomas are rare in all species, though most often seen in **dogs**, **cats**, and **cattle**.

The **neuroblastoma** can originate in the central nervous system, but the majority occur in the adrenal medulla. Wherever located, it occurs in the young and is highly malignant. The microscopic appearance is similar to that of the medulloblastoma, to which the neuroblastoma is embryonically related. **Ganglioneuroma** originates from nervous tissue capable of forming neurons. This tumour is related to **neuroblastoma**. However, neuroblastoma consists of undifferentiated or neoplastic cells. Ganglioneuroma is well differentiated into 'ganglion cells'. These tumours are rare in brain, and like the neuroblastoma, more likely to arise in the adrenal medulla. The **medulloblastoma** arises from primitive undifferentiated glial cells. Mitotic figures are numerous. Medulloblastomas are rare neoplasms and occur in young animals, particularly in **dogs** and **cattle**. They have also been reported in **cats**, **pigs**, and mice. It is usually located just dorsal to the fourth ventricle, where it appears as a spherical, discrete, reddish-grey mass.

Pinealoma is a rare neoplasm derived from the pineal body. It has been reported in **horses** and rats. **Meningiomas** arise from the cranial or spinal meninges. Unlike humans, **these tumours are rare in animals**. They arise from the mesothelial cells that form the surface of cranial and spinal meninges. In meningiomas, the cells are more plump and the nuclei more rounded than in the neurofibroma. Many tumours in the centre have a calcified body, suggestive grossly of a grain of sand. This form of meningioma is called **psammoma** (G. psammos = sand), and the granules brain sand. **Grossly**, the meningioma forms a spherical subdural mass. It compresses the underlying brain or cord, and may extend deep into the sulci. **Meningiomas** have been reported in **dogs**, **cattle**, and **horses**, and appear to be the most common intracranial neoplasm in the **cat**.

Schwannoma, also known as **neurilemmoma**, is a benign neoplasm, arising from Schwann cells (neurolemmal cells) surrounding the axon in peripheral nerves. **Neurofibroma** also arises from Schwann cells. Histologically, the tumours are distinct from one another. **Schwannomas are most common in cattle**. Cranial nerve schwannomas have been reported in **dogs**. A rather rare tumour involving the acoustic nerve is known as the **acoustic neuroma**, and has been reported in **cattle**. Neurofibromas also arise from Schwann cells, and therefore represent a histological variant of schwannomas. The neurofibroma is distinct from the ordinary fibromas. Malignant tumours are rare and are termed **neurofibrosarcomas**. They have been reported in **cattle**, in the heart.

Secondary or Metastatic Tumours

Tumours of the central nervous system that reach the brain by metastasis are not uncommon. They are mostly observed in the central hemispheres and are multiple, which indicates their metastatic nature. The majority of these metastatic tumours have their primary site in the lung. In the **dog**, the original tumour is usually located in the mammary gland. In **cats** and **cattle**, a malignant lymphoma is the most frequent of the secondary tumours, mostly located in the spinal cord. **Melanomas** and **haemangiomas** are also among the more frequent metastatic neoplasms.

Tumours of Epithelial Tissue

Epithelial tumours, on the surface, originate from the epidermis and hair follicles. Within the body, they originate from the mucous membranes, glands, and gland tubules and ducts.

Benign tumour of the stratified squamous epithelium of the skin or a mucous membrane is called a **papilloma**, or **wart**. **This is a very common tumour of domestic animals.** A malignant tumour of the stratified squamous epithelium of either the skin, or a mucous membrane, is called a **squamous-cell carcinoma**. Squamous-cell carcinomas occur mostly in older animals. A malignant tumour originating from the basal cells of the skin or hair follicle and sebaceous adnexa, is known as a **basal-cell carcinoma**. A benign epithelial tumour originating from the glandular epithelium is called an **adenoma**, and when malignant, an **adenocarcinoma**.

Papilloma

Macroscopic appearance: A papilloma is somewhat wart-like in shape and produces gross or microscopic finger-like (or nipple-like) processes, hence the name (L. papilla = nipple). Large papillomas may measure even up to 10 cm in diameter. Its surface is smooth, or may have a tuft (a small cluster or coiled mass), or be nodular. Occasionally, a papilloma may form horn-like process projecting from the skin. The base may be broad, or so small that the growth is pedunculated.

Microscopic appearance: A papilloma shows finger-like processes of stratified squamous epithelium that protrude above the surrounding epithelial surface and contains a connective tissue core. However, the epidermis is intact. There are no breaks in the basal layer, through which the epithelial cells infiltrate into the dermis and subcutaneous tissue, as they do in the malignant form (**squamous-cell carcinoma**). A papilloma originating from any stratified squamous mucous membrane is similar to that in the skin. The cells are of an adult type, and do not show any mitotic figures. With routine H & E staining, cells present normochromasia that indicates that the tumour is of a benign type.

Location: In **cattle, dogs**, and **rabbits** infectious papillomas are common. **In cattle**, papillomas also occur in the oesophagus and omasum. **In horses**, papillomas are located mostly on the skin of the prepectoral and shoulder regions, ears, eyelids, upper lip, and external genital organs.

Bovine Cutaneous Papillomatosis

Cutaneous papillomas are more common in **cattle** than in any other domestic animal, and are caused by the **bovine papilloma virus** (BPV), a DNA oncogenic virus. **The disease is characterized by the appearance of warts on various parts of the body**. Grossly, warts are rough, cauliflower-like mass of varying size and of irregular shape, attached by a narrow stalk, or a broad base. The lesions are first round and smooth, but soon become rough and horny. Papillomas are most frequent on the head, sides of the neck, shoulders and dewlap; and less common on the ears, eyelids, throat, and lips. **In cows**, they occur mainly on the teats and udder. **In calves**, the warts may become large and pendulous. The disease is generally self-limiting, and often papillomas disappear spontaneously. When lesions occur on the genitalia (see 'transmissible fibropapillomas of cattle'), they may interfere with reproduction. **Microscopically**, the finger-like lesions have a greatly thickened epidermis, showing both acanthosis (thickening of the epidermis from hyperplasia) and hyperkeratosis (thickening of the keratin layer, stratum corneum). The elongated processes have a core of richly cellular hyperplastic epidermis.

Equine Cutaneous Papillomatosis

Skin warts of horses are not as common as those affecting cattle. They are caused by equine papilloma virus. They develop mostly on the nose and around the lips, appearing as small, elevated, horny masses, varying from a few to several hundred. **Microscopically,** hyperplastic layers of squamous epithelium are supported by a thin core of connective tissue which is continuous with the dermis.

Canine Oral Papillomatosis

Canine papilloma virus induces **warts in the mouth of dogs**. The warts generally develop on the lips and spread to the buccal mucosa, tongue, palate, and pharynx. The papilloma may be single or confluent cauliflower-shaped masses with a rough surface. Mostly they are multiple, and in some dogs, they are so numerous as to interfere with mastication and deglutination. The warts are usually benign and disappear spontaneously after several months. Dogs recovered from the infection develop immunity to re-infection. **Microscopically**, the lesions present hyperplastic epithelium with mitotic figures and hyperkeratosis. A few plasma cells and lymphocytes may be seen in the underlying stroma.

Cutaneous and Oral Papillomatosis of Rabbits

In 1933, **Shope** isolated a virus from the natural cases of **papillomas of the skin in rabbits**. Therefore, the tumour is often referred to as the **Shope papilloma**. The warts occur on the inner surface of the thighs, abdomen, neck, and shoulders. The lesions are black or grey, and covered with a thick layer of keratin. They can be transmitted without difficulty from one rabbit to another by injecting, or applying filtered or unfiltered wart suspension to scarified skin. Once established, the papillomas can persist for long periods, undergo malignant transformation, and eventually kill animal by metastases.

In 1943, Parson and Kidd demonstrated a virus that produced **papillomas in the oral cavity of rabbits**. The viral agent is distinct from the Shope papilloma virus, which affects epithelium of the skin, but not mouth. Spontaneous papillomas are small, discrete, grey-white nodules, either sessile or pedunculated. They are usually multiple and mostly situated on the undersurface of the tongue.

Caprine Papillomatosis

Papillomatosis of **goats** occurs in two forms: (i) **cutaneous warts** on the head, face, shoulder, neck, and upper parts of the fore limbs, but not on the teats and udder, and (ii) **papillomatosis** limited to the teats and udder. Sometimes, the lesions undergo malignant transformation and metastasize. Caprine papillomatosis is caused by caprine papilloma virus.

Papillomatosis of Monkeys

This is extremely rare, and the papillomatous lesion does not show evidence of malignancy. The lesion has been experimentally transmitted from one monkey to skin site on another.

Squamous-Cell Carcinoma

A squamous-cell carcinoma is a malignant tumour of stratified squamous epithelium. It is the common form of carcinoma and occurs in all domestic species. It grows more rapidly than papilloma and the growth has no limit. **The tumour is therefore very destructive**.

Macroscopic appearance: The surface of a cutaneous carcinoma is not so densely keratinized as that of papilloma. The surface of a rapidly growing carcinoma is usually inflamed and ulcerated. Slowly growing tumours have a cauliflower head. A carcinoma usually has an offensive odour because of surface necrosis and the action of putrefactive bacteria. It has softer consistency than papilloma. The cut surface shows parenchyma and stroma, clearly contrasted. The parenchyma is in the form of nodules of white or grey, soft, homogeneous tissue; whereas stroma is in the form of white fibrous band of connective tissue, separating these nodules. There are often foci of haemorrhage and necrosis. The regional lymph nodes are swollen being the seat of secondary growth. On surgical removal, these tumours recur within a few weeks or months.

Microscopic appearance: A squamous-cell carcinoma differs from a papilloma in several ways. The epithelial cells are anaplastic as evidenced by their larger size, large nucleolus, and the presence of numerous mitotic figures. The tumour cells are not confined within the epidermis, or mucosa. They infiltrate the underlying tissues. The infiltrating cells grow at random. The proliferating cells appear in large groups without an admixture of stroma. However, the individual groups are separated from one another by strands of the stroma. **In sarcomas**, on the other hand, the parenchyma and stroma are uniformly mixed. **In cutaneous carcinomas**, the red-staining keratin of the stratum corneum, arranged concentrically, comes to lie at the centre of the epithelial mass. It becomes quite dense from the presence of growing cells, and forms a rounded, laminated structure known as an **'epithelial pearl'** or **'cell nest'**. Epithelial pearls, however, may be lacking in poorly differentiated squamous-cell carcinomas. The underlying tissue usually shows signs of a local chronic inflammatory reaction. Tumour cell emboli are often noticed in lymphatics and veins adjacent to the main tumour mass. Penetration into these vessels favours metastasis into the venous circulation, and to the lymph nodes.

The term **epidermoid carcinoma** is sometimes used for tumours derived from epidermis. The tongue, oesophagus, rumen, ocular surfaces, and vagina also bear cornifying squamous-cell carcinomas.

Squamous-cell carcinoma usually occurs in the skin, and at those places where the skin passes into a mucous membrane. **In horses**, the common sites are the membrana nictitans, the eyelid, and the external genitals; and **in cattle**, the lower eyelid and the membrana nictitans. The tumours are particularly common in areas of the skin where there is a deficiency of melanin, e.g., squamous-cell carcinoma of the eye is more common in the Hereford breed of cattle than those in which the pigment is more abundant. The pigment prevents part of the rays of the sun from penetrating into the skin. Another example of defective pigmentation in cattle is vulva in Ayrshire cattle, in which tumours of the vulva are quite common on sunlight exposure. Squamous-cell carcinomas of the skin are quite common in the Angora **goats**, usually in the perineum, and involve anus and vulva. In **sheep**, they are quite common in the frontal-parietal region of sheep. In **cattle**, these tumours metastasize to the regional lymph nodes by lymphatics. They also metastasize to the lungs through veins. Further metastasis to other organs may also occur.

Squamous-Cell Carcinoma of the Bovine Eye

Squamous-cell carcinoma of the eye is the most common malignancy in **cattle** in the United States. The epidermal eye tumours are divided into **four types** according to the degree of malignancy: (1) epidermal plaque, (2) epidermal papilloma, (3) early squamous-cell carcinoma, and (4) squamous-cell carcinoma. The **prognosis** is good if proper treatment is started early. The tumour usually metastasizes only after a long period of progressive growth.

Horn Cancer

An unusual form of **squamous-cell carcinoma** called **horn cancer** or **cancer of the horn** occurs at the junction of the skin and the horn. It is seen in **Zebu cattle in India** and Sumatra. It is most common in castrated bulls (bullocks), rare in cows, and almost non-existent in intact bulls. The aetiology is unknown.

Horn cancer arises from horn core epithelium. The cancerous growth begins from the middle or distal region of the core, and progresses towards the frontal sinus. **Macroscopically**, the tumour is pinkish in colour and polypoid like a cauliflower. It is friable and bleeds easily. **Microscopically, horn cancer is a squamous-cell carcinoma** characterized by the presence of **epithelial pearls**. **Metastasis** occurs mostly in regional lymph nodes and sometimes in visceral organs, such as lungs, heart, and pituitary gland. The

377

metastasis occurs by direct extension, through the lymphatic system, and sometimes haematogenously.

Usually one horn is affected. Clinical signs include frequent shaking of the head, rubbing of the horn on some hard object, bloody discharge from the nostril of affected horn, and slight bending of the horn. In the advanced stages, there is gradual loosening and marked bending of the horn, sloughing of horn, and development of highly vascular, foul-smelling, cauliflower-like neoplastic growth. The growth may acquire infection and bleed. Affected animals suffer from weakness, anaemia, acquire cachexia, and die. The neoplasm mostly recurs after surgical removal.

Immunological studies suggest **depression of cell-mediated immunity** in the affected animals. Horn cancer can be diagnosed on the basis of clinical signs and confirmed by histopathology. Prognosis is good, if the base is not affected.

Ethmoidal Neoplasms

Tumours arising from the mucosa lining the ethmoid bone are observed in **cattle, sheep, buffalo, goat, pig,** and **horse. In India**, they are **seen mainly in cattle**, particularly in the southern states of Kerala and Tamil Nadu. Their endemic nature in both **cattle** and **sheep** suggests involvement of an infectious agent. **In cattle**, both a herpesvirus and retroviral particles have been isolated and identified. Role of aflatoxin, a common feed contaminant, has been suspected.

Adenocarcinoma is the most common type **in sheep**; the types **in cattle** include squamous-cell carcinoma, adenocarcinoma, and undifferentiated carcinoma. **The tumour arises from mucosa of the ethmoid**, and then spreads. **Cattle** affected with ethmoid carcinoma usually do not show any **clinical signs**, until the tumour assumes a considerable size, fills up the sinuses, and blocks the nasal and pharyngeal passages. The earliest signs include sudden epistaxis (nosebleed), or blood-tinged mucus or mucopurulent nasal discharge, accompanied by sneezing and dyspnoea (difficult breathing). The other manifestations include protrusion of the eyeball (**exophthalmos**) of one or both eyes, with swelling of the submaxillary lymph nodes. **The affected animals eventually die in course of time.**

Grossly, tumour fills up the nasal cavity and the paranasal sinuses and destroys turbinates. It is fleshy and grey-white. It may invade the retrobulbar region, the pharynx, and the frontal bones and comes out as frontal swelling. Metastases occur usually in the regional lymph nodes, and very rarely in the lungs and liver. **Microscopically**, the tumour consists of irregular clusters of anaplastic cells with prominent mitotic figures along with neutrophilic infiltration, and stromal fibrosis. Tumour giant cells with multiple nuclei are present. Areas of necrosis and haemorrhage are also observed.

Basal-Cell Carcinoma

Basal-cell carcinomas originate from the basal or germinal layer (stratum germinativum) of the epidermis, and also from the basal cells of hair follicles, sebaceous glands, or sweat glands. It is an important tumour of humans, in which it arises from the basal cells of the pilosebaceous adnexa. In both animals and humans, these tumours remain localized and almost never metastasize. The tumour is also known as **'rodent ulcer'**. Most of them have been reported on the head and shoulder of **horses**, **dogs**, and **cats**. There is no sex or age predilection.

Macroscopically, tumours are slow growing, firm, nodular, and usually attached by a broad base. The skin over the tumour may be devoid of hair. They tend to ulcerate early, and the ulcerations are characteristically rimmed by a pearly border, as if gnawed by a rodent (hence the name **'rodent ulcer'**). There is a great tendency for the cells to infiltrate the surrounding tissues, but metastasis seldom occurs. **Microscopically**, the cells resemble the basal cells of the Malpighian layer. They are cuboidal or columnar, and stain deeply with haematoxylin. A large numbers fuse and have a concentric or alveolar arrangement. One or two nucleoli may be seen in the nucleus. Mitotic figures are not abundant. The stroma consists of collagen fibres present in variable proportions.

The **prognosis** is good. Although there is local destruction and invasion, they seldom metastasize to the regional lymph nodes or other organs. Ulceration, secondary bacterial infection, and extension into the surrounding tissue should not be interpreted as signs of malignancy.

Adenoma

An adenoma is a benign tumour of glandular epithelium. In the **dog**, sebaceous, mammary, and prostate gland adenomas are fairly common. In the **pig**, polypoid adenomatosis of the large intestine is more common. In the **horse**, thyroid adenoma is more common. In **other species of domestic animals**, there are no such favoured locations.

379

The **gross appearance** of adenomas varies considerably depending on their location and the tissue from which they originate. Generally, they are sharply circumscribed and encapsulated. In the stomach and intestine, they become polypoid in shape, and are known as **polypoid adenomas,** or **adenomatous polyps. Microscopically,** adenomas look very much like the gland from which they originate. However, the amount of glandular tissue is more and the acini are lined with more than one layer of cells, but they are held in place by the basement membrane. Sometimes secretions are retained in the acini, causing them distended, and their epithelium to undergo atrophy. Such an adenoma is called a **cystadenoma**. Cystadenomas are usually found in the thyroid glands of **older dogs** and **horses**. Occasionally, the proliferating epithelium grows into the lumen of acini and takes the form of branching papillae. Such an adenoma is known as a **papillary adenoma.**

The **prognosis** of adenoma is good. On surgical removal, there is little danger of recurrence. Some may become malignant, which is indicated by infiltration, metastasis, and extensive local tissue destruction.

Adenocarcinoma

An adenocarcinoma is a malignant tumour of glandular epithelium. Its gross appearance varies with its location, the glandular tissue from which it arises, and the age of the growth. On the mucous surfaces, it may be well-defined, rather flat, thickened area. At other places, it may even take the form of a cauliflower head. The metastatic adenocarcinomas may consist of several sharply defined nodules. **Microscopically**, these tumours are highly anaplastic epithelial cells of the acini or alveoli and are not confined by the basement membrane, but infiltrate into the tunica propria of the mucosa and the interstitial tissue of the gland. The cells possess the usual characteristics of malignancy, that is, large vesicular nuclei with large nucleoli, and mitotic figures.

Adenocarcinomas usually **occur** in **cattle, horses**, and **dogs**. In the **sheep**, the adrenal gland and liver appear to be the more common sites, although adenocarcinomas are rare in this species. **In cattle,** adenocarcinoma of the uterus is common, and metastasizes early. **In dogs**, adenocarcinomas of the mammary, thyroid, and prostate glands, and liver appear common. **In hens**, these tumours are common in the ovary. Their **prognosis** is always serious. Local invasion and metastasis make the surgical removal of all the tumour mass impossible. The rapidity with which adenocarcinomas spread varies with the species of animal and the type of tumour.

Having described adenomas and adenocarcinomas, let us consider these tumours briefly as they occur in different domestic animals.

Epithelial Tumours of the Female Genital Tract

Although these tumours are seen occasionally in all species of domestic animals, they are **important in cattle** and **dog**.

Adenocarcinoma of the Uterus of the Cow

This is **the most common malignant glandular neoplasm of the cattle**, and may be associated with sterility. It occurs in animals between 7 to 12 years of age. **Macroscopically**, the tumour may occur in the horn of uterus or in the body. It usually forms a sclerotic (hard) annular (ring-shaped) constriction of the anterior horn. It is yellow or grey in colour, and firm and dense due to the connective tissue. One characteristic of this tumour is that tumour cells from the serosa of the uterus are transplanted on the abdominal viscera, such as broad ligaments of the uterus, spleen, and liver. The tumour usually metastasizes to lymph nodes and the lung.

Microscopically, both in the primary and secondary sites, there are masses of cellular, often necrotic debris. The epithelial cells occur in islands in small solid nests, or in a distorted glandular pattern. The tumours have a very fibrous stroma. The growth is usually located deep in the endometrium and spreads laterally under an intact surface epithelium. The tumour also spreads through the myometrium. The tumour cells sometimes appear in the lymphatics, or veins. The regional lymph node involvement comes from lymphatic metastasis.

Ovarian Tumours

Granulosa-cell tumours are the most common ovarian tumours and are most frequent in the **cow**, **bitch** being the next common species. They are **less common in the ewe**, and occur **seldom in other species**. The other common group of tumours includes adenomas, cystadenomas, carcinomas, and cystadenocarcinomas. These have a definite glandular structure. The glandular tumours are commonly seen in the **bitch** and the **hen**, but only occasionally in other species. Both groups of tumours rarely metastasize. The arrhenoblastoma (resembling a Sertoli cell tumour), the dysgerminoma (arising in undifferentiated cells of the ovary), and the teratomas are rare tumours.

Granulosa-Cell Tumours of the Cow

Here, a theca-cell tumour, a granulosa-cell tumour, and a luteal-cell tumour, all are treated as one - granulosa-cell tumour. The tumour is seen in **younger cattle**, i.e., **heifers** and **2-5 year-old cows**. The outward symptoms may be nymphomania (abnormally excessive sexual desire), debility, and sterility. The tumours may be bilateral, or multiple in the same ovary. They are large, between 10 and 20 cm in diameter, or even larger. Usually they have a thick fibrous capsule. On incision, the growth is divided by thick fibrous bands into lobules which contain large cystic spaces filled with a reddish, watery fluid. **Microscopically**, the tumour consists of large, polyhedral cells with small nuclei and abundant cytoplasm. The cells may be arranged in large masses, or are present around fluid-filled space. There are often large areas of necrosis.

Mammary Gland Neoplasms

These are mostly seen in the **dog**. In other animals, they are relatively uncommon. **Surprisingly, cattle with a highly developed mammary gland have the lowest incidence of mammary tumours.**

Mammary Gland Tumour of the Dog

It is most common in **dogs** that are **10-14 years of age**. **Macroscopically**, the tumours may be single or multiple; most occurring on the posterior pair of mammary glands, fewer in the first two, and least in the central glands. The size varies greatly, from just palpable nodules of a cm or less, up to 8-10 inches in diameter. In consistency, they may be quite soft or oedematous, to firm and sclerotic, and may contain bone and cartilage. They may be solid, or contain numerous cysts filled with secretions. Colour also varies. The majority are grey or white, but may be red, yellow, orange, or brown, depending on the amount of haemorrhage and necrosis. Ulceration of the surface may occur.

The **microscopic appearance** of the tumour varies greatly. This is because the hormonal stimulation causes both glandular and connective tissue elements to proliferate. The amount of glandular or connective tissue varies with the individual tumour. At times the glandular tissue predominates and is relatively benign adenomatous, or may be extremely anaplastic. **The connective tissue proliferation may consist of fibrous tissue, cartilage, bone, and even muscle.** Cartilage and bone result from metaplasia. Areas of necrosis are very common. Also, on account of dead and degenerating tissue, calcification occurs.

These tumours are also called **mixed mammary gland tumours** due to the presence of both glandular and connective tissue in varying proportions.

Prognosis: In dog, they are not as malignant as in humans. If removed early, chances of recovery are very good. In the later stages, metastasis occurs to the regional lymph nodes and lungs.

Testicular Tumours

Testicular tumours of the **dog** are of **three types**: (1) adenocarcinoma (seminoma), (2) sustentacular-cell tumour, and (3) interstitial cell tumour (Leydig-cell tumour). These neoplasms are very common, particularly in cryptorchids (i.e., animals in which testicles have not descended into the scrotum).

Adenocarcinoma (Seminoma)

The seminoma arises from the germinal epithelium of the seminiferous tubules. They occur mostly in the **older dogs**, and vary from 1-3 cm in diameter. Most of the tumours are soft in consistency and grey in colour. Areas of necrosis and haemorrhage may give the tumour a yellow or red appearance. **Microscopically**, the seminoma is composed of polyhedral cells with prominent, hyperchromatic round nuclei. Mitotic figures are numerous. Multiple nuclei may be found within the cell. Fine trabeculae divide the masses of cells into compartments. **This is the most malignant of the testicular neoplasms**, and metastases occur in the regional lymph nodes and other organs. Early removal of both testicles is advised.

Sustentacular-Cell Tumour (Sertoli-Cell Tumour)

This tumour arises from the sustentacular or Sertoli cells of the seminiferous tubules. **It occurs almost exclusively in dogs**, and is the most frequent tumour in the cryptorchid testicle. It varies in size from being just visible to 3 cm in diameter, and may consist of one or more nodules. The tumours are grey in colour, round in shape, firm in consistency, and may contain areas of haemorrhage and necrosis. **Microscopically**, anaplastic areas consist of solid masses of round or polyhedral cells with central nuclei. However, in most areas continuity can be traced to seminiferous tubules of normal size and shape, but their lining is devoid of germinal cells, and contains only one or two layers of tall Sertoli cells.

This tumour is less serious than the adenocarcinoma, but more dangerous than the interstitial cell tumour, because it metastasizes and spreads to other organs. It commonly produces **oestrogen**. As a result the mammary glands enlarge, the hairs of the belly are thinned, and the dog becomes sexually attractive to other males.

Interstitial-Cell tumour (Leydig-Cell Tumour)

This tumour arises from the interstitial, androgen-secreting cells. **It is the most common of the testicular tumours in the dog.** They vary in size from 5 mm to 5 cm in diameter. The smaller tumours are usually yellow in colour and solid in consistency, while the larger tumours contain cysts and areas of haemorrhage. **Microscopically**, cells are larger and have more eosinophilic cytoplasm than the two previous testicular tumours. Their cytoplasm contains numerous fat droplets, which account for their foamy character and yellow colour grossly. The nuclei are small, and the nucleoli are not prominent. Mitotic figures are uncommon. The **prognosis** of this tumour is good. They are seldom malignant and rarely metastasize. Surgical removal prevents the spread of the neoplasm. Endocrine disturbances are not associated with this tumour.

Tumours of Melanoblasts

These tumours are of neuro-ectodermal origin, and therefore included under tumours of epithelial origin. A benign tumour of melanin-forming cells **melanoblasts** is a **melanoma**. The malignant tumour composed of melanoblasts is known as a **malignant melanoma**, or **melanocarcinoma**. Since melanoblasts arise in neuro-ectodermal tissues, it is advisable **not to use the term melanosarcoma.**

Macroscopically, melanoma is brown, black, or of grey colour. The intensity of pigmentation depends on the amount of melanin. The size is very variable. They may be barely visible, or up to 60 cm in diameter. In weight, they vary from a few mg to more than 20 kg. The shape is also variable depending on the degree of malignancy. Most of the melanotic tumour in **horses** and **cattle** are round in shape. In **pigs** and **dogs**, they are more flattened and wart-like. In consistency, they may be very soft, or dense and firm, depending on the amount of connective tissue and necrosis present.

Microscopically, clumps of brownish-black pigment granules are present, usually within the cells - either melanoblasts or macrophages. Melanoblasts are irregularly round, spindle-shaped, or stellate shaped (star-shaped). The phagocytes are round. The cells are closely packed with granules, and no nuclei or cytoplasm can be seen. However, the malignant tumours may contain little or no pigment. **The lack of pigment indicates that the tumour is probably quite malignant.**

Most of these tumours occur in grey and white horses, where they are located in the ventral surface of the tail, the recto-anal region, the external genitals of both sexes, the perineum, the head, and shoulders. Metastases are common in the lungs, spleen, liver, kidney, lymph nodes, and bone marrow. In **pigs**, they occur in the lower jaw, flank and the hind leg. Melanotic tumours are **not common in cattle**. In the **dog**, they are observed in the skin of the head, thorax, and extremities. **Prognosis**: Melanomas can be removed quite easily by surgical procedures. The malignant melanomas are extremely serious and metastasize early.

Sebaceous Gland Adenomas of Dogs

These adenomas originate in the sebaceous glands of the perianal region, the prepuce, and the skin of the back, loin, and tail. Majority of them occur in **aged male dogs**. **Grossly**, they are circumscribed, yellowish brown in colour, single or multiple, and vary from 0.5 cm to 6 cm in diameter. The cut surface has a slightly lobulated appearance. In some cases, the skin may be ulcerated and haemorrhagic. **Microscopically**, the cells appear very much like sebaceous and perianal glands. However, their arrangement is not that of a normal gland. The anaplastic cells are large, polyhedral, and contain numerous small droplets of fat. The nuclei have one or two nucleoli, and the mitotic figures are rare.

Sweat Gland Neoplasms

These tumours are derived from the epithelium of the sweat glands. They usually occur on the face, neck, and shoulders, and **are mostly adenomas.** The tumour measures 1-2 cm in diameter, is greyish-white in colour, and firm in consistency. **Microscopically**, it resembles the basal-cell carcinoma. The cells are small, and do not become large and irregular as in squamous-cell carcinoma. The nuclei are oval and the nucleoli are small. The **prognosis** is usually good.

The majority of the tumours are benign, and if removed early, they do not recur.

Tumours of the Adrenal Gland

The primary tumours of the adrenal originate either, in the **cortex** or **medulla**. Secondary tumours are infrequent in all species, except lymphosarcoma.

Adreno-Cortical Tumours: The cortical tumours are adenomas or adenocarcinomas.

Adenoma of the Adrenal Cortex (Adreno-Cortical Adenoma): This tumour occurs in almost all species of animals, and is usually functional, that is, it produces cortical steroid hormones. These tumours are usually unilateral, and arise within the cortex. They are circumscribed and grow by expansion. The cells are usually well-differentiated and resemble with some zone of the cortex. These tumours have been reported in **old cows** and **ewes**, and also **dogs** and **horses. In the dog,** they are of particular interest because they secrete enough adreno-cortical hormones and cause hyperadrenocorticism, a common problem in **dogs**.

Carcinoma of the Adrenal Cortex (Adreno-Cortical Carcinoma): The cells of this neoplasm resemble those of the cortical adenoma, but mitoses and anaplastic cells are more frequent. Also necrosis is more common, and the neoplastic cells invade adjacent adrenal cortex, blood and lymph vessels, and metastasize. They usually extend into the vena cava, and spread along its intima. Metastatic tumours are found in lungs, or other organs. **This tumour is commonly seen in cattle**. They may also produce enough corticosteroid hormones to cause hyperadrenocorticism.

Adrenal Medullary Tumours

In domestic animals, these comprise pheochromocytoma, ganglioneuroma, ganglioneuroblastoma, and neuroblastoma. However, **except pheochromocytoma, all others are extremely rare.**

Pheochromocytoma: This tumour originates from the chromaffin cells, and is the **most common tumour of the medulla in all species**. They are more common in **old ewes** and **older cows. Dogs** and **horses** are also commonly affected. **Grossly,** they are reddish-brown, and may be single or multiple, involving one or both adrenals. The tumour cells are large with abundant cytoplasm. Chromaffin granules can be demonstrated with appropriate techniques. The cells may be arranged in irregular cords, separated by rich vascular system. Some tumours secrete either adrenaline (epinephrine), noradrenaline (norepinephrine), or both (catecholamines), and have functional effects on the host.

The term **paraganglioma** is applied to chromaffin tumours outside the adrenal gland. Some call them as **nonchromaffin parangliomas**. These tumours are extremely rare, and have been reported only as an incidental finding.

Tumours of the Thyroid Gland

These may originate from: (i) follicular cells, (ii) parafollicular or C cells, and (iii) mesenchymal cells. **Thyroid tumours have been reported from all domestic animals.**

Follicular Adenoma and Follicular Carcinoma

Follicular adenoma occurs as single or multiple nodules in one or both lobes of the thyroid. The nodules are circumscribed, and are encapsulated by thin connective tissue. They grow by expansion. The epithelial cells form follicles or even cords, several cells in thickness. They resemble normal thyroid follicles. The cells are low cuboidal. In some cases, these cells form a papillary pattern called '**papillary adenoma**'. At times, it is extremely difficult to differentiate between hyperplasia of the thyroid, adenomas, and adenocarcinomas.

Follicular carcinoma appears to be the least malignant histological type, but local invasion into capsule and blood vessels has been reported, particularly in the **dog**. The cells are cuboidal or columnar, and form follicles that contain colloid.The follicular pattern is often mixed with papillary areas. The cells usually produce thyroxine, which results in clinical signs of thyrotoxicosis, or hyperthyroidism.

Compact cellular or solid carcinomas are firm masses. **Microscopically**, they contain solid sheets of closely packed cells, with a fine stroma dividing the tumour into lobules. The cells have a centrally placed nucleus, and eosinophilic cytoplasm. Mitoses are rare. However, the cells often invade the capsule, adjacent thyroid, and blood and lymph vessels.

Papillary carcinoma of the thyroid is characterized by the projections of epithelial cells supported by a fine stroma. The papillary type is more common in the **cat** than in the **dog**. **Squamous-cell**

carcinoma of the thyroid is an infrequent tumour in animals, but may occasionally be encountered. **Anaplastic (undifferentiated) carcinomas** are those in which cells are pleomorphic and undifferentiated.

Medullary carcinoma of the thyroid **develops from the parafollicular or C cell of thyroid**. They occur in the **dog, cattle** and **human**, and produce thyrocalcitonin. They usually invade one lobe of the thyroid. The cut surface is yellow and divided into lobules by septa. **Microscopically**, the lobules have rows of tall columnar cells. Hypocalcaemia has been described in the **dog** and **bull** with elevated levels of thyrocalcitonin.

Mesenchymal tumours, such as fibrosarcomas, osteosarcomas, and chondrosarcomas, are very rare. **Epithelial-mesenchymal tumours** have been described in **dogs**. They contain both elements of follicular carcinoma and undifferentiated sarcoma. **Secondary neoplasms** are also rare. Squamous-cell carcinoma and lymphosarcoma may occur as secondary tumours.

Parathyroid Tumours

These do not appear to have been much reported in animals. It is important to differentiate parathyroid hyperplasia from adenoma. Hyperplasia is seen commonly in the **dog** in kidney disease where the phosphorus metabolism is deranged.

Pituitary Tumours

Neoplasms of the pituitary commonly occur in the **dog**, but occasionally also in the **cat, horse, sheep,** and **cattle**.

Adenomas and adenocarcinomas

Adenomas are circumscribed, grow by expansion, and do not invade adjacent tissues. The cells have the staining features of acidophils, basophils, or chromophobes, and each of these three types may secrete hormones. **Chromophobe adenomas**, which may or may not secrete a hormone, are the most common in the **dog**. **Adenomas of the pars intermedia** are less frequent than chromophobe adenomas. **Adenocarcinomas** are those neoplasms whose cells invade and destroy neighbouring tissues, outgrow their blood supply and undergo necrosis, or metastasize by way of blood or lymphatics to lymph nodes, or other organs.

Secondary neoplasms are infrequent, and include lymphosarcoma (**dogs, cattle**), malignant melanoma (**dogs, cats, horses**), adenocarcinoma of the mammary gland (**dogs**), osteosarcoma and ependymoma (**dogs**).

Pancreatic Tumours

The two neoplasms of the exocrine cells of the pancreas are **adenoma** and **adenocarcinoma**.

Adenoma has been described **in several species**, and is recognized by its ductal or acinar pattern of cells and encapsulation. **Adenocarcinoma** is the most common neoplasm in all species, particularly in the **dog**, and also in the **cat, cattle, sheep**, and **pigs**. It is made up of epithelial cells, which form tubules or acini or are undifferentiated. The characteristic feature is the presence of zymogen granules in at least a few cells. These granules are eosinophilic with H & E stain. The tumour usually has a delicate connective tissue framework. Invasion of stroma and adjacent normal pancreas is extensive. Metastasis to duodenum, liver, spleen, lymph nodes, mesenteric fat, and lungs has been reported.

Neoplasms of the islets of Langerhans also comprise **adenoma** and **adenocarcinoma**. They often secrete insulin, causing hyperinsulinism. They have been mostly reported in the **dog**, but other species are susceptible. **Adenomas** appear as nodules in the pancreas with no evidence of invasion, or metastasis. The cells are polyhedral with centrally placed nucleus and abundant cytoplasm. **Adenocarcinomas** are usually multiple, invade the adjacent pancreas, and metastasize to the pancreatic lymph nodes and liver. All functional tumours secrete insulin, and induce hypoglycaemia. The affected **dog** suddenly collapses, and goes into convulsions or coma.

Adenomas and adenocarcinomas of **non-beta cells** have also been reported in **dogs**. The tumour cells secrete gastrin, which is believed to cause ulcers in jejunum. The clinical disease has been called **canine Zollinger-Ellison syndrome**, after the human disease to which it closely resembles.

Neoplasms of the Stomach

Tumours of the stomach in animals are rare. Adenomas project from the mucosa into the lumen. They consist of hyperplastic epithelial cells which form elongated villi (**papillary** or **villous form**), or irregular tubules (**adenomatous polyp**). **Adenocarcinoma** is mostly

389

seen in the **dog**, and rarely in the **cat** and **cattle**. **In dogs**, they arise in the pyloric antral segment along the lesser curvature. The tumour invades wall of the stomach and also produces metastasis in lymph nodes, liver, and lung. The tumour cells originate from columnar cells of the gastric mucosa. They invade the gastric submucosa and muscular layer and eventually metastasize by way of the lymphatics.

Squamous-cell carcinomas originate from the squamous epithelium of the stomach in the cardia in those species that have a large cardiac component to the stomach (**horse, pig, rat**). Mitoses are frequent. Metastasis occurs by way of the lymphatics.

Leiomyoma and **leiomyosarcoma** may occasionally originate from the muscular layer of the stomach. The tumour cells resemble those of the muscular layer except for irregular arrangement, mitoses, and immaturity. **Carcinoid tumours are extremely rare** and have been reported in the **dog**. They are more commonly found in the small intestine in **cat** and **cattle**. They originate from enterochromaffin cells. **Secondary tumours** of the stomach may include lymphosarcoma, mast cell tumours, and metastatic tumours from liver or pancreas.

Neoplasms of the Small Intestine

Adenoma is made up of cells that closely resemble those of normal intestinal mucosa, but is more cellular. Adenomas project toward lumen, and may be polypoid. **Adenocarcinoma** arises from the epithelial cells of the intestinal mucosa. Its important feature is that it grows through the muscularis mucosa into the submucosa, and then through the muscular layer to the serosa. Invasion of the lymphatics is common. It may also metastasize to regional (mesenteric) lymph nodes, and to lungs and liver. There are several morphological types, namely, papillary, tubular, mucinous, and signet ring. **Adenocarcinoma of the small intestine is an uncommon tumour in most animal species**. A remarkable exception is the more frequent occurrence in **aged sheep in New Zealand. After sheep, cat, cattle**, and **dog** are also subject to this tumour.

Carcinoid tumours of argentaffin or non-argentaffin types, as described for stomach, have been reported in the small intestine of the **dog, cat, cattle**, and **elephant**. **Leiomyoma** and **leiomyosarcoma** may originate from the muscular layer, and rarely from the muscularis mucosa. The tumour cells resemble smooth muscle cells. The malignant variety is characterized by its lack of cell differentiation and invasion of neighbouring structures, and metastasis. Other rare tumours of small intestine include cavernous haemangioma and mast cell tumours. **Secondary tumours** may involve the small intestine by direct extension from adjacent organs (pancreas), or by implantation on the serosa from seeding of the peritoneal cavity or by metastasis through the general circulation.

Neoplasms of the Large Intestine

Lymphosarcoma occurs in the **caecum**. **Adenocarcinoma** has been described in the caecum of **dog, cat**, and **horse**; and **leiomyosarcoma** in the caecum of **dog. Adenocarcinoma** of the **colon** has been reported in the **dog**, but is rare in other species. These tumours arise in the mucosa; invade the submucosa, muscular layer, and lymphatics; and metastasize to colonic lymph nodes, and lungs.

Neoplasms in the **rectum** and **anus** include **adenoma** and **adenocarcinoma**. Adenomas and adenocarcinomas of the **perianal glands** are important tumours in the **dog**. Adenomas are common particularly in **male dogs**. Adenocarcinomas are much less common and arise in aged spayed bitches (i. e., bitches with ovaries removed) in which the benign form is rare. The malignant form may metastasize to the lymph nodes, and from there to sublumbar and other lymph nodes. **Adenocarcinomas** of the rectal mucosa are the most frequent gastrointestinal tumour in the **dog**. Squamous-cell carcinomas originate at the mucocutaneous junction of the anus, and are more commonly reported in the **dogs**.

Neoplasms of the Liver

Liver Cell Adenoma (Hepatocellular Adenoma)

This tumour has been described in domestic animals. They are usually single and sharply circumscribed. They may reach a large size, but do not invade or metastasize. Most have an acinar pattern made up of cells resembling normal hepatocytes, but often contain glycogen and fat droplets. In young animals, tumours have been reported **in which extramedullary haematopoiesis was a prominent feature.**

Liver Cell Carcinoma (Hepatocellular Carcinoma)

This is made up of cells that resemble liver cells, but are anaplastic. The cells may be arranged in trabecular or acinar patterns, or mixtures of both. The tumour compresses and may invade adjacent liver. The undifferentiated cells vary in size, staining features, and cytoplasmic fat and glycogen content. Mitosis and enlarged nuclei are commonly seen. Some cells are so undifferentiated that it is difficult to identify their origin from liver cells. Occasionally, acini and cysts are formed. The cells may metastasize to hepatic lymph nodes and lung.

Intrahepatic Bile-Duct Adenoma (Cystadenoma)

This is a circumscribed tumour made up of irregular-sized tubules lined with cuboidal epithelium, which resembles epithelium of intrahepatic bile ducts. Cystic variety is very common. Cysts contain clear fluid, vary in size, and their lining cells may be flattened. Mitoses are rare.

Intrahepatic Bile-Duct Carcinoma (Cholangiocarcinoma)

This is made up of epithelial cells that resemble those of the intrahepatic bile ducts. These tumours occur in any part of the liver, and spread along the biliary tract. Mitoses occur through the lymphatics to the lungs. The tumour cells are cuboidal or columnar, and usually form acini. When less differentiated, they may appear in solid cords. Papillary arrangement of tumour cells may be seen. In some cases, proliferation of connective tissue (desmoplasia) gives the tumour dense fibrous consistency.

Other tumours of liver include hepatoblastoma, haemangiomas, and haemangiosarcomas. **Hepatoblastoma is rare. Haemangiomas** are benign and may be primary in the liver. They are solitary or multiple nodules of vascular architecture, with a fine supporting stroma between endothelial-lined vascular channels. The tumour compresses the adjacent liver cells, but does not invade or metastasize. **Haemangiosarcoma** (haemangio-endothelioma, angiosarcoma) is a malignant vascular tumour with many immature, pleomorphic, endothelial cells that form vascular spaces or solid masses of cells. The nuclei are hyperchromatic, and often, in mitosis. Haemorrhage frequently occurs, and even there may be necrosis. These tumours are invasive, and metastasize to lungs.

Secondary neoplasms of the liver in animals are more common than primary, and include pancreatic adenocarcinoma, lymphosarcoma, and mast cell tumours. Malignant tumours of the intestine and pancreas metastasize to liver through portal veins.

Neoplasms of the Gallbladder

These are uncommon in most animal species. Adenomas are localized and originate from the epithelium. The tumour cells form acinar or papillary patterns of tall columnar cells. Adenomas and adenomatous polyps in cattle characteristically possess parietal and chief cells similar to those of the gastric mucosa. **Adenocarcinoma** has a tendency to invade to gallbadder wall, to form incomplete tubules and undifferentiated cells, and to undergo necrosis. Extension to liver and adjacent peritoneum may occur, and in advanced cases the tumour metastasizes to the lungs.

Neoplasms of the Kidney

Embryonal Nephroma (Nephroblastoma, Wilm's Tumour)

This is the most common tumour in pigs, especially in the young, and occurs rarely in older species. It arises in the kidney, and occasionally outside. It originates from renal blastema, from which kidney is formed. The blastema is pluripotent, which explains why this embryonal tumour contains more than one kind of tissue. Structurally, it is gland-like acini or tubules, with large masses of cells, indistinguishable from anaplastic fibrosarcoma. This led to the earlier name **adenosarcoma**. It consists of highly cellular fibroblastic tissue. This tumour is comparable to Wilm's tumour of human, which typically contains smooth muscle, but this is rarely seen in animals. Both in humans and animals, the tumours are fatal at an early age, but pigs commonly thrive longer, and the tumour is discovered at postmortem examination. **Apart from pigs**, the tumour has also been reported in **cattle**, **sheep**, **chickens**, and **rabbits**. **In pigs**, it is more common in females than males. The growth is rapid, and usually metastasizes to the lungs or liver. Partially calcified bone and striated muscle (not smooth, as in human), have been demonstrated.

Adenoma and Adenocarcinoma

These tumours arise from tubular epithelium and resemble their tissue of origin. They are mostly seen in the **dog**, in which they are malignant. An undifferentiated form has been called **hypernephroma** (undifferentiated renal carcinoma). **Carcinoma of the kidney** usually metastasizes by blood vessels, metastases being found in the regional lymph nodes. **Transitional cell carcinoma** may originate in the renal pelvis and is morphologically similar to those that develop from the transitional epithelium of the ureter, urethra, or bladder.

Metastatic neoplasms in kidney are less frequent than in the liver and lungs, the most common being the malignant lymphoma (lymphoblastoma). Other tumours include malignant melanoma, squamous-cell carcinoma, and transitional cell carcinoma (from pelvis, ureter, urethra, or bladder).

Neoplasms of the Lung

Tumours of the lung may be **primary** or **secondary**. **Secondary (metastatic) neoplasms in the lung are more frequent than the primary neoplasms**. Secondary neoplasms include almost any malignant neoplasm of any part of the body. If malignant cells become detached from the primary growth and are swept into the lymphatics or veins, they soon reach the pulmonary circulation. The capillaries of the lungs form a fine screen through which all of the blood circulates. Tumour cells are readily trapped and often find the lung a suitable place in which to grow.

Primary tumours of the lungs in animals include: (1) adenocarcinoma, (2) squamous-cell carcinoma, (3) chondroma and chondrosarcoma, and (4) lipomas, fibrosarcoma, chondroma, and haemangioma.

1. Adenocarcinoma (bronchiolar-alveolar cell carcinoma) arises from the epithelial cells of the alveoli. However, some believe that its origin is in bronchiolar epithelium. The neoplastic cells grow into alveoli. The cells may be columnar or cuboidal, but are usually tall columnar with cilia. **Pulmonary adenomatosis of sheep (jaagsiekte)** is a viral-induced lesion that resembles adenocarcinoma of the lungs, and may be difficult to distinguish in some circumstances. Adenocarcinoma metastasizes to bronchial lymph nodes.

2. Squamous-cell carcinoma (bronchogenic carcinoma) is much less common than adenocarcinoma in most animal species. This tumour resembles the bronchogenic carcinoma (squamous-cell carcinoma) of humans. The tumour originates from the epithelium of the terminal bronchi, which undergoes squamous metaplasia and neoplasia. From its central position, it extends peripherally, involves much of the lobule, and then the lobe of the lung.

3. Chondromas and chondrosarcomas appear to arise from cartilage in the terminal bronchi, but are much less frequent than epithelial tumours.

Other rare tumours include lipoma, fibrosarcoma, teratoma, and haemangioma. **Mesothelioma of the pleura** is a primary tumour, and arises from the mesothelial lining of the pleural sac and resembles its parent cells. They are usually benign.

Epidermal Inclusion Cyst

It is a non-neoplastic cyst mostly seen in the dog. They appear as small nodules, firmly attached in the dermis. The skin usually remains covered with hair. Incision of the nodules reveals one or more spherical cysts with a thin wall and a grey, coarse, granular material. **Microscopically**, the cyst wall is made up of flattened squamous epithelium. The cysts contain concentrically laminated masses of keratin.

The origin of these cysts is not clear, but **in the dog** they appear to result from occlusion of the mouth of hair follicles.

Epidermold or Dermold Cyst

This is similar to the epidermal inclusion cyst, but is made up of epidermis supplied with skin adnexa. Sebaceous gland, hair follicles, and sweat glands may be present.

Teratomas

Teratoma is a true tumour composed of multiple tissues. Of these, at least two are foreign to the tissue where it is found. They may be **benign teratomas**, or undergo malignant transformation - **malignant teratomas**. In animals, they are seldom seen in sites other than the gonads. However, they are also seen in other tissues.

The benign teratomas are **seen commonly in** the **horse**; but are **less common in** the **cattle, dog,** and **chicken**; and **extremely rare in** the **cat, sheep,** and **pig. In the horse**, they occur in the testicle, and are usually unilateral. **In the dog, cattle, and pig**, they are found mostly in the ovaries, while in the **chicken** usually in the testicle. Many of the cysts contain hair, keratin, and sebaceous material. Some teratomas have nodules of cartilage, spicules of bone, and even teeth. **Malignant teratomas have not been described in animals.**

Chapter 9

Diseases of Immunity

The immune system is like a two-edged sword. On the one hand, organisms depend on this system for their survival, on the other they fall prey to its many disorders that could threaten their very existence. These disorders range from immunodeficiency states to hypersensitivity reactions. **In other words from 'too little' to 'too much' activity on the part of the immune system.** The various diseases of immunity are described under three headings: (1) hypersensitivity reactions, (2) autoimmune diseases, and (3) immunodeficiency diseases. The chapter will conclude with a discussion of acquired immunodeficiency syndrome (AIDS).

The **immune system** is composed of **two components** designed to protect the body against extracellular and intracellular pathogens (Fig. 60). The two components are: **(i) humoral immunity**, mediated by soluble **antibody** proteins, and **(ii) cellular immunity**, mediated by **lymphocytes** (discussed later). **B-lymphocytes** or **B-cells** are the source of antibodies. Antibodies participate in immunity either by directly neutralizing extracellular microbes, or by activating complement and certain effector cells (neutrophils and macrophages) to kill microorganisms. **T-lymphocytes** or **T-cells** can either directly lyse (destroy) targets (achieved by **cytotoxic T-cells**), or arrange for the antimicrobial immune response of other cells by producing soluble protein mediators called **cytokines** (made by **helper T-cells**, discussed later). While B-cells and their antibodies can recognize and bind to **intact antigens** (e.g., bacteria), T-cells can 'see' (recognize) only those antigens which have been **processed** (i.e., enzymatically broken into smaller pieces) and **presented** by other cells to T-cells in the context of major histocompatibility complex (MHC) molecules (discussed later). Thus, participation of T-cells in the immune response requires both **antigen-presenting cells (APCs),** such as macrophages and dendritic cells to exhibit the processed antigen to T-cells, and also a variety of effector cells (cells that carry out the action) to eliminate the processed antigen (such as, viruses). **Natural killer (NK) cells** are a separate class of lymphocytes that act as a **first line of defence.**

397

Cells of the Immune System

The most important cell of the immune system is the **lymphocyte.** Lymphocytes arise from stem cells in the bone marrow. After originating from stem cells, lymphocytes follow **two pathways** (Fig. 60). Those that travel through the thymus (both in mammals and birds), and are therefore differentiated here, are called **thymus-derived lymphocytes,** or **T-lymphocytes,** or **T-cells.** The T-lymphocytes are responsible for cellular or cell-mediated immunity. Those that travel through the bursa of Fabricius in birds (bone marrow in mammals) and are therefore differentiated here, are called **bursa-derived lymphocytes,** or **B-lymphocytes,** or **B-cells** (Fig. 60). B-cells

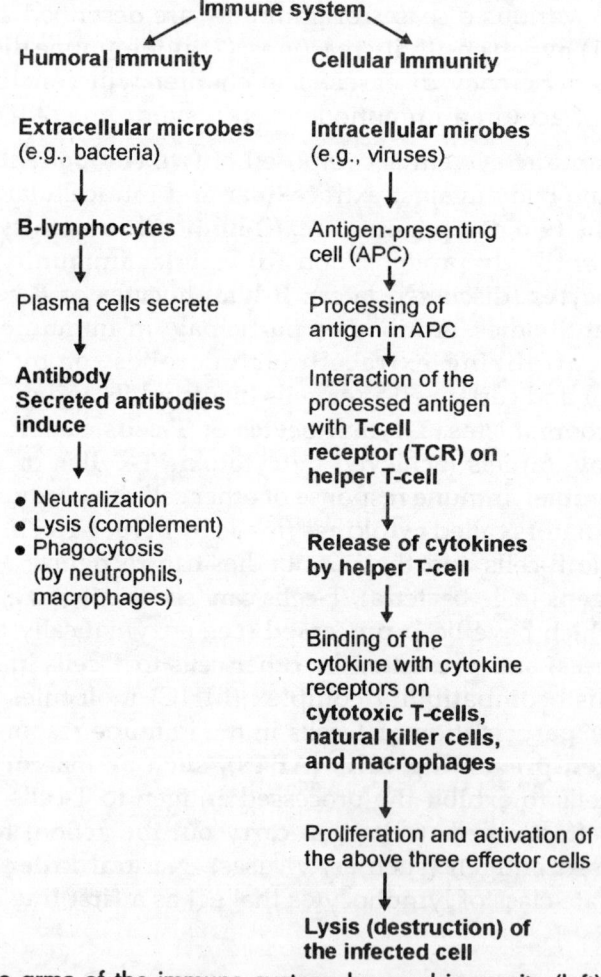

Fig. 60. Two arms of the immune system: humoral immunity (left), and cellular immunity (right).

are responsible for the humoral or antibody-mediated immunity. Thus, two populations of antigen-sensitive cells exist in the body: **(i) T-lymphocytes**, that are responsible for the cell-mediated immune responses, and **(ii) B-lymphocytes**, that produce antibodies and are responsible for antibody-mediated immune responses. The organs that regulate the production and differentiation of lymphocytes are called **primary lymphoid organs**, and include **thymus** (in both mammals and birds), **bursa of Fabricius** (only in birds) and **bone marrow** (in mammals).

T-Lymphocytes

Thymus-derived, or T-cells mediate cellular immunity. They are also essential for inducing the B-cell-derived humoral immunity. In humans, T-cells constitute between 60% and 70% of the lymphocytes in circulating blood, and in **domestic animals** up to 80%. In the chicken, T-cells constitute between 60% and 70% of the total lymphocyte population. Besides blood, T-cells are also found mainly in the splenic periarteriolar sheaths and lymph node inter-follicular zones.

Each T-cell is genetically programmed to recognize a specific processed antigen (a peptide fragment) by means of a **T-cell receptor (TCR)**. The TCR is a protein heterodimer that is made up of two different kinds of polypeptide chains (Fig. 61A). These two chains, alpha and beta, are linked by a disulphide bond. Each chain has a variable (antigen-binding) and a constant region. TCR diversity for billions (crores) of potential antigens (peptides) is generated by somatic rearrangement of the genes that encode individual chains of the TCR.

The TCRs, are non-covalently linked to a cluster of five constant polypeptide chains. These are composed of the gamma, delta and epsilon proteins of the **CD3 molecular complex** (CD = cluster of differentiation), and **two zeta chains** (Fig. 61A). The CD3 proteins and zeta chains do not themselves bind antigens (antigenic peptides), but they interact with the constant region of the TCR to transduce (transfer) signals into the T-cell after it has bound the antigen.

In addition to these signalling proteins (CD3 proteins and zeta chains) T-cells express a variety of other constant function-associated molecules, including **CD4** and **CD8** (Fig.61B). These two molecules are expressed on two different types of T-cells and serve as **co-receptors** for T-cell stimulation (discussed later). **CD4** is expressed on about 60% of mature T-cells (known as **'helper T-cells'**), whereas **CD8** is expressed on about 30% of T-cells (known as **'cytotoxic T-cells'**). In humans, in normal healthy individuals, the CD4/CD8 ratio is therefore about 2:1. The CD4- and CD8-expressing T-cells, called

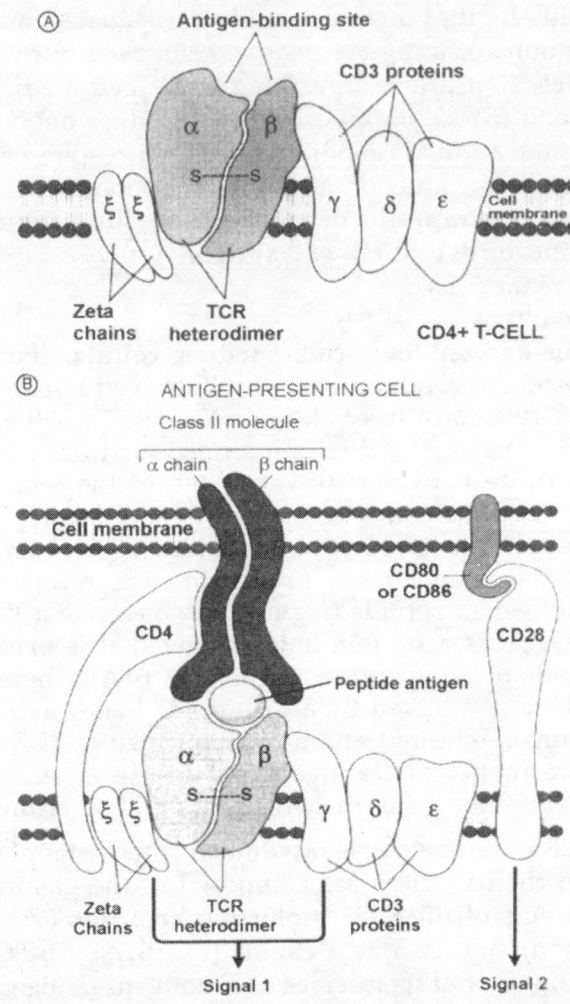

Fig. 61. The T-cell receptor (TCR) complex. (A) Schematic illustration of TCR-alpha and TCR-beta polypeptide chains linked to CD3 and zeta chain molecular complex. (B) TCR complex and its interaction with major histocompatibility complex (MCH) molecules on an antigen-presenting cell. The diagram represents **antigen recognition by CD4+ T-cells**. Note that the alpha-beta TCR heterodimer recognizes a peptide fragment of antigen bound to the **MHC class II molecule**. The **CD4** molecule binds to non-polymorphic portion of the class II molecule. The interaction between TCR and the MHC-bound antigen provides **signal 1 for T-cell activation**. **Signal 2 is provided by** the interaction of the **CD28** molecule with the **co-stimulatory molecules (CD80 or CD86)** expressed on antigen-presenting cells. **Similar interactions occur between MHC I molecules and the TCR on CD8+ T-cells**. In that case, the CD8 molecule binds to the non-polymorphic portion of the **class I molecule**.

CD4+ and **CD8+**, respectively, perform different but overlapping functions. **CD4+ T- cells are helper T-cells** because they secrete soluble molecules (**cytokines**) that influence almost all other cells of the immune system The CD8+ T-cells can also secrete cytokines, but they play a more important role in directly killing virus-infected or tumour cells (**cytotoxic T-cells**).

During antigen recognition, CD4 molecules on T-cells bind to portions of class II MHC molecules (discussed later) on antigen-presenting cells (APCs). Likewise, CD8 binds to class I MHC molecules. **It is important to note that T-cells require two signals for complete activation** (Fig. 61B). **Signal 1** is provided by the interaction between TCR and the MHC-bound antigen. The CD4 and CD8 co-receptors increase this signal. **Signal 2** is provided by the interaction between CD28 molecules on T-cells with the co-stimulatory CD80 or CD86 molecules (also called B7-1 and B-72, respectively) expressed on antigen-presenting cells (APCs) (Fig. 61B). **CD28 co-stimulation is essential, because in the absence of signal 2 the T-cells undergo apoptosis or become unreactive (anergic).** This two-signal arrangement may be a foolproof way to ensure that the normal individual successfully prevents autoreactivity (see 'immunological tolerance'). Because of the role played by the CD4 and CD8 co-receptors, **CD4+ helper T-cells respond to antigens only in the context of class II MHC molecules, whereas the CD8+ cytotoxic T-cells respond to antigens associated with only class I MHC molecules.**

CD4 T-cells are of two types with different functions determined by their cytokines. **Th1 (helper T1) CD4+ cells** secrete cytokines that direct cell-mediated immune responses, including macrophage and natural killer cell activation. **These Th1** cytokines include **interleukin-2 (IL-2)** and **interferon-gamma (IFN-gamma).** In contrast, **Th2 (helper T 2) CD4+ cells** secrete **cytokines IL-4, IL-5, and IL-10 that antagonize Th1 effects** and/or promote certain aspects of humoral immunity.

B-Lymphocytes

B-lymphocytes constitute 10% to 20% of the lymphocytes in human blood, and 15% to 40% in domestic animals. In the chicken, B-cells constitute between 30% and 40% of the total lymphocyte population. They are also present in the bone marrow, in peripheral lymphoid tissues (lymph nodes, spleen), and in non-lymphoid organs such as the gastrointestinal tract. In the lymph nodes, they are found in the cortex in lymphoid follicles and in the spleen in the white pulp. Stimulation by local infection leads to the formation of a central zone of large, activated B-cells in follicles called a **'germinal centre'**.

After antigenic stimulation, B-cells form **plasma cells** that secrete **immunoglobulins (antibodies)** (see Fig. 60). Immunoglobulins, in turn, mediate humoral immunity. Of the five immunoglobulin isotypes, **IgG, IgM,** and **IgA** constitute more than 95% of serum antibodies, whereas **IgE** and **IgD** occur in traces. Each immunoglobulin has characteristic ability to activate complement or recruit inflammatory cells, and have defined roles. For example, IgA is an important mediator of mucosal immunity, whereas IgE has special importance for helminthic infections and in allergic responses.

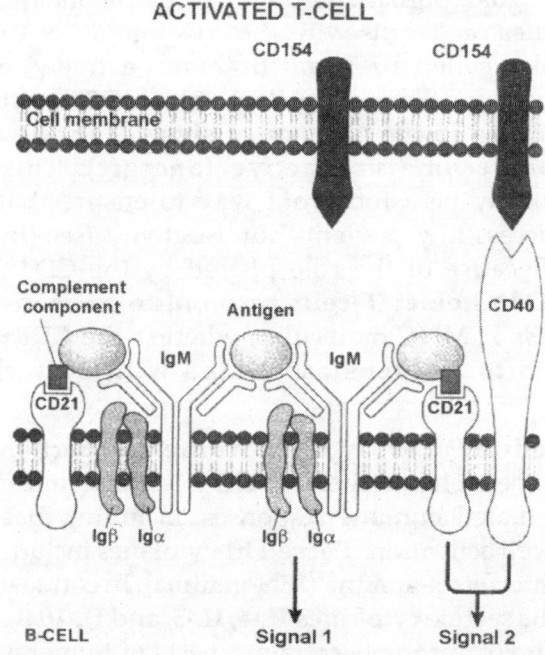

Fig. 62. The B-cell receptor (BCR) complex and its interaction with antigen and co-stimulatory molecules. Membrane-bound immunoglobulin (here shown as IgM) binds to exogenous antigen. Intracellular signal 1 for B-cell activation is then provided by interaction with BCR-associated Ig-alpha and Ig-beta heterodimers. **Signal 2** is provided by activated complement interacting with B-cell CD21 or by interaction of B-cell surface CD40 with CD154 on activated T-cells.

B-cells recognize antigen through monomeric surface IgM (i.e., IgM consisting of only one subunit), the so-called **B-cell receptor (BCR)**

(Fig. 62). (Note that IgM consists of five subunits linked by disulphide bonds. BCR consists of only one such subunit). As with T-cells, each BCR has a unique antigen specificity, derived from somatic rearrangement of immunoglobulin genes. Like TCR-CD3 complex, **BCRs interact with several constant molecules** that are **responsible for signal transduction** (i.e., conversion of signal from one form to another) **and for complete B-cell activation** (Fig. 62). For example, B-cell **CD40** molecule binds to **CD154** on activated T-cells. This is essential for B-cell maturation and secretion of IgG, IgA, or IgE antibodies. **CD21** (also known as CR2 complement receptor) is another important B-cell-associated co-stimulatory molecule. It is also the receptor by which Epstein-Barr virus (EBV) enters into the human B-cells.

Macrophages

Macrophages are part of the **mononuclear phagocyte system (MPS)**. Their role in inflammation was discussed in Chapter 4. However, macrophages also play important roles in the immune response.

1. **Macrophages** along with **dendritic cells** (described next) **express class II MHC molecules** (see later). Macrophages therefore play the central role in the **processing and presentation of antigen** to CD4+ helper T-cells. **This is essential because T-cells, unlike B-cells, cannot be triggered by free antigen.** Presentation of processed antigen by macrophages, or other antigen-presenting cells (APCs), therefore is a must for induction of cell-mediated immunity.

2. Macrophages **produce a large number of cytokines** and are therefore important effector cells in certain forms of cell-mediated immunity, for example, delayed-type hypersensitivity (discussed later). These cytokines not only influence T- and B-cell function but also affect other cell types, including endothelium and fibroblasts.

3. Macrophages **phagocytose and ultimately kill microbes** coated by antibody and/or complement (i.e., **opsonized**; see Chapter 4). Therefore, they are important effector elements in **humoral immunity.**

4. Macrophages **kill tumour cells** by producing reactive oxygen metabolites (free radicals), or by secretion of tumour necrosis factor (TNF) (see 'anti-tumour effector mechanisms').

5. Macrophages phagocytose and kill bacteria coated by antibody

and/or complement (opsonized, Chapter 4). Therefore, they are important effector elements in **humoral immunity**.

Dendritic Cells

Cells with dendritic morphology, that is, having free dendritic (branching like a tree) cytoplasmic processes, occur in two functionally **different types: (1) dendritic cells** (interdigitating dendritic cells): These are non-phagocytic cells and **express high levels of MHC class II and co-stimulatory molecules (B7 - CD80, CD86).** They are widely distributed, and occur in lymphoid tissues and in the interstitium of many non-lymphoid organs, such as the heart and lungs. Similar cells within the **epidermis** are called **Langerhans cells.** The distribution and surface molecule expression of dendritic cells make them best suited for presenting antigens to CD4+ T-cells. **(2) follicular dendritic cells:** These cells are present in the germinal centres of lymphoid follicles in the spleen and lymph nodes. They possess Fc receptors for IgG, that is, receptors that bind the Fc portion (constant portion) of antibodies. Therefore, they effectively trap antigen bound to antibodies.

Natural Killer (NK) Cells

NK cells are somewhat larger than small lymphocytes. Both in human and domestic animals, they comprise 10% to 15% of peripheral blood lymphocytes. These cells contain abundant azurophilic granules and **can lyse (destroy) a variety of tumour cells, virally infected cells**, and some normal cells, **without prior sensitization.** These cells are therefore called **'natural killer cells'** and are the **first line of defence.** They are part of the innate as opposed to acquired immune system. In the chicken, morphology of the NK cells is unclear, but they are probably large granular lymphocytes.

NK cells do not express TCR and are CD3 negative. Instead, **NK cells express two types of surface receptors** that enable them to kill neoplastic or virus-infected cells (Fig. 63). **(1)** One type is **an 'activating receptor'.** It recognizes certain unknown molecules on target cells. **(2)** The other type called **'killer inhibitor receptor (KIR)'** inhibits NK cytolysis (destruction) by recognizing self, class I MHC molecules. **NK cells do not lyse healthy nucleated cells because they all express class I MHC molecules. If virus infection or neoplastic transformation reduces normal MHC I expression, inhibitory KIR signals are interrupted and lysis occurs** (Fig. 63).

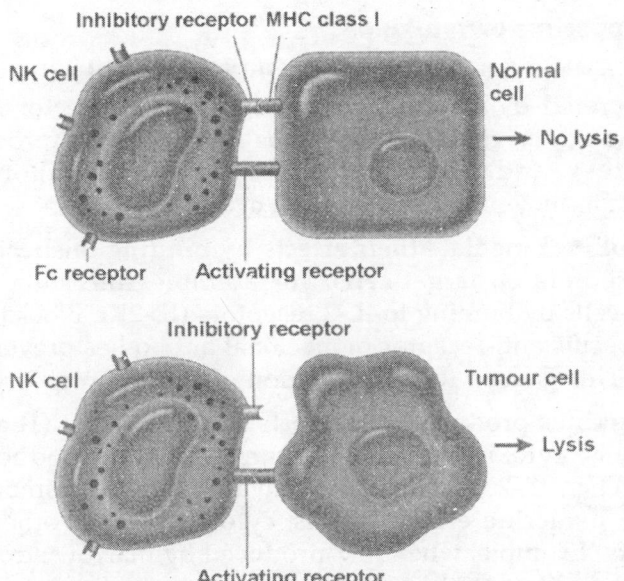

Fig. 63. NK cell receptors and killing. Normal cells are not killed because **inhibitory signals** from MHC class I molecules override (dominate) activating signals. In tumour cells or virus-infected cells, reduced expression or alteration of MHC molecules **interrupts the inhibitory signals,** allowing activation of NK cells and lysis of target cells.

NK cells are identified by the presence of **two cell-surface molecules: CD16** and **CD56. CD16** is of particular importance. It is an **Fc receptor for IgG** and gives NK cells **an extra ability to lyse IgG-opsonized target cells.** This process, known as **'antibody-dependent cell-mediated cytotoxicity (ADCC)',** is described under type II hypersensitivity. NK cells also secrete cytokines and are an important source of interferon-gamma (IFN-gamma).

Cytokines: Soluble Mediators of the Immune System

The induction and regulation of immune responses require that interactions of many cell types, including lymphocytes, monocytes, other inflammatory cells (neutrophils), and endothelium are properly organized and coordinated. Many interactions require cell-cell contact. However, others are mediated by short-acting soluble mediators called **'cytokines'.** They are so called because they are derived from cells (G. cytos = cell).

405

General Properties of Cytokines

Cytokines are low molecular weight **polypeptides** (10 to 40 kD) that are secreted by **lymphocytes** as well as by effector cells and APCs. Although originally classified as **lymphokines** (produced by lymphocytes) and **monokines** (produced by monocytes/ macrophages), they are all now called **cytokines**.

1. Cytokines mediate their effects by binding to specific high-affinity receptors on target cells. For example, interleukin-2 (IL-2) activates T-cells by binding to IL-2 receptors (IL-2R). Blockade of the IL-2R by specific anti-receptor monoclonal antibodies prevents T-cell activation. This is used to treat rejection of transplanted organ.

2. Cytokines produce their effects in three ways: (1) autocrine effect: In this, cytokines act on the same cell that produces them. Example: When IL-2 produced by activated T-cells promotes T-cell growth, **(2) paracrine effect:** In this, cytokines affect other cells in their vicinity. Example: when IL-7 produced by marrow stromal cells promotes the differentiation of B-cell progenitors (ancestors) in the bone marrow, and **(3) endocrine effect:** In this, cytokines affect cells systemically. Example: IL-1 and TNF that produce the **acute phase response** during inflammation (see Chapter 4).

3. Cytokines can act in amplifying sequences. For example, TNF induces IL-1 production, which in turn drives IL-6 synthesis.

4. Same cytokines are produced by different cell types. For example, IL-1 and TNF can be produced by virtually any cell.

5. The effects of cytokines are pleiotropic. That is, they act on many cell types, causing many different effects. For example, IL-2, initially described as a T-cell growth factor, regulates the growth and differentiation of B-cells and NK cells.

6. Many cytokines may produce similar effects. That is, they are redundant (superfluous). For example, IL-1 and TNF produce very similar effects.

7. Cytokines may be antagonistic, that is, have opposing effects. In this way, they can finely regulate the intensity and type of an immune response. For example, interferon-gamma activates macrophages while IL-10 prevents macrophage activation.

General Classes of Cytokines

Cytokines can be divided into **five categories** on the basis of their general properties.

1. Cytokines that mediate innate immunity: This group includes IL-1, TNF, IL-6, and type 1 interferons. Interferons protect against viral infections, while IL-1, TNF, and IL-6 initiate non-specific pro-inflammatory responses, such as the activation of endothelium and mononuclear inflammatory cells and induction of acute-phase reactant synthesis by the liver. **Macrophages are the major source of these cytokines.**

2. Cytokines that regulate lymphocyte growth, activation, and differentiation: These are IL-2, IL-4, IL-5, IL-12, IL-15, and transforming growth factor-alpha (TGF-alpha). Some, such as IL-2 and IL-4 favour lymphocyte growth and differentiation, while others, such as IL-10 and TGF-alpha down-regulate (decrease) immune responses. Some of these cytokines (e.g., IL-2) fall under the group of **Th1 cytokines**, which direct cell-mediated responses, whereas others (e.g., IL-4, IL-10) are **Th2 cytokines**, which antagonize Th1 effects and/or promote certain aspects of humoral immunity.

3. Cytokines that activate inflammatory cells: These include interferon-gamma (a Th1 cytokine), TNF lymphotoxin (TNF-beta), and migration inhibitory factor. Most of these cytokines are derived from **T-cells**.

4. Chemokines are cytokines that recruit inflammatory cells to sites of injury (Chapter 4). These occur in **two** structurally different **groups**: **C-C** and **C-X-C chemokines** based on the arrangement of certain cysteine (C) residues. The **C-X-C chemokines,** which include interleukin-8 are produced by activated macrophages and tissue cells such as endothelium. **C-C chemokines** are produced largely by T-cells and include monocyte chemoattractant protein 1 (MCP-1) and monocyte inflammatory protein 1 alpha (MIP-1 alpha).

5. Cytokines that stimulate haematopoiesis: Many cytokines derived from lymphocytes or stromal cells stimulate the growth and production of new blood cells by acting on haematopoietic progenitor (ancestor) cells. They are called **colony stimulating factors (CSFs)** because they were originally identified by their ability to promote the growth of haematopoietic cell colonies from bone marrow precursors. Lymphocytes and bone marrow stromal cells are the major sources of these cytokines. Examples: granulocyte-macrophage (GM)-CSF and granulocyte (G)-CSF.

Histocompatibility Molecules

General Properties

These were first detected as the antigens that caused rejection of transplanted organs. Hence the name 'histocompatibility' (Greek **histo** = tissue, i.e., tissue **compatibility**). However, histocompatibility molecules are now known to play an extremely important role in inducing and regulating the normal immune functions. **Remember, T-cells (unlike B cells) recognize only membrane-bound antigens, and only in the context of 'self' histocompatibility molecules.** This phenomenon is referred to as **MHC restriction. Thus, the main role of histocompatibility molecules is to bind peptide fragments of foreign proteins (i.e., antigens) for presentation to appropriate antigen-specific T-cells.** In addition, by engaging KIRs on natural killer cells, MHC class I molecules prevent lysis of normal cells by NK cells (see 'natural killer cell'). Several genes code for histocompatibility molecules, but the most important are clustered (grouped) on a small fragment of chromosome 6. This cluster (group) constitutes the **major histocompatibility complex (MHC).** Because MHC-encoded histocompatibility molecules were first detected on blood leukocytes they were indicated by the **initials of the species, followed by LA (leukocyte antigen).** Thus, **HLA** indicates the MHC antigens in **humans**; **DLA** those in **dogs**; and **BoLA** those in **cattle**.

Based on their chemical structure, tissue distribution and function, **MHC gene products are classified into three categories.**

1. Class I MHC molecules: Each of these molecules is a heterodimer. That is, it is composed of **two different molecules: alpha chain** and **beta-microglobulin** (Fig. 64). The extracellular portion of the **alpha chain contains a cleft where foreign peptides (i.e., antigens) bind to MHC molecules for presentation to CD8+ T-cells** (Fig. 64). In general, **MHC I molecules bind to antigens derived from proteins synthesized within the cells (e.g., viral antigens). Because MHC I molecules are present on virtually all nucleated cells, virally infected cells can be detected and lysed (destroyed) by cytotoxic T-cells.**

2. Class II MHC molecules: MHC II molecules are also heterodimers composed of two different molecules alpha and beta subunits. Like MHC I, the extracellular portion of the MHC II heterodimer contains a cleft for binding antigens (Fig. 64). However, MHC II molecules differ from MHC I molecules in several ways. Unlike MHC I molecules, **the tissue distribution of MHC II-expressing cells is quite restricted. They are expressed mainly on antigen-presenting**

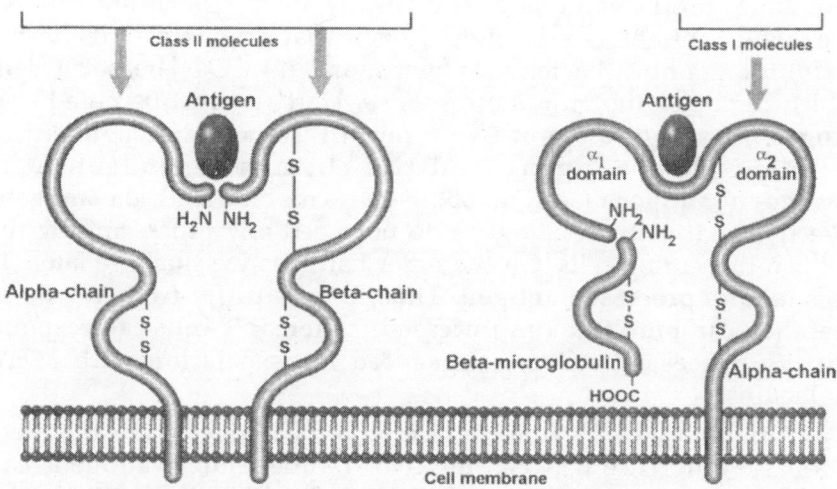

Fig. 64. Schematic representation of MHC I and MHC II molecules. Both have similar structure, but the subunit organization and origin of the peptides in the **antigen cleft** are different (see text).

cells (monocytes, macrophages, dendritic cells) and B-cells. In addition, other cell types such as vascular endothelial cells, fibroblasts, and renal tubular epithelial cells, are induced to express MHC II by interferon-alpha (IFN-alpha). **In general, MHC molecules bind to antigens derived from proteins synthesized outside the cell, for example, those derived from extracellular bacteria. This allows CD4+ T-cells to recognize the presence of extracellular pathogens and to organize a protective cytokine-mediated response.**

3. Class III Proteins: These include those **complement components** (C2, C3, and Bf) that are encoded within the MHC. Genes for tumour necrosis factor (TNF) and lymphotoxin (TNF-beta) are also encoded within the MHC. Although genetically linked to class I and class II antigens, **class III molecules and the cytokine genes do not act as histocompatibility (transplantation) antigens.**

Mechanisms of the Immune Responses

The major function of the **histocompatibility molecules (MHC molecules)** is to present foreign antigens to T-cells. Thus, histocompatibility molecules play an important role **in the induction of humoral and cellular immunity.**

1. **Humoral Immunity (Antibody Response)**

Two key cells are involved in the development of humoral immunity (antibody production). These are: **(1) B-lymphocyte or B-**

409

cell, which produces antibodies to destroy an exogenous antigen. An exogenous antigen is a foreign antigen that originates outside the body, for example, bacterial antigens, and **(2) CD4+ helper T-cell**, which regulates the immune response. Here, it must be noted that **exogenous antigens** are **of two types: (i) Thymus-independent** or **T-independent antigens**, and **(ii) Thymus-dependent** or **T-dependent antigens** (see Fig. 65). B-cells can bind both the antigens directly. That is, these antigens do not need any processing by the antigen-presenting cells. On the other hand, as we shall see later, T-cells require **processed antigen. Thus, B-cells differ from T-cells in that they can bind free (unprocessed), whereas T-cells can respond only to processed antigen presented in association with MHC molecules.**

Although B-cells can recognize both the antigens directly, there is a basic difference between the two. **T-independent antigens** can **produce antibodies** without help from helper T-cells, that is, **in the absence of helper T-cells. But, they trigger only IgM response in B-cells and cannot form IgG** (Fig. 65). This is because they fail to induce the formation of cytokines from helper T-cells and therefore **cannot trigger a class switch of antibody. T-dependent antigens**, on the other hand, need the help of helper T-cells (discussed later). **Without this help, they cannot form antibody.** Since these antigens induce formation of cytokines from helper T-cells, **they can trigger a class switch** and form IgM, IgG, IgA, and IgE (Fig. 65). Most antigens in the environment are T-dependent, that is, they require cytokine help from helper T-cells to produce antibody.

With this background, let us now understand the **mechanisms** involved in antibody production, **keeping Fig. 65 constantly in view.**

Mechanisms: After entry, the exogenous antigen binds to B-cell through cell's receptors. If the antigen is **T-independent** then, without help from helper T-cells, it triggers B-cells to produce antibodies. B-cells then form plasma cells, which, in turn, produce antibodies (of IgM type only) (Fig. 65). If the antigen is **T-dependent**, then it would require cytokine help from helper T-cells. **But helper T-cells bind and respond only to processed antigen in association with MHC class II molecules.** This means that, in the case of T-dependent antigens, two different processes must occur together for antibody production. **First**, the antigen must bind to B-cells. **Secondly**, the helper T-cells must also be activated simultaneously **by the same antigen**. As helper T-cells require **processed antigen**, the antigen is also picked up concurrently by the antigen-presenting cells

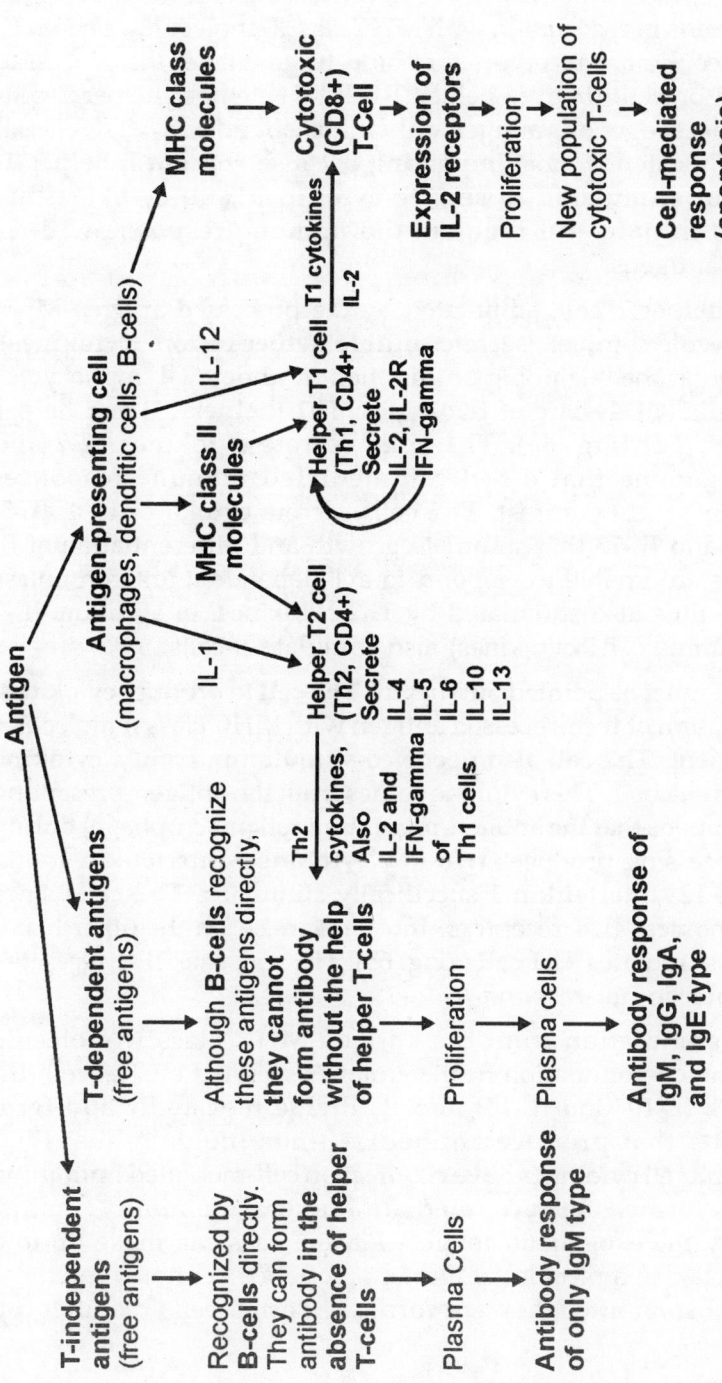

Fig. 65. Mechanisms involved in the development of humoral and cellular immunity. IL = interleukin; Th1 = helper T1 cell; Th2 = helper T2 cell; IFN-gamma = interferon-gamma; IL-2R = interleukin-2 receptor

411

(macrophages, dendritic cells, B-cells), **processed**, and then presented to helper T-cells in association with MHC class II molecules. The MHC class II molecules are receptors that bind fragments of the processed antigen and present them to helper T-cells. Remember helper T-cells recognize this exogenous antigen **only** if it is bound to a MHC class II molecule. **This step is most important, because without it helper T-cells are not stimulated to secrete cytokines**, and cytokines are required to initiate and regulate the immune response with T-dependent antigens.

Next, helper T-cell, stimulated by the processed antigen-MHC class II molecule complex, **secrete soluble helper factors (cytokines).** As described at the beginning of this chapter under 'T-lymphocytes', **helper T-cells (CD4+) are of two types: Th1 (helper T1) and helper Th2 (helper T2)** (Fig. 65). **Th1 cells** secrete cytokines IL-2 and interferon-gamma that direct cell-mediated immune responses (discussed next). In contrast, **Th2** cells secrete cytokines IL-4, IL-5, IL-6, IL-10, and IL-13 that stimulate growth and differentiation of B-cells. B-cells are unable to respond to a T-dependent antigen unless at the same time also stimulated by Th2 cytokines. In addition, IL-2 and IFN-gamma (Th1 cytokines) also stimulate B-cells.

Here, it must be pointed out that for **Th2 cell** to produce cytokines, just presentation of the processed antigen with MHC class II molecules is not sufficient. **Th2 cell also needs co-stimulation from a cytokine called interleukin-1**. This cytokine comes from the antigen-presenting cell. It so happens that the antigen-presenting cell (macrophage) during antigen processing produces **two key cytokines: interleukin-1**, and **interleukin-12**. **Interleukin-1** specifically stimulates **Th2 cells** since these cells possess IL-1 receptors. **Interleukin 12**, on the other hand, specifically stimulates **Th1 cells** (Fig. 65). Th1 cells lack IL-1 receptors and therefore do not respond to IL-1.

After stimulation from the antigen-MHC class II molecule complex, and co-stimulation from cytokines secreted by Th2 cell (IL-4, IL-5, IL-6, IL-10, and IL-13), **B-cells divide repeatedly and form plasma cells** that produce antibodies (immunoglobulins) (Fig. 65). These Th2 cell cytokines have no effect on cell-mediated immunity. **Antibodies formed, in turn, mediate humoral immunity**, that is, they destroy the exogenous antigen. Plasma cells can make up to a million (ten lakhs) molecules of immunoglobulins per hour, and these are secreted soon after they are formed. Plasma cells die after 3-6 days.

2. Cell-Mediated Immune Response (Cellular Immunity)

Three types of cells are involved in the development of a cell-mediated immune response (**cellular immunity**). These are: **(1)** a cell expressing **endogenous antigen** on its surface (the **target cell**). In fact, this is the **antigen-presenting cell** that processes and expresses the endogenous antigen on its surface and thus becomes the target cell for destruction by cytotoxic T-cell. An endogenous antigen is a foreign antigen synthesized within body cells, for example, newly formed virus proteins, **(2) a helper T-cell (Th1)** that regulates the immune response, and **(3) a cytotoxic T-cell (CD8+)** that destroys the endogenous antigen present inside the target cell. In other words, **cytotoxic T-cell is the cell that induces cell death (apoptosis)**. Note that cytotoxic T-cell responds to antigen **only** when it is presented by the antigen-presenting cell **in association with MHC class I molecules** (Fig. 65).

Mechanism: The cytotoxic T-cell needs **two signals** to destroy the target cell. The **first signal** comes when cytotoxic T-cell binds to **endogenous antigen** in association with **MHC class I molecules** through its receptors. The **second signal** comes **from helper T1 cell (Th1)** in the form of cytokines. For **Th1 cell** to secrete cytokines, it needs **two stimuli**. **First**, it must respond to the same antigen to which cytotoxic T-cell responds but in association with MHC class II molecules, and bind the antigen through its receptors. The **second signal** is **interleukin-12** that comes from the same antigen-presenting cell that processes the endogenous antigen. **Interleukin-12 acts as a co-stimulator** (Fig. 65). Following stimulation from the antigen-MHC class II complex and interleukin-12, **helper T1 cell (Th1) secretes two key cytokines: interleukin-2,** and **interferon-gamma** as well as **IL-2 receptors (Fig. 65). Interleukin-2 is the second signal for cytotoxic T-cell**. IL-2 is produced only by Th1 cell. IL-2, in turn, binds to IL-2 receptors (IL-2R) on the surface of cytotoxic T-cells and triggers them to produce more IL-2 receptors. **The combination of these signals** (antigen-MHC class I complex and IL-2) **activates cytotoxic T-cells**, which then undergo cell division and produce a new population of cytotoxic T-cells that bring about the cell-mediated cell response. **Thus, IL-2 is a key component of the immune response.**

The fully activated cytotoxic T-cells trigger apoptosis (cell death) in their target cells, through two pathways. One pathway involves the secretion of proteins called **perforins (perforin pathway)**. The **second pathway** is mediated through a cell surface receptor called

413

CD95 or **Fas** (**CD95 pathway**) (see 'T-cell-mediated cytotoxicity'). Both pathways require physical contact between cytotoxic T-cell and its target.

One of the important functions of cytotoxic T-cells is to eliminate virus-infected cells from the body. As viral antigens (endogenous antigens) by cytotoxic T-cells can be recognized only in association with **MHC class I molecules**, perhaps this may be the reason why nature has provided **widespread expression** of class I molecules, so that body can be adequately protected against viral infections.

Mechanisms of Immune-Mediated Injury (Hypersensitivity Reactions)

Although immune responses are usually protective against infections, and to some extent tumours, **such responses may also potentially damage host tissues**. When immune responses, humoral or cell-mediated to either exogenous or endogenous antigens, cause tissue-damaging reactions, all such forms of immune-mediated injury are collectively called **'hypersensitivity reactions'**, and the resultant tissue lesions as **'hypersensitivity diseases (or disorders)'**. The term hypersensitivity, however, is somewhat misleading. This is because it suggests abnormal or excessive sensitivity to an antigen, whereas **hypersensitivity disease** may result from a perfectly normal immune response to an antigen. For example, the rejection of tissue grafts from antigenically dissimilar donors.

Hypersensitivity diseases are best classified on the basis of the immunological mechanism initiating the disease (Table 19). This approach clarifies the manner in which the immune responses ultimately cause tissue injury and disease. **The hypersensitivity reactions are classified into four types: three are variations of antibody-mediated injury, whereas the fourth is cell-mediated (Table 19). Type I hypersensitivity reaction** results from IgE antibodies adsorbed (adhered) on mast cells or basophils. When these IgE molecules bind their specific antigens (allergens), they are triggered to release vasoactive amines and other mediators from mast cells or basophils, which in turn affect vascular permeability and smooth muscle contraction in various organs. **Type II hypersensitivity reaction** is caused by humoral antibodies that bind to fixed tissue or cell surface antigen. This leads to a pathological process by predisposing cells to phagocytosis, or to complement-mediated lysis (destruction). **Type III reactions** are best known as **'immune complex diseases'**. Antibodies bind antigens to form large antigen-antibody complexes that precipitate in various blood vessels and activate complement. The immune complexes and complement activation fragments attract neutrophils. Ultimately, it is the activated complement and the release of neutrophilic enzymes and other toxic molecules (oxygen metabolites, i.e., oxygen free radicals) that cause the tissue damage. **Type IV reactions**, also called **'delayed-type hypersensitivity'** are cell-mediated immune responses. Here, antigen-specific T-lymphocytes are the cause of cellular and tissue injury.

Table 19. Mechanisms of hypersensitivity reactions

Type	Immune mechanism	Typical example
I. Anaphylactic type	Allergen (antigen) cross-links antibody ⟶ release of vasoactive amines and other mediators from basophils and mast cells ⟶ recruitment of other inflammatory cells	Anaphylaxis, some forms of bronchial asthma
II. Antibody to fixed tissue antigen	IgG or IgM binds to antigen on cell surface ⟶ phagocytosis of target cell or lysis of target cell by complement or antibody dependent cell-mediated cytotoxicity (ADCC)	Autoimmune haemolytic anaemia, transfusion reactions, haemolytic disease of the newborn (erythroblastosis foetalis in humans)
III. Immune complex disease	Antigen-antibody complexes activate complement ⟶ attract neutrophils ⟶ release of lysosomal enzymes, oxygen free radicals, etc.	Arthus reaction, serum sickness, certain forms of acute glomerulonephritis
IV. Cell-mediated (delayed) hypersensitivity	Sensitized T-lymphocytes ⟶ release of cytokines and T-cell-mediated cytotoxicity	Tuberculin reaction, tuberculosis, contact dermatitis, transplant rejection

We shall now discuss each of these hypersensitivity reactions in some detail.

Type I Hypersensitivity (Anaphylactic Type Hypersensitivity, Immediate Hypersensitivity, Allergy and Anaphylaxis)
This is a rapidly occurring reaction (within minutes). It follows

interaction of allergen (antigen) with IgE antibody previously bound to the surface of **mast cells** and **basophils** in a sensitized host. Depending on the route of entry of allergen, type I hypersensitivity may occur as a **local reaction** or may end in a **fatal systemic disorder (anaphylaxis)**. Because mast cells and basophils are the most important cells in the development of type I hypersensitivity, let us first consider briefly some of their salient characteristics. We shall then discuss the immune mechanisms that underlie this form of hypersensitivity.

Mast cells are bone marrow derived cells. They are widely distributed in the tissues, and are found particularly near blood vessels

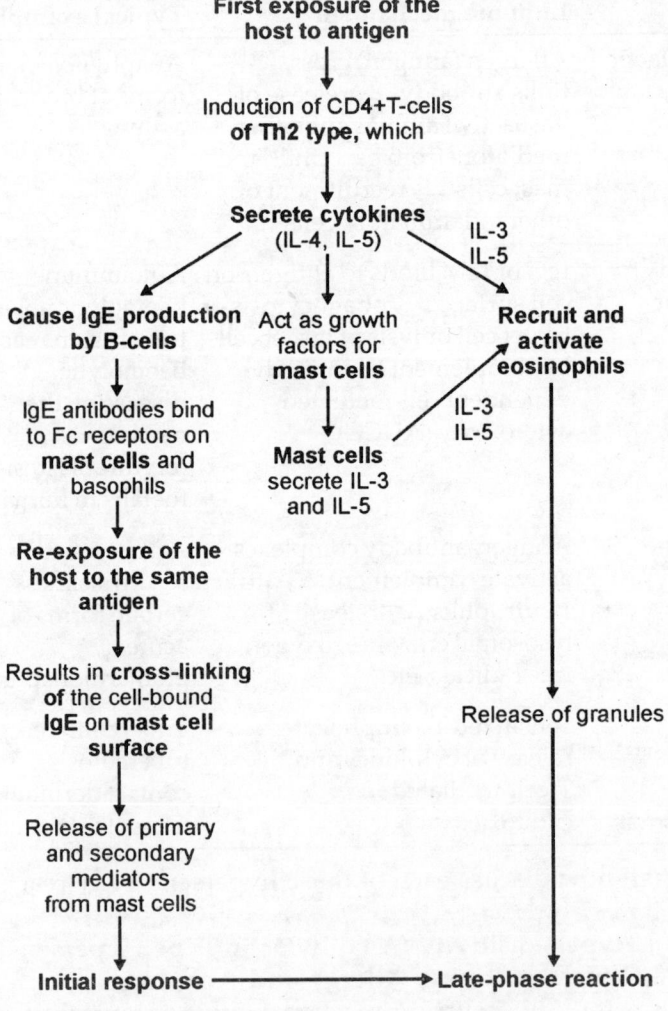

First exposure of the host to antigen

Induction of CD4+T-cells **of Th2 type, which**

Secrete cytokines (IL-4, IL-5)

IL-3
IL-5

Cause IgE production by B-cells

Act as growth factors for **mast cells**

Recruit and activate eosinophils

IgE antibodies bind to Fc receptors on **mast cells** and basophils

IL-3
IL-5

Mast cells secrete IL-3 and IL-5

Re-exposure of the host to the same antigen

Results in **cross-linking of the cell-bound IgE on mast cell surface**

Release of granules

Release of primary and secondary mediators from mast cells

Initial response ⟶ **Late-phase reaction**

Fig. 66. Sequence of events leading to type I hypersensitivity.

and in subepithelial locations. Their cytoplasm contains membrane-bound granules that possess a variety of biologically active mediators. As discussed later, mast cells and basophils are activated following cross-linking of IgE by the antigen (see Fig, 67). IgE is bound to the surface of these cells by high-affinity Fc receptors. Mast cells are also activated by the binding of complement components C5a and C3a (anaphylatoxins) to specific mast cell membrane receptors (Chapter 4). **Basophils** are similar to mast cells, but are not present in tissues. Instead, they circulate in the blood in very small numbers and, like other granulocytes, can be recruited to inflammatory sites.

Pathogenesis: Type I reactions are mediated by IgE antibodies. The sequence of events is as follows (Fig. 66). **First**, there has to be an **exposure** to certain **allergens** (antigens). The allergen stimulates the induction of CD4+ T-cells of the Th2 type. These CD4+ cells play an extremely important role in the pathogenesis of type I hypersensitivity because the cytokines secreted by them (IL-4 and IL-5 in particular)

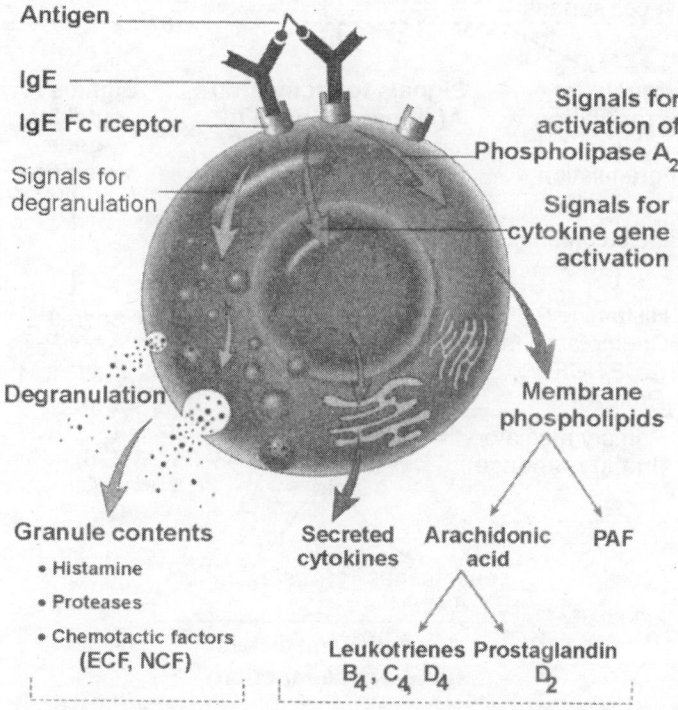

Fig. 67. Activation of mast cells in type I hypersensitivity following cross-linking of IgE by the antigen. This leads to release of their mediators. ECF = eosinophil chemotactic factor; NCF = neutrophil chemotactic factor; PAF = platelet-activating factor

cause IgE production by B-cells, act as growth factor for mast cells, and recruit and activate eosinophils. IgE antibodies bind to high-affinity Fc receptors expressed on mast cells and basophils. Once the mast cells and basophils are **'armed'** in this way, the individual is primed to develop type I hypersensitivity (Fig. 67). **Re-exposure to the same antigen** results in cross-linking of the cell-bound IgE and triggers a sequence of intracellular events that lead to the release of several powerful mediators (Fig. 67, 68). **One set of signals** leads to mast cell degranulation with discharge of **preformed or primary mediators** (Fig. 67, 68). **Another set** causes *de novo* (fresh) synthesis and release of secondary mediators, such as arachidonic acid metabolites and cytokines (Fig. 67, 68).

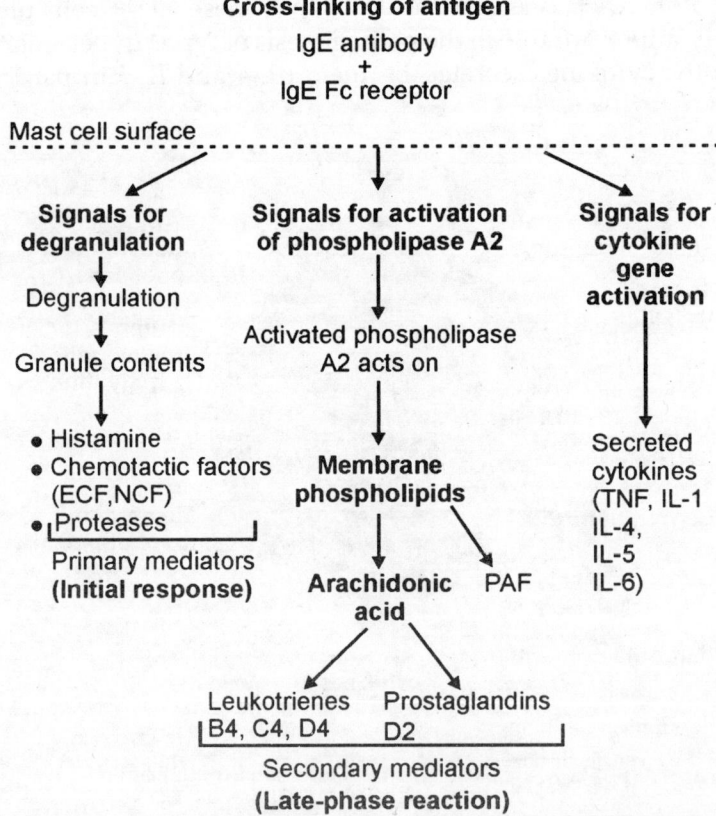

Fig. 68. Same as Fig. 67 presented in a flow chart. Activation of mast cells following cross-linking of IgE by the antigen leads to release of their mediators. ECF = eosinophil chemotactic factor; NCF = neutrophil chemotactic factor; PAF = platelet activating factor

Primary Mediators

These are preformed, that is, they are already present within mast cell granules. After IgE triggering, primary mediators are released. **Histamine**, the most important of these preformed mediators (Fig. 67, 68), causes increased vascular permeability, vasodilation, bronchoconstriction, and increased secretion of mucus. Other rapidly released mediators include **adenosine** (causes bronchoconstriction and inhibits platelet aggregation) and **chemotactic factors for neutrophils and eosinophils. Some mediators are found in the granule matrix** and include heparin and **neutral proteases** (e.g., **tryptase**). Neutral proteases generate kinins and cleave (split) complement components to produce **additional chemotactic and inflammatory factors**, that is, **C3a** and **C5a**, also called **anaphylatoxins** (see Chapter 4).

Secondary Mediators

These include **two classes** of components: (1) **lipid mediators**, and (2) **cytokines**. The lipid mediators are generated by activation of **phospholipase A2**, which cleaves mast cell membrane phospholipids to produce **arachidonic acid**. This is the parent compound from which **leukotrienes** and **prostaglandins** are synthesized (Fig. 67, 68).

(a) **Leukotrienes** result from the action of **5-lipoxygenase on arachidonic acid** (Fig. 68). Leukotrienes are extremely important in the pathogenesis of type I hypersensitivity. **Leukotrienes C4** and **D4** are the most powerful vasoactive and spasmogenic (produce spasms) agents known. **On a molar basis, they are several thousand times more active than histamine in increasing vascular permeability** and causing bronchial smooth muscle contraction. **Leukotriene B4** is highly chemotactic for neutrophils, eosinophils, and monocytes.

(b) **Prostaglandin D$_2$** is the most abundant mediator produced by the **cyclooxygenase pathway** in mast cells (Fig. 67, 68). It causes intense bronchospasm and increased mucus secretion.

(c) **Platelet activating factor (PAF**, see Chapter 4) is another secondary mediator. It causes platelet aggregation, **histamine release**, and bronchospasm. Although its production is initiated by the activation of phospholipase A2, **it is not a product of arachidonic acid metabolism**.

(d) **Cytokines**: Mast cell-derived cytokines (TNF, IL-1, IL-4, IL-

419

5, and IL-6) and chemokines play an important role in type I hypersensitivity reaction (Fig. 68). **They recruit and activate a variety of inflammatory cells. TNF** is an extremely powerful mediator for leukocyte adhesion, emigration, and activation. **IL-4** is also a mast cell growth factor and is required for IgE synthesis by B-cells.

To summarize, a variety of chemotactic, vasoactive, and bronchospasmic compounds mediate type I hypersensitivity reactions. Some, such as histamine, are released rapidly from sensitized mast cells and cause intense immediate reactions, such as in **systemic anaphylaxis** (described next). Many others, such as leukotrienes, PAF and cytokines cause late-phase reactions, including inflammatory cell recruitment. The secondarily recruited inflammatory cells not only release additional mediators, but also cause local epithelial damage.

Eosinophils are recruited by **eotaxin and other chemokines** released from TNF-activated epithelium. These are important effectors of tissue injury (i.e., cells that carry out), in the late-phase response. For example, eosinophils produce **major basic protein** and **eosinophil cationic protein**, which are toxic to epithelial cells. Similarly, **leukotriene C4** and **platelet-activating factor** produced by eosinophils directly activate mast cell mediator release. As a result, the recruited cells increase and sustain the inflammatory response **in the absence of any additional antigen exposure**. Since inflammation is a major component of the late-phase reaction, its control usually requires broad-spectrum anti-inflammatory drugs such as **corticosteroids**

Clinical Manifestations

Type I reaction may occur as a **systemic disorder, or** as a **local reaction**. This depends on the route of antigen exposure. Systemic (parenteral) administration of protein antigens (such as bee venom) or drugs (such as penicillin) results in **systemic anaphylaxis**. Within minutes of an exposure in a sensitized host, pruritus (itchiness), urticaria, and skin erythema appear, followed by profound respiratory difficulty caused by pulmonary bronchoconstriction and aggravated by hypersecretion of mucus. In addition, musculature of the entire gastrointestinal tract may be affected. This may cause vomiting, abdominal cramps, and diarrhoea. **Table 20 compares anaphylaxis in various species.**

Table 20. Anaphylaxis in the domestic species and human

Species	Shock organs	Symptoms	Pathology	Major mediators
Ruminants (cattle, sheep, goat)	Respiratory tract	Cough, dyspnoea, collapse	Lung oedema, emphysema, haemorrhage	Leukotrienes, kinins, histamine
Horse	Respiratory tract, intestine	Cough, dyspnoea, diarrhoea	Emphysema, intestinal haemorrhage	Histamine, 5-hydroxytrptamine, (serotonin), kinins
Pig	Respiratory tract, intestine	Cyanosis, pruritus, (itchiness)	Systemic hypotension	Histamine (uncertain)
Dog	Hepatic veins	Vomiting, diarrhoea, dyspnoea, collapse	Hepatic engorgement, visceral haemorrhage	Histamine, leukotrienes
Cat	Respiratory tract, intestine	Dyspnoea, vomiting, diarrhoea	Lung oedema, intestinal oedema	Histamine, leukotrienes
Chicken	Respiratory tract	Dyspnoea, convulsions	Lung oedema	Histamine, 5-hydroxytryptamine, leukotrienes
Humans	Respiratory tract	Dyspnoea, urticaria	Lung oedema, emphysema	Histamine, leukotrienes

Local reactions occur when antigen is confined to a particular site because of the route of exposure, such as **skin** (contact, causing urticaria), **gastrointestinal tract** (ingestion, causing diarrhoea), or **lung** (inhalation, causing bronchoconstriction). Common forms of skin and food allergies, hay fever, and asthma in humans are examples of localized anaphylactic reactions. **Susceptibility is genetically controlled.** The term **atopy** is used to indicate familial predisposition to such localized reactions. The genetic basis of atopy is not clearly understood. Recent studies suggest an association with cytokine genes that regulate the expression of circulating IgE.

Apart from the damaging role, IgE antibodies play an important protective role in parasitic infections. IgE antibodies are produced in response to many **helminthic infections**. Figure 69 provides a schematic representation of the process by which IgE antibodies inflict damage to schistosome larvae. IgE-sensitized mast cells, however, do not cause direct damage to the parasites. Instead, they attract

421

eosinophils by releasing chemotactic factors. In addition to mast cells, eosinophils, platelets, and some macrophages possess Fc receptors for IgE. IgE-armed leukocytes attach to the surface of parasites and inflict damage by a variety of mechanisms. For example, eosinophils are capable of mediating antibody-dependent cell-mediated cytotoxicity (ADCC) (described under type II reaction), while macrophages release toxic oxygen metabolites and lysosomal enzymes.

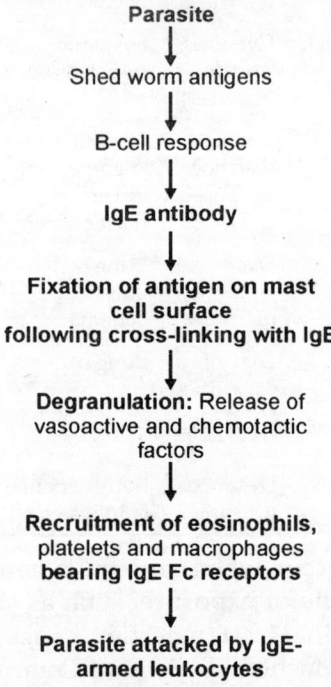

Fig. 69. IgE-mediated destruction of parasites.

Type II Hypersensitivity (Antibody-Dependent)

Type II hypersensitivity is mediated by antibodies. These antibodies are directed against target antigens on the surface of cells or other tissue components. The antigens may be normal molecules intrinsic to (i.e., part of) cell membranes or extracellular matrix, or they may be adsorbed (adhered) exogenous antigens, such as a drug metabolite. In either case, the **hypersensitivity response results from antibody binding followed by one of the following three different antibody-dependent mechanisms** (Fig. 70).

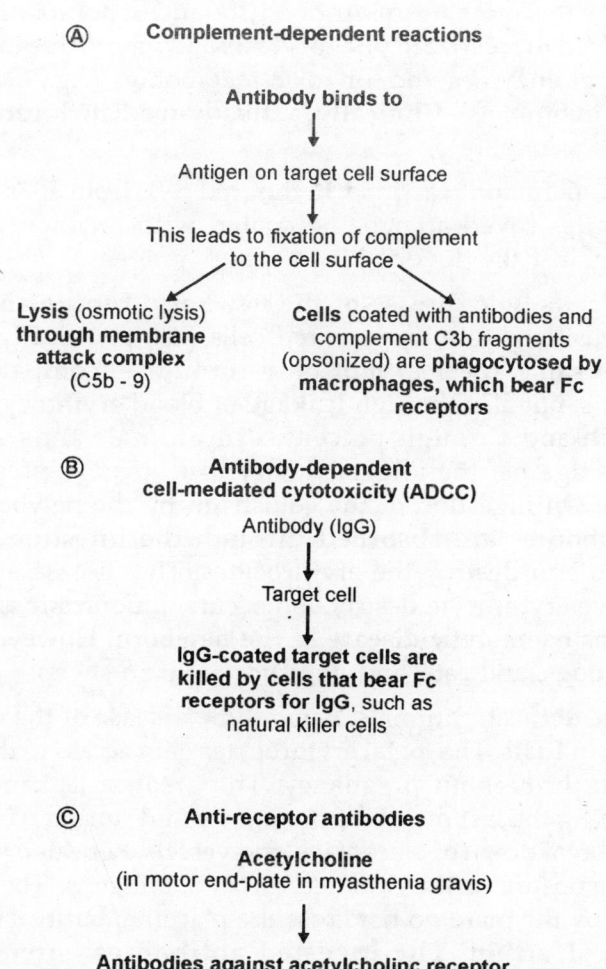

Ⓐ **Complement-dependent reactions**

Antibody binds to
↓
Antigen on target cell surface
↓
This leads to fixation of complement
to the cell surface

Lysis (osmotic lysis) **through membrane attack complex** (C5b - 9)

Cells coated with antibodies and complement C3b fragments (opsonized) are **phagocytosed by macrophages, which bear Fc receptors**

Ⓑ **Antibody-dependent cell-mediated cytotoxicity (ADCC)**

Antibody (IgG)
↓
Target cell
↓
IgG-coated target cells are killed by cells that bear Fc receptors for IgG, such as natural killer cells

Ⓒ **Anti-receptor antibodies**

Acetylcholine
(in motor end-plate in myasthenia gravis)
↓
Antibodies against acetylcholinc receptor

Fig. 70. Three different mechanisms of antibody-mediated injury in type II hypersensitivity.

1. Complement-dependent reactions: Complement can mediate type II hypersensitivity in **two ways**: (i) **direct lysis,** and (ii) **opsonization**. (i) **In direct lysis (complement-mediated cytotoxicity)** antibody bound to a cell surface antigen causes fixation of complement to the cell surface with subsequent lysis through the **membrane attack complex** (Fig. 70A). (ii) **Opsonization**: Cells coated with antibodies and complement C3b fragments (opsonized) become susceptible to **phagocytosis** (Fig. 70B). Mostly circulating blood cells are the ones

423

damaged by this mechanism. Antibody bound to non-phagocytosable tissue can lead to **frustrated phagocytosis** and injury, due to the release of lysosomal enzymes and/or toxic metabolites (e.g., Goodpasture syndrome in humans). **Clinically**, antibody-mediated reactions occur in:

(A) Transfusion reactions: In this, red cells from an incompatible donor are destroyed after being coated with recipient antibodies directed against the donor's blood group antigens.

(B) Haemolytic disease of the newborn: Female animals may become sensitized to allogeneic red cells (i.e., genetically dissimilar but of the same species), not only through incompatible blood transfusions, but also through **leakage** of blood erythrocytes into the maternal blood through placenta. **In animals** thus sensitized, antibodies against the allogeneic erythrocytes are present in the **colostrum**. On ingestion of the colostrum by the newborn animal, these antibodies are absorbed through the intestine, reach the circulation, and destroy the erythrocytes. The disease arising from this massive erythrocyte destruction occurs in **domestic animals** and is known as **haemolytic disease of the newborn.** However, it is rare in **calves, dogs**, and **cats**, and **does not occur in sheep.**

Of the domestic animals, haemolytic disease of the newborn is important in foals. The foetal erythrocytes gain access to the maternal circulation throughout pregnancy. The greatest leakage probably occurs during the last month of pregnancy and during parturition, as a result of breakdown of placental blood vessels. Repeated pregnancies result in exposure to the same erythrocyte antigens. The antibodies produced by the mare do not cross the placenta, but reach the blood through colostrum. **The ingested antibodies enter the foal's circulation and cause erythrocyte destruction.** The earliest signs are weakness and depression. They develop jaundice and haemoglobinuria, and may even die.

In humans, haemolytic disease of the newborn is due to alloimmunization against antigens of the Rhesus (Rh) system. **Rhesus incompatibility** occurs when an Rh-negative mother is sensitized by red cells from Rh-positive foetal red cells. The resulting syndrome is called **erythroblastosis foetalis** or **haemolytic disease of the newborn**, and is characterized by severe red cell destruction giving rise to haemolytic anaemia and jaundice, which if severe, may result in death.

(C) Drug reactions: In this, antibody is directed against a particular drug or its metabolite, which is non-specifically adsorbed (adhered) to a cell surface. Example: haemolysis that can occur after **penicillin** administration.

(D) Hypersensitivity to infectious diseases: We have seen that drugs adsorbed on red cells render them immunologically foreign. Likewise, viruses such as equine infectious anaemia virus, rickettsiae such as anaplasma, and protozoa such as trypanosomes and babesia, also make red cells immunologically foreign. These altered red cells, being taken as foreign, are either lysed by antibody and complement, or phagocytosed by mononuclear phagocytes. Therefore, these diseases are clinically characterized by severe anaemia.

2. Antibody-dependent cell-mediated cytotoxicity/injury (ADCC): This form of antibody-mediated injury involves killing through cells that bear receptors for the Fc portion of IgG (Fig. 70B). Target cells coated by antibody are lysed (destroyed) without phagocytosis or complement fixation. ADCC may be mediated by a variety of leukocytes, including neutrophils, eosinophils, macrophages, and **natural killer (NK) cells**. Although ADCC is mediated by **IgG antibodies**, in certain cases, for example, eosinophil-mediated killing of parasite (discussed under type I; see also Fig. 69), **IgE antibodies** are used.

3. Antibody-mediated cellular dysfunction: In some cases, antibodies directed against cell surface receptors damage or dysregulate function without causing cell injury or inflammation. For example, in **myasthenia gravis** in **humans**, **dogs**, and **cats**, antibodies against acetylcholine receptors in the motor end plates of skeletal muscle damage neuromuscular transmission with resultant muscle weakness (Fig. 70C).

Type III Hypersensitivity (Immune Complex-Mediated)

Type III hypersensitivity is mediated by the deposition of antigen-antibody (immune) complexes. This is followed by complement activation and accumulation of neutrophils. Immune complexes can involve **exogenous antigens** such as bacteria and viruses, or **endogenous antigens** such as DNA. It is important to note that just formation of immune complexes does not mean type III hypersensitivity. Antigen-antibody complexes form during many immune responses and it is a normal mechanism of antigen removal. Pathogenic immune complexes either form in the circulation, or form at extravascular sites when antigen has been deposited (*in situ* immune complexes).

425

Immune complex mediated injury can be **systemic** when complexes are formed in the circulation and are deposited in many organs, **or localized** to particular organs, such as kidneys, joints, or skin, if the complexes are formed and deposited in a separate site. The mechanism of tissue injury in both is the same. However, the sequence of events and the conditions that lead to the formation of immune complexes are different. Let us consider the **two patterns**.

(i) Systemic Immune Complex Disease

The pathogenesis of systemic immune complex disease can be divided into **three phases**, as shown in Figure 71.

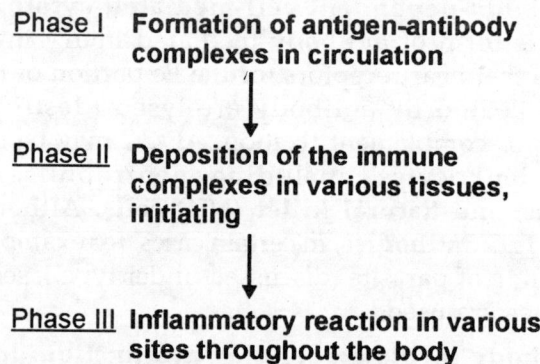

Phase I   **Formation of antigen-antibody complexes in circulation**

Phase II   **Deposition of the immune complexes in various tissues, initiating**

Phase III   **Inflammatory reaction in various sites throughout the body**

Fig. 71. Three sequential phases in the induction of systemic type III (immune complex) hypersensitivity.

Acute serum sickness is the typical example of a systemic immune complex disease. It was described first in humans when large amounts of foreign serum were administered for passive immunization, such as horse anti-tetanus serum. **It is now rare.** About 5 days after a foreign protein is injected, specific antibodies are produced. These react with the antigen still present in the circulation to form antigen-antibody complexes (Fig. 71, phase I). In the **second phase**, antigen-antibody complexes formed in the circulation deposit in various tissue beds (Fig. 71, phase II).

Two factors decide whether immune complex formation leads to tissue deposition and disease.

(i) **Size of the immune complex: Very large complexes** formed during antibody excess are rapidly removed from the circulation by mononuclear phagocytic cells and are therefore relatively **harmless**. The most pathogenic complexes are formed during antigen excess and are **small** or of **intermediate size**. These are cleared less rapidly by phagocytic cells and therefore **circulate longer**. (ii) **Status of the mononuclear phagocytic system**: Macrophages normally remove circulating immune complexes. Therefore, their overload or dysfunction leads to persistence of immune complexes in the circulation and increases the chances of tissue deposition.

In addition, several other factors influence whether and where immune complexes would deposit. The common sites of immune complex deposition are kidney, joints, skin, heart, serosal surfaces, and small blood vessels. For complexes to leave the circulation and deposit within or outside the vessel wall, an increase in vascular permeability must occur. This is mediated when immune complexes bind to inflammatory cells through Fc and C3b receptors and trigger release of vasoactive mediators and/or permeability-increasing cytokines. Once complexes are deposited in the tissue, the **third phase** (Fig. 71, phase III), inflammatory reaction, occurs. It is during this phase, about 10 days after antigen administration that clinical features such as fever, urticaria, arthralgia (pain in the joints), lymph node enlargement, and proteinuria appear.

Mechanism: Regardless of the site of immune complex deposition, tissue damage is similar. **Complement activation by immune complexes is the most important factor in the pathogenesis of injury** (Fig. 72). It releases active fragments such as **anaphylatoxins (C3a** and **C5a)**, which increase vascular permeability and are chemotactic for neutrophils (Chapter 4). Phagocytosis of immune complexes by the accumulated neutrophils results in the release, or generation of a variety of additional pro-inflammatory substances. These include prostaglandins, vasodilator peptides, and chemotactic substances as well as lysosomal enzymes capable of digesting basement membrane, collagen, elastin, and cartilage. Tissue damage is also mediated by oxygen free radicals produced by activated neutrophils. Immune complexes can also cause platelet aggregation and activate Hageman factor. Both of these reactions increase the inflammatory process and initiate microthrombi formation that contribute to tissue injury by producing local ischaemia (Fig. 72). The pathological lesion that occurs is called **vasculitis** if it occurs in blood vessels, **glomerulonephritis** if it occurs in renal glomeruli, **arthritis** if it occurs in the joints, and so on.

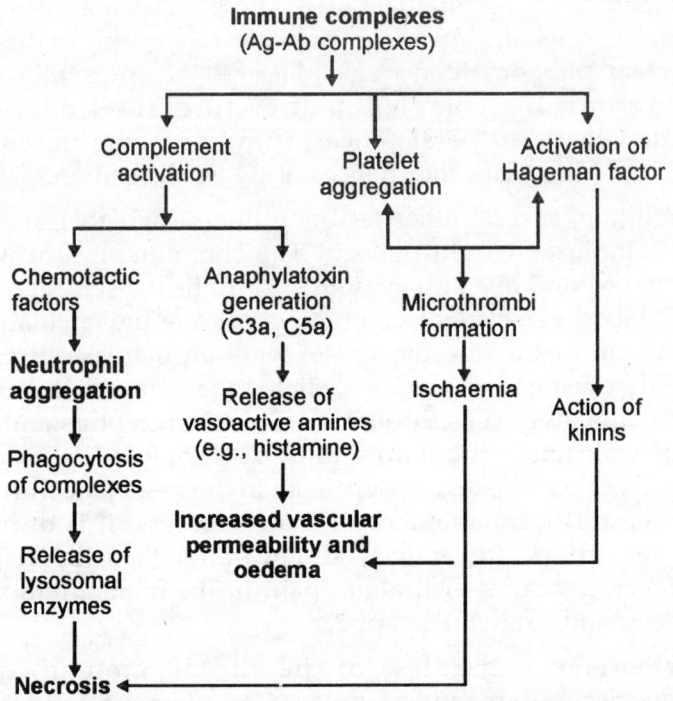

Fig. 72. The sequence of events in the pathogenesis of immune complex-mediated tissue injury. The effects are shown in bold letters.

Morphologically, the immune complex injury is characterized by **acute necrotizing vasculitis**, microthrombi, and iscahemic necrosis accompanied by acute inflammation of the affected organs. The necrotic vessel wall takes on an eosinophilic appearance called **'fibrinoid necrosis'** caused by protein deposition. Immune complexes can be seen in the vascular wall by both electron microscopy and immunofluorescence.

To conclude, only complement-fixing antibodies (IgG and IgM) are involved in type III hypersensitivity, and that complement and neutrophils play an extremely important role in its pathogenesis.

(ii) Local Immune Complex Disease (Arthus reaction)

The Arthus reaction is a localized area of tissue necrosis that results from acute immune complex vasculitis. The reaction is produced experimentally by injecting an antigen into the skin of a previously immunized animal. Antibodies against the antigen are therefore already present in the circulation. Because of the **excess of**

antibodies, immune complexes are formed as antigen diffuses into the vascular wall. These are precipitated at the site of injection, especially within vessel walls, and trigger the same inflammatory reaction and microscopic appearance already discussed for systemic immune complex disease. Arthus lesions take a few hours to appear and reach a peak 4 to 10 hours after injection, when the injection site develops visible oedema with severe haemorrhage occasionally followed by ulceration.

Type IV Hypersensitivity (Cell-Mediated)

Type IV hypersensitivity is mediated by specifically sensitized T-cells rather than antibodies. It is of two basic types: (1) delayed-type hypersensitivity, initiated by CD4+ helper T-cells, and (2) direct cell cytotoxicity, mediated by CD8+ cytotoxic T-cells. In delayed hypersensitivity, Th1 type CD4+ T-cells secrete cytokines. These cytokines recruit other cells, especially macrophages, which are the major effector cells, that is, they induce the changes. In contrast, in cell-mediated cytotoxicity, cytotoxic CD8+ T-cells themselves perform the effector function.

(i) Delayed-Type Hypersensitivity

The classical example of delayed hypersensitivity (DTH) is the **tuberculin reaction,** induced in an animal already sensitized to the tubercle bacillus by a prior injection, or infection. Eight to 12 hours after intradermal injection of tuberculin (a protein-lipopolyssacharide extract of the tubercle bacillus), a local area of erythema and induration (hardening) appears. It reaches a peak (typically 1 to 2 cm diameter) in 24 to 72 hours (hence the adjective, **delayed**), and then slowly subsides. **Microscopically,** the DTH reaction is characterized by perivascular accumulation ('**cuffing**') of **CD+ helper T-cells** and, to a lesser extent, **macrophages**. Local secretion of **cytokines** by these mononuclear inflammatory cells leads to an increase in vascular permeability and escape of plasma proteins. This gives rise to skin oedema and fibrin deposition. **Fibrin deposition is the main cause of tissue induration (hardening) in these responses.**

Pathogenesis

The sequence of events in DTH (typical example - tuberculin reaction) begins with the **first exposure** of animal to tubercle bacilli. **CD4+ lymphocytes** recognize peptide antigens of tubercle bacillus in association with **class II antigens** on the surface of macrophages or dendritic cells that have processed the mycobacterial antigens (Fig. 73A). This process leads to the formation of **sensitized CD4+ cells of**

429

the Th1 type that remain in the circulation for years. Why certain antigens preferentially induce a Th1 type response is not clear. **On subsequent intradermal injection** of tuberculin in such an animal, the **memory cells** (circulating **CD4+ T-cells** formed from the first exposure) respond to processed antigen on antigen-presenting cells and are **activated**, that is, they undergo blast formation and proliferation. This is accompanied by **secretion of Th1 cytokines**. It is these **Th1 cytokines,** that are ultimately responsible for the development of the DTH response (73A). Of the various cytokines, the most important in the process include:

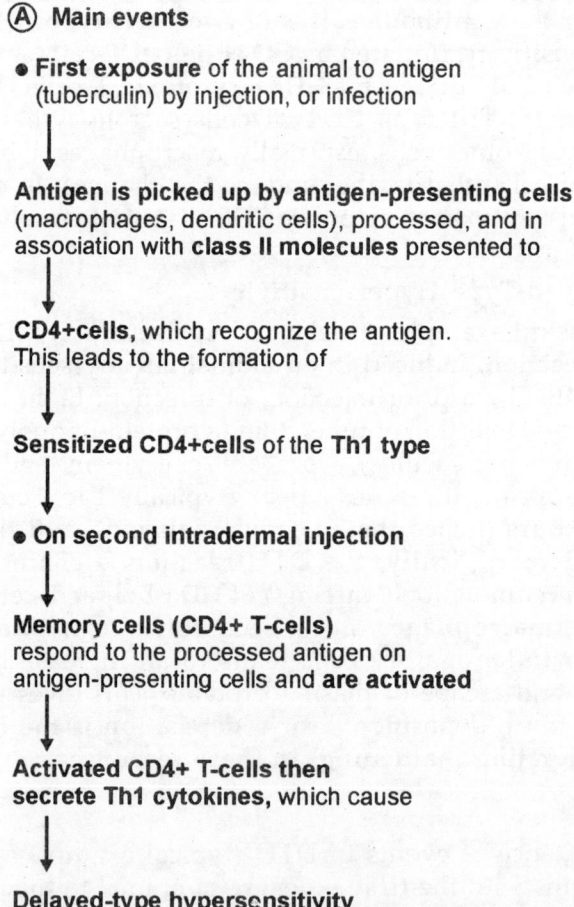

Ⓐ **Main events**

● **First exposure** of the animal to antigen
(tuberculin) by injection, or infection

↓

Antigen is picked up by antigen-presenting cells
(macrophages, dendritic cells), processed, and in
association with **class II molecules** presented to

↓

CD4+cells, which recognize the antigen.
This leads to the formation of

↓

Sensitized CD4+cells of the **Th1 type**

↓

● **On second intradermal injection**

↓

Memory cells (CD4+ T-cells)
respond to the processed antigen on
antigen-presenting cells and **are activated**

↓

Activated CD4+ T-cells then
secrete Th1 cytokines, which cause

↓

Delayed-type hypersensitivity

Fig. 73. Sequence of events in the pathogenesis of delayed-type hypersensitivity.
A. Main events. **B.** Role of various cytokines (see next page).

Ⓑ **Role of various cytokines**

Th1 T-cells
(CD4+Th1)

↓

Interferon-gamma (IFN-gamma)

↓

**Activates macrophages
Activated macrophages then produce**

↓

Interleukin 12

Induces T-cells
to secrete
IFN-gamma

Causes differentiation
of **Th1 cells**

Induces NK cells
to secrete
IFN-gamma

↓

**Th1 cells then
produce**

IFN-gamma

IL-2

**TNF and lymphotoxin
(TNF-beta) act on
endothelial cells and
cause :**

**Activated
macrophages**

**Causes
proliferation
of T-cells**

• Increased secretion of
nitric oxide and
prostacyclin

• More
expression
of class II
molecules

Secretion of several
growth factors
[PDGF, TGF-alpha]

• Increased expression of
E-selectin

• **Increased
phagocytic
and
microbicidal
activity**

Stimulate fibroblast
proliferation, **increase
collagen synthesis**

• Secretion of
chemotactic factors

Together these changes
cause **emigration of
lymphocytes and
monocytes**
at the site of DTH

• Increased
IL-2
production

1. Interleukin-12 (IL-12) (Fig. 73B): This cytokine is produced by **macrophages** after first interaction with the tubercle bacillus. It is a very important cytokine in the development of DTH, because it is the main cytokine that causes differentiation of **Th1 cells**. In turn, **Th1 cells produce other cytokines mentioned below**. IL-12 is also a powerful inducer of interferon-gamma secretion by T-cells and NK cells.

2. Interferon-gamma (IFN-gamma) (Fig. 73B): This cytokine has a variety of effects, and **is the most important mediator of DTH**. It is a powerful activator of macrophages and increases their IL-12 production. **Activated macrophages** express more class II molecules on the surface and this leads to their increased antigen presentation capacity. They also have increased phagocytic and microbial activity, and their capacity to kill tumour cells is increased. **Activated macrophages** secrete several **polypeptide growth factors**, including platelet-derived growth factor (PDGF) and TGF-alpha. These stimulate fibroblast proliferation and increase collagen synthesis. In brief, IFN-gamma activation increases the ability of macrophages to eliminate offending agents. If macrophage activation is sustained, fibrosis occurs.

3. Interleukin-2 (IL-2) (Fig. 73B): This cytokine causes proliferation of T-cells that have accumulated at sites of DTH. In the accumulation, there are about 10% antigen-specific CD4+ cells. However, majority of the cells are bystander T-cells, that is, they are present but are not specific for the original inciting agent.

4. Tumour-necrosis factor (TNF) and lymphotoxin (TNF-beta) (Fig. 73B): These cytokines produce important effects **on endothelial cells.** (1) They cause **increased secretion of nitric oxide** and **prostacyclin** and thus induce increased blood flow through local vasodilation and (2) They cause increased expression of **E-selectin**, an adhesion molecule promoting mononuclear cell attachment (Chapter 4), and (3) They induce and **make endothelial cells secrete chemotactic factors**, such as IL-8. **Together these changes facilitate emigration of lymphocytes and monocytes at the site of DTH responses.**

Granulomatous Inflammation

Granulomatous inflammation is a special form of delayed-type hypersensitivity. It is characterized by the formation of a **granuloma** (a granular nodule), which occurs in response to persistent and/or non-degradable antigens. The early perivascular **CD4+ T-cell infiltrate** is replaced by macrophages within 2 to 3 weeks. These accumulated macrophages show features of activation, that is, they become large, flat, and eosinophilic and resemble epithelial cells. Such cells are known as **'epithelioid cells'**. The epithelial cells sometimes fuse under the influence of certain **cytokines** (mainly **interferon-gamma**) to form multi-nucleated **giant cells** (Fig. 74). A microscopic aggregate of epithelial cells, characteristically surrounded by a collar (circular band) of lymphocytes is called a **'granuloma'**. This pattern of inflammation is known as **granulomatous inflammation**. The process is basically the same as described for other DTH responses. Older granulomas develop an enclosing rim of fibroblasts and connective tissue. Recognition of a granuloma is of diagnostic importance because of the limited number of conditions that cause it.

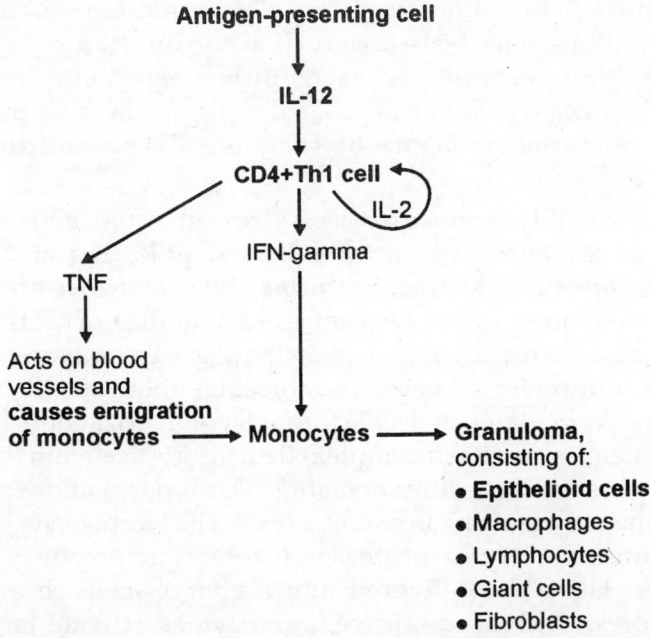

Fig. 74. Sequence of events in the formation of granulomas in type IV hypersensitivity reactions. Note the role of **CD4+ Th1** cell-derived cytokines. IL-12 = interleukin 12; TNF = tumour necrosis factor; IFN = interferon-gamma

DTH is a major mechanism of defence against a variety of intracellular pathogens, including mycobacteria, fungi, and certain parasites, and it may also be involved in transplant rejection and tumour immunity. The central role of **CD4+ T-cells** in delayed hypersensitivity is seen in human patients with acquired immunodeficiency syndrome (AIDS). Because of the loss of CD4+ T-cells, the patient's response against intracellular pathogens such as *Mycobacterium tuberculosis* is markedly damaged. The bacteria are engulfed by macrophages, **but are no killed**, and instead of granuloma formation, there is accumulation of **unactivated macrophages** poorly equipped to deal with the invading microbe.

433

2. T-Cell-Mediated Cytotoxicity

In this form of type IV hypersensitivity, **sensitized CD8+ T-cells** kill antigen-bearing target cells. As discussed earlier, **class I MHC molecules** bind to intracellular viral peptides (antigen) and present them to CD8+ T-lymphocytes (see Fig. 65). The CD8+ effector cells, called **cytotoxic T-lymphocytes** (CTLs) play a critical role in resistance to viral infections. **The lysis (destruction) of infected cells, before viral replication is completed, leads ultimately to elimination of the infection.** Many tumour-associated antigens are also presented on tumour cell surfaces (Chapter 8). Therefore, CTLs are also involved in tumour immunity.

Cytotoxic T-lymphocytes kill virus-infected cells by **two mechanisms: (1) perforin-granzyme-dependent killing,** and **(2) Fas-Fas ligand-dependent killing. Perforins** and **granzymes** are soluble mediators contained in the lysosome-like granules of CTLs. As its name indicates, **perforin** makes holes in the plasma membrane of target cells. First, a number of perforin molecules (between 12 and 18) combine and form a large molecule through polymerization. This large molecule (**membrane attack complex**) then inserts itself into the target cell and makes a pore (a tiny opening). These pores allow water to enter into the cell, resulting in **osmotic lysis**. The lymphocyte granules also contain a variety of proteases (proteolytic enzymes) called **granzymes**. These are delivered into the target cells through the perforin pores. Once inside the cell, **granzymes activate target cell apoptosis** (Chapter 3). Activated cytotoxic T-lymphocytes also express **Fas ligand** (a molecule similar to TNF), which **binds to Fas on target cells** (see Fig. 11). This interaction leads to **apoptosis** (see 'apoptosis'). In addition to viral and tumour immunity, CTLs directed against cell surface histocompatibility antigens also play an important role in **graft rejection**, discussed next.

Transplant Rejection

Rejection of transplanted organs (organ transplant), such as kidney, **is a complex immunological phenomenon**. It involves both cell-mediated and antibody-mediated hypersensitivity responses of the **host**. Both the responses are directed against **histocompatibility molecules (antigens)** on the donor graft (see Fig. 75). The identification and destruction of **foreign molecules** are central to the defence of the body. Transplanted organs are the major source of these foreign molecules.

T-Cell-Mediated Rejection

Classical acute rejection in a non-immunosuppressed host occurs within 10 to 14 days. It is **mainly the result of cell-mediated immunity,** involving both delayed-type hypersensitivity (DTH) and cytotoxic T-lymphocyte (CTL) mechanisms. **Since the only major antigenic difference between host and donor tissue is their histocompatibility molecules, rejection occurs as a response to MHC.** The host recognition and response to the donor MHC occurs by **two mechanisms.**

1. Indirect recognition: In this case, **host CD4+ T-cells** recognize **donor MHC antigens after they are processed** and presented by the **host's own APCs.** This involves taking in and processing by the host APC of MHC antigens shed from donor cells. This is similar to the physiological processing and presentation of other foreign (e.g., microbial) antigens. This form of recognition mainly activates DTH pathways.

2. Direct recognition: In this case, T-cells of the host recognize **directly** graft MHC molecules on the surface of an antigen-presenting cell **of the donor** (i.e. without any processing). But such a direct recognition is against the rules of MHC restriction (see 'histocompatibility molecules'). However, this is possible because **dendritic cells** (APCs) present in the donor organs do not only express high levels of both MHC I and MHC II molecules, **but also express co-stimulatory molecules B7-1 (CD80), and B7-2 (CD86)** (Fig. 75). **Dendritic cells are therefore the most important APCs in direct recognition.** Macrophages and endothelial cells are also potentially involved. The T-cells of the host come in contact with dendritic cells either within the grafted organ, or after these cells migrate to the draining lymph nodes.

Both CD4+ and CD8+ T-cells of the host are involved in this reaction. Host CD4+ helper T-cells are triggered into proliferation and cytokine production by recognition of **donor MHC II molecules,** and induce DTH response. At the same time, precursors of **CD8+ cytotoxic T-lymphocytes (CTLs)** recognize **MHC I molecules** and differentiate into mature CTLs. This process of differentiation is complex and incompletely understood. CD8+ cytotoxic T-cells can recognize MHC I molecules on any cell type, but naïve CD8+ T-cells also require the **co-stimulation** provided by 'professional' APCs (dendritic cells). Then, with the help of cytokine from CD4+ T-cells, CD8+ T-cells differentiate into **cytotoxic T-lymphocytes** (Fig. 75).

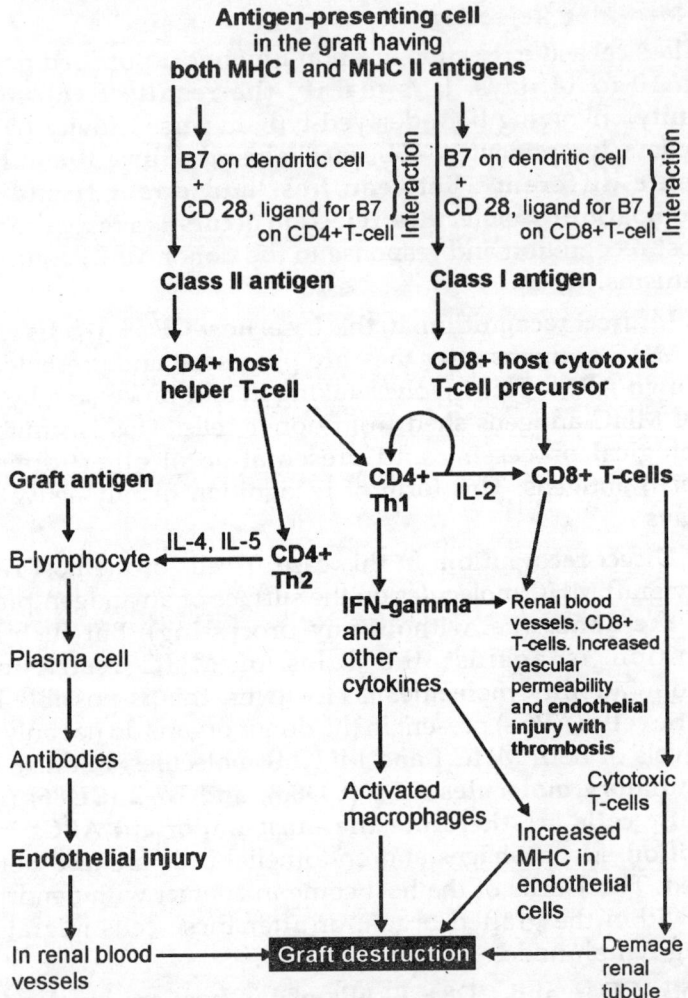

Fig. 75. Events that lead to the destruction of histo-incompatible grafts. Donor class I and class II antigens (i.e., present in the graft) along with B7 molecules (CD80, CD86) are recognized by CD8+ cytotoxic T-cells and CD4+ helper T-cells, respectively, **of the host**. The interaction of the CD4+ T-cells with antigens presented by class II antigens leads to proliferation of Th1-type CD4+ cells and the release of interleukin-2 (IL-2) from these cells. IL-2 further increases the proliferation of CD4+ cells and also provides helper signals for the differentiation of class I-specific CD8+ cytotoxic T-cells. In addition, activation of Th2-type CD4+ T-cells generates a variety of other soluble mediators (cytokines) that promote B-cell differentiation. The Th1 cells also participate in the induction of a local delayed-type hypersensitivity reaction. **Ultimately, several mechanisms join to destroy the graft**: (1) lysis of cells that bear class I antigens by CD8+ cytotoxic T-cells, (2) anti-graft antibodies produced by sensitized B-cells, and (3) non-specific damage caused by macrophages and other cells that accumulate as a result of the delayed hypersensitivity reaction.

Once the donor graft has been recognized as **foreign**, rejection proceeds through the effector mechanisms already discussed (Fig. 75). Mature CTLs lyse target cells in the grafted tissue, causing parenchymal and endothelial cell death, **resulting in thrombosis and graft ischaemia**. Cytokine-secreting CD4+ T-cells cause increased vascular permeability and local accumulation of mononuclear cells (lymphocytes and macrophages). The DTH response, accompanied by its microvascular injury, also results in tissue ischaemia, which along with the destruction mediated by accumulated macrophages, is an important mechanism in graft destruction.

Antibody-Mediated Rejection

Although T-cells are of greatest importance in the rejection of grafted organ, **antibodies also play a role. Anti-graft antibodies** produced by sensitized B- cells also contribute toward destruction of the graft, through type III and II hypersensitivity reactions. **The major target of antibody-mediated damage is the vascular endothelium (Fig. 75).** The bound antibody causes injury and secondary thrombosis through complement, immune complex, or ADCC-mediated pathways. Superimposed on the immunological vascular damage are platelet aggregation and coagulation (caused by complement activation), adding further ischaemic insult to injury. **Microscopically,** this form of rejection resembles the vasculitis described earlier for type III hypersensitivity.

To conclude, eventually, several mechanisms act together to destroy the graft: **(1)** lysis (destruction) of cells that bear class I antigens by CD8+ cytotoxic T-cells, **(2)** anti-graft antibodies produced by sensitized B-cells, and **(3)** non-specific damage inflicted by macrophages and other cells that accumulate as a result of the delayed hypersensitivity reaction (Fig. 75). Based on the mechanisms involved, rejection reactions have been classified as **hyperacute, acute,** and **chronic. Hyperacute rejection** occurs within minutes to a few hours after transplantation in a pre-sensitized host; **acute rejection** within days to weeks; and **chronic rejection** within months to years. **Immunosuppression** of the recipient is therefore a practical necessity in all organ transplantation, except in the case of identical twins.

Autoimmune Diseases

An immune reaction against **'self-antigens'**, that is, **autoimmunity** is the cause of certain human and animal diseases. A growing number of diseases have been placed under this category.

However, it must be noted that the simple presence of autoreactive antibodies or T-cells does not mean that it is an autoreactive disease. For example, non-pathological antibodies to self-antigens can be easily demonstrated in most healthy individuals. Moreover, similar harmless antibodies to self-antigens are frequently produced following other forms of injury (e.g., ischaemia), presumably serving a physiological role in the removal of tissue breakdown products. **The diagnosis of an autoimmune disease should therefore be based on**: (1) the evidence that specific immune responses are directed against one particular organ or cell type, and (2) that the specific immune responses result in localized tissue damage characterized by lesions in many organs and associated with a large number of autoantibodies or cell-associated reactions. The pathological changes occur mainly in the **connective tissue** and **blood vessels** of the various organs involved. Thus, although the reactions in these systemic diseases are not specifically directed against the constituents of connective tissue or blood vessels, they are usually referred to as **'collagen vascular disorders'** or **'connective tissue disorders'**.

Since autoimmunity means **loss of self tolerance**, the question arises as to how does this happen? To understand this, let us first consider the **mechanisms of normal immunological tolerance.**

Immunological Tolerance

Immunological tolerance is a state in which an individual is incapable of developing an immune response against a specific antigen. Self-tolerance specifically means a lack of immune responsiveness to one's own tissue antigens. Naturally, such self-tolerance is necessary if our tissues are to live in harmony with an army of lymphocytes that are constantly going around in search of antigens to be attacked.

Two major groups of mechanisms have been put forward to explain the tolerant state: **(1) central tolerance**, and **(2) peripheral tolerance** (see Fig.76, 77).

1. Central tolerance: This means deletion (removal) of self-reactive T-and B-lymphocytes during their maturation in central lymphoid organs (thymus for T-cells; bone marrow for B-cells in mammals and bursa of Fabricius in birds). Many self-protein antigens (autologous protein antigens) are processed and presented by the thymic antigen-presenting cells (APCs) in association with self-MHC. **Any developing T-cell that expresses a receptor for such self-antigen**

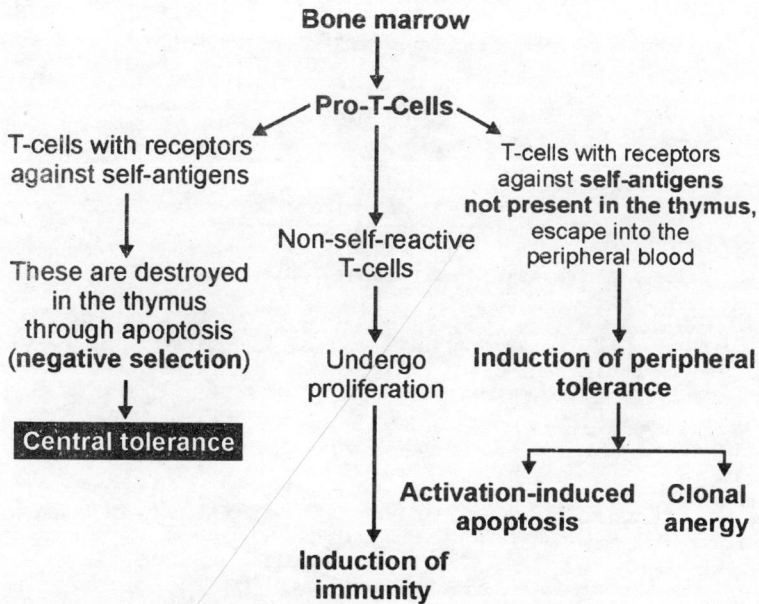

Fig. 76. Two major groups of mechanisms involved in central and peripheral tolerance of T-cells. Similar pathways occur for B-cells (see text). APC = antigen-presenting cell; MHC = major histocompatability complex.

is negatively selected (apoptosis), and the resulting peripheral T-cell pool thereby depleted of self-reactive cells (Fig. 76, 77). As with T-cells, deletion of **self-reactive B-cells** also occurs. When developing B-cells encounter a membrane-bound antigen during their development in the bone marrow (bursa of Fabricius in birds), they undergo **apoptosis**.

Explained simply, the **T-cells** and **B-cells** released into the circulation must be able to participate in immune responses, **yet they must not respond to normal body constituents**. This is achieved by both **positive and negative selection** of cells. Thus, thymus selectively destroys those T-cells, and bone marrow (bursa of Fabricius in birds) those B-cells that respond to self-antigens, while stimulate proliferation of those that respond to foreign antigens. The elimination of self-reactive T- or B-cells occurs through **apoptosis**. The killing of T-or B-cells that have the potential to react to self-antigen is called **'negative selection' or 'clonal deletion'**. It has been observed that up to 99% self-reactive B-cells are destroyed through apoptosis in the bursa of Fabricius. The increased proliferation of cells that respond to foreign antigen is called **positive selection**.

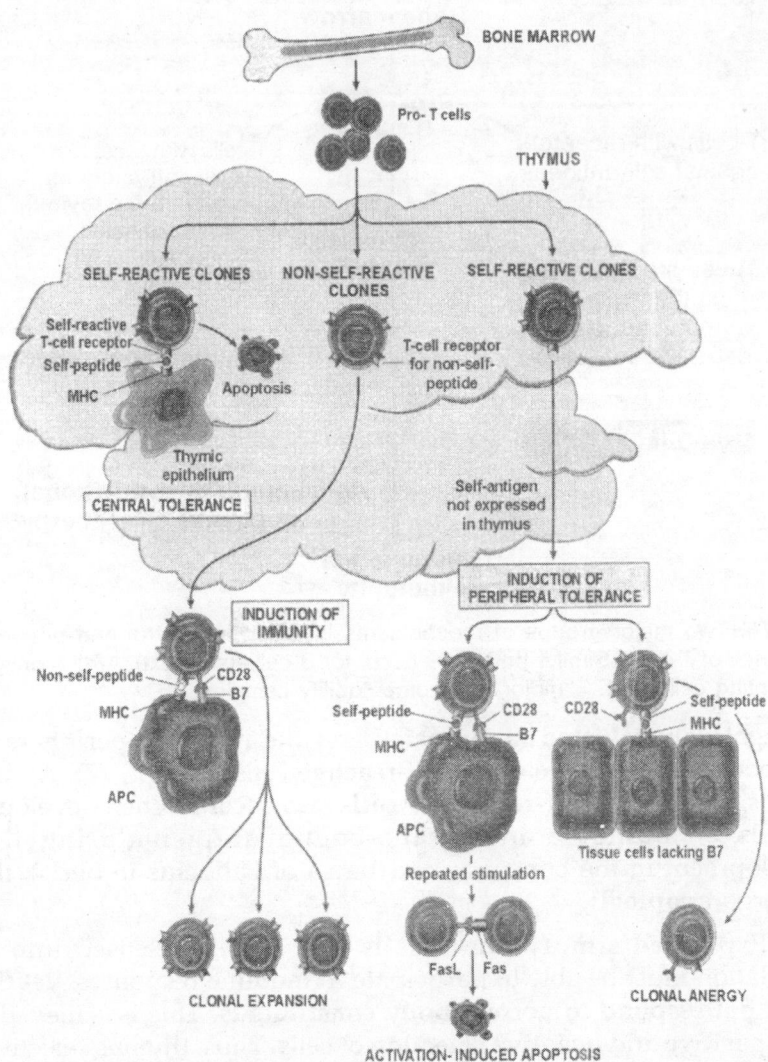

Fig. 77. Same as Fig.76, presented as a schematic illustration of the mechanisms involved in central and peripheral tolerance of T-cells. Similar pathways occur for B cells (see text). APC = antigen-presenting cell; MHC = major histocompatibility complex.

Unfortunately, the process of deletion of self-reactive lymphocytes is not perfect. For example, many self-antigens are not present in the thymus and therefore T-cells having receptors for such autoantigens escape into the periphery (i.e., circulation). There is

440

similar **'slippage'** (escape) in the B-cell system as well. For example, B-cells that have receptors for a variety of self-antigens, including collagen, DNA, and thyroglobulin, are easily found in the peripheral blood of healthy individuals.

2. Peripheral tolerance: Self-reactive T-cells that escape negative selection (destruction through apoptosis) in the thymus can potentially cause great damage, unless they are deleted or effectively kept under control. Several **backup mechanisms** in the **peripheral tissues,** that silence (keep under control) such potentially autoreactive T-cells, have been identified.

(i) Anergy: This is prolonged or irreversible **inactivation** of lymphocytes (**not apoptosis**). In other words, **lymphocytes become unreactive** (Fig. 76, 77). It occurs when lymphocytes come in contact with the antigens under certain conditions. Remember that activation of T-cells requires **two signals** (see 'lymphocytes'). **First** is recognition by T-cells of antigen in association with self-MHC molecules on APCs. **Second** is a set of co-stimulatory signals (via B7 molecules) provided by the APCs. **If the second co-stimulatory signals are not delivered, the T-cell becomes anergic (unreactive)** (Fig. 76, 77). **Such a T-cell will be unresponsive even if the relevant antigen is presented again by competent APCs that can deliver co-stimulation. Since co-stimulatory molecules are not strongly expressed on most normal tissues**, the contact between autoreactive T-cells and their specific self-antigens usually results in anergy. **B-cells** can also become anergic, if they encounter antigen in the absence of specific helper T-cells.

(ii) Activation-induced cell death: Another mechanism to prevent uncontrolled T-cell activation during a normal immune response is **apoptosis** of activated T-cells by the **Fas-Fas ligand system** (see 'apoptosis'). **Fas ligand is a membrane protein** that is structurally similar to the cytokine tumour necrosis factor (TNF) and is expressed mainly on activated T-lymphocytes. Its role in CTL-mediated killing has already been discussed (see 'T-cell-mediated cytotoxicity'). **Lymphocytes also express Fas, and Fas expression is markedly increased on activated T-cells**. As a result, binding of Fas by Fas ligand co-expressed (expressed together) on activated T-cells, suppresses the immune response by inducing apoptosis of these cells (Fig. 76, 77). Such activation-induced cell death can also cause peripheral deletion of autoreactive T-cells. Thus, abundant self-antigens may cause repeated and persistent stimulation of autoreactive T-cells in the periphery, leading eventually to their removal through Fas-mediated apoptosis (Fig. 76, 77).

(iii) Peripheral suppression by T-cells: Although anergy and activation-induced cell death are the most important mechanisms of peripheral self-tolerance, additional foolproof mechanisms (i.e., which cannot go wrong) exist. Recently it has been revealed that this is because of the **regulatory (suppressor) T-cells**, which regulate the function of other T-cells. It is now known that certain cytokines secreted by these cells, such as IL-10 and transforming growth factor-beta TGF-beta), can check or reduce a variety of T-cell responses. Regulatory T-cells also modulate T-cell activity by pathways involving direct cell-cell contact.

Mechanisms of Autoimmune Disease

Breakdown of one or more mechanisms of self-tolerance can result in an immunological attack on tissues and development of autoimmune diseases. Immunocompetent cells are involved in mediating the tissue injury. It is now clear that no single mechanism works for all autoimmune diseases and that self-tolerance can be bypassed (avoided) in a number of ways. More than one defect may be present in each disease, and the defects differ from one disorder to the other. Moreover, the breakdown of tolerance and initiation of autoimmunity involves interaction of complex immunological, genetic, and microbial factors. Here, the immunological mechanisms (mainly failure of peripheral tolerance) are discussed, followed by a brief consideration of the role of genetic and microbial factors.

Mechanisms Involved in the Breakdown of Self-Tolerance

1. Failure of activation-induced cell death: As discussed, persistent activation of T-cells may lead to their apoptosis through the Fas-Fas ligand system. This means that defects in this pathway may allow **persistence and proliferation of autoreactive T-cells in peripheral tissues**. It has been found that mice with **genetic defects in Fas or Fas ligand** develop chronic autoimmune diseases.

2. Breakdown of T-cell anergy: Remember that those autoreactice cells that escape central deletion (negative selection) become anergic (non-functional) when they come in contact with self-antigens **in the absence of co-stimulation. This means that such anergy may be broken if normal cells that do not usually express co-stimulatory molecules can be induced to do so**. Such induction may occur after **infections,** or where there is **tissue necrosis and local inflammation**. Up-regulation (increased expression) of the co-stimulatory molecule B7-1 has been observed in various tissues in several human autoimmune diseases, such as multiple sclerosis, rheumatoid arthritis, and psoriasis

3. Bypass of B-cell requirement for T-cell help: Many self-antigens have a large number of **antigenic determinants (epitopes)**. Some are recognized by B-cells, others by T-cells. **Antibody response** to such antigens occurs only when self-reactive B-cells receive help from T-cells (Fig. 78). Tolerance to such antigens may be associated with **deletion or anergy (unreactivity) of helper T-cells** in the presence of fully competent specific B-cells. Therefore, this form of tolerance can be broken if the requirement of tolerant (anergic, unreactive) helper T-cells is bypassed (avoided) or substituted. One way to achieve this is if the T-cell antigenic determinant of a self-antigen (autoantigen) is modified. This would allow recognition of the modified self-antigens (autoantigens) by helper T-cells that were not deleted (Fig, 78). Such helper T-cells could then cooperate with the B-cells, leading to the formation of **autoantibodies**. Such modification of the T-cell determinants of an autoantigen may result from complexing (binding) with **drugs** or **microorganisms**. For example, **autoimmune haemolytic anaemia**, which occurs after the administration of certain drugs, may result from drug-induced alteration in the red cell surface that create antigens that can be recognized by helper T-cells (Fig. 78).

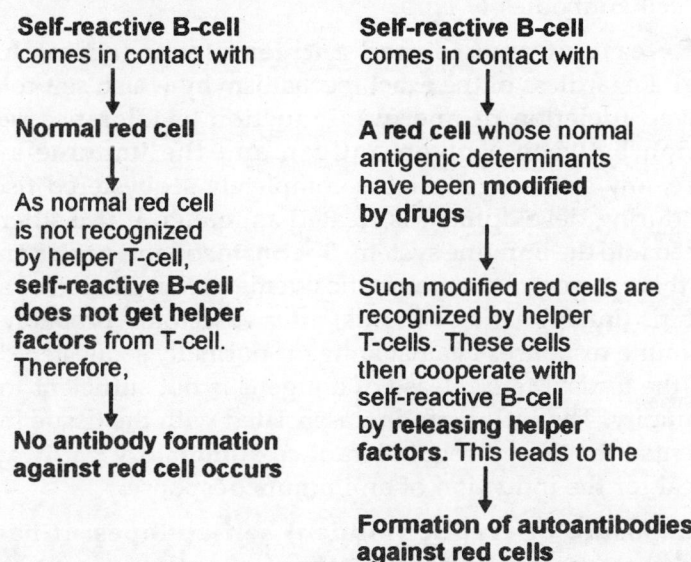

Self-reactive B-cell
comes in contact with
↓
Normal red cell
↓
As normal red cell is not recognized by helper T-cell, **self-reactive B-cell does not get helper factors** from T-cell. Therefore,
↓
No antibody formation against red cell occurs

Self-reactive B-cell
comes in contact with
↓
A red cell whose normal antigenic determinants have been **modified by drugs**
↓
Such modified red cells are recognized by helper T-cells. These cells then cooperate with self-reactive B-cell by **releasing helper factors**. This leads to the
↓
Formation of autoantibodies against red cells

Fig. 78. Flow chart showing how drug-induced modification of a red cell membrane protein may be recognized by helper T-cells and lead to formation of anti-erythrocyte autoantibodies.

4. Failure of T-cell-mediated suppression: Reduced regulatory (suppressor) T-cell function may result in autoimmunity. Recent studies have demonstrated a special type of antigen-specific CD4+ T-cell that secretes **IL-10**. This CD4+ cells can suppress antigen-specific proliferation of other T-cells, and may prevent autoimmune diseases. However, this is at present under investigation.

5. Molecular mimicry (resemblance): Some infectious agents share antigenic determinants (epitopes) with self-antigens. Therefore, an immune response against such microbes will produce similar responses to the cross-reacting self-antigens. For example, rheumatic heart disease in humans sometimes follows streptococcal infection because antibodies to streptococcal M protein cross-react with cardiac glycoproteins.

6. Polyclonal lymphocyte activation: As discussed earlier, tolerance in some cases is maintained by anergy of autoreactive T-cells. Autoimmunity may occur if such self-reactive but anergic (unreactive) clones are stimulated by antigen-independent mechanisms. Several microorganisms and their products are capable of causing **polyclonal** (i.e., antigen-nonspecific) activation of B-cells. The best example is bacterial lipopolysaccharide (endotoxin), which induces mouse lymphocytes to form anti-DNA, anti-thrombocyte, and anti-red cell antibodies *in vitro*.

7. Release of sequestered antigens (exposure of hidden antigens): Regardless of the exact mechanism by which self-tolerance is achieved (deletion or anergy), induction of tolerance requires interaction between a given antigen and the immune system. Therefore, any self-antigen that is completely sequestered (isolated, hidden) during development is treated as foreign if it is afterwards introduced into the immune system. **Spermatozoa** and **ocular antigens** fall into this category. Post-traumatic uveitis (inflammation of a uvea) and orchitis (inflammation of testis) after vasectomy probably result from immune responses against antigens normally sequestered in the eye and the testis. Mere release of antigens is not sufficient to cause autoimmunity. The **inflammation** associated with the tissue injury is also essential for the up-regulation of **co-stimulatory pathways** that are critical for the induction of an immune response.

8. Exposure of cryptic (hidden) self-epitopes: It has been observed that '**molecular sequestration**' of antigens is much more common, than is anatomic sequestration discussed under item 7. From the many present, each self-protein has only a few antigenic determinants (epitopes) that are effectively processed and presented to T-cells. During development most T-cells capable of reacting to such dominant epitopes are either deleted in the thymus, or made anergic in the periphery. By contrast, a large number of self-determinants are not processed and therefore are not recognized by the immune system. **Thus, T-cells specific for such 'cryptic self-epitopes' are not deleted. Therefore, such T-cells could cause autoimmune diseases, if the cryptic epitopes are somehow afterward presented to them in an immunogenic form.** The molecular basis of epitope crypticity and the unmasking of such epitopes is not fully understood.

Genetic Factors in Autoimmunity

Genetic factors play a significant role in the predisposition to autoimmune diseases. However, the precise role of MHC genes in autoimmunity is not entirely clear.

Infection and Autoimmunity

A variety of microbes, including bacteria, mycoplasmas, and viruses have been shown to be involved in the triggering of autoimmunity. Microbes may trigger autoimmune reactions in several ways.

1. Viruses and other microbes, particularly certain bacteria like streptococci, **may share cross-reacting epitopes with self-antigens.**

2. Microbial antigens and autoantigens may become associated to form immunogenic units **and bypass T-cell tolerance**, as described earlier.

3. Some viruses and bacterial products are non-specific polyclonal B-cell or T-cell mitogens and thus may induce formation of autoantibodies and/or break T-cell anergy.

4. Microbial infections with resulting tissue necrosis and inflammation can cause up-regulation (increased expression) of co-stimulatory molecules on resting APCs in tissue. This favours a breakdown of T-cell anergy.

5. Local inflammatory response may facilitate presentation of cryptic antigens.

Against this background, we shall now consider very briefly some of the **more important single organ and systemic autoimmune diseases of domestic animals,** as per Table 21.

Table 21. Autoimmune diseases of domestic animals

Single organ	Systemic
Autoimmune endocrine disease	Systemic lupus erythematosus
Autoimmune neurological disease	Discoid lupus erythematosus
Autoimmune ocular disease	Sjögren's syndrome
Autoimmune reproductive disease	Autoimmune polyarthritis
Autoimmune skin disease	Erosive polyarthritis
Autoimmune nephritis	Rheumatoid arthritis
Autoimmune haemolytic anaemia	Non-erosive polyarthritis
Autoimmune thrombocytopaenia	Dermatomyositis
Autoimmune muscle disease	Immune vasculitis

Autoimmune Endocrine Disease

Although domestic animals suffer from autoimmune endocrine diseases, they differ from humans in that these tend to present as single organ disorders, rather than involving many endocrine glands. **Dogs, humans,** and **chickens** suffer from a naturally occurring **autoimmune thyroiditis. In dogs**, it is associated with the presence of **autoantibodies against thyroglobulin and a thyroid colloid antigen.**

Microscopically, affected thyroids are infiltrated with plasma cells and lymphocytes to such an extent that germinal centre formation may occur. The infiltrating cells probably cause epithelial cell destruction through antibody-dependent cell-mediated cytotoxicity (ADCC) and T-cell cytotoxicity. The other autoimmune endocrine diseases include **hyperthyroidism in cat,** and **insulin-dependent diabetes mellitus and autoimmune adrenalitis in dogs.**

Autoimmune Neurological Disease

Because brain antigens are normally sequestered (isolated) behind the blood-brain barrier, it is easy to produce autoimmune brain disease in animals in the laboratory, known as **experimental allergic encephalomyelitis (EAE).** An **encephalitis,** similar in many ways to EAE, used to occur after administration of rabies vaccines containing phenolized brain tissue to humans. Signs of this **post-vaccinal encephalitis** appeared between 4 and 15 days after vaccination. For this reason, the use of adult brain tissue was stopped, and suckling mouse brain tissue is used in the production of rabies vaccines. Post-distemper demyelinating leukoencephalopathy is also thought of as autoimmune in origin. Naturally occurring autoimmune neurological diseases in domestic animals include **equine polyneuritis of horses**, and **canine polyneuritis, steroid-responsive meningitis** and **degenerative myelopathy of dogs.**

Autoimmune Ocular Disease

An eye disease of horses, known as **equine recurrent uveitis** or **periodic ophthalmia**, which can cause complete blindness, is believed to be of an autoimmune origin. Affected horses possess circulating antibodies against *Leptospira interrogans*. By gel diffusion and ELISA, it is possible to show partial antigenic identity between equine cornea and *L. interrogans*. It is likely therefore that disease may be due to an autoimmune attack on ocular tissues as a result of molecular mimicry (cross-reactivity) with *L. interrogans*.

Autoimmune Reproductive Disease

Tolerance to self-antigens develops during foetal life. At the onset of puberty new antigens appear in the developing testes, antigens to which the immune system is not tolerant. **These antigens are recognized by the adult immune system as foreign.** If the testes are damaged and these antigens are released into the body, **an autoimmune response** may occur that results in the development of an **orchitis. Autoantibodies to sperm** may also be detected in the serum of some animals following injury to the testes. A typical example of this occurs in **male dogs** infected with *Brucella canis*. These animals suffer from a chronic epididymitis and become sensitized by sperm antigens carried to the circulation after phagocytosis by macrophages. These sperm antigens stimulate the production of IgG or IgA autoantibodies. The autoantibodies agglutinate and immobilize sperm, and as a result, affected animals may be **infertile. In cows,** antibodies to sperm have been reported to arise as a result of absorption through the vagina, uterus, Fallopian tube, or peritoneum. If these antibodies reach high levels, they may cause **infertility.**

Autoimmune Skin Disease

This disease complex usually involves **blister** or **vesicle formation** in the skin. The terms **pemphigus** or **pemphigoid** are used to describe them, after the Greek word **pemphix** meaning **'a blister'.**

447

The **pemphigus complex group of diseases**, all result from the formation of **autoantibodies** against intercellular cement in the skin. The complex consists of **four rare skin diseases** that have been described in **humans, dogs, horses**, and **cats**: (i) **pemphigus vulgaris**, (ii) **pemphigus vegetans**, (iii) **pemphigus foliaceous**, and (iv) **pemphigus erythematosus**. The most severe of this is **pemphigus vulgaris** and is characterized by the development of bullae (vesicles or blisters) around the mucocutaneous junctions, especially of the nose, lips, eyes, prepuce, and anus. The bullae rupture easily, leaving weeping, denuded areas that may become secondarily infected. **Microscopically**, bullae show a separation of the skin cells (**acantholysis**) in the lower epidermis. The formation of bullae results from an autoantibody attack on the protein in the desmosomes called desmoglein-3 (i.e., intercellular cement), which is responsible for squamous cell adhesion. The combination of antibody with **desmoglein-3** triggers keratinocytes to secrete proteases such as **plasminogen activator**. As a result, the **adhesion proteins are digested and the keratinocytes separate from each other**. Eventually, this loss of cellular adherence leads to acantholysis and to bullae formation. **Pemphigus vegetans** is a very rare and mild variant of pemphigus vulgaris. **Pemphigus foliaceous** is a milder and commoner disease than pemphigus vulgaris. It has been described in **humans, dogs, cats, goats**, and **horses**. It is also a vesicular disease, but the bullae are rarely confined to mucocutaneous junctions. The lesions in **pemphigus erythematosus** are usually confined to the face and ears.

Autoimmune Nephritis

There are **two immunopathogenic types of glomerulonephritis.** In the immune-complex type (type III hypersensitivity), immune complexes containing complement are deposited in a **lumpy, granular fashion** on glomerular basement membranes (GBMs). In contrast, if autoantibodies are produced against GBM antigens, they are deposited in a **smooth, linear fashion**. These anti-GBM antibodies may be produced experimentally in animals, but they may also arise spontaneously in a condition known as **Goodpasture's syndrome** in humans. In this syndrome, the autoantibodies react not only with the GBM but also with the basement membrane of pulmonary alveolar septa and capillaries. No condition similar to Goodpasture syndrome has been observed in domestic animals. However, **horses** may develop antibodies to GBMs, which may provoke a glomerulonephritis. Clinically, the condition is characterized by signs of renal failure.

Autoimmune Haemolytic Anaemia

Autoantibodies to antigens on red blood cells cause their destrúction and thus induce autoimmune haemolytic anaemia (AIHA). Such haemolytic anaemias are well recognized in **humans** and **dogs**, and have been recorded in **cattle, horses, cats,** and **rabbits.** The affected dogs show pallor (paleness), weakness, and lethargy accompanied by fever, jaundice, and hepatomegaly. The destruction of red cells is due either to **intravascular haemolysis through complement,** or more commonly, to **removal of antibody-coated red cells by macrophages** in the spleen and liver. **In the dog,** the disease is more common in females by a 2:1 ratio. The average age of onset is around 4 to 5 years. **AIHA in dogs are divided into five classes** depending on the class of antibody involved, the optimal temperature for antibodies to react, and nature of the haemolytic process.

Class I AIHA: This is caused by autoantibodies that agglutinate red cells **at body temperature.** In these cases, the antibodies cause direct agglutination, which may be seen when blood is withdrawn and a drop is placed on a glass slide. Both IgG and IgM antibodies are involved. **Since IgG does not activate complement effectively,** intravascular haemolysis is not a feature of this form of AIHA. **The red cells,** however, **are destroyed by phagocytosis in the spleen.** In severe cases, a blood smear may show extensive erythrophagocytosis by neutrophils and monocytes.

Class II AIHA: This is usually **mediated by IgM antibodies** acting **at body temperature. Because IgM activates complement, affected red cells are destroyed by intravascular haemolysis.** This results in haemoglobinaemia, haemoglobinuria, jaundice, and development of a very severe anaemia. **Affected dogs** become anaemic, weak, and possibly jaundiced, and haemoglobin may appear in the urine. Red cells with complement on the surface are removed by the Kupffer cells in the liver and in lymph nodes. As a result, most of these animals have hepatomegaly and lymphadenopathy.

Class III AIHA: Most cases of AIHA in **dogs** and **cats** are mediated by IgG antibodies, which although can react with red cells at 37° C, cannot activate complement or agglutinate the red cells. IgG antibodies can form bridges between cells only 15 to 25 mm apart. As a result, they are unable to counteract the zeta potential of the red cells, and therefore do not cause direct agglutination. IgM antibodies, in contrast, can bridge cells 30 to 50 mm apart and so can agglutinate cells despite their zeta potential. The immunoglobulins on these red

449

cells, however, opsonize them, and they are phagocytosed by mononuclear phagocytes mainly in the spleen. Splenomegaly is a consistent feature of this form of disease.

Class IV AIHA: Some IgM anti-red cell antibodies cannot agglutinate red cells at body temperature but agglutinate them when the blood is chilled. These antibodies are called **cold agglutinins.** As blood circulates through the extremities (e.g., tail, toes, ears) of animals, it may be cooled sufficiently to permit erythrocyte agglutination within capillaries. This can lead to vascular stasis, tissue ischaemia, and eventually, necrosis. This form of AIHA is more severe during winter.

Class V AIHA: The fifth class of AIHA is usually mediated by **IgM antibodies.** These may combine with red cells when chilled to 4° C, but will not agglutinate them. These antibodies can only be identified by **antiglobulin test conducted in the cold.** They do not produce necrosis of extremities but can activate complement, leading to intravascular haemolysis.

Diagnosis: IgG-mediated AIHA is diagnosed by demonstrating the presence of **non-agglutinating** or **incomplete antibodies** on the animal's red cells (class II, III, and IV). This is done by means of a **direct antiglobulin test** or **Coomb's test**. The erythrocytes of the affected animal are collected in the anticoagulant, washed to remove free serum, and then incubated in an antiglobulin serum. The best antiglobulin is one with activity against IgM, IgG, and complement. Erythrocytes coated with autoantibody or complement, will be cross-linked and agglutinated by the antiglobulin serum.

AIHA due to **direct-acting agglutinins** (class I) or to haemolysis (class II) is usually of acute onset, is rapidly progressive, and has a poor prognosis.

Autoimmune Thrombocytopaenia

Autoimmune thrombocytopaenia (AITP), due to the development of antiplatelet autoantibodies, has been reported in **horses, dogs,** and **cats.** Affected animals show many petechiae in the skin, gingiva, other mucous membranes and conjunctiva. **Epistaxis** (nose bleeding) may occur and the **dog** may show melena (blood in faeces) and haematuria. Blood examination shows a severe thrombocytopaenia. The main cause of death in these dogs is severe gastrointestinal haemorrhage. Antibodies against platelet surface antigens lead to a shortened life span as a result of extravascular destruction of opsonized platelets in the spleen. These antibodies may also interfere with normal platelet function. The condition is usually observed as a primary disease along with AIHA and systemic lupus erythematosus. A secondary thrombocytopaenia is observed in animals with multiple myeloma or other lymphoid tumours, or following certain drug treatments. It may be due to the non-specific binding of IgG to platelets.

Autoimmune Muscle Disease

Myasthenia gravis (MG) in **humans, dogs**, and **cats** is **a disease of skeletal muscle** characterized by abnormal fatigue and weakness after even mild exercise. A dog with MG will collapse after trotting for only a few yards. MG results from a **failure of transmission of nerve impulses** across the motor end plate of striated muscle due to **a deficiency of acetylcholine receptors**.

In young dogs, a congenital form of the disease occurs from an inherited deficiency in the acetylcholine receptors. **In adult dogs**, on the other hand, an acetylcholine receptor deficiency results from the production of autoantibodies to the receptor proteins. These antibodies cause increased degradation of the receptors as well as functional blockage of the acetylcholine-binding sites. They also trigger complement-mediated damage to the receptors. As a result, the number of available effective acetylcholine receptors in each neuromuscular junction is greatly reduced.

Systemic Autoimmune Diseases

Animals also suffer from several autoimmune diseases **in which many organ systems are involved**. This group of diseases includes systemic lupus erythematosus (SLE), rheumatoid arthritis, non-erosive polyarthritis, various vasculitis, dermatomyositis, and Sjögren's syndrome. **All of these diseases have some form of autoimmune component**. Unlike the conditions affecting single organ, they are not simply diseases in which a hypersensitivity reaction leads to tissue destruction. Most are associated with the presence of circulating immune complexes or the presence of chronic deposition of immune complexes and complement in tissues. This **immune complex deposition** leads to the gradual development of chronic inflammatory lesions. The initiating antigens are unknown, but may be infectious agents.

Systemic Lupus Erythematosus

Systemic lupus erythematosus (SLE) is a generalized

451

immunological disorder that has been described in **humans, horses, dogs,** and **cats**.

Pathogenesis: SLE results from a **loss of contact over the B-cell response**. This leads to polyclonal gammopathy and the production of **autoantibodies. Gammopathy** is an abnormal increase in gamma globulin levels. As a result of this loss of control, affected animals make autoantibodies against a great range of normal organs or tissues. These autoantibodies, in turn, initiate a wide spectrum of pathological lesions and clinical manifestations.

One characteristic feature of SLE is the development of autoantibodies against antigens in the cell nucleus (anti-nuclear antibodies, ANAs). About 16 different nuclear antigens have been described in humans. **Dogs** differ from humans in that they develop autoantibodies against a restricted group of nuclear antigens, mostly **histones**. These ANAs can cause damage by several mechanisms. They can combine with free antigen to form immune complexes. These immune complexes may be deposited in the glomeruli causing a **membranous glomerulonephritis**. The complexes may also be deposited in arteriolar walls, where they cause local fibrinoid necrosis and fibrosis, or in synovia, where they provoke arthritis. ANAs also bind to the nuclei of degenerating cells. In tissues, this produces round or oval bodies of DNA bound to antibody known as **haematoxylin bodies**. They are found in the skin, kidney, lung, lymph nodes, spleen, and heart. Within the bone marrow these opsonized nuclei may be phagocytosed, giving rise to **lupus erythematosus (LE) cells**. LE cells are found mainly in bone marrow and less commonly in blood.

Although ANAs are characteristic of SLE, many other autoantibodies are also produced, such as autoantibodies against red cells that cause haemolytic anaemia, and antibodies against platelets that cause thrombocytopaenia. Anti-lymphocytic antibodies interfere with immune regulation, anti-muscle antibodies cause myositis, anti-myocardial antibodies cause myocarditis or endocarditis, and antibodies against skin components cause dermatitis.

In horses (equine lupus) the disease occurs mainly as a generalized skin disease. Affected horses show alopecia (loss of hair), dermal ulceration, and crust formation. The affected horses may become almost totally hairless. **In dogs (canine lupus)** the disease affects middle-aged dogs and is characterized by the occurrence of non-erosive, polyarthritis. **In cats (feline lupus)** SLE is rarely diagnosed. It usually occurs as an antiglobulin-positive anaemia

Diagnosis depends on either a positive test for antinuclear antibodies (ANA) or a positive test for LE cells. ANAs are demonstrated by immunofluorescence. LE cells are neutrophils that have phagocytosed nuclei from dead and dying cells. They therefore look somewhat like binucleated cells. Their presence is detected in the bone marrow. However, LE cells are not a reliable diagnostic feature of SLE in domestic animals, since there is a high incidence of both false-positive and false-negative results.

Discoid Lupus Erythematosus

This is a mild, uncommon variant of SLE characterized by the occurrence of facial skin lesions. It occurs in **dogs, cats, horses**, and **humans**.

Sjögren's Syndrome

In this syndrome, which occurs in both **humans** and **dogs**, autoimmune attack on salivary and lachrymal glands leads to the conjunctival dryness (**kerato-conjunctivitis sicca**) and mouth dryness (**xerostomia**). Affected animals later develop gingivitis, dental caries, and excessive thirst.

Autoimmne Polyarthritis

Animals suffer from a variety of immunologically mediated joint diseases. Most are associated with the **deposition of immunoglobulins, or immune complexes within joint tissues.** They are divided into **two distinct groups** on the basis of the presence or absence of **joint erosion**.

I. Erosive Polyarthritis

Rheumatoid Arthritis

This is the commonest immune-mediated erosive polyarthritis. Rheumatoid arthritis (RA) is a common, crippling disease in **humans**, and is also seen in domestic animals, especially in **dogs**. Besides joints, other body systems are also affected. Affected dogs may have depression, anorexia, pyrexia, and lameness. RA causes severe joint erosion and deformities. In advanced cases, the joints may even fuse as a result of the formation of the bony ankyloses (unions of separate bones).

Pathogenesis: Rheumatoid arthritis commences as a synovitis with extensive infiltration of lymphocytes in the synovia and neutrophils in the joint fluid. As the disease progresses, synovia swell and proliferate. The outgrowths eventually extend into the joint cavities, where they are known as **pannus**. Pannus consists of fibrous vascular tissue. When it invades the joint cavity, it releases **proteases** that érode (eat away) the articular cartilage, and ultimately the neighbouring bony structures.

A variety of different stimuli especially infectious agents, initiate the disease. **In domestic animals**, mycoplasmas such as *Mycoplasma hyorhinis* and bacteria such as *Erysipelothrix rhusiopathiae* produce a chronic non-suppurative arthritis that resembles rheumatoid arthritis in humans. **Dogs** with rheumatoid arthritis have significantly higher than normal levels of antibodies against canine distemper in their synovial fluids. These antibodies are not present in dogs with osteoarthritis. This suggests that in dogs canine distemper virus may be present in rheumatoid joints and that it may play a role in the pathogenesis of the disease.

Although RA is considered as an autoimmune disease, the identity of the autoantigens involved is unclear. **Two autoantigens** involved may be **IgG** and **collagen**. The development of **autoantibodies against IgG** is characteristic of RA. These autoantibodies are called **'rheumatoid factors, RFs'**. They can belong to any immunoglobulin class including IgE, but IgG RFs are the most common. In **dogs**, although RFs are usually associated with rheumatoid arthritis, they are also found in the serum and synovial fluid of some dogs with osteoarthritis or infective arthritis.

Autoantibodies against collagen may also contribute to the development of RA. **Type II collagen** is the main form of collagen in articular cartilage and so may serve as an autoantigen. Antibodies against type II collagen can be detected in the serum and synovial fluid of dogs with rheumatoid arthritis, infective arthritis, and osteoarthritis. Whatever the inciting factors, the first stage in the development of RA involves **activation of T-cells within the synovial membrane**. Local cytokine production by   macrophages results in the formation of new blood vessels. Circulating lymphocytes from these vessels emigrate into the tissues. These infiltrating lymphocytes are mainly **activated CD4+ T-cells**. In addition, there is some B-cell emigration into the tissues and this leads to local RF production. These RFs form large immune complexes and activate the complement system.

As inflammation develops within synovia, large quantities of **cytokines** are produced. These cytokines are mainly secreted by macrophages and include **IL-1, IL-6, GM-CSF,** and **TNF-alpha.** There are much lower levels of the T-cell-derived cytokines, namely, interferon-gamma (IFN-gamma) and IL-2. The presence of **C5a, leukotriene B4,** and **platelet-activating factor** (PAF) causes accumulation of large numbers of neutrophils within the synovial fluid. **Activation by phagocytosis of immune complexes and tissue debris leads to protease escape and the release of free radicals.** This, together with activation of **kinins** and **plasmin,** leads to **intense inflammation.** The released neutrophil proteases degrade the articular cartilage and ligaments.

The progressive development of inflammation within the joint leads to stiffness. The animal may show signs of depression and fatigue from the systemic effects of IL-1 and TNF-alpha. If the joints develop effusions, they become swollen. As the disease progresses, the extremely inflamed synovia invades the cartilage, ligaments, and bone and results in the **destruction of articular cartilage.** Synovial lining cells, small blood vessels, and fibroblasts proliferate. Large numbers of macrophages are found in the pannus.

II. Non-Erosive Polyarthritis

In this group of immune-mediated polyarthritis, **the joint cartilage is not eroded** and the inflammatory lesion is largely confined to the joint capsule and synovia. Many of these resemble rheumatoid arthritis clinically but may be differentiated by their non-erosive character.

Equine polyarthritis has been reported in the **horse.** Affected **foals** (up to 3 months of age) have many swollen joints involving all four limbs and a persistent fever. **Canine arthritis** has been reported in the **dogs. Feline polyarthritis** occurs as a chronic progressive arthritis of **male cats.** Affected cats are usually infected with feline syncytia-forming virus or feline leukaemia virus, or both.

Dermatomyositis: It is a familial disease of **dogs,** that resembles dermatomyositis (inflammation of the skin and muscles) in humans. It is mainly a clinical syndrome of dermatitis and less of myositis. The onset and progression of the disease correlate with a rise in circulating immune complexes and serum IgG, but the reason for these increases is unclear. Circulating immune complexes and IgG levels return to normal as the disease resolves, suggesting a causative association.

Immune vasculitis: Several forms of immune vasculitis have been described in domestic animals. Their exact relationships are unclear,

455

and as a result they have been given several different names. These include **canine juvenile polyarteritis** in **dogs**, **polyarteritis nodosa** in **humans, pigs, dogs**, and **cats**, and leukocytoclastic vasculitis.

Immunodeficiency Diseases

These are disorders of the immune system that result in an immunological deficiency. Immunodeficiency diseases may be caused by **inherited defects** affecting immune system development (**primary immunodeficiencies**) or they may result from secondary effects of other diseases (**secondary immunodeficiencies**), such as infection, malnutrition, aging, immunosuppression, autoimmunity, or chemotherapy. Clinically, animals with immunodeficiency show **increased susceptibility to infections or parasitic agents** as well as to certain forms of cancer. Animals with defect in immunoglobulin, complement, or **phagocytic cells** typically suffer from recurrent infections with pyogenic bacteria. On the other hand, those with defects in cell-mediated immunity are prone to infections caused by viruses, fungi, and intracellular bacteria.

PRIMARY IMMUNODEFICIENCIES

The **primary immunodeficiency diseases** are genetically determined and affect either specific immunity (humoral or cellular), or non-specific host defence mechanisms mediated by **complement proteins** and cells such as **phagocytes** or **natural killer (NK) cells**.

1. Inherited defects in phagocytosis: There are two important congenital deficiency syndromes associated with **phagocytic failure**. **In one**, there is a **failure of opsonization**. This has not been recorded in the domestic animals, with the exception of **canine C3 deficiency in dogs**. Such dogs show increased susceptibility to infections. **In the other**, there is a **failure of intracellular killing**.

Chédiak-Higashi syndrome is an inherited disease of cattle, cats, rats, and humans. It is associated with an **increased susceptibility to infection**. This syndrome results from a defect that produces **abnormally large granules in neutrophils**, monocytes, and eosinophils. The enlarged neutrophil granules result from the fusion of primary and secondary granules. In other words, **they are abnormal lysosomes.** The leukocyte granules of affected animals are more fragile than, those of normal animals. They rupture spontaneously and cause tissue damage, such as cataracts. These leukocytes have defective chemotactic responsiveness, reduced motility, and reduced intracellular killing as a result of defective granule fusion and a deficiency of elastase. The syndrome also influences the development of natural killer (NK) cells. As a result, affected animals may show an increased susceptibility to tumours and some viruses. NK cells are present but have a reduced ability to kill their targets. Platelet function may also be abnormal.

Pelger-Hüet anomaly (P-H anomaly) is also an inherited condition characterized by a **failure of neutrophil nuclei to segment into lobes**. As a result, nuclei remain rounded. Thus, the neutrophils appear on the first sight to be very immature (a left shift). This anomaly has been observed in **humans, dogs, cats,** and **rabbits**.

Canine leukocyte adherence deficiency (LAD): For neutrophils to leave inflamed blood vessels, they must adhere to the endothelial cells. Adherence is mediated through **integrins** (adhesion proteins) on the neutrophil surface that bind ligands on vascular endothelial cells. In other words, integrins are required to bind neutrophils to blood vessel walls. This permits neutrophils to emigrate to sites of bacterial invasion. **In the absence of integrins**, neutrophils cannot adhere firmly to the vessel walls and neutrophil emigration fails to occur. As a result, invading bacteria can grow freely without fear of attack by neutrophils. **Affected dogs suffer from recurrent infections** and at the same time have large numbers of neutrophils in their bloodstream.

Bovine leukocyte adherence deficiency: An inherited integrin deficiency has been observed in **calves**. Clinically, it is characterized by **recurrent bacterial infections**, delayed wound healing, and a persistent extreme neutrophilia. **Affected calves** usually die between 2 and 7 months of age. Such calves have large numbers of intravascular neutrophils, but very few extravascular neutrophils even in the presence of invading bacteria. **In the absence of integrin**, neutrophils fail to attach firmly to endothelial cells and cannot emigrate from blood vessels.

2. Inherited defects in the immune system: If both cell-mediated and antibody-mediated immune responses are defective, the genetic lesion lies at a point before thymic and bursal cell processing, that is, **a stem-cell lesion**. A defect that occurs only in thymic development will result in an inability to mount a cell-mediated immune response, although antibody production may be normal. Similarly, a lesion restricted to the B-cell system will result in an absence of antibody-mediated immune responses.

Immunodeficiencies of Horses

The most important is the **'severe combined immunodeficiency syndrome (SCID)'** that occurs in **foals**. Affected foals fail to produce functional T- or B-cells and have very few circulating lymphocytes. As a result, **these foals cannot produce antibodies** and eventually become **agammaglobulinaemic**. Affected foals are born healthy but fall sick within two months. All die by 4 to 6 months from severe infection by a variety of low-grade pathogens.

On necropsy, the spleen lacks germinal centres and periarteriolar lymphoid sheaths. The lymph nodes lack lymphoid follicles and germinal centres. The thymus is so hypoplastic that it may be difficult to find on necropsy. The **diagnosis** requires that at least two of these criteria be met (1) an absence of circulating lymphocytes, (2) gross hypoplasia of the primary and secondary lymphoid organs, and (3) an absence of IgM from pre-suckle serum. As a result, a normal newborn foal will always have some IgM in its serum, but a SCID foal will have none.

Agammaglobulinaemia: Primary agammaglobulinaemia is a rare disease of **foals**. Affected animals have no B-cells and very low levels of all immunoglobulins. Their lymphoid tissues contain no primary follicles, germinal centres, or plasma cells. Affected foals suffer from recurrent pyogenic bacterial infections but can survive for 17 to 18 months. The condition should be suspected in a foal having a normal lymphocyte count but lacking both IgM and IgG. In addition to these two conditions, **foals** also suffer from **selective IgM deficiency**, **selective IgG deficiency**, and **transient hypogammaglobulinaemia**.

Immunodeficiencies of Cattle

A **'severe combined immunodeficiency'** has been described in a **calf**. Other immunodeficiencies include **selective IgG2 deficiency** and **hereditary parakeratosis (Trait A-46)**. Trait A-46 is characterized by thymic and lymphocytic hypoplasia. **Affected calves** are born healthy, but by 4 to 8 weeks suffer from severe skin infections, and die a few weeks later. None survives for longer than 4 months. There is atrophy of the thymus, spleen, and lymph nodes, and depletion of lymphocytes in the gut-associated lymphoid tissue (GALT). These animals are deficient in T-cells and have depressed cell-mediated immunity but normal antibody responses. If these calves are treated by oral **zinc oxide** or **zinc sulphate**, they recover the ability to mount normal cell-mediated responses. Zinc is an essential component of the thymic hormone **thymulin** and is therefore required for a normal T-cell response.

Immunodeficiencies of Dogs

An **X-linked severe combined immunodeficiency (SCID)** has been described in **dogs**. The disease is characterized by **increased susceptibility to infections** and a lack of palpable lymph nodes. Affected dogs have low lymphocyte counts, the major drop being in CD8+ T-cell numbers. The dogs have normal level of B-cells. The puppies are hypogammaglobulinaemic with normal levels of IgM, but lack in IgG and IgA. The dogs do not mount antibody responses against antigens.

On necropsy, the thymus is about 10% of the normal weight. The lymph nodes are very small and may be very difficult to find. The spleens contain large periarteriolar lymphoid nodules with occasional small lymphocytes and few plasma cells. About 42% of the thymocytes of these dogs are CD4-CD8 - compared with 16% of the thymocytes of normal dogs.

The **other immunodeficiencies of dogs** include **selective IgM deficiency, selective IgA deficiency, transient hypogammaglobulinaemia, T-cell deficiency,** and **acrodermatitis.**

Immunodeficiencies of Chickens

In certain strains of chicken, **selective IgA and IgG deficiencies** have been reported. IgG deficiency is also known as **hereditary dysgammaglobulinaemia.**

SECONDARY IMMUNODEFICIENCIES

The immune system, like any other body system, is subject to destruction and dysfunction from infection by a variety of pathogenic agents. Among the most important of these agents are **microorganisms** especially viruses, the other agents being toxins, stress, and malnutrition. As a group, the secondary immunodeficiencies are more common than the disorders of genetic origin.

Virus-Induced Immunosuppression

Viruses that affect the immune system may be divided into those that **affect primary lymphoid tissues,** and those that **affect secondary lymphoid tissues.** For example, in **poultry,** the virus of **infectious**

bursal disease (IBDV) destroys lymphocytes in the bursa of Fabricius (primary lymphoid organ) and causes bursal necrosis. The bursa then atrophies. As a result, **young birds** infected soon after hatching **are unable to make antibodies.**

The most important virus-induced immunodeficiency disease is **acquired immunodeficiency syndrome (AIDS) of humans,** a disease that results from infection with the human immunodeficiency virus (HIV). **There are many viruses, which cause similar disease in animals.** Two that closely resemble human AIDS are **simian AIDS of monkeys** and **feline AIDS of cats.** Another animal virus that infects and destroys **secondary lymphoid organs** is **canine distemper virus.** Apart from many different types of cells, canine distemper virus has a predilection for cells of lymphoid tissues. **In infected dogs,** the virus spreads from tonsils and bronchial lymph nodes to the spleen, lymph nodes, and bone marrow, where it replicates, **causing lymphoid destruction.** Canine distemper virus destroys lymphocytes and produces lymphopaenia. It depresses activities of macrophages and lymphocytes. **Thus, canine distemper virus depresses production of IL-1 and IL-2 while it also stimulates prostaglandin release by macrophages.** As a result, lymphocyte blastogenesis is depressed, immunoglobulin levels fall, and immediate hypersensitivity and skin graft rejection are suppressed. This **immunosuppression** accounts, in large part, for the clinical signs of canine distemper.

Depletion of lymphoid tissues occurs in **feline panleukopaenia, canine parvovirus-2 infection, feline leukopaenia,** and **African swine fever,** where the virus localizes in germinal centres. **Bovine virus diarrhoea** can cause lymphopaenia and destruction of both B- and T-cells in the lymph nodes, spleen, thymus, and Peyer's patches. As in canine distemper, surviving B-cells fail to make immunoglobulins. Bovine virus diarrhoea virus also exerts a generalized immunosuppressive effect. Infected cattle show depressed neutrophil function.

Herpesvirus infections are also immunosuppressive. For example, **equine herpesvirus-1** causes a T-cell lymphopaenia and depresses cell-mediated responses in **foals. Bovine herpesvirus-1** also causes a drop in T-cells and in the responses to T-cell mitogens.

The results of virus-induced lymphoid tissue destruction are readily seen. Animals show a lymphopaenia (deficiency of lymphocytes in blood), or a reduced response of blood lymphocytes to mitogens (substances that induce mitosis/cell division) such as phytohaemagglutinin (PHA) and concanavalin A (ConA). For example, the responses of peripheral blood lymphocytes to PHA is depressed in **canine distemper, Marek's disease, Newcastle disease (Ranikhet disease), feline leukaemia, and bovine virus diarrhoea.** **Thymic atrophy and lymphopaenia are common manifestations of many virus infections.**

Retrovirus Infections in Cats

Feline leukaemia: Feline leukaemia virus (FeLV) is an oncogenic retrovirus that causes many different syndromes in **cats**. The virus first replicates in the oral lymphoid tissues, **and then infects all the other lymphoid tissues.**

Cats have a higher incidence of lymphoid tumours than any other domestic animal. Most of these lymphoid tumours are due to FeLV. A **lymphosarcoma** caused by FeLV is usually a T-cell neoplasm. In young cats, FeLV-induced tumours are mainly of T-cell origin. In older cats, they tend to be both T- and B-cell in origin.

Immunosuppression: FeLV is profoundly immunosuppressive. It causes **two major immunopathological lesions. (1)** destruction of lymphocytes and suppression of their function, leading to immunodeficiency, and **(2)** production of large amounts of immune complexes, leading to severe glomerulonephritis. Infected cats suffer from severe lymphopaenia, neutropaenia, or both. The lymphopaenia in FeLV-infected cats is due to a loss of circulating T-cells, especially CD4+ T-cells. In contrast to the severe T-cell dysfunction, B-cell activities in FeLV-infected cats are only mildly impaired.

FeLV-AIDS: During natural FeLV infection, a form of the virus may develop that is **profoundly immunosuppressive**. This isolate, called FeLV-AIDS, causes fatal immunodeficiency in nearly 100% of infected cats. There is a **drastic drop in CD4+ T-cells**, while CD8+ T-cell and B-cell numbers remain normal. The immunological defect is an **inability to mount antibody responses.** The loss of CD4+ T-cells results in the production of lower levels of B-cell stimulatory cytokines. **This virus selectively impairs T-helper cell function.**

Feline immunodeficiency virus: Feline immunodeficiency virus (FIV) occurs mainly in **older male cats**. FIV causes **three syndromes**: (1) lymphoproliferative (lymphomas, squamous-cell carcinomas, and myeloproliferative disease), (2) immunodeficiency, and (3) neurological disease. In the **primary stage**, cats develop generalized lymphadenopathy and lymphoid hyperplasia. Cats then develop

461

leukopaenia, which is due to a drop in CD4+ T-cells. Most cats recover from this stage. In the **second stage**, there is a progressive drop in CD4+ T-cell numbers. The cat's lymph nodes show gradual hyperplasia leading to aplasia. There is also bone marrow suppression, suggesting that bone marrow stem cells are destroyed by the virus. The gradual onset of progressive generalized lymphadenopathy marks the **third stage** of the disease. In the fourth stage, the cat suffers from secondary bacterial infections.

The **final stage** is **a severe AIDS-like disease**. The cat may suffer from many opportunistic infections. The animals show major immunological defects as well as anaemia, lymphopaenia, and neutropaenia. Malignancies also occur. **Mortality is greater than 50%, and no cats have been seen to recover.**

Immunosuppression: FIV-infected cats have lower numbers of neutrophils, lower percentage of T-cells, and a higher percentage of B-cells compared with uninfected animals. FIV infects feline T-cells. **Most of the infected cats have a significant drop in the numbers of CD4+ T-cells**. They may also show an increase in CD8+ T-cells. As a result, the CD4+: CD8+ ratio drops significantly.

Retrovirus Infections in Cattle

Bovine immunodeficiency virus (BIV) infected cows show lymph node hyperplasia, lymphocytosis, central nervous system lesions, loss of weight, and weakness. BIV can also infect **sheep**.

Retrovirus Infections in Dogs

Canine immunodeficiency virus (CIV) has been isolated from dogs. Another retrovirus also has been isolated from a dog with a severe acquired immunodeficiency syndrome. The dog had depressed humoral and T-cell-mediated immune responses. On necropsy, the dog showed depletion of lymphoid organs and bone marrow hypoplasia.

Other Causes of Secondary Immunodeficiency

1. Microbial and parasitic infections: Immunosuppression usually accompanies infestation with **Toxoplasma** or **trypanosomes**, helminths such as *Trichinella spiralis*, arthropods such as **Demodex** and bacteria such as *Pasteurella haemolytica*, the actinobacilli, and some streptococci.

2. Toxin-induced immunosuppression: Many environmental toxins, such as dieldrin, iodine, lead, cadmium, methyl mercury, and

DDT are immunosuppressive. **Mycotoxins** are important immunosuppressants when **cattle** and **poultry** are fed feed containing mouldy grain. These include **T-2 toxin** from **Fusarium** that depresses the respcnse of calf lymphocytes to mitogens and decreases the chemotactic migration of neutrophils. T-2 toxin also reduces IgM, IgA, and C3 levels in **cattle**. **Aflatoxins** increase the susceptibility of chickens to **Salmonella** as a result of decreased phagocytic activity. **Ochratoxins** and trichothecenes are also immunosuppressive in **pigs** and **poultry**.

3. **Malnutrition and the immune response**: In general, severe nutritional deficiencies reduce T-cell function and **therefore impair cell-mediated responses**. At the same time, they spare B-cell function and humoral immunity. Thus, starvation rapidly induces thymic atrophy and a reduction in the level of thymic hormones. **The number of circulating T-cells drops** and cells are lost from the T-cell areas of secondary lymphoid tissue. However, severe starvation has little effect on B-cell functions. Serum immunoglobulin of all classes may remain normal or even rise. **Starvation**, however, results in depressed complement levels and impairment of neutrophil and macrophage chemotaxis, the respiratory burst, release of lysosomal enzymes, and microbicidal activity.

Specific nutritional deficiencies have range of effects. **Deficiencies of some B vitamins, vitamin A**, and **polyunsaturated fatty acids** can depress immunoglobulin levels through effects on regulatory T-cells. **Magnesium deficiency** causes a similar effect by a direct action on B-cells. **Vitamin E deficiency in dogs and lambs** results in decreased lymphocyte blastogenesis. **Deficiencies of vitamin A, vitamin B12,** and **folic acid** can depress cell-mediated immune responses. **Vitamin D** is responsible for proper macrophage development. Zinc is especially critical for proper functioning of the immune system. **Zinc-deficient pigs** have reduced thymus weight, depressed cytotoxic T-cell activity, depressed B-cell activity, and depressed NK cell activity. If pregnant animals are deprived of **zinc, their offspring have severely depressed immune function. Copper deficiency** can reduce neutrophil numbers and function, reduce responsiveness to mitogens, reduce T and NK cell numbers, and increase mast cell histamine release. **Selenium deficiency** reduces neutrophil activity, T-cell blastogenesis, and IgM production. **Chromium** supplementation may increase some aspects of immune function. Therefore, its deficiency may be immunosuppressive.

4. Exercise and the Immune Response

Regular moderate exercise increases immune function. Exercise raises blood neutrophil levels, increases NK cell activity, promotes responses to mitogens, and increases blood levels of IL-1, IL-6, and TNF-alpha. However, strenuous exercise is stressful and increases susceptibility to infectious diseases. This is due to raised steroid levels due to stress. Thus, although mild exercise is good for immune function, intensive prolonged exercise may induce a functional immunodeficiency.

5. Trauma and the Immune Response

Severely injured animals (e.g., from trauma, burns) usually die from sepsis as a result of an immunodeficiency. Corticosteroids, prostaglandins from damaged tissues, and a small protein called **suppressive active peptide,** that appears in serum following a burn all have immunosuppressive properties. Although surgery can result in some suppression of lymphocyte responses to mitogens, routine surgery has no significant effect on the response of healthy animals to vaccination.

6. Age and the Immune Response

Both cell-mediated and humoral immune responses decrease with advancing age.

T-cells: As an animal ages, there is a significant drop in the numbers of CD4+ cells as a result of thymic involution (atrophy) and a decline in the export of T-cells from the thymus.

B-cells: The bone marrow is relatively unaffected by age. Also, antigen processing and presentation are not affected by the aging process. However, **aged macrophages** show reduced cytokine production and responses to activating agents such as interferon-gamma. Despite this, young animals may show relatively poorer resistance to infections than mature animals. This is especially important in **sheep**. Thus, lambs are more susceptible than mature sheep to parasitic and infectious diseases during the first year of life. Older sheep show greater resistance to internal parasites. There is thus clear evidence of a mild immunodeficiency in lambs than in mature adults. This may be due to immaturity of the immune system during the first year of life.

Acquired Immunodeficiency Syndrome (AIDS)

Although AIDS is a human disease, its pathogenesis is briefly described as an exercise in comparative immunopathology, and also because the disease has assumed epidemic proportions in recent years threatening the world population. AIDS is caused by the **human immunodeficiency virus (HIV),** a human **retrovirus** (i.e., it contains enzyme reverse transcriptase) belonging to the lentivirus family. Other members of this group are feline immunodeficiency virus, bovine immunodeficiency virus, equine infectious anaemia virus, simian (monkey) immunodeficiency virus, and visna/maedi virus of sheep. AIDS is characterized by **profound immunosuppression** leading to **opportunistic infections, secondary neoplasms**, and neurological manifestations.

Pathogenesis: There are **two major targets of HIV infection:** the **immune system** and the **central nervous system.** We shall discuss **only the immunopathogenesis** of AIDS.

The most important pathological event in AIDS is **profound immunosuppression, mainly affecting cell-mediated immunity.** This results from infection and **severe loss of CD 4+ helper T-cells** as well as damage to the function of surviving helper T-cells. Macrophages and dendritic cells (important in CD4+ T-cell activation) are also targets of HIV infection. **The CD4 molecule is a high-affinity receptor for HIV. This explains the selective tropism (affinity) of the virus for CD4+ T-cells and its ability to infect other CD4+ cells, particularly macrophages and dendritic cells.** However, binding to CD4 is not sufficient for infection. The HIV envelope glycoprotein gp120 must also bind to other cell surface molecules (**co-receptors**) to facilitate cell entry. Two cell surface chemokine receptor molecules, **CCR5** and **CXCR4**, serve this role (see 'chemokines'). After fusion, the virus core containing the HIV genome enters the cytoplasm of the cell. **The co-receptors are critical components of the HIV infection process.**

Once inside the cell, the viral genome undergoes **reverse transcription,** leading to formation of complementary DNA (cDNA). In quiescent T-cells the cDNA enters the nucleus and becomes integrated into the host genome. After integration, the provirus may remain non-transcribed for months or years and the infection becomes **latent**. Alternatively, proviral DNA may be transcribed to form complete viral particles that bud from the cell membrane. Such **productive infections,** associated with extensive viral budding **lead to cell death.**

T-cells in HIV infection: HIV infections are characterized by a **profound loss of CD4+ cells from blood**. Approximately 100 billion new viral particles are produced every day, and 1 to 2 billion CD4+ T-cells die each day. (One billion is one thousand million(s); one million is ten lakhs). Thus, **productive infection** of T-cells is the mechanism by which HIV causes **CD4+ T-cell depletion**. However, recently it has become known that loss of CD4+ T-cells occurs by both increased destruction and reduced production. This leads to a reversal of CD4 - CD8 ratio in the blood. Although marked reduction in CD4+ T-cells is a typical feature of AIDS and accounts for much of the immunodeficiency, qualitative defects in T-cell function also play an important role. Such defects include reduced antigen-induced T-cell proliferation, impaired Th1 cytokine production, and abnormal intracellular signalling. There is also a loss of memory CD4+ helper T-cells.

Monocytes / macrophages in HIV infection: In addition to loss of CD4+ T-cells, **infection of monocytes and macrophages is also extremely important in the pathogenesis of HIV**. Like T- cells, most of the HIV-infected macrophages are found in the tissues and not in blood. In contrast to CD4+ T-cells, macrophages are quite resistant to cytopathic effects of HIV. The initial infection of macrophages (or dendritic cells) is **critical for HIV transmission**. Besides providing a means for initial transmission, monocytes and macrophages are viral reservoirs. Macrophages also provide a vehicle for HIV transport to various parts of the body, particularly the nervous system. In late stages of the disease, when CD4+ T-cells are massively lost, **macrophages** remain a major site of continued viral replication.

Dendritic cells in HIV infection: In addition to macrophages, two types of dendritic cells are also important targets for maintenance of HIV infection: (1) mucosal, and follicular dendritic cells. Mucosal dendritic cells, also called **Langerhans cells**, capture the virus and transport it to regional lymph nodes, where CD4+ T-cells are infected. Follicular dendritic cells in the germinal centres of lymph nodes are important reservoirs of HIV. **To summarize**, CD4+ T-cells, macrophages, and follicular dendritic cells contained in peripheral lymphoid tissues are the major sites of HIV infection and persistence. Low-level chronic or latent infection of T-cells and macrophages is an important feature of HIV infection. Latent infection can persist within cells for **months to years**.

B-cells and other lymphocytes in HIV infection: Apart from T-cells and macrophages, patients with AIDS also show severe abnormalities of B-cell function. Patients with AIDS are unable to mount an antibody response to a new antigen. **This is not only due to deficient T-cell help, but antibody responses against T-independent antigens are also suppressed, indicating additional B-cell defects.**

To conclude, CD4+ helper T-cells play a central role in the immunopathogenesis of AIDS. As is known, helper T-cells are extremely important in regulating the immune response. They produce a large number of cytokines such as IL-2, IL-4, IL-5, IFN-gamma, and macrophage chemotactic factors, which activate CD8+ cytotoxic T-cells, B-cells, and macrophages. Therefore, loss of this **'master cell'** has ripple effects on almost every other cell of the immune system. **These effects include** decreased response to soluble antigens, decreased cytokine secretion by CD4+ helper T-cells, decreased specific cytotoxicity by CD8+ cytotoxic T-cells, decreased killing of tumour cells by NK cells, decreased antibody production by B-cells in response to new antigens, and reduced cytotoxic ability, decreased chemotaxis, reduced interleukin-1 secretion, and poor antigen presentation by macrophages.

Chapter 10
Nutritional Diseases

An appropriate diet should provide: (1) **sufficient energy** in the form of carbohydrate, fat and protein for body's daily metabolic needs, (2) **essential** (as well as non-essential) **amino acids** and **fatty acids** to be used as building blocks for synthesis of structural and functional proteins and lipids, and (3) **vitamins** and **minerals** that function as co-enzymes or hormones in vital metabolic pathways, or in the case of calcium and phosphate, as important structural components.

Deficiency of a single nutrient is rare as a natural disease, although several examples can be cited such as iodine deficiency leading to goitre and iron deficiency leading to anaemia. **But, in general, nutritional diseases in both animals and humans are multiple deficiencies.** This creates complex disease states that are more difficult to analyze.

Nutritional deficiencies may be primary or secondary. In **primary deficiency**, one or all of the nutrients are missing from the diet. **Secondary deficiency**, on the other hand, results from nutrient malabsorption, poor nutrient utilization or storage, excess nutrient losses, or increased need for nutrients. Nutritional deficiency can arise from several different causes. These include:

1. The diet may be of a poor quality (e.g., mainly roughage), or the amount may be inadequate (starvation). There may also be a lack of specific ingredients in commercially prepared diets, or a diet may be specifically lacking in one or more essential nutrients.

2. Interference with intake due to anorexia, mechanical obstruction, dental disease, or parasitism. It has the same effect as inadequate supply.

3. Interference with absorption of nutrients due to lack of digestive secretions from hepatic or pancreatic disease, enteritis, hypermotility of the intestinal tract, or parasitism.

4. Interference with storage or utilization of a nutrient. For example, in thyroiditis, insufficient normal tissue may be available for the proper utilization of iodine.

5. Increased excretion or retention of nutrients. Examples include loss of potassium in diarrhoea, and calcium loss in hyperparathyroidism.

6. Increased requirements in pregnancy, lactation, or hyperthyroidism may cause deficiency states if the diet is not adjusted.

VITAMIN DEFICIENCIES

Thirteen vitamins are necessary for health; four **A, D, E,** and **K** are **fat-soluble**, and the **remaining water-soluble**. The difference is important because, although the fat-soluble vitamins are more readily stored in the body, they are poorly absorbed in gastrointestinal disorders of fat malabsorption. Certain vitamins can be synthesized in the body - vitamin D from precursor steroids, vitamin K and biotin by the intestinal microflora, and niacin from tryptophan, an essential amino acid. Despite this endogenous synthesis, a dietary supply of all vitamins is essential for health.

Fat-Soluble Vitamins

Vitamin A

Vitamin A is actually a group of related natural and synthetic chemicals that exert a hormone-like activity. **Retinol** is the most important form of vitamin A. It is the transport form, the storage form being **retinol ester**. Retinol ester in body is oxidized to the aldehyde **retinal** and **retinoic acid**. The term **retinoids** refers to both natural and synthetic chemicals that are structurally related to vitamin A, but do not necessarily possess vitamin A activity. Yellow and leafy green vegetables such as carrots contain large amounts of **carotenoids**. Many of these are **provitamins** that can be metabolized to active vitamin A in the body. The most important of these is **beta-carotene**.

Important dietary sources of vitamin A are animal-derived foods, such as eggs, butter, milk, fish, and liver. The vitamin A is fat-soluble and, since certain fishes store large amounts of it, cod liver oil and shark-liver oil are concentrated sources of this vitamin. Herbivorous animals obtain their vitamin A in the form of carotenoids from plants, whereas carnivorous animals from animal tissues, liver being especially rich. As with all fats, digestion and absorption of carotenes and retinoids requires bile and pancreatic enzymes. Retinol is transported to the liver for esterification and storage as retinol ester. **More than 90% of the body's vitamin A reserves are stored in the liver.**

Functions: The best-defined functions of vitamin A are: **(1)** To maintain normal vision in reduced light, **(2)** To bring about differentiation of mucus-secreting cells, and **(3)** To increase immunity against infections. In addition, retinoids and beta-carotenes function as photoprotective and antioxidant agents.

The visual process involves four forms of vitamin A-containing pigments: **rhodopsin** (visual purple) in the rods and three **iodopsins** in cone cells. Rhodopsin is the most light-sensitive pigment and therefore important in reduced light. The synthesis of rhodopsin from retinol involves: (1) oxidation of retinol derived from the blood to all-**trans**-retinal, (2) conversion of all-**trans**-retinal to 11-**cis**-retinal, and (3) interaction of 11-**cis**-retinal with the rod protein, **opsin**, to form **rhodopsin**. When light falls on the dark retina, rhodopsin undergoes a sequence of changes to yield all-**trans**-retinol and opsin. In the process, a nerve impulse is generated which is transmitted from retina to the brain, through neurons. During dark adaptation, some of the all-**trans**-retinal is re-converted to 11-**cis**-retinal, but most is reduced to retinol and lost to the retina. **Therefore, a continuous supply of retinol is required for the visual process in reduced (dim) light.** George Wald received the Nobel Prize for elucidating this visual process.

Vitamin A plays an important role in the differentiation of mucus-secreting epithelium. During deficiency, the epithelium undergoes **squamous metaplasia** and differentiation to a keratinizing epithelium (see 'metaplasia', Chapter 7). The mechanism is not precisely understood. In addition, vitamin A plays some role in **host's resistance to infections**. This beneficial effect of vitamin A is due to its ability to stimulate immune system through the formation of a metabolite called **14-hydroxyretinol**.

Deficiency states: One of the earliest signs of deficiency is impaired vision, particularly in reduced light (**night blindness or nyctalopia**). The animal is unable to see well in partial darkness. Night blindness occurs in all domestic animals, but is most commonly observed in **horses and cattle**. If the deficiency persists, this condition is followed by a sequence of physical changes referred to as **xerophthalmia**, which means dryness of the eye. First, there is dryness of the conjunctivae (**xerosis conjunctivae**) as the normal lachrymal and mucus-secreting epithelium is replaced by keratinized epithelium. Dryness of the eye exposes animals, especially horses and cattle, to recurrent episodes of conjunctivitis and keratitis (inflammation of

471

cornea). Xerosis is followed by the development of keratin debris in small opaque plaques (**Bitot spots**) and, eventually erosion of the roughened corneal surface with softening and destruction of the cornea (**keratomalacia**) and total blindness.

In addition to the ocular epithelium, **squamous metaplasia** is most evident in mucosa of the alimentary, respiratory, and genitourinary tract. This metaplastic change has many adverse consequences. In birds, the epithelial linings of the mucous glands in the oesophagus and pharynx undergo squamous metaplasia and hyperkeratosis (overgrowth of the keratin layer). This blocks their ducts and causes their distension with inspissated secretion. **The spherical nodules, 1-2 mm in diameter, are pathognomonic of hypovitaminosis A**. Accompanied by coryza and other respiratory infections, and by general malaise and inanition (weakness from lack of food), the condition in birds is called **nutritional roup**.

When respiratory airways are affected, the loss of mucus secretion and the defensive **'mucociliary apparatus'**, predisposes the lungs to infections. The most important effect of squamous metaplasia is found in the urinary tract. In renal pelvis or other urinary surfaces, the desquamated keratinized squamous cells **provide a nidus for stone formation**, on which mineral salts precipitate. Practically all **male cattle, sheep**, and **goats** in severe deficiency of vitamin A **die of urinary obstruction caused by urinary calculi** lodged at the sigmoid flexure. Females escape the effects of this **urolithiasis** because of less constricted urethra.

Vitamin A deficiency also interferes with **maternal reproduction**. Squamous metaplasia in vagina leads to excessive cornification, which upsets the cycle of epithelial changes. This defect, based on imperfect endometrial function, is an important cause of **infertility in cattle**. Severe deficiency of this vitamin also alters normal bone growth and remodelling, especially of cranial bones, resulting in a disparity of growth of the nervous system and its bony closure. This may lead to **foetal malformations**, such as failure of the optic foramina to grow to sufficient diameter. This may cause, through constriction of the optic nerve, blindness in newborn calves. Hypovitaminosis A also impairs immune function. Deficiency in animals is associated with increased susceptibility to infection. Increased cerebrospinal fluid pressure regularly follows vitamin A deficiency.

To conclude, except through the secondary development of some fatal disorder such as urinary obstruction, deficiency of vitamin A does not cause death. Vitamin A is toxic when, consumed or administered in large doses.

Vitamin D

Vitamin D is formed from **two steroid precursors** or **provitamins** found in nature: (1) **ergosterol** (provitamin-D2) found in plants, and (2) **7-dehydrocholesterol** (provitamin-D3) found in animal tissues. Humans and animals have **two sources of vitamin D**: (1) **endogenous synthesis** in the skin, and (2) the **diet**. The main source of vitamin D is endogenous synthesis in the skin. Skin contains the precursor 7-dehydrocholesterol, and ultraviolet light in the sunlight converts it to **vitamin D3 (cholecalciferol)**. The remainder is obtained from the dietary sources, such as plants, grain, and fish. In plants and grains, vitamin D is present in its precursor form **ergosterol**, which is converted to **vitamin D2 (ergocalciferol)** in the body. Since **D3 and D2** undergo similar metabolic changes and have similar functions, **both from now will be referred to as vitamin D.**

Metabolism: The metabolism of vitamin D can be outlined as follows: (1) First, there is absorption of vitamin D from the gut, or synthesis from precursor in the skin. (2) Vitamin D then binds to plasma alpha-1-globulin (D-binding protein) and is transported to the liver. (3) In the liver, vitamin D is converted to 25-hydroxyvitamin D by the enzyme 25-hydroxylase. (4) 25-hydroxyvitamin D is then converted to 1, 25-dihydroxyvitamin D by alpha-1-hydroxylase in the kidney. **Biologically, this is the most active form of vitamin D.**

Functions: Biologically, active form of vitamin D functions as a **steroid hormone**. Its **major function is to maintain normal plasma levels of calcium and phosphorus**. This function involves actions on the intestine, bones, and kidneys. **To summarize**: (1) **vitamin D stimulates intestinal absorption of calcium and phosphorus,** (2) it works with parathyroid hormone (PTH) in the mobilization of calcium from bone, and (3) it stimulates PTH-dependent reabsorption of calcium in the distal renal tubules.

Vitamin D has two opposing actions on the bone, which depend on the plasma levels of calcium. On the one hand, with hypocalcaemia (low blood calcium) vitamin D works with PTH in the resorption (removal) of calcium and phosphorus from bone to support blood levels. On the other hand, vitamin D is required for normal mineralization of epiphyseal cartilage and osteoid matrix. It is still not clear how the resorptive function is mediated. Equally unclear is

473

the role of vitamin D in renal reabsorption of calcium. The main function of vitamin D may be to maintain calcium and phosphorus at supersaturated levels in the plasma.

Deficiency states: Very little vitamin D is transferred from mother to the foetus. Because of this, the newly born individual must have an adequate supply of vitamin D that must be provided through the feed or by exposure to sunlight. In confined or dark-skinned animals, all of the vitamin D must be provided through the feed because its synthesis in the skin by ultraviolet light is prevented due to confinement, or by melanin pigment in the skin. Vitamin D deficiency in young animals, causes **rickets** and in adults **osteomalacia**. Both forms of skeletal disease may result either from dietary deficiency or from delayed vitamin absorption or metabolism. Whatever the cause, a deficiency of vitamin D causes **hypocalcaemia** and also **hypophosphataemia** (low blood phosphorus). This is due to deficient absorption of calcium and phosphorus from the gut. When hypocalcaemia occurs, parathyroid hormone production is increased, which: (1) activates renal alpha-1-hydrolase, thus increasing the amount of active vitamin D and calcium absorption from the gut, (2) mobilizes calcium and phosphorus from the bone, (3) decreases renal calcium excretion, and (4) **increases renal excretion of phosphate**. Thus, the serum level of calcium is restored to almost normal, **but hypophosphataemia persists**, and therefore mineralization of bone is impaired.

Young chickens are hatched with enough vitamin for the first two weeks of life. If more is not received from the food, that is, when dietary intake is inadequate, chicks kept in darkness die between the 18th and 21st days of life from **leg weakness**. Skeletal mineralization is defective giving rise to **rickets** in the young (from reduced bone mineral deposition) and **osteomalacia** in adult birds (from bone mineral loss). **Rachitic deformities** develop especially in the legs, producing painful, hard, joint swelling, and lameness. The head of the ribs (capitula) and occasionally the costochondral junctions may be enlarged. The bones, beak, and claws become soft and pliable. Growth is retarded and feather development is poor. In the laying bird, egg production decreases, with thin or soft-shelled eggs and reduced hatchability. Osteomalacia gives rise to brittle bones of reduced density and strength. Such bones are light, porous, and fragile **(osteoporosis)**. Common feed ingredients contain little or no vitamin D, and therefore it should be incorporated in the feed, the common form being D3. D2 is also commercially available but should not be used for birds because it is poorly utilized. Excessive levels of vitamin D are toxic, leading to tissue calcium deposition.

Vitamin E

Vitamin E consists of **eight** closely related fat-soluble compounds. Of these, **four** are **tocopherols** and **four tocotrienols**. All show vitamin E biological activity, but **alpha-tocopherol is the most active and the most widely available**. Tocopherols were so named because they were believed to maintain pregnancy (G. tokus = childbirth; phero = to carry). Vitamin E is abundant in many foods - vegetables, grains, nuts, and their oils, dairy products, fish, and meat. The absorption of tocopherols, like all fat-soluble vitamins, requires normal biliary tract and pancreatic function. After absorption, vitamin E is transported in the blood in the form of chylomicrons, which rapidly combine with plasma lipoproteins, mainly low-density lipoproteins (LDLs). Thus, disorders that derange fat absorption and chylomicron formation are the main causes of vitamin E deficiency. Unlike vitamin A, which is stored mainly in the liver, vitamin E accumulates throughout the body, mostly in the fat depots, but also in liver and muscle.

Functions: Vitamin E is a naturally occurring antioxidant and plays an important role in scavenging (removing) free radicals formed in redox (reduction + oxidation) **reactions throughout the body** (see 'Cell injury and cell death', Chapter 3). It helps in termination of free radical-generated lipid peroxidation chain reactions (Chapter 3), particularly in cellular and organellar membranes that are rich in polyunsaturated lipids. **Thus, vitamin E protects the cell and therefore the tissue against damage by free radicals**. This action supports that of **selenium**, which as a component of **glutathione peroxidase**, also metabolizes (destroys) peroxides before they cause membrane damage. The nervous system is a particular target of vitamin E deficiency. It is speculated that neurons with long axons are particularly vulnerable because of their large membrane surface area. **Mature red cells** are also vulnerable to vitamin E deficiency because they are exposed to oxidative injury caused by superoxide free radicals generated during oxygenation of haemoglobin.

Deficiency states: In domestic animals, vitamin E was originally regarded as being important only as an **anti-sterility factor**. Later on it was shown that it was much more important as an **antioxidant**, and that it prevented diseases of the brain, muscle, and fat. Deficiencies

475

of vitamin E and selenium have been associated with **white muscle disease (nutritional myopathy)** in several species, but it is important in **cattle, sheep, pigs,** and **horses**. It is mainly a disease of young animals. In suckling lambs, the condition has been called as **stiff-lamb disease** due to stiffness. The disease is prevalent in nursing animals because milk is a poor source of vitamin E. **Lambs**, not more than 1-2 months of age, and **calves** from a few days to a year, are involved. The clinical signs include locomotor disturbances, namely, a reluctance to move, stiffness, inability to stand, and death.

Acute hepatic necrosis or **hepatosis dietetica (dietary hepatic necrosis)** of rapidly growing **young pigs** has been clearly related to vitamin E deficiency, although selenium and sulphur-containing amino acids give protection. Again, in **pigs**, a condition characterized by a yellowish-brown pigmentation of fat known as **'yellow fat disease'** or **'steatitis'** (inflammation of adipose tissue) is associated with feeding of a ration low in tocopherols and high in fish meal. The discoloration of fat (mainly subcutaneous and mesenteric) is due to the accumulation of an oily or waxy pigment known as **ceroid**. It is insoluble in fat solvents, does not stain for iron, and is basophilic with H and E stain. Its presence in tissue indicates mild inflammatory reaction (**steatitis**), characterized by accumulation of macrophages, neutrophils, and an occasional foreign-body giant cell. Formation of **ceroid** and the discoloration of fat are usually prevented by increased amounts of alpha-tocopherol in the diet. Steatitis also occurs in **cats** fed on certain fish diets.

Poultry: Inadequate vitamin E levels give rise to several conditions in poultry that may occur separately or together, depending on age, degree of deficiency, or other factors. Most grain storage lead to loss of natural vitamin E and therefore increase the supplementation requirement, as do stressful conditions, such as overcrowding, transportations, poor ventilation, and disease. Since the primary function of vitamin E is protection of cell membranes as an intracellular antioxidant, its deficiency results in damage to blood vessels and changes in capillary permeability. Deficiency in breeders may give rise to early embryonic mortality associated with vascular lesions, usually around 4th day of incubation. In **young growing birds**, deficiency condition include: (1) **encephalomalacia**, (2) **exudative diathesis**, and (3) **nutritional muscular dystrophy** (or **myopathy**).

1. Encephalomalacia (Crazy chick disease): Encephalomalacia is a nervous disorder. It is seen in birds, usually in good condition, up to the age of 5 weeks (often between 2 and 3 weeks). Symptoms include muscular weakness, progressive muscular incoordination with frequent falling, backward or downward retraction of the head, and/ or rapid contraction and relaxation of the legs, torticollis (twisting of the neck), and finally paralysis, and death. Vascular lesions give rise to oedema and petechial or even larger haemorrhages in the **cerebellum**, with ensuing neuron degeneration. **These lesions, with appropriate clinical signs, are almost pathognomonic**. The reason why cerebellum is affected and not cerebrum, is because of the increased polyunsaturated fatty acid levels, which occur in the second and third week in the cerebellum, but not in the cerebrum.

2. Exudative diathesis: Exudative diathesis is an oedema of the subcutaneous tissue. Capillary wall lesions cause increased vascular permeability, with resulting plasma leakage. Plasma accumulates subcutaneously, particularly over the breast and under the wings. It also accumulates in the pericardial sac and between the muscles. The condition is prevented by vitamin E and selenium

3. Nutritional muscular dystrophy (or myopathy): This condition usually occurs with exudative diathesis. It occurs when vitamin E deficiency is accompanied by sulphur-containing amino acids (methionine and cysteine) in chicks. Micro-thrombosis of smaller vessels causes occlusion, which gives rise to degeneration and necrosis of muscle fibres. This is seen as **pale (white) streaks** mainly in breast and thigh muscles (hence the name **white muscle disease**).

Vitamin K

Vitamin K was discovered in chickens, by Henrik Dam in 1943, who was awarded the Nobel prize. Vitamin K consists of a group of compounds that exhibit **anti-haemorrhagic activity**. Vitamin K is abundant in green plants, vegetables, and fruits. It is also synthesized in the body by the intestinal flora. **Therefore, vitamin K requirements of animals are easily satisfied and no clinical deficiency occurs in healthy animals**. Its absorption in the small intestine requires adequate bile flow and pancreatic function.

Functions: Vitamin K is anti-haemorrhagic and is indispensable for blood coagulation. In its absence blood cannot clot. This is because vitamin K is required for synthesis of prothrombin. In the absence of vitamin K, an abnormal type of **prothrombin** is released into the blood by the liver. Since prothrombin plays an important role in blood-clotting mechanism, deficiency of vitamin K results in markedly prolonged blood-clotting time. **Mechanism**: Vitamin K is a required cofactor for a liver microsomal carboxylase that is necessary to convert glutamyl residues in four clotting factors (factor II (**prothrombin**), factor VII, factor IX, and factor X) to gamma-carboxyglutamates (carboxylation). **That is, these four factors require vitamin K for carboxylation**. Carboxylation provides calcium-binding sites and thus allows calcium-dependent interaction of these clotting factors with a phospholipid surface involved in the generation of thrombin.

Deficiency states: Deficiency occurs in: (1) fat malabsorption syndrome, particularly with biliary tract disease, (2) following destruction of the intestinal vitamin K synthesizing flora, particularly with ingestion of sulpha drugs and broad-spectrum antibiotics, (3) in the neonates, where liver reserves are small and the bacterial flora are not yet developed, and (4) in diffuse liver disease, because hepatocyte dysfunction interferes with the synthesis of vitamin K-dependent coagulation factors.

The major result of vitamin K deficiency is the development of a **bleeding diathesis** (bleeding tendency). A **haemorrhagic syndrome** is observed in **commercial broilers** when birds are fed a restricted ration, deficient in vitamin K. The addition of chemical compounds, such as sulphaquinoxaline to the ration to control or treat coccidiosis, may prevent the synthesis of vitamin K in the intestine by destroying bacterial flora. The resulting deficiency causes multiple haemorrhages throughout the body. A similar bleeding tendency occurs in pigs that are fed rations containing sulphonamide drugs, or are medicated excessively with these drugs. The animals bleed from the nose, and excessive haemorrhage occurs from any wound. Postmortem examination reveals haemorrhages throughout the carcass and should be differentiated from those of septicaemic disease, such as swine fever. Newborn animals tend to have a deficiency of vitamin K. For example, litter of pigs may bleed excessively from the umbilical cord or from any injury received at the time of birth, or shortly thereafter.

Water-Soluble Vitamins

This category includes B group vitamins and vitamin C. **Most of the water-soluble vitamins are widely available and readily absorbed, mainly in the small intestine**. A variety of foods are rich sources of B vitamins, especially cereals, leafy green vegetables, yeast, liver, and milk. Vitamin C is widely available in citrus fruits, vegetables, and some meats. Moreover, **in ruminants**, several members of vitamin B group are synthesized by microorganisms in the rumen. **Thus, deficiency states of water-soluble vitamins are not problems like fat-soluble vitamins, except in small animals and poultry.**

Thiamine (Vitamin B1)

Thiamine (vitamin B1) was also discovered in chickens, in 1929, this time by Christian Eijkman who received the Nobel prize. Vitamin B1 is present in adequate amounts in normal rations containing whole grain and green feed. However, refined foods such as polished rice and white flour ('maida'), and milk and meat, contain little. During absorption from the gut, thiamine undergoes phosphorylation to produce **thiamine pyrophosphate**, the functionally active co-enzyme form of the vitamin.

Functions: Thiamine plays an important role in carbohydrate metabolism. **Thiamine pyrophosphate** has three major functions: (1) it plays an important role in the synthesis of adenosine triphosphate (ATP), (2) it acts as a cofactor in the pentose phosphate pathway, and (3) it maintains normal nerve conduction, chiefly of peripheral nerves. **The major targets of thiamine deficiency are peripheral nerves, heart, and brain.**

Deficiency states: Deficiency may result when: (1) the diet may lack sufficient thiamine, (2) the vitamin may be destroyed by thiamine analogues (i.e., chemical compounds similar in function, but different in structure), such as amprolium, (3) destruction may result from the action of thiaminases (thiamine-splitting enzymes) in the diet, such as found in flesh of certain fishes. In **dogs, cats**, and **foxes** deficiency usually results from lack of thiamine in the diet, or from feeding certain thiaminase-containing fish. **Birds** are also susceptible to a deficient diet. **Adult ruminants**, such as **cattle, sheep**, and **goat** do not require thiamine in the diet, because the vitamin is produced by bacteria in the forestomachs. **Calves** and **lambs**, however, have no such activity in early life, and are therefore susceptible to dietary deficiency at this time. **Thiamine deficiency is important only in poultry and pigs.**

Poultry: Thiamine deficiency appears when there are inadequate levels of this vitamin in the feed. The signs are loss of appetite and weight, weakness, polyneuritis, paralysis, and even death. The bird characteristically sits on its flexed legs and retracts its head, called 'stargazing' or 'ophisthotonus'. These nervous symptoms are the result of degenerative changes in the peripheral nerves (peripheral neuropathy) with myelin degeneration and disruption of axons.

Pigs: Thiamine deficiency in pigs causes acute cardiac dilatation, which results in sudden death (a cardiovascular syndrome). Microscopic areas of necrosis are present in the myocardium.

Riboflavin (Vitamin B2)

Riboflavin is abundant in green grass, vegetables, meat and milk, but is rather low in grains and grain by-products. It is synthesized in rumen and absorbed in small intestine. In birds (adult birds not young chicks), it is synthesized in the caeca and large intestine, both being the sites of microbial activity. However, as the absorption of vitamin B2 occurs from the small intestine, this is of no use to the bird. Therefore, coprophagy (eating of faeces) appears to be the useful source. The vitamin is not stored in the body but it is stored in the eggs, particularly in yolk. Absence of body storage means that daily supply is required in the feed.

Functions: Riboflavin is essential in normal cell metabolism. (1) It is an important component of the coenzymes flavin mononucleotide (FMN) and flavin adenine dinucleotide (FAD) that participate in a wide range of oxidation-reduction reactions, metabolism of carbohydrate, amino acid and fat, and the regulation of cellular metabolism. The vitamin is therefore essential for growth and health. (2) In addition, flavin in covalent linkage is incorporated into succinic dehydrogenase and monoamine oxidase as well as into other mitochondrial enzymes.

Deficiency states: The appearance of signs of riboflavin deficiency does not always mean inadequate supply, because antagonists (e.g., mycotoxins, mainly aflatoxin) may interfere with absorption or body transport. In breeders, riboflavin is required for optimum hatchability. Reduced egg production occurs in severe deficiency, but with marginally low deficiency, there is greatly reduced hatchability with embryonic deaths in mid or late incubation (dead-in-shell). Hatched chicks may be dwarfed and oedematous, show 'clubbed down', poor feathering, and leg paralysis. Often there is inward curling of the toes and resting on the hocks (curled-toe paralysis). Clubbed down is produced by a failure of the feathers to rupture their sheaths, producing a club shape. Curled-toe paralysis and clubbed down are diagnostic of the lack of available riboflavin in the yolk of the incubated eggs.

Curled-toe paralysis may be seen in chicks around 10-14 days of age. Birds may be unable to rise from their hocks, and the legs are outstretched with flaccid paralysis and in-curling of the toes. The bird's head, wings and tail feathers droop, growth is retarded, birds are recumbent, emaciated, and die. The sciatic and brachial nerves are swollen and discoloured, histologically showing Schwann cell proliferation. They show degenerative changes in the myelin sheath and swelling and fragmentation of the axis cylinder.

Pigs: The clinical signs include rough, thin, and dry hair coat, ulceration of the skin at various places, particularly on the snout, ridging and thickness of the hoof wall, diarrhoea from catarrhal enteritis, mild anaemia. Eye lesions comprise conjunctivitis, oedema of the eyelids, vascularization of the cornea, and corneal opacities.

Niacin (Nicotinic acid)

Niacin is composed of nicotinic acid and nicotinamide. It is widely available in green grass, vegetables, grains, legumes and seed oils, but in much smaller quantity in meat and milk. Niacin can be obtained from diet, or may be synthesized endogenously from the amino acid tryptophan. In birds, only a small amount is synthesized from tryptophan. Most of it is synthesized by microbial action in the caeca and large intestine, **but as there is no absorption beyond small intestine, this is of limited value.**

Functions: In the form of nicotinic acid, it is **an essential component of two enzymes: nicotinamide adenine dinucleotide (NAD) and nicotinamide adenine dinucleotide phosphate (NADP)**, both of which have central roles in cellular intermediary metabolism. NAD functions as a coenzyme for a variety of dehydrogenases involved in the metabolism of fat, carbohydrate, and protein. NADP participates in a variety of dehydrogenation reactions, particularly in the hexose-monophosphate shunt of glucose metabolism.

Deficiency states: Niacin deficiency is important in the pig and dog. Both when fed on maize suffer, **because maize is deficient in niacin**. Maize is also deficient in **tryptophan**. Therefore, when maize is the main ingredient of the diet, there is niacin deficiency in the body. Since human pellagra (Italian pelle = skin; gra = rough) has a similar cause, the names **'swine pellagra'** and **'canine pellagra'** are applied to niacin-deficiency disease in animals. **Thus, pellagra may result from either a niacin or a tryptophan deficiency.**

Pig: In **young pigs**, the deficiency causes a type of nutritional deficiency. The pigs develop a chronic diarrhoea, have diminished appetite, become emaciated and anaemic, show dermatitis, and grow very poorly. There is severe degeneration of the colon and rectum. The mucosa may be invaded by *Salmonella choleraesuis*, *Fusobacterium necrophorum* (earlier *Sphaerophorus necrophorus*) and *Balantidium coli*, and develop diffuse necrotic enteritis.

Dog: Dogs develop a niacin deficiency disease called **blacktongue** or **'canine pellagra'**, characterized by cyanosis of the distal portion of the tongue, which in severe cases, makes it almost **black**. Petechial and ecchymotic haemorrhages and inflammation occur throughout the alimentary tract. The symptoms include anorexia, bloody diarrhoea, vomiting, emaciation, convulsions, fever from bacterial infection, and death.

Poultry: There is loss of appetite, poor growth, skin and feather disorders, inflammation of the oral cavity, dermatitis, poor feathering, and enlargement of the hock joints. In young growing birds, niacin deficiency can cause **chondrodystrophy**, a generalized disorder of the epiphyseal growth plates of long bones.

Pyridoxine (Vitamin B6)

Three naturally occurring substances: (1) pyridoxine, (2) pyridoxal, and (3) pyridoxamine possess vitamin B6 activity, **and are collectively referred to as pyridoxine**. All are equally active metabolically, and are converted in the tissues to the coenzyme form, pyridoxal 5-phosphate. Vitamin B6 is present in virtually all foods. It is abundant in most cereal grains, and therefore a deficiency is not likely to occur with normal rations.

Functions: Pyridoxine, as pyridoxal 5-phosphate coenzyme, participates as a cofactor for a large number of enzymes involved in transaminations, carboxylations, and deaminations in the metabolism of lipids and amino acids and in the immune response.

Deficiency states: **Pigs**: A severe microcytic anaemia is present. Dermatitis is also a constant feature. There is haemosiderosis of the spleen, liver, and bone marrow. Involvement of the central nervous system is manifested by a stiff jerky movement and convulsions. Peripheral nerves reveal demyelination and degeneration of the axis cylinder.

Other species: Ataxia (muscular incoordination) and convulsions are described in **puppies** and **calves**. In **kittens**, necrosis of renal tubular epithelium develops.

Poultry: Chicks show reduced appetite, weakness, poor feather growth, anaemia, inability to coordinate muscle movements (ataxia), chondrodystrophy, and death.

Pantothenic Acid

It has been referred to as vitamin B5 in USA, and also as **'chick anti-dermatitis factor'**. Pantothenic acid is an unstable hydroscopic oil (i.e., readily taking up and retaining moisture), and is widely distributed in plant and animal tissues. It is found in adequate amounts in most cereals, **but is deficient in maize**. Since pigs are fattened on maize, a deficiency is often a problem in this species.

Functions: It is an essential component of coenzyme A. Coenzyme A is a vital element of energy and participates in the metabolism of carbohydrate, fatty acids and amino acids, in antibody formation, and in the function of nerves. It is also precursor of cholesterol and thus of steroid hormones. Poultry do not benefit from its bacterial synthesis in the intestine.

Deficiency states: **Pigs**: The clinical signs are thin and rough hair coat, patchy alopecia, diarrhoea, muscular weakness, and jerky goosestep gait. The pigs eventually drag themselves with their forelegs. They develop catarrhal, haemorrhagic, and necrotic enteritis. Necrosis of neurons in the dorsal spinal ganglia and degeneration of myelin and axons in brachial and sciatic nerves result in an ataxic gait and terminal recumbency.

Poultry: There is loss of appetite and reduced growth, dermatitis with inflammatory changes in the corners of the beak and the eyelids, roughening, and loss of feathers. In breeders, there is lowered egg production and impaired hatchability, with embryo death in early, mid, or late incubation, depending on the extent of deficiency. Embryos are oedematous and haemorrhagic; those that hatch are stunted and weak. However, these signs have been determined mostly experimentally and pantothenic acid deficiency in poultry occurs rarely as a clinical condition in the field.

Biotin

Biotin is believed to be a member of vitamin B group. It is widely distributed in foods of plant and animal origin. Moreover, biotin is synthesized by microbial flora and so natural deficiency does not occur in animals, **except poultry**. In poultry, it is synthesized by bacteria in the caeca and large intestine. **Since the absorption is from the small intestine, this is of no use to the bird**. Moreover, in feed, much of the biotin is in a bound form and thus biologically unavailable to the bird. Also, the feed may contain biotin binders and antagonists, such as mycotoxins, mainly aflatoxin.

Functions: It is a cofactor (coenzyme) for several carboxylase enzymes; two of the most important being pyruvate carboxylase (gluconeogenesis), and (2) acetyl coenzyme A carboxylase (lipogenesis). **That is, biotin is essential in carbohydrate and lipid metabolism, as well as in protein synthesis.**

Deficiency states: In **poultry**, biotin deficiency leads clinically to reduced growth rate, and skin and sometimes bone lesions. In growing chicks, there is impaired feathering, dermatitis around the eyes, encrustations and fissures in the angles of the beak and eyelids and on the footpads and toes, growth depression, poor feathering, deformed **'parrot' beak**, and sometimes bone abnormality (**chondrodystrophy**). **Fatty liver and kidney syndrome (FLKS)** (see FLKS), a metabolic disorder causing death of young broilers and sometimes layer pullets, responds to biotin treatment. It is usually associated with diets that have marginal levels of biotin.

Folic Acid (Folacin)

It is also a member of vitamin B group, and is particularly abundant in green leaves, fresh vegetables, and fruits. Chemically, it is a complicated compound. Several related compounds with similar activity in amino acid metabolism are grouped under this heading. Folic acid is necessary for growth, muscle formation, blood formation, and feather growth. Diets are rarely low in this vitamin.

Functions: Folic acid is a part of the enzyme system involved in single carbon metabolism. It is involved in the synthesis of methyl groups (CH_3) of such important metabolites as choline, methionine, and thymine. **Folic acid is therefore required for cell mitosis.**

Deficiency states: In livestock, deficiency is important only in poultry. In birds, the clinical signs are poor appetite and growth, diarrhoea, a severe macrocytic megaloblastic anaemia, defective feather development, and chondrodystrophy,

Vitamin B12 (Cobalamin)

Vitamin B12 has the most complex structure of all the vitamins. It is abundant in all animal foods, including eggs, dairy products, **but plants and vegetables contain very little**. Ruminants do not require dietary source because it is synthesized by bacteria growing in the rumen. These bacteria require cobalt to produce vitamin B12. Lack of cobalt in the diet leads to vitamin B12 deficiency. However, the **deficiency is important only in poultry.**

Functions: Vitamin B12 is involved in the metabolism of protein, carbohydrate, and fat. In this action, it is closely associated with folic acid. Vitamin B12 is also involved in nucleic acid and methyl group synthesis, along with folic acid.

Deficiency states: **In poultry**, the deficiency is associated with slow growth, decreased efficiency of feed utilization, mortality, and reduced egg size and hatchability. Chondrodystrophy may occur in chicks when their diets lack choline and methionine as source of methyl groups. In laying birds, hatchability may drop to zero in about 6 weeks. Vitamin B12-deficient embryos have maximum mortality on the 7th day of incubation.

Choline

Choline is sometimes referred to as vitamin B4 or B7, and is at times classed as a necessary food substance rather than as a vitamin. It forms a part of the actual cell structure (in lecithin) and is therefore required in considerably greater quantities than vitamins. **The chick's requirement for choline is high**.

Functions: The primary role of choline is as a component of lecithin and other lipids. Lecithin is a main component of cell structure. As such, choline is needed for the structure of cell membranes. In tissues, choline forms the important neurotransmitter acetylcholine. Acetylcholine plays an important role in the transmission of nerve impulses in the body. It also acts as a **methyl donor. Choline has essential roles in fat metabolism. In liver, for transformation of neutral fat to phospholipids, choline is needed**. In choline deficiency, this transformation is interfered with and results in accumulation of neutral fat in the hepatic cell (**fatty change**). Choline is therefore called a **'lipotropic factor'** or **'lipotrope'**, because it promotes mobilization of lipids out of the liver. **Fatty livers** in **newborn pigs** and **calves** that have been deprived of colostrum may be due to choline deficiency. The choline requirements of these young animals are very high, and

485

colostrum is an excellent dietary source of choline.

Deficient states: Poultry: In chicks, apart from poor growth, the most important symptom of choline deficiency is **chondrodystrophy,** a bone disorder, earlier known as **'perosis'.** In egg-laying hens, choline deficiency causes fatty liver. In livers of chickens, **fat content is higher in females than males.**

Vitamin C

Vitamin C is abundant in green leafy plants, green vegetables, and fresh fruits. Citrus fruits contain the greatest amount of vitamin C. It is also present in milk and some animal products (liver, fish). **Most animals and birds synthesize sufficient amounts of vitamin C from glucose, because they possess the required enzyme gluconolactone oxidase.** Humans, monkeys, and guinea pigs lack this enzyme and therefore cannot synthesize this vitamin. In mammals, ascorbic acid is synthesized in the liver, but in the chicken, it is synthesized in the kidneys. Because domestic animals consume an abundance of green feed, and since they and poultry are capable of synthesizing vitamin C, a deficiency is seldom observed.

Functions: Ascorbic acid functions in a variety of biosynthetic pathways **by accelerating hydroxylation and amidation reactions.** The most clearly established function of vitamin C is the **activation of prolyl and lysyl hydroxylases from inactive precursors,** which in turn, **bring about hydroxylation of the amino acids proline and lysine,** respectively (see 'tissue repair (healing)'; Chapter 5). Collagen has the highest content of hydroxyproline in the body. Hydroxylation of proline and lysine imparts structural stability and tensile strength to collagen. Procollagen having unhydroxylated proline is unstable. Vitamin C also has **antioxidant properties.** Vitamin C can scavenge free radicals directly in aqueous phases of the cell and can act indirectly by regenerating the antioxidant form of vitamin E. **Thus, vitamin E and C act together.**

Deficiency states: Deficiencies are important in humans, monkeys, and guinea pigs. **In animals and birds, deficiency is seldom observed.** However, even the high rate of synthesis of **vitamin C in the chicken may be inadequate during periods of severe stress of heat and physical trauma, and in infections.** Also, there are no stores of vitamin C that are able to protect chicken against prolonged dietary deficiency. Moreover, in the chicken, vitamin C is not transported to the egg, but it is synthesized by the young embryo.

MINERAL DEFICIENCIES

A number of minerals are essential for health. The most important in the rations of domestic animals and poultry are calcium, phosphorus, sodium chloride, magnesium, iodine, iron, selenium, zinc, copper, and cobalt. Causes for the deficiency of minerals may be similar to those of vitamin deficiency, mentioned earlier. Their deficiency may result in various structural and functional changes in the body.

Calcium

Calcium is found in the soil and is absorbed by plants. The leaves and stems of plants contain an abundance of calcium, but grains are deficient. Calcium is the most common mineral in the body, and is required in the diet in a greater amount than any other mineral. About 99% of the body's calcium is in bones, with the remainder in extracellular fluid. Optimum serum calcium levels are maintained by the interaction of parathyroid hormone, thyrocalcitonin, and the active form of vitamin D.

Functions: Calcium is essential for the ossification of bone and calcification of cartilage. It gives not only bones their mechanical strength, but acts as a mineral reserve. Calcium has important functions as electrolyte in body fluids - calcium ions activating several hydrolytic enzymes, and acting in nerve cell excitation, neuromuscular transmission, muscular contractions, and blood clotting. VitaminD is necessary for its absorption from the intestine.

Deficiency states: The amount of calcium in the blood fluctuates between 10 and 11 mg per 100 ml (10-11 mg percent), depending on the species of animal. If this is reduced to 8 mg percent, tetany and incoordination result, and at 6 mg percent or lower, tetany, paralysis, coma and death occur. **Calcium deficiency (hypocalcaemia)** may occur from deficient dietary intake; disturbances in absorption due to diarrhoea, malabsorption, vitamin D deficiency; excessive excretion from kidneys; and parathyroid deficiency.

Normally, a balance exists between calcium in the blood and that in the bone. This balance is under the direct control of parathyroid and is closely associated with vitamin D. **The calcium content of the bones is in a state of constant flux (change) during both physiological and pathological conditions.** In deficiency, the reserve supply in the bones is withdrawn. This leads to softening of bones called **osteomalacia**. During pregnancy, large amounts of calcium are required. When the requirements are not met calcium is mobilized from bones, making them softer and softer. During lactation, the animal is prone to deficiency due to elimination of large amounts in milk. Again, calcium is removed from the bones. This may result in multiple fractures of the bones, their distortion, bowing of the legs, and abnormal curvatures of the back.

Milk fever (post-parturient paresis, parturient hypocalcaemia, eclampsia): It is a disorder of **dairy cows** and sometimes **sheep**. It occurs at or shortly after parturition, resulting from acute hypocalcaemia. A rapid depletion of calcium from the blood at the beginning of lactation in **cows**, and to a lesser extent in **ewes**, **goats**, **sows**, and **bitches**, may result in tetany, incoordination, muscular spasms, unconsciousness, and death. The animal lies with the head characteristically turned toward the flank. The condition is known as **milk fever**. It is especially common in **heavy milking cows**, particularly those not fed sufficient amount of calcium and phosphorus during pregnancy. Blood supply is regained by withdrawal from bones, for which parathyroid hormone is necessary. In animals suffering from milk fever, blood calcium is not regained because of low parathyroid activity, and therefore hypocalcaemia develops.

Poultry: When dietary supplies of calcium are inadequate, the skeleton is depleted. As a result, the young growing birds suffer from **rickets**, or **osteomalacia** leading to **osteoporosis** in adult or laying birds. Because sufficient calcium for eggshell production is no longer available, an early sign of calcium deficiency in the laying hen is the production of thin or soft-shelled eggs. **'Cage layer fatigue'** is seen in caged hens, which suddenly become recumbent (sometimes paralysed) with legs extended. **Excess of calcium**: Calcium in the ration must be in a definite proportion to phosphorus, for most species calcium: phosphorus ratio is 2:1. With excessive amount of calcium along with excessive amount of vitamin D, calcification of many tissues other than bone may occur throughout the body (see 'pathological calcification'). The calcium in the blood is already maintained in a supersaturated solution. If it exceeds 10 mg percent, it cannot be maintained in a supersaturation and is deposited. **In poultry**, excess calcium in the feed of young growing birds may give rise to nephropathy and visceral gout.

Phosphorus

In the bones and tissues, phosphorus and calcium are closely linked. Like calcium, most (about 80%) of the body's phosphorus is in bones, and disorders in phosphorus metabolism are reflected in skeletal disease similar to calcium or vitamin D deficiency. **Ruminants are most likely to suffer from phosphorus deficiency because roughages and forage plants are low in phosphorus.**

Functions: Phosphorus not only gives bones the mechanical strength, but also acts as a mineral reserve. Phosphate has important functions as electrolyte in body fluids. Phosphate is a component of nucleic acids, phospholipids, certain proteins, and coenzymes, as well as part of acid-base balance and other biochemical processes, such as metabolic energy transfer, protein synthesis, and carbohydrate metabolism.

Deficiency states: The clinical signs in **cattle** include poor growth and development, lamenesses of various types, bone diseases, reproductive disorders, and depressed appetites. In **dairy cows**, the quality of milk decreases and the period of lactation is shortened. Deficiency may cause **rickets** and **osteomalacia**, because phosphorus like calcium is replenished in the blood by reducing the amounts in the bone. Because cattle with depraved appetites chew bones or eat dirt to obtain phosphorus, the symptom is known as **pica**. However, pica is not a synonym for phosphorus deficiency. In fact, pica also occurs in other deficiencies (calcium, iron, salt, protein, etc.), or even from anaemia such as that caused by strongyle worms. In South Africa, a disease known as **lamsiekte** occurs in certain areas due to soil being deficient in phosphorus. The animals suffer from lameness (hence the name 'lamsiekte' = lame sickness), develop depraved appetites and chew bones of dead animals on the fields. Some of these bones have the toxins of *Clostridium botulinum* that thrive in the bones. Animals ingesting the toxins die of botulism.

In poultry, when dietary supplies of phosphorus are inadequate, the skeleton is depleted. As a result, the young growing birds suffer from rickets or osteomalacia, leading to osteoporosis in adults.

Excess of phosphorus: Concentrate feeds, particularly of **cottonseed meal and wheat bran, contain an abundance of phosphorus**. When too much phosphorus is present in the ration, the calcium phosphorus ratio is altered. To balance excessive amount of blood phosphorus (hyperphosphataemia), calcium is removed from the bone. This results in osteomalacia, and has been observed in **cattle** fed large amounts of cottonseed meal or cake. In **bran disease of horses** also, symptoms and lesions are those of osteomalacia; the jaw and limb bones are weakened. Hyperphosphataemia also occurs as the secondary effect of severe nephritis

Sodium Chloride

Sodium and chlorine ions in the body perform vital functions in the **maintenance of osmotic pressure and water and acid-base balance**. The sodium ion is the main cation of the extracellular fluid, and is involved in metabolic transfer across cell membranes and nerve impulse transmission. Chloride is a component of intra- and extracellular fluids and occurs as hydrochloric acid in gastric secretion. Deficiencies of these ions therefore produce widespread disturbances in cellular function and water distribution.

Deficiency states: Usually, with balanced diets salt deficiency does not occur. Carnivorous animals obtain sufficient sodium chloride from the animal tissues that they eat. **But sometimes in herbivore (horses, cattle, sheep, and goats) deficiency arises if ration is not supplemented by salt, since plants are usually deficient in this salt; they contain mainly potassium, not sodium. Deficiency may also occur in: (1) excessive vomiting and diarrhoea**. This may cause excessive loss of salt, which may lead to dehydration. Salt is lost because sodium chloride is present in secretions of the gastrointestinal tract; chlorine ions in the gastric juice and sodium ions in the intestinal secretions. (2) **excessive sweating. Horses** sweat profusely while at hard work during hot seasons and lose excessive amounts of sodium chloride. The resulting sodium chloride depletion causes the symptoms associated with heat exhaustion. (3) **excessive loss through milk**. This is observed in **sows** nursing large litters of pigs. Sows secrete a large amount of milk and thus lose considerable salt, and depletion occurs. The sows show anorexia, agalactia (absence of milk secretion after parturition), and loss of weight.

Clinical signs in **herbivore** include poor growth, general unthriftiness, rough coat, and poor reproduction. In **poultry**, signs are retarded growth, reduced egg production, dehydration, neuromuscular dysfunction, and death. Poultry feed must be supplemented to meet sodium requirements by adding common salt (sodium chloride). In **laying birds**, salt deficiency causes an abrupt fall in egg production and also increased pecking behaviour and intense cannibalism, especially at everted cloaca of the other bird.

Salt poisoning: This is important in **pigs** and **poultry**. The **pigs** have a catarrhal gastroenteritis and an eosinophilic meningo-encephalitis. In **poultry**, clinical signs include diarrhoea, excessive thirst, loss of appetite, progressive muscular weakness, inability to stand, convulsions, and death. Ascites may be present. Severe kidney damage occurs in young birds, with renal failure and death. Postmortem findings present visceral gout and ureters impacted with urates.

Magnesium

Magnesium is usually present in adequate amounts in the soil, water, and plants. About 70% of the body's magnesium is present, along with calcium and phosphorus, in bone. It is important in bone development and is also concerned with muscle contractability. Magnesium is essential for carbohydrate metabolism and for activation of a large number of enzymes. Eggshells contain about 0.4% magnesium.

Deficiency states: Two clinical syndromes are associated with hypomagnesaemia: (1) hypomagnesaemia in **calves**, and (2) grass tetany in **adult cattle**. Clinically, the two syndromes are similar, but differ in pathogenesis. **Hypomagnesaemia in calves** occurs in animals raised on a low magnesium diet, usually milk. Thus, the disease is due to a nutritional deficiency. Serum magnesium falls. Clinical signs comprise excitement, tetany, convulsions, and death. When **cattle**, **sheep**, and rarely **horses** are fed for some time exclusively on lush and succulent grasses, they suffer from tetanic convulsive seizures. The syndrome has been variously described as **grass tetany**, **grass-staggers**, or **wheat poisoning**, when apparently the cause is young growing wheat. The condition is characterized by **hypomagnesaemia**. **Cows** in advanced pregnancy and early lactation are first to show the symptoms. No postmortem lesions are seen, and the cause of the disease is not exactly known. High dietary intake of potassium by ruminants leads to reduced absorption of magnesium. Also consumption of forage, with high potassium content, inhibits the absorption of magnesium and can lead to hypomagnesaemia and tetany. In chicks, signs of magnesium deficiency include slow growth, dullness, brief convulsions, accompanied by gasping, and finally periods of coma, sometimes ending in death.

Manganese

Natural feeds contain an adequate amount of this mineral. Rice bran is a very good source of manganese. Small amounts of manganese are essential for several mechanisms of the body. However, deficiency of this element does not occur clinically except in birds. **Birds are much more susceptible to deficiency than mammals because their requirement is much higher (up to 100 times in some cases).** This is

491

due to **relatively poor duodenal absorption**. Absorption is inhibited also by excessive dietary calcium and phosphorus.

Functions: Manganese is an activator of several enzymes. It is necessary for formation of normal bones. Manganese deficiency interferes with the growth of bones. Manganese is also necessary for maximum eggshell quality, egg production, and hatchability.

Deficiency states: In **young growing birds**, growth is retarded and there is deformity of bone growth called **'chondrodystrophy'**, earlier known as **'perosis'**. However, apart from manganese, deficiency of choline, biotin, niacin, folic acid, zinc, and pyridoxine can cause chondrodystrophy. In **laying** or **breeder birds**, the eggshells become thin, porous, and soft, and the production falls with greatly reduced hatchability in incubated eggs. Embryos usually die, showing gross skeletal and other defects, including chondrodystrophy.

Iodine

Iodine is necessary for proper functioning of the thyroid gland. In thyroid, it is converted into the active principle of thyroid hormone, **thyroxine**. In some areas a deficiency of this element occurs in the soil, and therefore in the water and plants.

Deficiency states: Deficiency of iodine causes goitre. **Normal thyroid stores extremely small amounts of iodine**. A deficiency of iodine leads to a decrease in the iodine content of the thyroid, which in turn results in an enlargement of this gland (**simple goitre**). Goitre is a hyperplasia and hypertrophy of the thyroid gland. Newborns of mother deficient in iodine may suffer from goitre, alopecia, weakness, and high mortality. The thyroid gland in the foetus may be so enlarged that at parturition a dystocia results. In **poultry** iodine deficiency also results in goitre, and in some cases lower body weight in growing chicks. Other symptoms include mortality late in incubation. Embryo size is reduced and yolk sac resorption is retarded.

Iron

The soil usually contains adequate amounts of iron for the needs of animals. Absorption and excretion of iron occur through mucosal cells of the small intestine. Iron is stored in the form of either ferritin (a protein-iron complex) or haemosiderin, particularly in liver, spleen, bone marrow, and the skeletal muscles.

Deficiency states: Dietary deficiency of iron causes **anaemia**, which is **hypochromic** and **microcytic**. Deficiency means either the amount in the diet is inadequate, or absorption may be seriously impaired by long-standing diarrhoea. In **domestic animals, anaemia** due to insufficient iron is **seldom seen, except in baby pigs raised without access to the soil**. In the production of haemoglobin not only iron is necessary but also a minute quantity of copper. Since sow's milk does not contain iron or copper, baby pigs obtain it from soil. When raised on concrete or wooden floors, iron is not available, body's reserve is depleted, and anaemia occurs when pigs are about 21 days of age (**iron deficiency anaemia**). Pneumonia and enteritis are common in anaemic pigs. Excess of iron in humans causes a condition known as **haemochromatosis** (pigment cirrhosis), which is characterized by progressive accumulation of iron in the liver and its consequent damage.

In poultry, iron deficiency results in anaemia. A deficiency in laying hens also causes anaemia in the developing chick embryo and reduced hatchability.

Selenium

Selenium is an essential nutrient for animals and birds. Its deficiency may result from lack of selenium in soil, water, and feed.

Functions: Selenium is a component of the enzyme **glutathione peroxidase**, which like vitamin E, is involved in the removal of peroxides (free radicals) from the cells; and thus protects the cells against peroxidative damage (oxidative damage) of membrane lipids (see 'Vitamin E', and Chapter 3).

Deficiency states: Lack of dietary selenium limits production and function of **glutathione peroxidase**, leading to lipid hydroperoxide production in oxygen-laden cells with subsequent cell wall damage. The clinical effects include myopathy, microangiopathy, and capillary fragility. In **ruminants** and **pigs**, deficiency produces **muscular dystrophy (white muscle disease)**. In **poultry**, selenium deficiency leads to nutritional muscular dystrophy, exudative diathesis, and encephalomalacia (see 'Vitamin E').

Toxicity of selenium: Selenium is the most toxic of the trace minerals. Toxicity in animals may occur from eating plants containing a high percentage of selenium, when grown on selenium rich soils. **Acute toxicity** occurs in herbivorous animals, and is largely an acute congestive and enteric disease, with gastrointestinal symptoms and collapse from respiratory and cardiac failure. Lesions include haemorrhagic enteritis, congestion of lungs, and toxic changes in the

493

liver and kidneys. **Chronic toxicity** has been described under two syndromes: **'blind staggers'** and **'alkali disease'**. **Blind staggers occurs in cattle**. The animal tries to walk through obstacles and presses his head forward. Great weakness and paralysis occur, followed by dyspnoea, cyanosis, and death from respiratory failure. The second form **'alkali disease'** was once thought to be due to excessive ingestion of soil alkali (sodium carbonate, sulphate). However, it occurs from consumption of mildly seleniferous plants over a long period. It is characterized by falling hair on mane and tail (**bob-tail disease**), and malnutrition of the hoofs. Walking becomes difficult, and the animal may die from inability to get food and water. Lesions in both the syndromes are basically similar, and comprise necrosis in the heart muscle, oedema of the lungs, brain, and lymph nodes, hepatic damage, and mild gastroenteritis. Selenium may be deposited in the foetus and therefore malformations are common. In **poultry**, excess selenium interferes with sulphur metabolism due to the formation of sulphur-selenium complexes. This reduces protein synthesis. The developing embryo is particularly affected by high selenium.

Zinc

Zinc is an essential element for animals and poultry. It is abundant in plants (more in roots and stems than leaves), legumes, whole-grain cereals, meat, and fish. Zinc has a very large number of functions and **is an activator, or a cofactor, of more than 200 enzymes**. It is among the most metabolically active of the trace minerals. Zinc is required for skeletal growth and development, for epithelial tissue formation and maintenance, and for egg production. In animals, zinc affects growth, development, reproduction, and through its involvement in many enzymes, is concerned with almost every metabolic function.

Deficiency states: These **occur in pigs and poultry only**. A deficiency of zinc in **pigs** results in an imperfect keratinization (**parakeratosis**) of the skin. The disease occurs in pigs when excessive amounts of calcium and phosphorus are added to the ration in the form of mineral mixture. It is believed that excessive dietary calcium and phosphorus interfere with zinc absorption. Calcium in the presence of phytic acid or phosphate forms an insoluble complex with zinc, making it unavailable for absorption. The affected animals are young and show circumscribed erythematous areas, particularly in the skin of the abdomen and thighs. In **poultry**, deficiency gives rise to poor growth and appetite, poor feathering, scaly skin especially on the legs and feet, and in young growing birds chondrodystrophy. Egg production is reduced and hatchability is impaired. Embryonic mortality is highest around mid-incubation. **Recently it has been revealed that zinc deficiency affects immunocompetence of the birds.** For example, chickens maintained on a zinc-deficient diet are unable to produce antibodies against T-cell-dependent antigens, even though lymphocytes are capable of antibody production.

Copper

Copper is found in adequate amounts in most soils, but there are areas where copper deficiencies exist. **Cattle** and **sheep** grazed on poorer land suffer. Trace amounts of copper are critical to health, but an excess is harmful.

Functions: Copper functions as a trace mineral in a number of ways: (1) Copper is a component of many enzymes that participate in redox (oxidation-reduction) reactions. (2) Copper is essential for formation of haemoglobin. In the absence of copper, although dietary iron is absorbed and deposited in the liver, haemoglobin synthesis does not occur. Copper is necessary for iron utilization when haemoglobin is formed. Therefore, when absent from the diet, anaemia results. (3) Most of the blood copper is found as a component of **ceruloplasmin**, a copper-binding protein with enzymatic activity. Ceruloplasmin is necessary for iron transport and also plays a role in the acute phase of the immune response. It protects the bird by reducing the formation of free radicals. (4) Copper and its enzymes are also involved in **myelin synthesis** or its maintenance. Therefore, impaired myelination is seen in animals with a lack of copper. (5) Copper is critical to the function of several central nervous system enzymes. (6) The copper metalloenzyme - **lysyl oxidase** - is required for the formation of cross-linkage in elastin and collagen (see 'tissue repair (healing)', Chapter 5). Copper deficiency may cause impairment of vascular integrity and skeletal growth and maintenance, and (7) Tyrosinase is a copper-dependent enzyme and with its deficiency little or no melanin is produced.

Deficiency states: As discussed, minute amounts of copper are essential for the utilization of iron in haematopoiesis. Thus, anaemia usually occurs in copper deficiency and is mostly microcytic hypochromic. Other clinical signs include unthriftiness, and disorders of hair and central nervous system. **Baby pigs**, raised on wooden or concrete floors and thus deprived of soil, suffer from **severe anaemia**.

Sow's milk does not contain copper and the copper reserves of the baby pigs become depleted in about three months.

In **sheep**, a disorder characterized by changes in hair and wool has been described as **steely wool**. The wool becomes more hair-like. Disorders of the central nervous system also follow copper deficiency. In England and Australia, **sheep**, sometimes **goat**, suffer from a disease called **enzootic ataxia** or **swayback**, characterized by incoordination and weakness of the hind legs. Spastic paralysis and sometimes blindness occur. The lesions are most pronounced in **newborn lambs**, and consist of demyelination and extensive softening and necrosis in cerebral hemispheres. A disease also due to copper deficiency in Australia and USA is known as **'falling disease'**, because the cows fall and die suddenly. Anaemia and loss of weight occur. Copper deficiency may also result in extensive skeletal changes.

In poultry, copper deficiency symptoms include anaemia, haemorrhages, lameness, and poor feather pigmentation. Anaemia is due to low levels of ceruloplasmin, which causes poor iron utilization. In **laying hens**, deficiency of copper causes reduced egg production, infertile eggs, increased egg size, and abnormal eggshell calcification. Eggshell abnormalities include shell-less eggs, misshapen eggs, wrinkled eggshells, and reduced eggshell thickness.

Excess of copper: Acute copper poisoning may occur in **sheep** from drenching copper sulphate for stomach worms. Copper sulphate causes severe gastritis and enteritis, and death. **In poultry**, signs of poisoning are depression, convulsions, coma, and death in severe cases.

Cobalt

Cobalt is necessary in ruminants only, and is usually provided by soil and plants that grow upon it. Cobalt is essential for the maintenance of normal rumen flora. Since cobalt is an important constituent of vitamin B12, and since vitamin B12 is synthesized by rumen flora, cobalt deficiency is harmful to the bacteria preventing their growth that, in turn, leads to a vitamin B12 deficiency. Vitamin B12 is essential for erythropoiesis.

Deficiency states: **Deficiency of cobalt, and therefore of vitamin B12, results in anaemia.** Dairy cattle lose their appetites, become progressively emaciated and weak, hair coat becomes rough, waste away, and die. Blood examination reveals anaemia. The disease has been variously named as **'hill sickness'** in New Zealand, **'wasting**

disease' and 'enzootic marasmus' in Australia, 'pine' in England (because animals pine away and die), and 'Grand Traverse disease' in USA.

Fluorine

Fluorine is found in the soil and is made available to animals through water and plants. **There is no evidence to indicate that fluorine deficiency is an important problem in domestic animals and poultry,** although it is generally accepted that fluorine is an essential nutrient in the development of teeth and bones, if normal hardness is to be attained. On the other hand, it is the fluorine poisoning which is more important.

Fluorine poisoning (fluorosis): Fluorosis may occur when the water or vegetation consumed by the animals comes from soil that contains an abundance of fluorine, or when rock phosphate, which contains considerable fluorine is fed to animals to correct phosphorus deficiency. Rock phosphate is used because it is cheap, while bonemeal, the usual source, is very expensive. Fluorosis may occur in chronic or acute forms, and is characterized by **lesions in bone and teeth**. **Chronic poisoning** occurs over a long period of time and the lesions include enamel defects in teeth. Teeth show 'chalky' areas, and 'mottling'. Once the teeth are formed, they are not affected by excessive amounts of fluorine. The bones become shorter, thicker, heavier, and broader than normal, the marrow cavity being diminished in size. The bones may be hard with exostoses, or may show osteomalacia and osteoporosis. Due to bone changes, lameness and stiffness are often observed. **Acute poisoning** may occur when sodium fluoride is administered to **pigs** and **poultry** to control ectoparasites and endoparasites. Sodium monofluoroacetate (a rat poison) can also pose a serious problem, when eaten by domestic animals, particularly dogs. It produces repeated attacks of excitement, vomiting, and convulsions, leading eventually to death.

Other Nutritional Diseases

Ketosis (Ketonaemia)

Ketosis, also known as **ketonaemia,** is a condition in which 'ketone bodies' appear in the blood, and from there in the urine. The ketone bodies are acetone, acetoacetic acid, and beta-hydroxybutyric acid. Ketosis, in all species, develops in response to a decrease in the availability of blood glucose, whether from hypoglycaemia or inability

497

to utilize glucose as in diabetes mellitus. To compensate for the lack of glucose, oxidation of fatty acids provides an alternative source of energy. This is accompanied by production of ketone bodies, which serve as a source of cellular energy.

Causes: The usual cause in animals is **starvation**. Other causes include diabetes mellitus, because of an inability to utilize glucose, and pregnancy and lactation, which place an increased demand for glucose. The animal then derives necessary energy by oxidation of its stored fats, and later proteins of the muscles. In **cattle**, it may also result from loss of appetite and failure to eat, from some other disorder like ruminal indigestion or atony. Digestive disorders that prevent assimilation cause it in any species. Thus ketosis, whether in **cattle** or **monogastric animals** is termed **primary nutritional ketosis** (simple starvation) and **secondary ketosis** (starvation on account of some other disease).

Symptoms: These include anorexia, depression, and terminal coma. The animal often has a sickly sweet smell derived from ketone bodies. **Lesions**: Lesions are mainly chemical. The ketone bodies are detected in the blood by appropriate tests. But the usual procedure is a test for acetone in the urine. If this is strongly positive, it can be assumed that acetoacetic acid and beta-hydroxybutyric acid are also present. In **cows**, it is convenient to test milk for acetone than the urine. There is also **hyperlipaemia** and this leads to accumulation of neutral fat in the hepatocytes, that is, fatty change. **Acidosis**, a depletion of the body's reserve for alkali ions, results from neutralization of the two ketone acids. **Hypoglycaemia** and a reduction in hepatic glycogen are also consistent findings in bovine ketosis.

Pregnancy Toxaemia of Ewes

Also known as **'pregnant ewe paralysis'**, it is a good example of ketosis. It occurs only in the last weeks of pregnancy and usually in ewes carrying twins or triplets. The **causes** are a combination of toxic waste products of mother and foetuses, plus those dietary factors that cause ketosis. Sometimes these are plain starvation. The **symptoms** include depression, sleepiness, and coma, but not true paralysis. The disease is usually fatal in a few days. The **lesions** are severe fatty change in the liver, kidneys, and heart (ketosis) with terminal subepicardial petechiae and ecchymoses (toxaemia).

Fatty Liver-Haemorrhagic Syndrome

This is a metabolic disorder characterized by a very fatty liver, accompanied by haemorrhages. The condition is sometimes seen in **older laying hens** kept in cages, particularly in hot weather. There is usually a fall in egg production in the affected flock. Death occurs occasionally and is due to massive liver haemorrhages.

Pathogenesis: **There are important basic differences in carbohydrate and fat metabolism between birds and mammals.** Birds have several times (3-4 times) higher blood glucose levels than mammals. Mammalian embryos obtain glucose through the placental circulation, whereas the chicken embryo develops on yolk nutrients, the energy source being almost all fat, not carbohydrate. The chicken embryo therefore has high levels of gluconeogenic enzymes, that is, enzymes that form glucose from substances other than carbohydrates, such as proteins and fats. These enzymes decrease after hatching as carbohydrate intake becomes available. Moreover, in contrast to mammals, where lipogenesis (fat formation) is mostly in adipose tissue, in birds, it almost all occurs in the liver. Fat formation increases in the first week or two after hatching from almost zero in the embryo (due to high yolk fat content) to much higher levels. As chickens reach sexual maturity and start laying, there is a further great increase in liver lipogenesis. The laying hens then attain high blood lipid levels to supply the developing ova, and the storage of fat in the liver enormously increases at this time.

It is this lipogenic function of liver in the birds that forms basis for the occurrence of conditions that involve excessive accumulation of fat in the liver, for example, **fatty liver and kidney syndrome (FLKS) in young broiler birds and fatty liver-haemorrhagic syndrome (FLHS) in older laying hens**. FLHS is characterized by pronounced fatty liver accompanied by haemorrhages. It occurs sporadically in older caged hens of heavier breeds in hot weather. There is usually a drop in egg production. The fat content of liver is usually greater than 40% dry weight and may reach 70%. Death only occasionally occurs and is due to massive liver haemorrhage. The kidneys are pale and swollen, and the abdomen contains large accumulation of fat. The exact cause of FLHS is not known, but **contributory factors** include high carbohydrate and low-fat feed leading to **fattiness**; lack of exercise, for example, in caged birds; stress, toxins, high egg production, high oestrogen, low thyroid blood hormone levels; and strain of bird. **Microscopically**, hepatocytes are greatly distended with fat globules, which eventually rupture cell

499

membranes. There is also secondary inflammation, necrosis, and regeneration.

Fatty Liver and Kidney Syndrome

Fatty liver and kidney syndrome (FLKS) is a metabolic disorder **causing death of young broilers**, and sometimes growers (pullets) between 10-30 days of age. It is usually associated with diets that have **marginal levels of biotin.**

Pathogenesis: FLKS arises **from a failure of hepatic gluconeogenesis** (metabolic synthesis of glucose from fat) and results in extensive fatty infiltration of body tissues with enlarged liver, kidneys, and heart, but not inflammatory or degenerative changes. Decreased hepatic gluconeogenesis is caused by decreased pyruvate carboxylase activity, and this leads to severe hypoglycaemia. Biotin is a cofactor for both pyruvate carboxylase (gluconeogenesis) and acetyl CoA carboxylase (lipogenesis). High-fat feed decreases the need for lipogenesis (and, therefore, for biotin by acetyl CoA carboxylase), so that biotin is available for pyruvate carboxylase and gluconeogenesis. However, on low-fat feed, there is insufficient biotin for both the enzymes, but acetyl CoA carboxylase has a greater access to biotin than pyruvate carboxylase. This means that fat formation (lipogenesis) will continue, but glucose formation (gluconeogenesis) will suffer. Therefore, if normal fat intake is interrupted for even a short period of time, **hypoglycaemia develops**, and may become serious due to low glycogen reserves of the young chick. In response to the low blood glucose level, there is mobilization of free fatty acids into the liver, from body tissues, for fat formation. The purpose being that fat so formed can be utilized to produce glucose to correct the low blood level. However, as pyruvate carboxylase is a biotin-containing enzyme, its activity is decreased in biotin deficiency. **Biotin deficiency** therefore prevents conversion of fat into glucose. This leads to increased conversion of pyruvate to fatty acids. **The net result is marked accumulation of fat in the liver.**

Clinical signs are sudden in onset. Well-grown birds become dull and depressed, lose appetite, lie down, and may die. Mortality may range between 5-30%. **Postmortem findings** include enlarged, pale, fat-rich liver and kidneys, and pink adipose tissue due to congestion of blood vessels. Crop and intestine usually contain blackish fluid due to blood content. The paleness of the liver and kidneys is due to the presence of excessive amount of fat (two to four times the normal). This is mostly **triglycerides (neutral fat).**

500

Chapter 11
Physical and Chemical Injuries

(A) Injury by Physical Agents

Injury caused by physical agents is divided into: (1) physical influences, (2) thermal injury, (3) injuries due to light, (4) electrical injury, (5) injuries from changes in atmospheric pressure, and (6) injury produced by ionizing radiation.

1. Physical Influences

Physical influences of a mechanical nature can injure the body in four ways: (i) mechanical trauma, (ii) pressure, (iii) obstruction, and (iv) malposition.

(i) Mechanical Trauma

Mechanical forces may inflict damage in several forms. The type of injury depends on the shape of the striking object, the amount of energy discharged at impact, and the tissue or organs that bear the impact. If large vessels are cut or pulled apart, severe haemorrhage occurs which may cause death. When the injury is located internally, the blood collects in the body cavities or in hollow organs. **Shock** may follow severe injury. **Bacterial infection** of the site is a common complication of traumatic injury. One of the most common causes of mechanical injury is automobile accidents. All soft tissues react similarly to mechanical forces, and the pattern of injury can be as follows:

Abrasion: An abrasion is a wound produced by scraping or rubbing, resulting in removal of the superficial layer. Skin abrasions may remove only the epidermal layer.

Contusion: A contusion, or **bruise**, is a wound usually produced by a blunt object. The skin is not broken but the underlying tissues are injured. Contusion is characterized by damage to blood vessels and escape of blood into tissues.

Laceration: A laceration is a pulling apart (tear) or disruptive stretching of tissue caused by the force of a blunt object. In contrast to an incision, most lacerations have intact bridging blood vessels and irregular edges.

Incised wound: Incised wound is a long, narrow, clean wound produced by a sharp object, such as a knife. Tissue damage is minimal, but the bridging blood vessels are cut.

Puncture wound: A puncture wound is caused by a long narrow instrument. It is called **'penetrating'** when the instrument pierces the tissue, and **'perforating'** when it passes through a tissue and creates an exit wound. For example, the type of wound produced by a bullet or nail.

Rupture: Is an injury in which the tissues are stretched until the fibres break. It is caused by a severe crushing blow or excessive distension.

Fracture: A fracture is an injury of bone, cartilage, tooth, hoof, horn, or claw in which the continuity of the hard structure is broken.

Concussion: Is a term used to describe a functional disturbance of the central nervous system, which may or may not be associated with loss of consciousness following severe injury to head.

Sprain or strain: Is an injury of a joint in which the supporting ligaments around the joint, have been stretched or torn slightly.

Luxation or dislocation: Is an injury of a joint in which the anatomical relation of the bony structure is not maintained and ligaments supporting the joint are torn.

(ii) **Injuries due to Pressure**

A pressure injury is caused by a less violent physical force acting over a considerable period of time. If the pressure is extended slowly over a long time, the main tissue alteration is **atrophy**. Lesions of this type are seen near tumours, abscesses, and cysts. When animals are recumbent and certain points (stifle, wing of the ileum, point of the shoulder, or wherever bone is close to the surface of the body) are pressed against the floor or the bedding, ischaemia occurs and the tissue dies. These focal areas of necrosis are known as **bed sores**.

(iii) **Injuries due to Obstruction**

An obstruction is the type of mechanical injury produced when the lumen of a hollow organ is closed and the normal flow of fluids through the part is prevented. Some of the obstructions arise from foreign bodies, such as concretions (hair balls in the intestine, calculi in the ureters), parasites (lungworms in the bronchi, roundworms in the bile ducts of pigs), objects that enter by accident (rubber ball in dog's stomach), objects that are introduced by someone (broken urinary catheter), or ones that are aspirated into the respiratory passages (feed, water, exudates, and medicine). Their presence may lead to **stenosis** (narrowing) of the lumen of the organ from inflammation and the contracting scar tissue. The stenosis caused by connective tissue is called a **stricture**.

(iv) Injuries due to Malposition

Through physical influences the position of organs, or parts of the body, may become displaced. Among the malposition of this nature are:

Volvulus: Is rotation of small intestine around its mesenteric attachment.

Torsion: Is a twisting of an organ upon itself as occurs with the large intestine of the horse, or the uterus of a cow.

Intussusception: Is a telescoping or invagination of one portion of the intestine into immediately posterior portion of the gut.

Prolapse: Is the appearance of an organ, or a portion of an organ, at a natural or artificial body opening.

Eversion: When the rectum turns inside out and protrudes through the anus, or when the vagina turns inside out and protrudes through the vulva, the malposition is called an eversion.

Eventration: When a portion of the intestine or other organ protrudes through a tear in the ventral abdominal wall, the protrusion of the viscera is called an eventration. It may be produced by a horn thrust.

Hernia: Is the protrusion of an organ, or a part of an organ, through the wall of the cavity, which normally contains it, e.g., inguinal, ventral, umbilical, or diaphragmatic hernia.

2. Thermal Injury

Both excess heat and excess cold are important causes of injury.

Excess Heat

Heat produces varying degrees of injury, depending on its intensity and duration, and the percentage of total body surface involved. A lesion produced from excessive application of heat is called a **thermal burn**, whereas excessive heat retention results in **heat stroke**.

Thermal burns: These are of **two types**: (i) **surface burns**, and (ii) **inhalation burn injuries** (internal thermal injury).

(i) Surface burns: The size of the burn and its depth are of critical importance. Any burn exceeding 50% of the total body surface, whether superficial or deep, is grave; and when it exceeds 70%, very often fatal. The depth of the burn modifies this outlook. To express depth two terms are used: **full-thickness burn** and **partial-thickness burn**. **Full-thickness burn** involves total destruction of the entire skin, with loss of the dermal appendages. As a result, no epithelial regeneration can occur except from the margin. The full-thickness burn may extend deep into the underlying muscles, viscera, and even bone, but with such penetration, death is often immediate. Both third and fourth-degree burns are in this category.

In **partial-thickness burn**, at least the deeper portions of the dermal appendages are spared. Partial-thickness burns imply a low intensity heat, and include first-degree burns (epithelial involvement only) and second-degree burns (involving both epidermis and superficial dermis). The area becomes reddened as small blood vessels dilate, This is soon followed by increased vascular permeability with exudation of serous or protein-rich fluid, creating the typical 'burn blister'. **Microscopically**, devitalized tissue shows coagulative necrosis. Nearby vital tissue quickly develops inflammatory changes with an accumulation of inflammatory cells and marked exudation.

(ii) Inhalation burn injuries (internal thermal injuries): Animals trapped in a burning building, who inhale heated air and noxious gases in the smoke may develop **inhalation injury** at any level of the respiratory tract from nose and mouth to the lungs. Water-soluble gases such as chlorine, sulphur oxides, and ammonia, may react with water to form acids or alkalies, particularly in the upper airways, and thus produce inflammation and swelling, which may lead to partial or complete airway obstruction. Lipid-soluble gases, such as nitrous oxide and products of burning plastics, are more likely to reach deeper airways, producing pulmonary oedema and bronchopneumonia from secondary infection. Unlike shock, which develops within hours, pulmonary manifestations may not develop for 24 to 48 hours.

Grading of burns: Burns are graded according to the extent of damage produced. **(1) First-degree burn**: There is simply reddening of skin due to hyperaemia or erythema and mild inflammatory reaction. This is followed later by a slight peeling of the superficial layers of the skin. **(2) Second-degree burn** is characterized by the formation of a **blister** (or **vesicle**). The epidermis appears coagulated (coagulative necrosis) and there is also inflammation. There is much destruction of epidermis, but living cells around and beneath it regenerate and fill the gap, so that complete recovery soon occurs. **(3) Third-degree burn**: There is complete necrosis and severe inflammation. The dead tissue sloughs, leaving an ulcer that heals slowly by granulation tissue formation. It later shrinks and leaves a scar. **(4) Fourth-degree burn**: The tissue is completely charred and blackened.

Significance and results: If burns are extensive, involving one-fourth to one-third of the body surface, then even if only a first- or second-degree burn is present, death occurs within 24 hours; and in most severe burns, even within an hour. The animal shows difficult respiration, fall in blood pressure and body temperature - symptoms of hypovolaemic shock (see 'shock', Chapter 6). With burns of more than 30 to 40% of the body surface, shock is the most life-threatening complication.

Organ system failure from **burn sepsis (septicaemia)** is the main source of death in burned patients. The burn site is ideal for the growth of microorganisms; the serum and debris provide nutrients, and the burn injury impairs blood flow, blocking effective inflammatory responses. Moreover, cellular and humoral defences against infections are damaged. Both lymphocyte and phagocytic functions are impaired.

Heat stroke: Animals react differently to increasing environmental temperatures than do humans. In **humans**, body temperature and rate of breathing are little affected but the pulse rate increases, whereas in animals the immediate effect is a rise in body temperature, while pulse rate is little affected. Humans tolerate heat better because their heat-dissipating mechanism from the skin is most efficient. **Most animals**, on the other hand, depend on cooling by evaporation from the **respiratory tract**. To increase heat loss many of them resort to panting. Ventilation from the tongue increases the rate of evaporation. It is believed that the blood flow in the tongue of dog increases six times during hyperthermia (i.e., prolonged exposure to elevated ambient temperature).

Heat stroke is associated with high ambient (surrounding) temperatures and high humidity. Thermoregulatory mechanisms fail, sweating ceases, and core body temperature rises. The early symptoms are dullness and depression, staggering, palpitation of the heart, rapid and weak pulse, difficult respiration, and rise in temperature. The

505

animal trembles, later falls, and dies in convulsions. Necrosis of the muscles and myocardium may occur. The postmortem changes are not particularly characteristic, and are indicative of circulatory failure and shock.

Excess Cold

The effects of hypothermia (prolonged exposure to low ambient temperature) depend on whether there is whole body exposure, or exposure only of parts. Death may result when the whole body is exposed, without causing necrosis of cells or tissues. This is because the systemic homeostatic mechanisms are more vulnerable to hypothermia than are individual cells.

Local effects: The local effects of low temperatures vary according to the duration and degree of cold. **Chilling** or **freezing** of cells and tissues, causes injury in two ways: **(i) Direct-effects**: Upon freezing, water within the cell and outside undergoes crystallization. This results in high salt concentrations inside the cell. Moreover, the ice crystals cause physical dislocations within cells. Together, they produce direct effects. **(ii) Indirect effects**: These are exerted by circulatory changes. With slowly developing chilling, first there is vasoconstriction and increased vascular permeability causing oedematous changes. Atrophy and fibrosis may follow. With sudden sharp drops in temperature, the vasoconstriction and increased viscosity of the blood in the local area may cause ischaemic injury and degenerative changes in peripheral nerves. Ischaemia, in turn, causes hypoxic changes and infarction (coagulative necrosis) of the affected tissues. The dead or necrotic areas are sharply demarcated from healthy tissue. This dead tissue may later become dehydrated (dry necrosis), or may putrefy from invasion by saprophytic bacteria (gangrene). Local freezing (**frostbite**) is usually confined to the extremities, e.g., feet, teats, scrotum, tails, fetlocks, pasterns and coronary bands; combs, wattles, and toes of fowl.

Systemic effects: Cooling of the peripheral blood soon causes depression of the body temperature in the vital organs with slowing of metabolic processes, particularly in the brain. The usual cause of death appears to be circulatory failure. Sudden acute chilling may cause death in a short time without producing tissue changes.

3. Injuries due to Light

In general, domestic animals do not suffer from **sunburn**. Most animals have heavily pigmented skin. Moreover, animals are usually covered with hair, feathers, or wool that protect them from sun's rays. However, when animals do show an unusual reaction to sun's rays, the phenomenon is called **photosensitization** or **light sickness**. It occurs in domestic animals and can be a serious problem.

Photosensitization

There are several substances called **photodynamic pigments** or **agents** that, when present, make tissues more sensitive to light. This is because they absorb certain wavelengths in sunlight. Photosensitization occurs when ultraviolet light or sometimes, even visible light, is absorbed by a photodynamic pigment in the skin. This results in activation of the photodynamic agent, producing necrosis and oedema of exposed tissues in all species of domestic animals. Skin lesions are limited to hairless skin, and to lightly or non-pigmented areas of skin.

Photosensitization usually involves teats, udder, ears, and eyelids in cows, and ears, eyelids, lips, and coronets in sheep. Sunburn is a reaction of unprotected skin produced by ultraviolet radiation of wavelengths shorter than 320 μm. The wavelengths involved in photosensitization usually lie in the range of 540 to 600 μm. Since these longer light waves readily pass through ordinary window glass, sensitized animals may develop characteristic lesions if exposed to sunlight naturally, or even through glass.

Diseases resulting from photosensitization are classified into **three types**, based on the origin of photodynamic agent, or the means by which it reaches the peripheral circulation.

(i) Primary photosensitization: This is due to the ingestion of **preformed** (already formed) photodynamic agents present in a variety of plants, when the plant is in the lush green stage and is growing rapidly. The photodynamic agent is deposited in tissues following its absorption into the blood after ingestion. When such animals are exposed to sunlight, photosensitization occurs. Animals are affected within 4-5 days of going onto pasture. Administration of phenothiazine, tetracycline, and sulphonamides also may cause primary sensitization.

(ii) Photosensitization from abnormal porphyrin metabolism: Porphyrins are pigments normally present in haemoglobin. In a disease called **congenital porphyria**, there is excessive production of two porphyrins in the body, which are themselves photodynamic. It is a metabolic disorder that occurs in several species, including **cattle** and

507

cats. The two porphyrins include uroporphyrin and coproporphyrin. Uroporphyrin is deposited in bones (**osteohaemochromatosis**) and teeth (**pink tooth**) and causes discoloration of these tissues.

(iii) **Hepatogenous (hepatotoxic) photosensitization**: This type results from a hepatic disease, which interferes with normal excretion in the bile of phylloerythrin. **Phylloerythrin** is a normal end-product of chlorophyll metabolism, contained in ingested plants, and **is a photodynamic agent**. When biliary excretion is obstructed by a hepatic disease, phylloerythrin accumulates in the body and may reach levels in the skin which make skin sensitive to light. Hepatogenous photosensitization is more common in animals grazing green pasture, but can occur in animals fed entirely on hay or other stored feeds. A large number of plants containing hepatotoxins, chemicals such as poisoning with carbon tetrachloride, and infectious diseases such as leptospirosis, are common causes of hepatogenous photosensitization.

4. Electrical Injury

Electrical injuries can arise from **low-voltage currents, high-voltage currents** from high-power lines, or **lightning. Injuries are of two types: (i) burns**, and (ii) **cardiac or respiratory arrest** resulting from disruption of normal electrical impulses. The type of injury and the severity and extent of burning depend on the amperage (strength of current expressed in amperes) and path of the electric current within the body. Animals may come in contact with high-tension wires torn from severe wind or storm. The effects of electrical currents and lightning are the same, except that in lightning, there are usually **lightning marks** or **figures** that are either tree-shaped, branching, or as reddish or reddish-blue streaks on the skin.

Severe electric shock usually causes death (**electrocution**). If the current is continuously applied, the muscles gradually relax and the animal is dead in less than a minute. Local effects may be absent, or at these places the skin and subcutaneous tissues show deep burns. General effects comprise pinpoint haemorrhages on the serous membrane of the internal organs. If the animal lives after electrical shock, there may be pulmonary oedema and dilatation of the right side of the heart. The blood is black and liquefied. Blood vessels, being good conductors of electricity, are severely injured. Some are ruptured, while others contain thrombi. **Death is from cardiac and respiratory failure.**

5. Injuries from Changes in Atmospheric Pressure

In general, the body withstands increases of pressure better than decreases. Changes in atmospheric pressure cause injuries in **three ways**: **(i)** with sudden decrease in pressure, free gaseous bubbles may be released in the blood and act as emboli; already described as **caisson disease** (see 'air or gas emboli'), **(ii)** in low atmospheric pressures, lowered oxygen tension in the inspired air causes systemic hypoxia as seen in high altitude reactions. In animals, it occurs as **brisket disease ('high-altitude illness'** in humans), and **(iii)** sudden increases or decreases of pressure may produce mechanical damage.

Brisket disease: When animals are moved from lower altitudes, where they have been raised, to an altitude of 8,000 feet or more, they suffer from **brisket disease**. In response to the lowered atmospheric pressure and the associated deficiency of oxygen, respiration is increased due to systemic hypoxia. This increases the cardiac function. The myocardium of the right side increases in thickness (hypertrophy) and later undergoes dilatation. Eventually, general passive hyperaemia occurs and causes oedema in the body cavities and in the subcutaneous connective tissue, particularly of the **brisket** (hence the name), the throat region, the neck, and the legs. Death may occur from cardiac exhaustion within 1-3 months.

6. Injury produced by Ionizing Radiation

Ionizing radiation occurs in **two forms**: **(1) electromagnetic waves** (x-rays and gamma rays), and **(2) high-energy neutrons and charged particles** (alpha and beta particles and protons). All types of ionizing radiation exert their effects on cells by displacing electrons from molecules and atoms with which they collide (strike). This causes ionization and induces a sequence of events that may alter the cell temporarily or permanently. **The most important target in living cells is DNA**. Ionizing radiation may directly damage DNA (**direct target theory**), but more often it indirectly damages DNA by inducing formation of **free radicals**, particularly those that form from the radiolysis of water (**indirect target theory**). Radiolysis is chemical decomposition by the action of radiation.

Absorbed radiant energy leads to **radiolysis** of cell water and formation of the ionized water molecules H_2O^+ and H_2O^-. These dissociate to form the free radicals $H^{\cdot}$ and $OH^{\cdot}$ (see 'free radical-induced cell injury'), which in turn initiate a chain of reactions with themselves, their own reaction products, and tissue water to form

509

other reactive radicals, such as $H_2O_2^\bullet$ and $HO_2^\bullet$ (latter is perhydroxyl radical). Ultimately, these free radicals interact with critical cell components, among which lipids in cell membranes, DNA, and proteins that function as critical enzymes, are the most important. In this manner, a crucial biochemical change takes place, causing inhibition of cell division or cell death. The transfer of energy to a target atom or molecule occurs within microfractions of a second, yet its harmful effect may not become apparent for minutes, and if the effect is on DNA, for even decades.

The biological effects of radiation depend on the following factors:

1. Since the primary target of ionizing radiation is DNA, rapidly dividing cells are more vulnerable to injury. During mitosis, cells that incur irreparable DNA damage die, because chromosome abnormalities prevent normal division. Therefore, **tissues with a high rate of cell turnover, such as bone marrow, lymphoid tissue, and mucosa of the gastrointestinal tract, are extremely vulnerable to radiation**. Tissues with slower turnover rates, such as liver and endothelium are not affected immediately, but are depopulated slowly, because cell division is interrupted. Tissues with non-dividing cells, such as brain and heart, do not show radiation effects except at doses that are very high.

2. Since tissues are made up of many types of cells, the effects of radiation are complex. For example, vascular injury can cause changes that interfere with repair. Endothelial cells, which are moderately sensitive to radiation, may be damaged. This results in narrowing or occlusion of the blood vessels, which may lead to impaired healing.

3. The rate of delivery modifies the biological effect. Although the effect of radiant energy is cumulative, delivery in divided doses allows cells to repair some of the damage in the intervals. **Radiotherapy of tumours** explains the fact that normal cells are capable of more rapid repair and recovery than tumour cells, and therefore do not sustain as much cumulative radiation damage.

4. Radiant energy may interact with molecular oxygen to form **free radicals**, such as **superoxide**, which interact with atoms and molecules to intensify the cellular injury.

5. Even at low doses, radiation can alter gene expression, for example, increased expression of proto-oncogenes, such as *MYC* or *FOS*; induction of cytokines such as TNF; or activation of the tumour

suppressor gene *TP53* (formerly *p53*) which causes cell cycle arrest and apoptosis.

Effects on Organ Systems

The **haematopoietic** and **lymphoid systems** are extremely susceptible to radiant energy. With high dose levels, **lymphopaenia** may appear within hours of irradiation, along with shrinkage of the lymph nodes and spleen. Radiation directly destroys lymphocytes, both in the circulating blood and in tissues (lymph nodes, spleen, thymus, gut). The circulating **granulocyte count** begins to fall towards the end of the first week. Levels near zero may be reached during the second week. **Platelets** are similarly affected. **Haematopoietic cells** in the bone marrow are also quite sensitive to radiant energy, including red cell precursors. **Erythrocytes** are radio-resistant, but even then, anaemia appears after 2 to 3 weeks and persists for months because of bone marrow damage. The **gonads** in both male and female, particularly the germ cells, are highly vulnerable to radiation injury, usually resulting in sterility.

Another very important effect of radiation on organ systems is **malignant transformation. Any cell capable of division that has sustained a mutation has the potential to become cancerous**. Thus, an increased incidence of neoplasms may occur in any organ after radiation. Radiation in very large doses kills cells and therefore is not associated with occurrence of tumours. Sub-lethal, but relatively high doses are associated with an increased risk. Also, prolonged exposure to low-dose radiation imposes risks.

Total-body irradiation: Exposure of large areas of the body to even very small doses of radiation may have devastating effects, and induce **'acute radiation syndrome'**. Three often fatal 'acute radiation syndrome' have been identified: (1) haematopoietic, (2) gastrointestinal, and (3) cerebral.

(B) Injury by Chemical Agents

There is an almost endless list of chemical agents, which can be injurious when inhaled, ingested, injected, or absorbed through the skin. All chemicals, including therapeutic drugs, are capable of causing injury or even death. The most toxic are **poisons**, others are relatively harmless. Poisoning occurs mostly accidentally, when **animals** ingest poisonous substances. Criminal poisoning does occur sometimes and is of medico-legal importance. However, before we take up the chemical agents important in animals, let us first consider the basic principles of chemical injury.

1. Dose: In general, the higher the dose, the greater the toxicity. However, small doses may cause serious problems, particularly over a long period.

2. Requirement for metabolic conversion: Some agents, such as certain alkaline cleaning materials are directly toxic to cells, and when swallowed injure mucosa of the oral cavity, oesophagus, and stomach. In contrast, many drugs, including alcohol (in humans), are converted in the liver to compounds that are more toxic than the parent compound. Thus, there may be no injury at the site of entry, whereas the liver may suffer the maximum damage.

3. Sites of absorption, accumulation, or excretion: These sites may be the targets of maximum injury.

4. Individual variation: An important factor that determines the rate of drug metabolism is inherited polymorphisms in enzymes that metabolize the drugs.

5. The capacity of the chemical to induce an immune response: Many chemicals are not directly toxic, but inflict injury by inducing an immune response. For example, **penicillin** may induce an immunoglobulin E (IgE)-mediated anaphylactic response or an IgG-mediated haemolytic anaemia in those who are genetically prone to develop type I or type II hypersensitivity reactions to this drug.

Chemical Poisons

Chemicals, poisonous in animals, may be either inorganic or organic substances. **Inorganic poisons** comprise acids (sulphuric acid), bases (potassium hydroxide), and salts (mercuric chloride). **Organic poisons** are derived from plants, moulds, fungi and bacteria, and from certain parasitic and venomous animals. These toxic agents may exert a corrosive (tending to corrode) or caustic action, or act as organ poisons, or nerve poisons, or they alter the blood.

1. Corrosives include the caustic alkalies, e.g., sodium hydroxide (caustic soda), potassium hydroxide (caustic potash), calcium oxide (quick lime) and barium chloride; the corrosive salts of heavy metals, e.g., mercuric chloride and zinc sulphate; and corrosive acids, e.g., nitric, sulphuric, oxalic, acetic, and carbolic. These substances act locally by producing burns that vary in their intensity from simple hyperaemia to severe inflammation, even to necrosis and ulceration, depending on the quantity, the concentration, and the place of contact of the particular agent.

2. Organ poisons produce degenerative changes in the organs, mainly liver, kidneys, and heart, e.g., phosphorus, arsenic, lead, mercuric chloride, and silver nitrate.

3. Nerve poisons either overstimulate, depress, or paralyze nerve cells. Some of these act as nerve stimulants at first but later as paralyzers. Among these poisons are the narcotics, strychnine, atropine, pilocarpine, physostigmine, the toxins of *Clostridium tetani* and *Clostridium botulinum*, and snake venoms.

4. Poisons affecting the blood prevent red cells from carrying oxygen, either by forming stable compound with haemoglobin or by inducing haemolysis, or by inhibiting coagulation of the blood, or by causing agglutination of erythrocytes (haemagglutination). Carbon monoxide is an example of a poison that combines with haemoglobin.

Carbon monoxide (CO): This is a non-irritating, colourless, tasteless and odourless gas produced by imperfect oxidation of carbonaceous materials. Its sources include industrial processes and automotive (self-propelled) engines. CO acts as a systemic asphyxiant. **Haemoglobin has a 200-fold greater affinity for CO than oxygen.** The resultant carboxyhaemoglobin is incapable of carrying oxygen. Moreover, it interferes with the release of oxygen for oxyhaemoglobin. Systemic hypoxia appears when haemoglobin is 20% to 30% saturated with CO, and unconsciousness and death occur with 60% to 70% saturation.

Occurrence of Poisoning

Livestock, in general, are exposed to the risk of various toxic chemicals used in mass treatment of animals for parasites; to toxic fresh water algae from drinking water of certain lakes; to alkaloids, glucosides, and saponins from eating poisonous plants; to hydrocyanic acid from eating sorghums during certain seasons; to lead or arsenic from drinking various dips and insect sprays; and from nitrate or chlorate of sodium or calcium from eating fertilizers or seed killers.

Cattle and sheep may suffer from **lead poisoning** by licking lead from freshly painted surfaces and from eating the contents of discarded paint pails. Cattle may also suffer from fluorine poisoning from raw rock phosphate as a mineral supplement. Sheep may also suffer from copper poisoning, following mass treatment for stomach worms with copper sulphate in grain. Dogs may suffer from phosphorus, arsenic, alphanaphthyl thiourea (antu) and thallium used in rodent baits.

Lead poisoning: Lead is absorbed through the gastrointestinal tract. Most of the absorbed lead (80% to 85%) is taken up by bone; the blood accumulates about 5% - 10%, the remainder is distributed throughout the soft tissues. Clinically, lead lines may occur in the gums, where excess lead stimulates hyperpigmentation of the gum tissue adjacent to the teeth (see 'plumbism'). Excretion of lead occurs through the kidneys, thereby exposing these organs to potential damage. Lead causes injury by binding to disulphide groups in proteins, including enzymes, altering their tertiary structure. The major targets of lead poisoning are the blood, nervous system, gastrointestinal tract, and kidneys.

Insecticides: Even in sufficient amounts, insecticides are harmful to animals and birds. They fall into two broad classes: (i) chlorinated hydrocarbons, e.g., DDT, dieldrin and lindane, and (ii) organo-phosphorus compounds, e.g., malathion and parathion. Both types accumulate in fat stores. Most are absorbed through the respiratory, skin, or gastrointestinal route. Since they are very resistant to degradation in the environment, they persist in soil and water and contaminate all levels of the food chain. DDT has been found in fruits, vegetables, milk, and meats. The chlorinated hydrocarbons affect the central nervous system and may induce depression, paralysis, coma, and death. The organo-phosphorus compounds are basically inhibitors of acetylcholinesterase. Thus acetylcholine accumulates at synaptic junctions, induces muscle twitching, flaccid paralysis, cardiac arrhythmias, respiratory depression, and death.

Poisonous plants may contain alkaloids, glycosides (glucosides), organic acids, minerals (nitrates, selenium, molybdenum), resins or resinoids, phytotoxins and substances causing photosensitization (porphyrins). Poisons from industrial plants include fluorine (fluorosis).

Body Defences against Poisons

To a certain extent, body can defend itself against poisonous substances. Vomiting, increased peristalsis resulting in diarrhoea, production of large amounts of mucus by mucous membranes, and excretion by way of the kidneys and lungs are examples of this defensive function. In addition, the body has special means of defence against some poisons. This falls under immunology.

Chapter 12

Concretions

A concretion is a **calculus**, that is, **'stone'** (L. calculus = stone). Commonly called **'stone'**, calculus is any abnormal concretion within the animal's body usually composed of mineral salts. Formation of calculi and concretions is called **'lithiasis'**. For example, formation of calculi in the urinary tract is called **'urolithiasis'**, that in biliary tract **'cholelithiasis'**, in the salivary duct or gland **'sialolithiasis'**, and in the pancreatic ducts as **'pancreolithiasis'**. A description of various concretions in domestic animals follows.

1. Uroliths

Uroliths or urinary calculi are concretions (stones) formed in the urinary tract. The formation of uroliths is called **'urolithiasis'**. Uroliths are usually found in the bladder (**cystic calculi**) and in the renal pelvis.

Uroliths may be of any **size** from sand-like particles to a single stone filling the bladder or renal pelvis. They may be hard or relatively soft, white or yellowish, smooth or rough, and rounded or faceted (i.e., with flattened sides). The **composition** of uroliths varies greatly. Chemically, the usual urinary stone of **herbivorous animals** contains mainly **silicates**, accompanied in some cases with phosphates, carbonates, or oxalates of calcium, ammonium, and magnesium. Sometimes calculi in herbivore may contain mixtures of both silicates and calcium salts. In **carnivorous** and **omnivorous animals**, the chemical constituents are quite different. The uroliths of these animals are much like those of the humans because of the acid urine, which is in contrast to the alkaline urine of herbivore.

The **oxalate stone** is very hard and heavy, white or light yellow, and covered with sharp, hard spines. It is usually found as a single stone in the bladder. It forms in acid urine and consists mainly of **calcium oxalate**. **Uric acid calculi** consist mainly of ammonium and sodium urates and uric acid. They are of small or medium size, firm or hard, yellow to brown in colour, and spherical or irregular in shape. Like the oxalate calculi, they form in acid urine. They are especially common in **dogs**. **Phosphate calculi** are more like the calculi of herbivore. They are white or grey, soft and friable. They are often multiple and may exist as sand-like granules. **They are the most common form of uroliths in dogs**, despite the acidity of the urine.

Bacterial infection with breakdown of urea to ammonia resulting in rise of urine pH favours precipitation of phosphates. Magnesium ammonium sulphate (struvite) is the commonest form of phosphate calculi in dogs. **Xanthine stones** are rare. **Cystine stones** are small, soft and yellow. Cystine, an amino acid, is relatively insoluble and may precipitate in the bladder of animals that excrete an increased amount through the kidney, which results from failure of tubular resorption of cystine. Cystine stone in the dogs have a tendency to occlude the urethra at the point where it enters the os penis. **Siliceous calculi** are rare in carnivore, but may develop if the diet contains a large amount of silicic acid.

Incidence: Uroliths occur in all species of animals. They are **least common in horses and pigs**, and are mostly seen in **cattle, dogs**, and **cats**. In **dogs**, the incidence of uroliths is between 0.6% to 2.8% of all canine illnesses with struvite calculi accounting for 40% to 85% of all stones; cystine, 7% to 22%; urate, 2% to 8%, and oxalate, 3 to 30%.

Causes

An organic matrix, nucleus or nidus is required for deposition of inorganic crystals and stone formation. This nucleus is usually a mucopolysaccharide or mucoprotein. The nucleus may consist of dead leukocytes, fibrin, cellular debris, or agglutinated bacteria. Crystallization on or within the nucleus then occurs. However, crystallization does not always occur, but results when there is disruption of the colloidal system that supports the supersaturated solution of crystalloids of urine. This may occur from an excess of crystalloids over protective colloids, or the presence of hydrophilic colloids. Some specific conditions include:

1. Bacterial infection of the urinary tract. This allows nidus formation and changes urine pH. This is the main cause of phosphate calculi in dogs.

2. Metabolic defect in uric acid metabolism in dogs leads to urate calculi.

3. Vitamin A deficiency causes **uroliths** through squamous metaplasia of urinary epithelium and increased nidus formation.

Effects

Calculi are irritating. In the renal pelvis, the stone is usually moulded to fit the **calyx** in which it is formed. These calculi predispose to pyelitis and pyelonephritis. The main damage caused by uroliths is due to the obstruction when they lodge at the uretero-pelvic orifice, in the ureter, or in the urethra. These changes may cause difficult or painful urination called **'stranguria'** or **'dysuria'**, and **haematuria** (blood in urine). Calculi in the bladder are usually passed out in the urine, but may lodge in the narrow male urethra, usually at the sigmoid flexure in **ruminants**, causing fatal obstruction unless relief is provided. The female usually escapes this problem because of the larger (in diameter) and shorter (in length) urethra.

One or more uroliths may lodge in the ureter, producing severe pain known as **ureteral colic**. However, if the calculus is small enough to enter the ureter, it is ultimately forced into the bladder, after which the colic is relieved. Otherwise, the involved kidney is reduced to small size by pressure and disuse atrophy, or it undergoes hydronephrosis (collection of urine in the kidney pelvis).

Choleliths

Choleliths, **gallstones**, or **biliary calculi** are rare, but occur in all the domestic species, including chicken. They are especially well described in **ruminants**. Formation of choleliths is called **'cholelithiasis'**. They may be of minute size like grains of sand. Several hundreds have been found in the bile ducts of **horse**. Or they may be few or single, a length of 11.5 cm has been reported. Choleliths differ in their chemical composition. The **cholesterol stone** is large, white, and light in weight, and contains crystals of cholesterol. However, the most common choleliths in animals are **'pigment stones'**, which are yellow to dark brown or black. They vary in weight and are composed of mixtures of materials, that include **salts of bilirubin, calcium carbonate, calcium phosphate**, and **glycoproteins**.

The **cause** of this type of cholelith is cholecystitis (inflammation of gallbladder) of infectious origin. **The mechanism of formation** is similar to that for urinary calculi. That is, solid particles of dead cells or inspissated material serve as the starting point for the process of crystallization. In the case of choleliths, however, changes in the water content and colloidal state are of great importance. It is likely that some constituents of bile are resorbed more easily than others when there is biliary stasis, leaving behind highly desiccated (dried up) residues.

Sialoliths

Sialoliths or **salivary calculi** form in a duct or in the salivary gland itself as a result of chronic inflammation. The formation of sialoliths is called **'sialolithiasis'**, and is **a rare disorder of cattle, dogs, monkeys, and humans**. Sialoliths are chalky yellow or white calcium concretions that form in the ducts of either the parotid or the submandibular salivary glands. The nidus (nucleus) could be bacteria, clumps of mucus, or desquamated epithelial cells. Inflammation provides desquamated cells or consolidated exudate on which calcium salts precipitate. Foreign bodies may also initiate precipitation of salts. Sialoliths have high calcium phosphate content, a lesser amount of calcium carbonate, other soluble salts, organic matter, and water. Since salivary secretions contain little dissolved material, the process of formation of salivary calculi is more similar to calcification of tissue than it is to the formation of urinary or biliary stones (i.e., uroliths or choleliths). Sialoliths may become quite large. Parotid calculi several centimetres in diameter and length have been found in the **horse**.

Affected animals salivate excessively, and **dogs** may injure the area in an attempt to deal with the discomfort resulting from distension and pressure within the occluded duct. When the duct is occluded for a long time, the salivary gland undergoes atrophy, but before this occurs, a **cyst** may form in the obstructed duct due to the dilating effect of the trapped secretions. Such a cyst in the sublingual duct, located in the frenulum of the tongue, is referred to as **ranula**. A **salivary fistula** sometimes forms when an injury creates an opening from the duct to the outside of the body. Proper healing is prevented by the flow of saliva through the opening.

Pancreoliths

Pancreoliths or **pancreatic calculi** are rare. They are sometimes seen in the pancreatic ducts of **cattle**. The formation of concretions or **'stones'** within the pancreatic duct system is called **'pancreolithiasis'**. It is usually an incidental finding at slaughter. No clinical signs or other pathological changes are found except for some inflammation in the wall of ducts containing calculi. **Pancreoliths** are usually hard, white and numerous, but small. They consist of carbonates and phosphates of calcium and magnesium, along with organic substances. Older cattle are more often affected.

Enteroliths

Enteroliths are hard, round concretions that form in the **large colon of the horse** and sometimes in other species. Animals between 6 to 14 years of age are affected.

Enteroliths form around a nidus (nucleus), usually an ingested particle or object. Items found at the centre include nails, pins, needles, coins, pebbles, grit, metal fragments, horse hair, and cloth. Ammonium magnesium phosphate (struvite) is deposited around the nidus, thus enlarging the calculus. A mass, the size of fist, may be produced in one year's time. Diets with high concentrations of magnesium and phosphorus increase enterolith formation.

Enteroliths may be **single** and round, **or multiple** and faceted. They usually weigh between 200 to 1500 gram, but enteroliths weighing up to 12 kg have been recorded. Enteroliths produce recurrent colic by causing obstruction. The next common sites for lodgement in **horses** are the small colon and pelvic flexure.

Faecaliths

These are discrete concretions of faeces, often mixed with long hairs. They are usually found in the small colons of **foals** or **young horses**. They usually become impacted in the small colon.

Phytobezoars

These are **fibre balls**. They occur rarely in **horses**. Fibre balls may cause obstruction of the large intestine and usually result in recurrent attacks of colic. They usually form in the small colon.

Chapter 13
Genetic Diseases

It is now well known that all diseases involve changes in gene structure or expression.

The **classification of animal diseases** falls into **three categories (1)** those that are genetically determined, **(2)** those that are environmentally determined, and **(3)** those to which both genetics and environment contribute. However, progress in understanding the molecular basis of many environmental disorders has tended to blur these distinctions. At one time infectious diseases were considered as examples of disorders arising wholly from environmental influences. But it is now clear that, to a great extent, an individual's genetic make-up influences one's immune response and susceptibility to microbial infections. Despite the complexities and the interplay between genetics and environment, it is now well established that the genetic component plays a major role in the occurrence and severity of many animal diseases.

However, before proceeding any further, it would be helpful to clarify three commonly used terms: hereditary, familial, and congenital. **Hereditary disorders** are derived from one's parents and are transmitted through the gametes to subsequent generations. They are therefore **familial**, that is, they tend to occur in more members of a family than expected by chance alone. The term **congenital** simply means 'present at birth'. It should be noted that some congenital diseases are not genetic, and that not all genetic diseases are congenital.

It is beyond the scope of this book to review normal animal genetics, but it would be helpful to discuss briefly certain fundamental concepts that have a bearing on the understanding of genetic diseases.

Mutations

The term **mutation** refers to a permanent change in the DNA. Those that affect germ cells are transmitted to the progeny and may give rise to inherited diseases. Mutations in somatic (body) cells are not transmitted to the progeny.

Point mutations result from the substitution of a single nucleotide base by a different base. This alters the meaning of the genetic code, resulting in the replacement of one amino acid by another in the protein product. **Frameshift mutations** occur when one or two base pairs are inserted or deleted from the DNA. This alters the reading frame of the DNA strand.

Genetic Disorders

Genetic disorders (genetic diseases) fall into **three categories**: **(1)** those related to mutant genes of large effect, **(2)** diseases with multi-factorial (polygenic) inheritance, and **(3)** those arising from chromosomal aberrations (abnormalities). The **first category**, also referred to as **'Mendelian disorders'**, includes many uncommon conditions such as the storage diseases and inborn errors of metabolism. All result from **single-gene mutations** of large effect. Most of the conditions are hereditary and familial. The **second category** includes hypertension and diabetes of humans. Multi-factorial or polygenic inheritance means that both genetic and environmental factors influence the expression of a disease. The **third category** includes disorders that are due to numerical or structural abnormalities in the chromosomes.

Disturbances caused by Single-Gene Defects (Mendelian disorders)

Single-gene defects (mutations) follow Mendelian pattern of inheritance. Therefore, the conditions they produce are often called **'Mendelian disorders'**. Mutations involving single genes follow any one of these patterns of inheritance: (1) autosomal dominant, (2) autosomal recessive, and (3) X-linked. However, before we discuss these three categories of genetic diseases, let us understand certain basic terminology used in genetics.

Genes are located on chromosomes. Chromosomes carry genetic information, since each is a long strand of DNA consisting of numerous genes strung together like a string of pearls. Genes that are carried on autosomes, that is, chromosomes other than the sex (X and Y) chromosomes, are called **autosomal genes**. Those carried on sex chromosomes are called **sex-linked genes**. The chromosomes in an organism, derived from each of the two parents, are always present in pairs. Morphologically similar chromosomes, having the same allelic genes with loci arranged in the same order, are called **homologous chromosomes** (G. homologos = agreeing, similar). Each member of such a pair is the homologue of the other. As chromosomes are present in pairs, the genes also occur in pair at the **same site (locus)**, except for X and Y chromosome. An alternative form of a gene on the same locus is called an **allele**. A gene that masks the effect of its alternative allele is called **dominant**, and the gene that is being masked is known as **recessive**. Individuals having similar genes at a locus (either both dominant or both recessive) are called **homozygous**, and the ones having different genes at a locus (one dominant and the other recessive) are called **heterozygous** for that particular locus.

If the gene is dominant, then its characteristics will be shown in the animal, regardless whether the arrangement is homozygous or heterozygous. If it is **recessive**, the characteristics will be shown only in a homozygous arrangement. Heterozygous are the carriers of the recessive genes. **The recessive genes express themselves in progeny only when they occur in a homozygous state.** As stated earlier, mutations involving single genes may follow any of the three patterns of inheritance: **autosomal dominant, autosomal recessive,** and **X-linked**. Each of these **three categories** will now be discussed.

1. Autosomal Dominant Disorders

In autosomal dominant disorders, the affected individuals are **heterozygous**. Every individual carrying the abnormal dominant gene suffers from the disease. Both males and females are affected, and both can transmit the condition.

Autosomal dominant diseases are not important in animals, but in human several important conditions are recognized. These include:

(i) Familial hypercholesterolaemia: This is perhaps the most common of all autosomal dominant disorders **in humans**. It is caused by a mutation in the gene that specifies the receptor for low density lipoprotein (LDL). LDL is the form in which 70% of total plasma cholesterol is transported. The affected persons develop excessive levels of serum cholesterol and premature atherosclerosis, resulting in myocardial infarction and even death.

(ii) von Willebrand disease: This disease is characterized by spontaneous bleeding from mucous membranes, excessive bleeding from wounds, and a prolonged bleeding time in the presence of a normal platelet count. Besides **human**, this disease has also been recognized in **dogs, cats, horses, pigs, and rabbits.**

(iii) Hereditary spherocytosis: This disorder is characterized by an inherited (intrinsic) defect in the red blood cell membrane that makes erythrocytes spheroidal (spherical), less deformable, and vulnerable to splenic destruction. A probable case of hereditary spherocytosis has been recorded in a **goat**.

(iv) Polycystic kidney disease: This occurs in adults and is characterized by multiple expanding cysts of both kidneys.

(v) Marfan syndrome: It is a disorder of connective tissue.

2. Autosomal Recessive Disorders

These disorders are **more common**, and are **also important in animals**. Autosomal recessive diseases make up the largest group of Mendelian disorders. These disorders, express themselves **only in homozygous recessive condition**, that is, when both the genes at a locus are recessive. In other words, these diseases occur when both the alleles at a given gene locus are **mutant.**

Before proceeding any further with autosomal recessive disorders, let us first consider the possible mechanisms by which an enzyme deficiency may give rise to an autosomal recessive disorder. Normally, a substrate is converted to an end product through intermediates by a series of enzyme reactions. An **enzyme defect** in such a reaction has **two major biochemical effects:**

(i) Accumulation of the substrate and intermediates

Depending on the site of the block, there may be accumulation of substrate and the intermediates. Tissue injury may result if the substrate or the intermediates are toxic in high concentrations. For example, in **galactosaemia** in humans, deficiency of enzyme galactose-1-phosphate uridylyltransferase leads to accumulation of galactose, with consequent tissue damage. Again, in humans, deficiency of enzyme phenylalanine hydroxylase results in accumulation of phenylalanine, resulting in **phenylketonuria**. Deficiency of degradative enzymes in lysosomes results in the accumulation of complex substrates in excessive amounts within lysosomes, producing a group of diseases, both in **humans and animals**, known as 'lysosomal storage diseases'.

(ii) Metabolic block: The enzyme defect can lead to a metabolic block, resulting in decreased amount of an end product than may be necessary for normal function. For example, a deficiency of melanin may result from lack of **tyrosinase**, which is necessary for the biosynthesis of melanin from its precursor, tyrosine. This results in a clinical condition called **albinism. Albinism occurs in both humans and animals.** In animals, it has been reported in occasional individuals of any species.

Enzyme deficiencies may also act in other ways. For example, **alpha-1-antitrypsin** is a protease inhibitor and inactivates neutrophil elastase. In patients with alpha-1-antitrypsin deficiency, elastic tissue in the walls of lung alveoli is destroyed by neutrophil elastase, leading eventually to emphysema in humans.

With this background, let us briefly discuss some of the **more common autosomal recessive disorders in animals.**

Lysosomal Storage Diseases

Lysosomes contain a variety of hydrolytic enzymes that are involved in the breakdown of complex substrates, such as sphingolipids and mucopolysaccharides, into **soluble end products**. With an inherited lack of a lysosomal enzyme, catabolism of its substrate remains incomplete, leading to accumulation of the **partially degraded insoluble metabolites** within the lysosomes. **These missing-enzyme syndromes are inherited as autosomal recessive disorders**. The storage of insoluble intermediates occurs mainly in cells of the mononuclear phagocyte system, since they ingest and degrade old and worn-out (senescent) red cells, leukocytes and other tissue breakdown products.

In lysosomal storage diseases lipid metabolites, usually glycolipids and phospholipids (**lipidoses**), or mucopolysaccharides (**mucopolysaccharidoses**) accumulate in cells. Neurons are most often affected in lipidoses, probably due to the high lipid content of the nervous system. The mucopolysaccharides also involve neurons, but liver, spleen, connective tissue and other organs are also affected. A large number of lysosomal enzyme deficiency diseases have been recognized in humans (about 35), **but only a few have been described in animals**. These are listed in **Table 22.** Their classification is based on the biochemical nature of the substrates and the accumulated metabolites, each resulting from the deficiency of a specific enzyme. Since most of the diseases are very rare, only a few of the more common conditions are mentioned.

1. GM1-Gangliosidosis: This has been described in **cats, dogs, sheep,** and **cattle**. It results from an inherited deficiency of the lysosomal enzyme **beta-galactosidase** and leads to the accumulation of **GM1-ganglioside** in lysosomes of neurons. Neurons throughout the brain, spinal cord, ganglia, and retina are distended with finely granular, faintly basophilic material. It is intensely PAS-positive.

2. GM2-Gangliosidosis: This results from a deficiency of **beta-hexosaminidase**, leading to an accumulation in lysosomes of GM2-

Table 22. Lysosomal storage diseases of the domestic animals

Disease	Enzyme deficiency	Major accumulating material	Species affected
Sphingolipidoses			
GM1-gangliosidosis	Beta-galactosidase	GM1-ganglioside	Cat, dog, sheep, cattle
GM2-gangliosidosis or Tay-Sachs disease	Beta-hexosaminidase	GM2-ganglioside	Dog, cat, pig
Sulphatidoses			
Gaucher disease	Glucocerebrosidase	Glucocerebroside	Dog, sheep, pig
Niemann-Pick disease	Sphingomyelinase	Sphingomyelin	Cat, dog
Mucopolysaccharidoses			
Type I or Hurler's syndrome	Alpha-L-iduronidase	Dermatan sulphate, heparan sulphate	Cat, dog
Type VI or Maroteaux-Lamy syndrome	Arylsulphatase B	Dermatan sulphate, chondroitin-6-sulphate	Cat, dog
Mannosidoses			
Alpha-mannosidosis	Alpha-mannosidase	Mannose-rich oligosaccharides	Cattle, sheep, cat
Beta-mannosidosis	Beta-mannosidase	Mannose-rich oligosaccharides	Cattle, goat
Neuronal glycoproteinosis or LaFora's disease	Enzymes involved in degradation of oligosaccharide side chains of glycoproteins	Glycoproteins	Dog
Leukodystrophies			
Globoid cell leukodystrophy or Krabbe's disease	Galactocerebroside beta-galactosidase	Galactocerebroside	Dog, cat sheep
Metachromatic leukodystrophy	Arylsulphatase A	Galactosyl-sulphatides	Cat
Glycogenoses			
Type II or Pompe's disease	Alpha-glucosidase (acid maltase)	Glycogen	Cattle, dog, cat, sheep
Type III or Cori-Forbes' disease	Amylo-1, 6, -glucosidase	Glycogen	Dog, cat

ganglioside, a glycolipid. It has been reported in **dog**, **cat**, and **pig**. Neurons in the brain, spinal cord, spinal ganglia, and retina have a foamy, vacuolated appearance. The material is PAS-positive. There is no involvement of visceral tissues, in contrast to the disease in humans.

3. Gaucher disease: This results from a deficiency of **glucocerebrosidase** and leads to the accumulation of **glucocerebroside**. It has been reported in **dog, sheep**, and **pig**. The accumulated material results in large foamy cells (Gaucher cells) which are slightly eosinophilic and PAS positive. Gaucher cells occur in liver, lymph nodes, and neurons. The spleen is spared in contrast to the disease in humans.

4. Niemann-Pick disease: This results from a deficiency of **sphingomyelinase**, leading to accumulation of **sphingomyelin** within lysosomes. It has been reported in **cat** and **dog**. There is vacuolation of neurons, hepatocytes, and mononuclear phagocytes of the liver, spleen, and lymph nodes. The stored material stains moderately with PAS.

5. Mucopolysaccharidoses: These are a group of diseases resulting from deficiencies of one or more enzymes necessary for mucopolysaccharide degradation. This leads to storage of mucopolysaccharide in various tissues. Mucopolysaccharides form a part of ground substance, and are synthesized in the connective tissues by fibroblasts (see Chapter 5). Most of the mucopolysaccharide is secreted into the ground substance, **but a certain fraction is degraded within lysosomes**. Several forms are recognized **in humans**, each resulting from the deficiency of one specific enzyme.

In animals, mucopolysaccharidosis has been recognized in **cats** and **dogs** as 'Type I or **Hurler's syndrome'**. It is due to deficiency of **alpha-L-iduronidase** and leads to the accumulation of **dermatan sulphate** and **heparan sulphate** within lysosomes. A 'Type VI or **Maroteaux Lamy Syndrome'** due to deficiency of **arylsulphatase B**, leads to accumulation of **dermatan sulphate** and **chondroitin-6-sulphate**. It has been reported in **cats and dogs**.

6. Mannosidosis is of **alpha** and **beta types**. Alpha occurs in **cattle, sheep,** and **cat**, and is characterized by deficiency of **alpha-mannosidase** leading to storage of **mannose-rich oligosaccharides** in lysosomes. There is vacuolation of mononuclear phagocytes in liver and lymph nodes, pancreatic cells, and neurons. The stored material stains with PAS, but is easily washed out from tissue sections. **Beta-**

mannosidosis has been reported in **cattle** and **goats** and is due to deficiency of **beta-mannosidase**.

7. **Neuronal glycoproteinosis (LaFora's disease)** is a rare disorder that has been reported in **dogs**. It is characterized by a deficiency of **enzymes involved in degradation of oligosaccharide side chains of glycoproteins**, resulting in accumulation of **glycoproteins** in neurons and skeletal muscle cells.

8. **Leukodystrophies**: These are diseases of white matter, in which the inborn defect is in the pathway of **myelin metabolism** due to the deficiency of a specific lysosomal enzyme. Pathologically, the main process is **demyelination**. In animals, two forms are recognized.

(i) **Globoid cell leukodystrophy (Krabbe's disease)** results from a deficiency of the lysosomal enzyme **galactocerebroside beta-galactosidase** and leads to accumulation of **galactocerebroside**. It has been reported in **dogs, cats, sheep, and monkeys**. The primary lysosomal defect appears to be in the **oliodendrocytes**, and not in neurons. This results in their destruction. Since oligosaccharides produce myelin, their destruction leads to disturbance of myelin formation and maintenance and accumulation of **globoid cells**. Globoid cells are macrophages that accumulate to phagocytose the galactocerebroside.

(ii) **Metachromatic leukodystrophy** is another disorder of myelin metabolism and has been reported in **cats**. It results from the deficiency of **arylsulphatase A** and leads to the accumulation of **galactosyl-sulphatides**.

Glycogen Storage Diseases (Glycogenoses)

An inherited deficiency of any one of the enzymes involved in glycogen synthesis or degradation can result in excessive accumulation of glycogen in various tissues. The glycogen is mostly stored within the cytoplasm, or sometimes within nuclei. About a dozen forms of glycogenoses have been described in humans on the basis of specific enzyme deficiencies. At least two forms are recognized in animals.

(i) **Type II** or **Pompe's disease**: This has been described in **cattle, dog, cat**, and **sheep**. It results from a deficiency of lysosomal **alpha-glucosidase (acid maltase)**, leading to **glycogen storage in brain, muscle, and liver**. The glycogen is stored within **lysosomes**. It is therefore a form of **lysosomal storage disease**. In other forms of glycogen storage disease, the glycogen is stored within the **cytoplasm**.

(ii) Type III or **Cori-Forbes' disease**: This has been reported in **dogs** and **cats**. It results from a deficiency of the **glycogen debranching enzyme amylo-1, 6-glucosidase**, an enzyme involved in the breakdown of glycogen to glucose. Glycogen is stored diffusely throughout the **cytoplasm** of liver, myocardium, skeletal and smooth muscles, and **nerve cells**.

X-Linked Disorders

All sex-linked disorders are X-linked. This is because so far no Y-linked diseases are known. Most X-linked disorders are X-linked recessive. They are transmitted by heterozygous female carriers. Little is known about the X-linked diseases in animals.

Diseases due to Abnormalities of Chromosomes

Diseases resulting from abnormalities of chromosomes are called **'chromosomal disorders'** or **'chromosomal aberrations'**. Chromosomal disorders are much more common than is generally realized. Earlier we have seen that defects of even single gene can cause disease. Therefore, chromosomal abnormality, which involve hundreds or thousands of genes are usually incompatible with life. Chromosomal abnormality can be seen with light microscope.

Chromosomes are best studied at **metaphase**, at which time individual chromosomes are greatly condensed and morphologically distinct. Rapidly multiplying cells are treated with **colchicine** to arrest them in metaphase stage of mitosis. **Karyotyping** is the basic tool of the cytogeneticist in studying chromosomal abnormality. A **karyotype** is a photographic representation of a stained metaphase spread, in which the chromosomes are arranged in order of decreasing length.

Detection of chromosomal abnormalities has been greatly improved by the use of **banding techniques**. These are special stains that pick out chromosomes very clearly. With the widely used Giemsa stain (**G-banding technique**), each chromosome set can be seen to possess a distinctive pattern of alternating light and dark bands of variable widths. The use of banding techniques allows certain identification of each chromosome, as well as precise localization of structural changes in the chromosomes.

Chromosomal abnormalities may result from (i) alterations in the **number** of chromosomes, or (ii) alterations in the **structure** of chromosomes, and may affect **autosomes** or **sex chromosomes**.

529

Numerical Abnormalities

The number of chromosomes for a particular animal is constant, and is therefore characteristic for each species. The total number of chromosomes (2n) in some species is:

Human	46	Dog	78	Fowl	77-78
Cattle	60	Cat	38	Duck	79-80
Horse	64	Sheep	54	Rabbit	44
Ass	62	Goat	60	Guinea pig	64
Mule	63	Pig	36/38	Mouse	40

As stated, each somatic cell in the body contains the number of chromosomes characteristic of that species. Thus, for example, in humans, each somatic cell will contain 46 chromosomes (**diploid 2n**), in 23 homologous pairs. Of the 46 chromosomes, 23 are derived from each parent. This is because following meiosis, each germ cell happens to contain half the **diploid** number, and is therefore **haploid** (n), and the diploid condition is restored in zygote after fertilization. Having understood the terms haploid and diploid, let us now consider the abnormalities in the number of chromosomes.

If the number of chromosomes in the gamete or zygote is different from the normal, the condition is called **heteroploidy**. Any exact multiple of the haploid number (n) is called **euploid**, and the condition **euploidy**. The affected animals die within the first days of embryonic life. Chromosome numbers such as 3n and 4n are called **polyploid**. **Polyploidy** generally results in spontaneous abortion. Any number that is not an exact multiple of 'n' is called **aneuploid**. The main cause of **aneuploidy** is **non-disjunction** of a homologous pair of chromosomes at the stage of meiosis when DNA strands separate to form gametes. **Non-disjunction** means that a chromosome pair fails to separate and that as a result the gametes will contain either both sex chromosomes, or neither. Aneuploidy may involve specific chromosomes in triple number (**trisomy**) (2n + 1), or single number (monosomy) (2n minus 1), rather than the normal double dose. Several of these are known in humans, involving either autosomes or sex chromosomes, **and a few have been found also in animals**. These will be described later.

Monosomy involving an autosome is incompatible with life, whereas **trisomies** of certain autosomes and monosomy involving sex chromosomes are compatible with life. These are usually associated with variable degrees of phenotypic abnormalities. (**Phenotype** means the visible properties of an organism that are produced by interaction of the genotype and the environment). **Mosaicism** is a term used to describe the presence of two or more diverse population of cells in the same individual. Regarding chromosome number, postzygotic mitotic non-disjunction would result in the production of a trisomic and monosomic daughter cell; the descendants of these cells would then produce a **mosaic**. Mosaicism affecting sex chromosomes is common, whereas autosomal mosaicism is not. **Chimerism** is mosaicism in which one cell type is acquired in uterus from a heterosexual twin. **Chimera** may be an individual, an organ, or a part consisting of tissues of diverse genetic constitution. In case of **chromosomal chimerism**, both the XX and XY type of cells are present in the same individual. **Freemartins** are the best examples of chromosomal chimerism having 60, XX/60, XY chromosomal complement (see 'freemartinism', described later).

Structural Abnormalities

Structural changes in the chromosomes usually result from chromosome breakage followed by loss or rearrangement of material. The patterns of chromosomal rearrangement after breakage are: **(1) Translocation** implies transfer of a part of one chromosome to another chromosome. The process is usually reciprocal, that is, fragments are exchanged between two chromosomes. Transfer of the segments leads to one chromosome being very large and other extremely small. It takes place during meiosis. **(2) Deletion** involves loss of a portion of a chromosome. The isolated fragment, which lacks a centromere does not survive and thus many genes are lost. Chromosomal deletion, like non-disjunction and translocation, takes place during meiosis. **(3) Inversions** occur when there are two breaks in a chromosome, and the segment reunites after a complete turnaround. **(4)** A **ring chromosome** is a variant of a deletion. After the loss of segments from each end of the chromosome, the arms unite to form a ring.

Against this background, we can turn first to **some general features of chromosomal disorders,** followed by some specific examples of diseases involving changes in the karyotypes.

1. Chromosomal disorders may be associated with absence (deletion, monosomy), excess (trisomy), or abnormal arrangements (translocations) of chromosomes.

2. In general, loss of chromosomal material produces more severe defects than does gain of chromosomal material.

3. Imbalances of sex chromosomes (excess or loss) are tolerated much better than similar imbalances of autosomes.

4. Sex chromosomal disorders often produce subtle abnormalities, sometimes not detected at birth. Infertility, a common manifestation cannot be diagnosed until adolescence.

Autosomal Disorders (Anomalies in Autosomal Chromosomes)

These are due to anomalies in autosomal chromosomes, as opposed to sex chromosomes. Since autosomes are more in number than sex chromosomes, theoretically, abnormalities in the autosomes should be more than the abnormalities of sex chromosomes. But in reality this is not so, because autosomal anomalies cause death of the zygote.

Down syndrome (Trisomy 21) or **mongolism** in children was the first autosomal abnormality identified, and is the most common of the chromosomal disorders. It consists of an extra chromosome in the pair 21. Patients with Down's syndrome therefore have 47 chromosomes, as against the normal of 46, and are said to exhibit **trisomy 21**. The most common cause of trisomy, and therefore of Down syndrome, is non-disjunction of the 21 chromosome pair at meiosis. Down syndrome is a leading cause of mental retardation in children. The physical abnormalities, including the heavy folds of skin over corners of eyes and flat facial profile, led to the term mongolism.

Trisomy of a small autosomal chromosome has been described in chimpanzee. Interesting alterations in autosomal chromosomes have been found in cases of bovine lymphosarcoma, canine lymphosarcoma, and in malignant lymphoma in **cats**. The way in which chromosomal abnormalities induces changes is less clear than in the case of point mutations involving single genes, where a biochemical explanation is available.

Sex Chromosome Disorders (Anomalies in Sex Chromosomes)

These are more common than disorders of autosomal chromosomes, because abnormal karyotypes involving the sex chromosomes are compatible with life. In fact, some of the best studied chromosomal disturbances affect the sex chromosomes. The anomalies are due to non-disjunction. This means that a chromosome pair fails to separate and that as a result the gametes will contain either both sex chromosomes, or neither. For example (see Table 23), the sperm of a male parent showing non-disjunction will contain either an X plus a Y chromosome (XY), two Ys (YY), or no sex chromosomes at all (0). All normal sperms will have either one or more Y chromosome. A female parent similarly affected will produce ova with two X chromosomes (XX), or no sex chromosomes (0). All normal ova will have only one X chromosome. The different combinations, and therefore disorders of sex chromosomes in the gamete of offspring showing non-disjunction, are best understood by **Table 23**.

Table 23. **Some sexual abnormalities resulting from chromosomal non-disjunction**

Normal ova	Abnormal sperm	Offspring	Clinical condition
X	XY	XXY	Klinefelter syndrome
X	XX	XXX	Super-female
X	YY	XYY	Super-male
X	O	XO	Turner syndrome
Abnormal ova	**Normal sperm**		
XX	Y	XXY	Klinefelter syndrome
XX	X	XXX	Super-female
O	X	XO	Turner syndrome
O	Y	OY	Non-viable

Abnormalities of sex chromosomes are important in medical genetics, **but are also of much significance in animals**. Three disorders arising in alterations of sex chromosomes are described briefly.

(i) Klinefelter syndrome: This syndrome occurs in **males**, and develops when there are two X and one Y chromosome, i.e., XXY karyotype. Patients have 47 chromosomes, one more than the normal number of 46. As already stated, this karyotype results from non-disjunction of sex chromosomes during meiosis. The extra chromosome may be of maternal or paternal origin. Patients exhibit small testes, subfertility or even sterility, and gynecomastia, that is, abnormally large mammary glands in the male, sometimes even with milk secretion. Abnormalities of sex chromosomes, similar to Klinefelter syndrome in humans, have been reported in **cat, dog, sheep, cattle, horse, and pig**.

(ii) Turner syndrome: This syndrome is found in **human females**. It develops when one entire chromosome is missing, resulting in X0 karyotype. Patients have only 45 chromosomes, one less than the normal number of 46. Cases of Turner syndrome have small external genitalia, and the ovaries are rudimentary. Many other abnormalities may be present, e.g., significant growth retardation, inadequate breast development, and primary amenorrhoea. In animals, Turner syndrome has been reported in **horse**, **pig**, **cat**, and **monkey**.

(iii) Super-females and **super-males** differ little from normal.

Intersexes

An **intersex is an animal or person** with some ambiguity in genitalia or secondary sexual characteristics, suggesting being both male and female. **Hermaphroditism** means having both male and female genitalia, external and internal. **True hermaphrodites**, that is, with gonads of both sexes, have either: (i) normal XX karyotype, (ii) a normal XY karyotype, or (iii) XX karyotypes in some of their cells, and XY karyotypes in others. This last condition is known as **mosaicism**, and is an important aspect of medical genetics. A **pseudohermaphrodite** has the external genitalia of one sex and the gonads of the opposite sex. Thus, a male pseudohermaphrodite has female genitalia and male gonads (testes). It is not unusual for both an ovary and testis to be present in some intersexes. Most states of intersexuality are due to causes other than chromosomal abnormalities. Intersexuality has been studied at some length in **pigs** and **horses**.

Freemartinism

A problem of continued interest is the arrested development of sex organs and sterility in **female calves** that are carried in uterus with a male twin. These **sterile heifers** have been recognized for many years and have been called 'freemartins'. The phenomenon of freemartinism is not clearly understood, but is explained as follows. In **cattle**, in twin pregnancy, the male and female co-twins share a common placental circulation in the uterus (chorio-vascular anastomosis), which allows them to exchange cells. The cells from one twin establish themselves in the other, producing **chimerism**. The presence of XX cells in gonads and other tissues of male calves, which are twins of females, appears to reduce fertility. And the presence of XY cells in the female co-twin is associated with sterility. The earlier theory postulated that sex hormones appear earlier in the male foetus than in the female, and that when one foetus is a male and the other female, the male hormone circulating in the blood of the female twin had a harmful effect on the development of the female gonads. The result is a sterile female. This theory, however, has still to be proved.

Diseases with Multi-Factorial Inheritance

Multi-factorial inheritance is also called **'polygenic inheritance'**, and is involved in many physiological characteristics of humans, such as height, weight, blood pressure, and hair colour. Whereas the effects of single-gene inheritance, described earlier, are due to the action of a single gene of large effect, polygenic inheritance is due to the additive effect of two or more genes of small effect, but **conditioned by the environmental, non-genetic influences**. For example, even monozygous (identical) twins reared separately may achieve different heights because of nutritional or other environmental influences.

Recent Advances in Genetic Diseases

Genetics has now permeated virtually every branch of medicine. The **'classical genetics'** has been revolutionized by the spectacular advances in molecular biology. The **'modern genetics'** has provided penetrating insights into common disorders such as diabetes and cancer. Much of the recent progress in medical genetics has resulted from application of **recombinant DNA techniques**. It is possible, for example, to cut human genes and insert them into appropriate animals, such as mice. The human gene when recombined with DNA of the mice can be replicated, transcribed, and translated. This technique has made piece-by-piece analysis of human genetic material possible. In fact, completion of the **human genome project** has been a landmark event in the study of human diseases. We now know that **humans have about 30,000 genes**. Let us therefore consider some examples of the impact of recombinant DNA technology in the understanding and diagnosis of human diseases. **An understanding of this new technology is essential, since similar advances in animal diseases are in progress**. For example, DNA probes have been developed for the early and effective diagnosis of Johne's and other diseases in animals.

Molecular Basis of Disease

Recombinant DNA technology has been applied to study genetic diseases. First, the relevant normal gene is isolated, cloned, and then the molecular changes that affect the gene in patients with the disorder, are determined. For example, cloning of haemoglobin gene revealed that **a single base substitution** changes haemoglobin A to sickle haemoglobin and produces changes in the physico-chemical properties of haemoglobin, giving rise to sickle cell anaemia in humans.

The **'modern genetics'** has made it possible to insert molecularly cloned human DNA into the genome of mice. These mice are called **'transgenic mice'**. The technique involves microinjection of a cloned gene into the pronucleus of mice embryo. The zygote is implanted into the oviducts of pseudo-pregnant female mice. Then by certain techniques, it is possible to target expression of the introduced gene in specific tissues such as beta cells of the islets of Langerhans in pancreas. Transgenic mice are proving extremely useful in the study of diseases such as diabetes mellitus, viral hepatitis, and even cancer.

Genetically Engineered Products

A large number of extremely pure biologically active agents can now be produced in unlimited quantity by inserting the requisite gene into bacteria, or other suitable cells in tissue culture. Some examples of **genetically engineered products** already in use include: tissue plasminogen activator (tPA) for the treatment of thrombotic patients, growth hormone for the treatment of deficiency states, erythropoietin in anaemia, and myeloid growth and differentiation factors to increase production of monocytes and neutrophils in states of poor marrow function.

Gene Therapy

This aims in treating genetic diseases by transfer of somatic cells transfected with the normal gene.

Disease Diagnosis

Molecular probes are proving extremely useful in the diagnosis of **both genetic and infectious diseases**. A DNA probe is a single-stranded labelled complementary DNA sequence of the cloned gene. In simple terms, presuming DNA to be an antigen, the DNA probe can be considered as its labelled antibody. DNA based diagnosis is finding wide application in many infectious diseases in humans, and also cancer. As stated, DNA probes are proving extremely useful for the early and effective diagnosis of Johne's and other infectious diseases of animals.

Diagnosis of Genetic Diseases

The conventional cytogenetic analysis in the diagnosis of genetic diseases used to involve examination of entire chromosomes (karyotyping). Recently two novel techniques have been evolved as additional tools to routine karyotyping. These are **'fluorescence *in situ* hybridization (FISH)'** and **'molecular detection of genetic disorders (molecular analysis)'**. The basic principles involved in these techniques are briefly presented.

Fluorescence *in situ* Hybridization (FISH)

FISH has become an important addition to routine karyotyping. A major limitation of karyotyping is that it is applicable only to cells that are dividing. This problem can be overcome with **DNA probes** that recognize chromosome-specific sequences. Such probes are labelled with **fluorescent dyes** and applied to metaphase spreads or interphase nuclei. The probe binds to its complementary sequence on the chromosome and thus labels the specific chromosomal region that can be visualized under a fluorescent microscope. FISH has been used for detection of numerical abnormalities of chromosomes (**aneuploidy**).

Molecular Detection of Genetic Disorders

Many genetic diseases are caused by changes in individual genes that cannot be detected by routine karyotyping, **or even FISH**. Traditionally, the diagnosis of single-gene disorders has depended on the identification of abnormal gene products. **Now, it is possible to identify mutations at the level of DNA and offer diagnosis for several genetic disorders.**

The **molecular diagnosis** of inherited diseases has definite advantages over other techniques: **(1) It is remarkably sensitive.** Moreover, use of technique like **polymerase chain reaction (PCR)** allows several million-fold amplification of DNA or RNA, making it possible to utilize as few as 1 or 100 cells for analysis. Tiny amounts of whole blood, or even dried blood, can supply sufficient DNA for PCR amplification. **(2) DNA-based tests are not dependent on a gene product.**

There are **two approaches** to the molecular diagnosis of single-gene diseases (1) **direct detection** of mutations, and (2) **indirect detection** based on linkage of the disease gene with surrogate (substitute) markers in the genome.

537

1. Direct Gene Diagnosis

Direct gene diagnosis has been appropriately called **'diagnostic biopsy of the genome'.** Such diagnosis depends on the detection of an important qualitative change in the DNA. Two techniques used are **(i) Southern blot analysis,** and **(ii) PCR analysis.** Southern blot analysis consists of a nitrocellulose sheet containing spots of DNA for identification by a suitable molecular probe. PCR analysis has been already explained.

2. Indirect Gene Diagnosis (or Linkage Analysis)

Direct gene diagnosis is possible only if the mutant gene and its normal counterpart have been identified and cloned and their nucleotide sequences are known. **In several diseases that have genetic basis, direct gene diagnosis is not possible,** because either the sequence of the suspected gene is unknown or the disease is multi-factorial (polygenic) and **no single gene is involved.** In such cases, surrogate markers in the genome are used to localize the chromosomal regions of interest, based on their linkage to one or more suspected disease-causing genes. Linkage analysis facilitates localization and cloning of the disease allele. The most commonly employed link analysis technique is **'restriction fragment length polymorphism (RELP) analysis.'**

Chapter 14
Disturbances in Development

Disturbances in development include anomalies, monstrosities, or serious deviations from the normal type. Developmental anomalies usually have their origins during embryonic life, when the development of most body structure begins. A **'teratogen'** is a substance which, when administered to the pregnant female, causes developmental malformations in the young. The study of **malformations** occurring during embryonic or foetal life constitutes the science of **'teratology'**.

Anomalies

An **anomaly** is a disturbance of development that involves an organ, or a portion of an organ. The causes of anomalies are not always known. Most of them have their origins within the first few weeks after fertilization. Some, however, may develop later in pregnancy. Many even have their inception in the germplasm, that is, they are hereditary.

Anomalies occur as **congenital malformations**. They are structural defects present at birth. The term **'congenital'** means 'born with', that is, **present at birth**. It does not suggest or rule out a genetic basis for birth defects. The term **'congenital diseases'** and **'inherited diseases'** are often used synonymously, **but they are different**. As stated, a **congenital disease** is one in which the individual is born with the disease, whereas an **inherited disease** is one which is because of factors present in the genetic material received from one's ancestors (genetic transmission). An inherited disease may not become noticeable until after several years, and is therefore not truly congenital. Only some of the congenital anomalies are genetic in origin, others are due to environmental influences, such as foetal exposure to viral infections, or teratogenic drugs during pregnancy. However, causes of the majority of birth defects remain unknown.

Aetiology

The causes of many congenital anomalies are unknown. Known causes of errors in malformations can be grouped into **two major categories**: (1) **genetic**, and (2) **environmental**. However, almost half

539

have no recognized cause. Malformations of genetic origin, again can be divided into two groups: (i) those associated with **chromosomal aberrations**, and (ii) those arising in **single-gene mutations**. Virtually all **chromosomal disorders** (e.g., Klinefelter syndrome in humans and animals, and Down and Turner syndrome in humans) are associated with congenital malformations (Chapter 13). Most chromosomal disorders arise during gametogenesis. **Single-gene mutations**, characterized by Mendelian inheritance, may underlie major malformations (see Chapter 13). In addition, malformations may arise from **multi-factorial inheritance**, which means the interaction of environmental factors with two or more genes of small effect. This is believed to be the most common genetic cause of congenital malformation.

Environmental influences, such as viral infections, drugs, and irradiation to which the matter was exposed during pregnancy, may cause malformations in the foetus and neonates (newborns). **With viruses**, the gestational age at which the infection occurs in the mother is most important. The risk is greater if infection occurs in the first eight weeks, than when it occurs in the second or third month of gestation. The important known causes of anomalies in animals include panleukopaenia (cerebellar hypoplasia), Newcastle disease of chickens (ocular or auditory anomalies), bovine viral diarrhoea infection of calves, bluetongue of sheep, and rickettsial infection. Most of these are associated with anomalies of the central nervous system.

A variety of **drugs** and **chemicals** have been suspected to be **teratogenic**, but perhaps less than 1% of congenital malformations are caused by these agents. More information is available in humans. The list, in humans, includes thalidomide, folate antagonists, androgenic hormones, alcohol, anticonvulsants, and warfarin (oral anticoagulant). Thalidomide, once a popular tranquillizer, causes an extremely high incidence (50% to 80%) of limb malformations. **Alcohol**, perhaps the most widely used agent **in humans** today, is **an important environmental teratogen**. Affected infants show growth retardation and facial anomalies, such as microcephaly (abnormal smallness of head) and maxillary hypoplasia. These together are known as **'foetal alcohol syndrome'**.

Radiation, in addition to being mutagenic and carcinogenic, is **teratogenic**. Exposure to heavy doses of radiation during the period of organogenesis leads to malformations, such as microcephaly, blindness, skull defects, spina bifida, and other deformities.

Pathogenesis

The pathogenesis of congenital malformations is complex and still poorly understood. Here, two important general principles of human developmental pathology are briefly discussed that may perhaps also apply to animals, regardless of the aetiological agent.

1. The intrauterine development of humans can be divided into two phases: **(i) the embryonic period,** occupying the first nine weeks of pregnancy, and **(ii) the foetal period**, which terminates at birth. In the **early embryonic period** (the first 3 weeks after fertilization), an injurious agent damages either enough cells to cause death and abortion or only a few cells, allowing the embryo to recover without developing defects. Between the third and ninth weeks, the embryo is extremely susceptible to teratogenesis, and the peak sensitivity during this period is between fourth and fifth weeks. It is during this period that organs are being made out of the germ cell layers. This process of organogenesis is extremely susceptible to insult, regardless of its nature. **The foetal period** that follows organogenesis is accompanied by further growth and maturation of the organs, **with greatly reduced susceptibility to teratogenic agents**. However, the already formed organs in the foetus remain susceptible to growth retardation or injury. Thus, the same teratogenic agent may produce different effects if exposure occurs at different times of gestation. To conclude, **the timing of the prenatal insult (i.e., before birth) has an important impact on the occurrence and the type of malformations produced.**

2. Since many congenital malformations reflect failure of normal **morphogenesis** during development, it is believed that alterations of genes that control these events might cause birth defects. **That is, genes that regulate morphogenesis may be the target of teratogenesis.** Two such classes of genes have been recently discovered. (1) **Homeobox (*HOX*) genes**: *HOX* genes regulate transcription of several other genes. It has been shown in **experimental animals** that agents which alter *HOX* gene expression produce malformations. It is now thought that at least some of the teratogenic effects of certain agents are mediated by *HOX* gene modulation. **(2)** *PAX* **genes**: Another class of developmental genes are the *PAX* genes. Mutations in two of the *PAX* genes cause human malformations, namely, *PAX-3* and *PAX-6*.

Malformations (Anomalies)

In this section, it is not possible to do more than introduce the terms used for the most commonly met **malformations**, and to indicate the type of structural defect the term implies. No attempt has been made either to be comprehensive, or to discuss what is known of the aetiology or pathogenesis of the malformation described.

Classification of Anomalies

Disturbances in Development

A. **Arrest of Development**

1. Agenesis (agenesia) refers to the complete absence of an organ, whereas **aplasia** is used to indicate incomplete development or underdevelopment of an organ.

Abrachia is absence of the forelimbs.

Abrachiocephalia is absence of forelimbs and head.

Acrania is absence of cranium.

Adactylia is absence of digits.

Agnathia is absence of the lower jaw.

Amelia is absence of one or more legs.

Amyelia is absence of spinal cord.

Anencephaly is absence of brain.

Anophthalmos (anophthalmia) is absence of both eyes.

Exencephaly (exencephalia) indicates that brain is outside the cranial cavity.

Hemicrania is absence of half of the head.

Hypocephalia is incomplete development of the brain.

2. Fissures on the median line of the head, thorax, and abdomen. The suffix **'schisis'** at the end of words is Greek and means a **'cleft'**.

Cranioschisis is fissure of skull.

Cheiloschisis is cleft lip, often referred to as **'harelip'**.

Palatoschisis is **'cleft palate'**.

Rachischisis is cleft spine (spinal column), often referred to as 'spina bifida'.

Schistocelia (schistosomus) is fissure of the abdomen.

Schistocormus is fissure of the thorax, neck, or abdominal wall.

Schistorrhachis is cleft in lower vertebral column. It is also called 'spina bifida'.

Schistothorax is fissure in thorax or sternum.

3. Fusion of paired organs

Cyclopia is only one eye in the middle of the forehead.

Ren arcuatus is fusion of both kidneys forming a horseshoe mass, often referred to as **horseshoe kidney**.

B. Excess of Development

Increase in the number of a part:

Polydactylia is the state of having supernumerary digits.

Polymastia is the state of having more mammary glands.

Polymelia is the presence of more legs.

Polyodontia is the presence of supernumerary teeth.

Polyotia is the presence of more than two ears.

Polythelia is the presence of more teats on mammary gland.

C. Displacements during Development

(i) Displacements of organs

Dextrocardia is presence of heart on the right side of the body.

Ectopia cordis cervicalis is displacement of heart into the neck.

(ii) Displacements of tissues

Teratoma: A teratoma is a neoplasm that contains cells or tissues representative of more than one germ-cell layer and sometimes all three, namely, endoderm, mesoderm, and ectoderm. At least two of the tissues are foreign to the tissues where it is found. A teratoma may contain skin, hair, teeth, nervous tissue, skeletal muscle, cartilage, bone, and/or other material.

Dermoid (Dermoid cyst): A dermoid or dermoid cyst is a non-malignant cystic tumour, which contains elements derived from the ectoderm, such as hair, feathers, teeth, or skin, depending on the species. It usually occurs in the subcutaneous connective tissue at places where foetal clefts or fissures occurred, and in the testicles and ovaries.

Odontoid cyst is a mass of dental enamel and cement. The tissues are found in the mandible or maxilla, and are usually present where a tooth is missing.

Dentigerous cyst is a cyst containing one or more imperfectly formed teeth.

(iii) Persistence of foetal structures

These include the foramen ovale, ductus arteriosus, and urachus.

(iv) Fusion of sexual characters

Hermaphrodite is an animal having both testicular and ovarian tissue, either in the form of a combined gonad (ovotestis) or as separate organs. Hermaphroditism occurs most often in **pigs** and **goats**. **Pseudohermaphrodite** is an animal with gonads of only one sex, either testes or ovaries, but the external genitalia have features of the opposite sex. They are classified as male or female depending on the type of gonad present. Several types of pseudohermaphrodites have been described in humans and animals. **Freemartin** is a **female calf** having arrested development of the sex organs. This female calf is among the set of male or female twins. The condition results from fusion of placental vessels and the sharing of blood between twins during early embryonic development. This allows the male blood cells to invade and colonize the female. A freemartin is characterized by a lack of development of sex organs. The gonads are so underdeveloped that they can hardly be identified as ovaries. There is a rudimentary vagina and uterus, the vulva is small or absent, clitoris is enlarged, and the **udder** small. **The male twin is least affected.**

Monsters

A monster is a malformed foetus. Monstrosity is a disturbance of development that involves sexual organs and causes great distortion of the individual. Usually monsters possess a duplication of all or most of the organs and other parts of the body. **They develop from a single ovum.** They are therefore the product of incomplete twinning. The pair, joined together, has a single chorion and is of the same sex.

Classification of the Monsters

Twins Entirely Separate

Although separate, these twins are in a **single chorion**. One twin as a rule is well developed; the other is malformed (**acardius**, i.e., without heart). In the malformed foetus, there is arrested development of the heart, lungs, and trunk. Such monsters may lack head (**acephalus**), limbs, and other recognizable features (amorphous), or the trunk (**acormus**).

Twins United

These twins are more or less completely united and are of symmetrical development.

A. Anterior twinning: The anterior part of the individual is double, the posterior single.

(i) **Pygopagus** - United in the pelvic region with the bodies side by side.

(ii) **Ischiopagus** - United in the pelvic region with the bodies at an obtuse angle (i.e., exceeding 90 degrees, but less than 180 degrees).

(iii) **Dicephalus**: Two separate heads. Doubling may also affect the neck, thorax, and trunk.

(iv) **Diprosopus**: Doubling in the cephalic region without complete separation of heads. Only the face is doubled.

B. Posterior twinning: The posterior part is double, the anterior single. The position of human monsters in relation to each other may be dorsal (back to back), lateral (side by side), or ventral (abdomen to abdomen). The position of monsters of domestic animals is practically always ventral.

(i) **Craniopagus**: Brains are usually separated. Bodies as a rule are at an acute angle.

(ii) **Cephalothoracopagus**: Union of head and thorax.

(iii) **Dipygus**: Doubling of posterior extremities and posterior part of the body.

C. Twinning almost complete: Duplication of the whole trunk, or the anterior or posterior extremities with parallel, ventral arrangement of the foetuses. The pair is joined in the region of the thorax, and also often in abdominal region.

(i) **Thoracopagus**: United only by the thorax.

(ii) **Prosopothoracopagus**: Besides union of the thorax, the abdomen, the head, and neck are united.

(iii) **Rachipagus**: Thorax and lumbar portion of the spinal column are united.

All the double monsters mentioned usually have symmetrical development. However, they may also have asymmetrical growth, that is, one of the pair may be smaller and less well developed than the other. The less well developed is called the **parasite** and the more normally developed **autosite**. Often the parasite is partially embedded in the autosite.

545

Chapter 15

General Pathology of Infectious Diseases

The purpose of this chapter is to discuss the **mechanisms by which infectious organisms cause disease**. But, first, let us consider briefly the various categories of infectious agents.

Various Categories of Infectious Agents

Organisms that cause infectious diseases range in size from the 23 nm foot-and-mouth disease (FMD) virus to the 33 feet long tapeworm *Taenia saginata*.

Various categories of infectious agents and their size are presented in Table 24.

Table 24. Various categories of infectious agents and their size

Category	Size
Viruses	18 - 450 nm•
Mycoplasmas	300 - 800 nm
Chlamydiae	200 - 1500 nm
Rickettsiae	490 - 2700 nm
Bacteria, spirochaetes, mycobacteria	0.8 - 30 μm••
Fungi	5 - 300 μm
Protozoa	1 - 50 μm
Helminths	3 mm - 10 m

• One nanometre = One billionth of a metre

•• One micrometer = One millionth of a metre

Prions

'Prions' are the most recent addition to the class of infectious agents causing diseases in domestic animals and humans. Since prions are composed of only a **modified host protein**, they are not included in Table 24. **'Prion' is a proteinaceous infective particle**. Recent work has revealed that prion is a heavily glycosylated specific protein (a polypeptide) of 30 kilodaltons (30-kD), called **'prion protein (PrP)'**. As it is a proteinaceous particle closely associated with infectivity, the term **'prion'** was coined from **'prot**einaceous **in**fective particle'. The word **'proin'** thus formed from **'pro'** and **'in'** was changed to **'prion'** to sound rhythmic.

Although both **'prions'** and **'viruses'** replicate, their properties, structure, and modes of replication are fundamentally different. **Prions lack nucleic acid (RNA or DNA)**, and also do not produce any inflammatory or immune reaction in the host. **Thus, prions are the most unconventional agents**. Because they lack nucleic acids, prions are remarkably resistant to many agents that normally inactivate viruses, such as ultraviolet light, standard sterilizing procedures, and many common disinfectants. In fact, they can be classified as entirely separate category. **For his discovery of 'prions', Stanley Prusiner,** Professor of Biochemistry at the University of California, San Francisco, USA, **won the 1997 Nobel Prize in Physiology and Medicine.** The diseases caused by prions are called **'prion diseases'.** Both in domestic animals and humans, prions cause a group of diseases known as **'transmissible spongiform encephalopathies (TSEs)'.**

In animals, prions cause **bovine spongiform encephalopathy in cattle (mad cow disease), scrapie in sheep,** and **transmissible feline encephalopathy in cat;** and **in humans** prions cause **Creutzfeldt-Jakob disease (CJD,** associated with corneal transplants) and **kuru** (associated with human cannibalism). In England, more than 100, 000 cattle have died of prion-associated bovine spongiform encephalopathy, better known as **'mad cow disease',** and several cases of atypical CJD have occurred in humans.

Infectious prion proteins (PrPsc) are not viruses, because they lack RNA and DNA. PrPsc proteins are protease-resistant and combine with normal protease-sensitive host proteins (PrPc) that are present on the surface of neurons. **Infectious PrPsc proteins then induce a conformational change on the normal PrPc proteins and abnormal complexes are internalized (taken) into neurons. These complexes damage the cells and produce spongiform encephalopathy.**

Viruses

Viruses are obligate intracellular agents that depend on the host's metabolic machinery for their replication (multiplication). They are the most common causes of animal and poultry diseases. Viruses are classified by the type of nucleic acid they contain - **either DNA or RNA,** but not both, and also by the shape of their **protein coat,** or **capsid.**

Each **virion** (virus particle) has a central core of **DNA** or **RNA**, surrounded by a **protein coat** called **capsid**. The capsid is composed of a large number of units called **capsomeres**. The nucleic acid core and its capsid, together, are referred to as **nucleocapsid**. The nucleocapsid may be surrounded by a lipoprotein envelope (peplos), or may lack this envelope ('naked'). **Virions** range in size from the large poxvirus, measuring 300 nm by 250 nm by 100 nm to the parvoviruses, which are only 20 nm in diameter (Table 24). **Viruses multiply only in living cells**.

Because viruses are only 18 to 450 nm in size, the individual viruses are best seen with the electron microscope, where they may appear spherical or cylindrical. Some virus particles aggregate within the cells they infect and form characteristic **'inclusion bodies'**, which may be of diagnostic importance with the light microscope. For example, characteristic cytoplasmic inclusion body in rabies (Negri body) and in fowl pox (Bollinger body); or they may be present in the nucleus as in infectious laryngotracheitis and inclusion-body hepatitis in the chicken; and also in infectious bovine rhinotracheitis and feline panleukopaenia (feline distemper). In canine distemper, they are present in both cytoplasm and the nucleus.

Bacteria

Bacteria lack nuclei and endoplasmic reticulum. However, bacteria synthesize their own DNA, RNA, and proteins. **They reproduce by binary fission**. One cell divides into 2, 2 into 4, 4 into 8, 8 into 16, and so forth. Soon the numbers are so large that they produce disease. Most bacteria multiply outside the cells. They do not require host-cell machinery for multiplication, like viruses. On the basis of Gram's staining, bacteria are divided into **two groups: Gram-positive** and **Gram-negative**. Cell walls of bacteria are composed either of **two phospholipid bilayers** (inner and outer) with a **peptidoglycan layer sandwiched in between** as in **Gram-negative** bacteria, or of a **single bilayer** (only inner layer) covered by peptidoglycan in Gram-positive bacteria (Fig.79). Peptidoglycan is an organic compound composed of polysaccharide and peptide chains. **The cell wall of Gram-positive bacteria is composed largely of peptidoglycan**, whereas that of Gram-negative is a polysaccharide-lipid protein **(lipopolysaccharide) structure**. The cell wall polysaccharides of Gram-negative bacteria are toxic, and are called **endotoxins**.

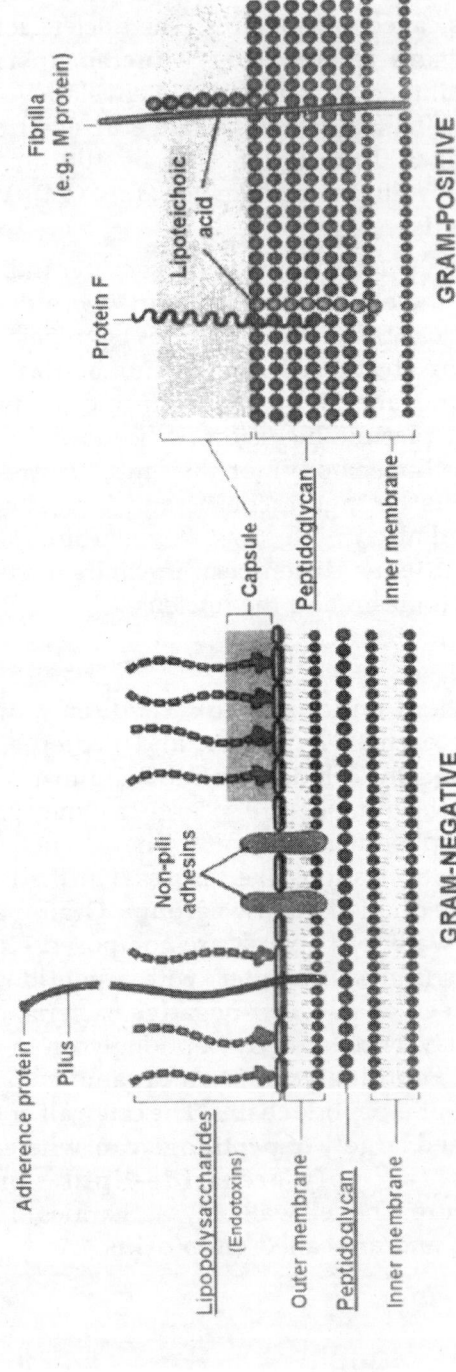

Fig. 79. The structure of bacterial cell walls. The cell wall of **Gram-negative bacteria** is composed of **two phospholipid bilayers** (inner and outer) with a **peptidoglycan layer** in between. Their cell wall is composed mainly of **lipopolysaccharides (endotoxins)**. The cell wall of **Gram-positive bacteria** is composed of only a **single phospholipid bilayer** (inner). Note that it is covered by **peptidoglycan. Lipopolysaccharides are not present.**

Fungi

Fungi (5-300 µm) are larger than bacteria and possess thick, **ergosterol**-containing cell walls.

Fungi can produce the whole range of bacterial pathology from acute pyogenic to chronic granulomatous inflammation, and they may not reveal their presence until identified by laboratory methods. However, their sturdy cell walls make fungi detectable microscopically in tissues, even in the midst of necrosis.

Pathogenic fungi elaborate mycotoxins and enzymes, but their role in disease is still not entirely clear. Some species have anti-phagocytic capsules; others have wall components resistant to phagolysosomal attack. Phagocytic competence of the host plays an important role in antifungal defence. Leukopaenic patients are as vulnerable to fungi as to bacteria. Corticosteroids and immunosuppressive drugs favour fungal infections. Fungal pathogens are of two types: those that remain **superficial** (restricted to the epidermal surface) and those that invade organs and tissues (**deep fungi**).

Mycoplasma

Mycoplasmas (300-800 nm) **are the smallest free-living organisms**. Like bacteria, they divide by binary fission, but do not have a rigid cell wall, instead are bounded by a plasma membrane. Mycoplasmas occur in various forms, and cause many important diseases in livestock and poultry. They spread from animal to animal in aerosols, bind to the surface of epithelial cells in the airways, and cause an atypical pneumonia characterized by peribronchiolar infiltration of lymphocytes and plasma cells.

Chlamydia

Chlamydiae (200-1500 nm) are obligate intracellular organisms. Like bacteria and rickettsiae (discussed next), they divide by binary fission, and multiply in phagosomes (phagocytic vacuoles) of epithelial cells. They are **Gram-negative** and possess DNA and RNA, and form their own cell walls, much like bacteria. By an unknown mechanism, chlamydiae inhibit the fusion of lysosomes with primary phagosomes, **and are thus protected from attack by proteases and oxygen-derived free radicals.** Both humoral and cellular immunity are induced, but neither seems to cope effectively with established chronic infections.

Rickettsia

Rickettsiae (490-2700 nm) are also **obligate intracellular organisms**, similar to chlamydiae. Like bacteria and chlamydiae, they divide by binary fission. They are small and **Gram-negative**, and normally inhabit ticks, mites, fleas or lice, where they seldom cause any damage, and are passed from generation to generation by transovarian infection. **Both in humans and animals, rickettsiae multiply mainly in the endothelial cells of small vessels**. By injuring the endothelial cells, rickettsiae cause a haemorrhagic vasculitis that is usually seen as a skin rash. However, they may also cause a transient pneumonia or hepatitis, or injure the central nervous system and cause death.

Rickettsial infections are usually acquired by exposure to arthropod vectors. Once inside the host, they adhere to the cell membrane, enter the cell by endocytosis, and begin dividing by binary fission. Rickettsiae generate no distant-acting toxins and their Gram-negative endotoxins are relatively feeble. T-lymphocytes dependent immune responses are important in the pathogenesis of rickettsial diseases. As in the case of viral infections, antigen-specific cytotoxic T-cells destroy rickettsia infected cells.

Protozoal Parasites

Parasitic protozoans (1-50 μm) are motile, single-celled eukaryotes (organisms with a distinct nucleus). **They are much more complex than viruses or bacteria** with a rich diversity of their life cycles and pathogenetic mechanisms. Their life cycles revolve between a specific mammalian host and a specific vector.

Following their entry into the host, protozoa localize to a site appropriate for their reproduction, which can be: (1) **luminal**, that is, in the cells lining lumen of a vessel, (2) **haemic**, that is, in the bloodstream, or (3) **intracellular**. However, our knowledge of their virulence factors remains incomplete. Haemic and intracellular parasites kill cells only after entering them, either actively or passively. Once taken up, they usually damage cells after multiplying sufficiently to interfere with cell metabolism, or destroy vital organelles. In addition to such **direct effect**, parasitic invasion can trigger the same non-specific inflammatory host mediators that potentiate bacterial tissue damage.

Host immune responses have the same importance in protozoal, as in bacterial pathogens. Host immunity also serves an important protective function. Usually, individuals with the heaviest parasitic loads or with defective immune or phagocytic functions, suffer from the disease clinically. In addition, protozoan parasites have developed many mechanisms of different kinds that permit them to escape the immune system of the host.

Helminths

Parasitic helminths, or **worms**, are highly differentiated **multi-cellular organisms**. Their life cycles are complex. The life cycle alternates between **definitive host**, in which **sexual reproduction** takes place, and **intermediate host** or **vector**, in which **asexual reproduction** occurs. Once adult worms come to live within the host, they do not multiply, but they produce eggs or larvae for the next phase of the cycle. Lack of multiplication by the adult worms leads to two important effects: (1) Disease is usually caused by inflammatory responses against the eggs, rather than the adult worms (e.g., schistosomiasis), and (2) the severity of the disease is proportional to the number of organisms that infected the host. For example, 10 hookworms have little effect, whereas 1000 hookworms cause severe anaemia by consuming 100 ml of blood per day.

Parasitic worms are of **three classes**: **(1) Roundworms** (Nematodes), **(2) Tapeworms** or flatworms (Cestodes), and **(3) Flukes** (Trematodes). **Intestinal helminths (adult worms) can cause disease by**: (1) competing for essential host nutrients (e.g., vitamin B12 depletion by *Diphyllobothrium latum*, (2) mechanically obstructing or perforating the gastrointestinal tract (*Ascaris lubricoides*), (3) blood-sucking (hookworms, **Ancylostoma**); (4) inducing inflammatory changes in the gut (*Strongyloides stercoralis*), or (5) inducing host hypersensitivity reactions (many helminths). **Hypersensitivity reactions** are often caused by the migratory larval stages of those helminths that must invade tissues and undergo several moults in order to reach maturity in the gut.

Eosinophils are characteristically found in inflammatory sites around parasitic infections. Eosinophil-specific granules contain **major basic protein (MBP),** a highly charged cationic protein that is **toxic to parasites.**

Ectoparasites

Ectoparasites are insects (lice, fleas) or arachnids (mites, ticks) that attach and live on or in the skin. These insects may cause itching and excoriations (abrasions of the epidermis), e.g., pediculosis caused by lice attached to hair shafts, or scabies caused by mites burrowing into the stratum corneum. At the site of the bite, mouthparts may be found in association with a mixed infiltration of lymphocytes, macrophages, and eosinophils.

How Infectious Agents Cause Disease

After reviewing the various categories of infectious agents, let us now examine the manner by which they injure cells and cause tissue damage. There are three general mechanisms:

1. Infectious agents may enter host cells and **directly cause cell death.**

2. Pathogens can release **endotoxins** or **exotoxins** that kill cells at a distance, **release enzymes** that destroy tissue components, or damage blood vessels and cause ischaemic injury.

3. Pathogens can **induce host cell responses** that may cause additional tissue damage, usually **by immune-mediated mechanisms.**

Mechanisms of Virus-Induced Injury

Viruses cause damage by entering into the cell and **replicating (multiplying) at the host's expense.** Viral replication cycle begins with **viral attachment** to the host cell. Viruses have specific surface viral proteins (**ligands**) that bind to particular host proteins (**receptors**), many of which have known functions. For example, neurons have the acetylcholine receptors for rabies virus. The **presence or absence of receptors** that allow the virus to attach is one reason for **viral tropism**, the tendency of certain viruses to infect specific cells but not others. For example, influenza viruses replicate in respiratory epithelial cells, which express a **protease** necessary for cleaving and activating the haemagglutinin present on the surface of the virus. A second major cause of viral tropism is the ability of the virus to replicate inside some cells, **but not in others**. For example, a member of the papovavirus group (JC virus), which causes a disease called leukoencephalopathy in humans, is restricted to oligodendroglia in the central nervous system. This is because JC virus promoter and enhancer DNA sequences, up-stream from the viral genes, are active in glial cells but not in neurons or endothelial cells.

Once attached, the entire virion, or a portion containing the genome (DNA or RNA) and essential polymerases, **penetrates the**

cell membrane by: **(1)** translocation (transfer) of the entire virus across the cell membrane, **(2)** fusion of the viral envelope with the cell membrane, or **(3)** receptor-mediated endocytosis and fusion with endosomal membranes. **After penetration**, the **virus uncoats**, that is, it separates its genome from its structural components and loses its infectivity. **Viruses then replicate** (multiply) using enzymes that are separate for each virus family. For example, **RNA polymerase** is used by negative-sense (negative-strand) RNA viruses to generate positive-sense (positive-strand) messenger RNA (mRNA), while **reverse transcriptase** is used by retroviruses to generate DNA from their RNA template. These **virus-specific enzymes** provide points at which drugs may be used to inhibit viral replication. **Viruses also use host enzymes for viral synthesis**. However, such enzymes may be present in some but not all tissues. Viral DNA synthesis occurs in the nucleus, whereas RNA and protein synthesis take place in the cytoplasm. Newly synthesized viral genomes (DNA or RNA) and capsid proteins are then assembled into **progeny virions** in the nucleus or cytoplasm, and are either released directly (**unencapsulated viruses**) or bud through the plasma (cell) membrane (**encapsulated viruses**).

Viruses kill host cells and cause tissue damage in a number of ways:

1. Viruses may inhibit host cell DNA, RNA, or protein synthesis.

2. Viral proteins may enter into the host cell's plasma membrane and directly damage its integrity, or promote cell fusion (herpesvirus).

3. Viruses replicate efficiently and lyse host cells. For example, respiratory epithelial cells are killed by explosive influenza virus multiplication and neurons by rabies virus.

4. Viral proteins on the surface of the host cells may be recognized by the immune system, and the host lymphocytes may attack the virus-infected cells (e.g., liver cells infected with hepatitis B virus in humans).

5. Viruses may also damage cells involved in antimicrobial defence, leading to secondary infections. For example, viral damage to respiratory epithelium predisposes to the subsequent development of pneumonia.

6. Viral killing of cells of one type may cause damage to other cells that are dependent on their integrity. For example, denervation caused by the attack of poliovirus on motor neurons in humans produces atrophy and sometimes death of skeletal muscle cells.

7. Slow viral infections result in severe, progressive disease after a long latency period. The precise mechanism of injury under these conditions remains unknown.

8. In addition to killing cells, **viruses can cause cell proliferation and transformation, resulting in cancer** (Chapter 8).

Mechanisms of Bacteria-Induced Injury

Bacterial damage to host tissues depends on the ability of bacteria to adhere and enter into the host cells, or to deliver toxins. The coordination of bacterial adherence and toxin delivery is extremely important to bacterial virulence. It is so important that the genes encoding adherence proteins and toxins are usually co-regulated by specific environmental signals. For example, the virulence of enterotoxic *Escherichia coli* depends on the expression of adherence proteins that allow the bacteria to bind to the interstitial epithelial cells and coordinate synthesis and release of heat-labile or heat-stable toxins that cause interstitial cells to secrete isotonic fluids.

Bacterial Adhesins

Bacterial adhesins are molecules that bind bacteria to host cells. They are limited in type, but have a broad range of host cell specificity. The surface of **Gram-positive cocci**, such as streptococci, is covered with **two molecules** that **mediate adherence of bacteria to host cells** (Fig. 79). **(1) lipoteichoic acids**. These molecules bind streptococci to the surface of **all** cells, and **(2) protein F** (Fig. 79), an adhesin that binds to **fibronectin**, an extracellular matrix protein, also **found on most host cells. M proteins,** which form fibrillae (singular 'fibrilla' and means 'a small fibre') on the surface of Gram-positive bacteria and their carbohydrate capsules, **prevent phagocytosis by host macrophages.**

Fimbriae or **pili** are filamentous (thread-like) structures on the surface of **Gram-negative** bacteria, **which mediate adherence of bacteria to host cells** (Fig. 79). At the tips of the pili (singular 'pilus') are **'adherence proteins'** that determine to which host cells the bacteria will attach (**bacterial tropism**). For example, in *Escherichia coli*, adherence proteins are antigenically separate and are associated with particular infections. Thus, type 1 proteins bind mannose and cause lower urinary tract infections, type P proteins bind galactose and cause pyelonephritis, and type S proteins bind sialic acid and cause meningitis. A single bacterium can express more than one type of pilus, as well as adhesins not located in pili (non-pili adhesins). Other molecules on the surface of Gram-negative bacteria important for virulence are **lipopolysaccharides** and **a carbohydrate capsule** (discussed later).

Unlike viruses, which infect a broad range of host cells, **intracellular bacteria are more restricted** and infect epithelial cells (entero-invasive *E. coli*), macrophages (*Mycobacterium tuberculosis*), or both (*Salmonella typhi* in humans). A **'type III secretory machine'** present in bacteria transports the bacterial proteins involved in attachment and invasion across the bacterial envelope and injects them into the cytoplasm of the target cells. Most of the bacteria attach to host cell integrins, plasma membrane proteins that bind complement, or extracellular matrix proteins, including fibronectin, laminin, and collagen (Chapter 5). For example, *M. tuberculosis* bind to CR3, the cell receptor for complement C3bi. Enteropathogenic *E. coli* secretes a protein that inserts into the target plasma membrane and is used as an additional attachment site by the bacterium. Once in the cytoplasm, *E. coli* inhibit host protein synthesis, rapidly replicate, and within 6 hours lyse (destroy) the host cells. In contrast, **Salmonella** and **Yersinia** organisms replicate within the phagolysosomes of the macrophage, while **Mycobacteria** organisms inhibit the acidification that normally occurs after endosome's (phagosome's) fusion with the lysosome. **In the absence of a host cellular immune response, many replicating organisms persist within the macrophages** (*M. avium-intracellulare* infection in AIDS patients), **but activated macrophages can kill these organisms or limit their growth.**

Bacterial Endotoxins

Bacterial endotoxin is a lipopolysaccharide (LPS). It is a structural component of the outer cell wall of Gram-negative bacteria (Fig. 79). Lipopolysaccharide is composed of a long-chain toxic fatty acid (**lipid A**) connected to a **core sugar chain**. Both of these are the same in all Gram-negative bacteria. Attached to the core sugar is a carbohydrate chain (**O antigen**), which is used to serotype and differentiate various bacteria. Endotoxins have many systemic effects, including induction of fever (Chapter 4), septic shock (Chapter 6), disseminated intravascular coagulation, and a variety of effects on cells of the immune system. **All the biological activities of endotoxin**

come from lipid A and the core sugars. They are mediated both by **direct effects of endotoxins** and by the induction of **host cytokines such as interleukin-1, tumour necrosis factor, and others.**

Bacterial Superantigens

Bacterial superantigens (e.g., **Staphylococcus** enterotoxins) cause fever, shock, and multi-system organ failure by a **mechanism different from that of endotoxin.** Superantigens are powerful microbial proteins that have the ability to stimulate an extremely large number of CD4+ T-cells by interacting with T-cell receptors (TCR). Bacterial superantigens bind to the major histocompatibility complex (MHC) class II molecules on the surface of many antigen-presenting cells (APCs), **without the usual internal processing.** These superantigen-containing APCs then stimulate numerous T-cells to secrete excess **interleukin-2** (IL-2), which in turn causes overproduction of **tumour necrosis factor** (TNF) and other cytokines **responsible for the systemic disturbances.**

Bacterial Exotoxins

Bacterial exotoxins are proteins secreted by bacteria that directly cause cell injury. Example: **lethal factor,** that is, exotoxin of *Bacillus anthracis* (cause of anthrax). Because *B. anthracis* forms spores, which are heat resistant and infect by aerosols, this bacterium has great potential as a biological weapon. *Clostridium perfringens,* cause of gas gangrene, digests host tissues, including the relatively resistant collagens. Its **alpha-toxin** is a **lecithinase** that disrupts plasma membranes, including those of red and white blood cells. *Clostridium tetani,* a wound contaminant, secretes an exotoxin called **tetanospasmin.** This toxin interferes with the release of inhibitory transmitter substances from pre-synaptic terminals of the spinal neurons. This results in violent muscle contractions that characterize tetanic spasm. *Clostridium botulinum* toxins block the release of cholinergic neurotransmitters, particularly at the neuromuscular junctions, resulting in progressive paralysis of the limbs, respiratory muscle, and cranial motor neurons

Mechanisms of Prion-Induced Injury

As already stated, prions cause **spongiform encephalopathies in both animals and humans.** They are called 'spongiform encephalopathies' because of the presence of microscopic vacuolation (**spongiosis**) that develops within the cell bodies of neurons and in the surrounding neuropil in most cases. For his discovery of prions, Dr. Stanley Prusiner received the 1997 Nobel Prize for Medicine. From the study of prions and the diseases caused by them, the following **four fundamental concepts** have emerged.

1. Prions are the only known class of infectious agents that **lack nucleic acids - RNA or DNA.**

2. Prion diseases may manifest as infectious, sporadic, or genetic disorders.

3. **Prion diseases result from accumulation of an abnormally folded form of the normal prion protein.**

4. Pathogenic prions can have a variety of conformations, each of which is associated with a specific disease.

Infectious prions are the modified form of a normal structural protein found in the mammalian nervous system. The **normal prion protein** is designated by the abbreviation **PrPc.** It is a 30 kD (kilodalton), membrane-associated protein encoded by a gene on chromosome 20. However, function of normal prion protein remains unknown.

Prion-associated diseases develop when **PrPc** undergoes a conformational (structural) change to form a structurally abnormal protein known as **PrPsc.** The **'sc'** designation is derived from the sheep disease 'scrapie'. Once present, PrPsc is capable of inducing other **normal PrPc molecules** to undergo conformational change to the **PrPsc form, resulting in the generation of extremely large numbers of abnormal molecules.** The polypeptide chains of PrPc and PrPsc are exactly similar to their chemical composition, **but differ in their three-dimensional conformations.** PrPc is rich in alpha helices, whereas the **PrPsc has much fewer alpha helices and many more beta sheets** (for 'beta sheets' see 'amyloidosis'). **This structural change is the fundamental event in the pathogenesis of prion disease.** In cases of **sporadic** bovine spongiform encephalopathy (BSE, mad cow disease), the most common and important form of animal spongiform encephalopathy, the initial conformational **change in PrPc to form PrPsc occurs slowly and spontaneously.** This conversion is greatly accelerated if there is a **mutation** in the prion gene. Inoculation of PrPsc from an infected animal into a normal animal of the same species also initiates a similar sequence of conformational changes in the recipient. **This explains the fact that spongiform encephalopathies are transmissible.**

Evasion of the Immune Response by Microbes

Humoral and cellular immune responses protect the host from infections (Chapter 9). Here, we focus on the ways in which microorganisms escape the host immune system by: (1) remaining inaccessible (unreachable), (2) cleaving antibody, resisting complement-mediated lysis, or surviving in phagocytic cells, (3) varying or shedding antigens, and (4) causing specific or non-specific immunosuppression.

Bacteria that thrive and multiply in the lumen of the intestine, for example, toxin-producing *Clostridium difficile* are inaccessible to the host immune defences, including secretory IgA. Viruses shed from the luminal surface of epithelial cells, for example, cytomegalovirus in urine or milk, or those that infect the keratinized epithelium (poxviruses that cause molluscum contagiosum) are also inaccessible to the host humoral immune system. Some organisms establish infections by rapidly involving host cells before the host humoral response becomes effective, for example, malaria sporozoites entering liver cells (in humans) and **Trichinella** and *Trypanosoma cruzi* entering skeletal and cardiac muscles, respectively. Some larger parasites, for example, the larvae of tapeworms, form cysts in host tissues that are covered by a dense fibrous capsule that walls them off from host immune responses.

The **carbohydrate capsule** on the surface of all the major pathogens that cause pneumonia or meningitis (**Haemophilus**, *E. coli*, **Klebsiella**, *Streptococcus pneumoniae*) makes them more virulent by covering bacterial antigens and preventing phagocytosis of the organisms by neutrophils. **Pseudomonas** bacteria secrete a **leukotoxin** that kills neutrophils. Some *E. coli* have antigens that prevent activation of complement by the alternative pathway and lysis of the cells. In contrast, some Gram-negative bacteria have very long polysaccharide O antigens that bind host antibody and activate complement at such a distance from the bacterial cells that the organisms fail to lyse. Staphylococci are covered by protein-A molecules that bind to the Fc portion of the antibody and so inhibit phagocytosis. **Haemophilus** and **Streptococcus** spp. secrete proteases that degrade antibodies.

Viral infection induces **neutralizing antibodies**, which prevent viral attachment, penetration, or uncoating. This highly specific immunity is the basis of antiviral vaccination, but it cannot protect against viruses with many antigenic variants, for example, influenza viruses. Pneumococci (infect humans) are capable of more than 80 permutations (variations) of their capsular polysaccharides, so that in repeated infections the host is unlikely to recognize the new serotype. Successive clones of African trypanosomes also change their major surface antigens to escape host antibody responses.

Inflammatory Response to Infectious Agents

This section discusses the most common microscopic patterns of host responses caused by infectious agents. Despite the vast molecular diversity of infectious agents, **the patterns of inflammatory response to these agents are limited**, even if the inflammatory mediators are different. At the microscopic level therefore many pathogens produce similar reaction patterns, and few of the features are unique or pathognomonic of each agent. Broadly speaking, there are five **histological patterns of tissue reaction.**

1. Suppurative (purulent) inflammation: The neutrophils are attracted to the site of infection by release of chemoattractants from the **rapidly dividing 'pyogenic' bacteria that produce this response. These bacteria are mostly extracellular Gram-positive cocci and Gram-negative rods**. The bacterial chemoattractants include secreted bacterial peptides. All of these contain **N-formyl methionine residues** at their amino terminals that are **recognized by specific receptors on neutrophils**. Also, bacteria attract neutrophils indirectly by releasing **endotoxin**. Endotoxin, in turn, stimulates macrophages to secrete interleukin-1 (IL-1) or tumour necrosis factor (TNF), or by cleaving complement into the peptide C5a. C5a is highly chemotactic for neutrophils. Accumulation and lysis of neutrophils result in the formation of pus.

2. Mononuclear inflammation: Diffuse, mainly mononuclear interstitial infiltrations (lymphocytes, plasma cells, macrophages) are common in all chronic inflammatory processes. However, when they occur in acute inflammation, they are **usually a response to viruses, intracellular bacteria, or intracellular parasites**. Moreover, helminths and spirochaetes cause chronic inflammation. Which mononuclear cell predominates depends on the host immune response to the organism. For example, in some cases plasma cells predominate, in others lymphocytes. **Lymphocytes represent cell-mediated immunity** against the pathogen, or the pathogen-infected cells. At the other extremes, macrophages predominate.

Granulomatous inflammation (Chapter 4) is a distinctive form of mononuclear inflammation. It is usually produced by relatively slowly dividing infectious agents (e.g., *Mycobacterium tuberculosis*, fungi), and by agents of relatively large size (e.g., schistosome eggs). **Granulomatous inflammation almost always reflects a cell-mediated immune reaction** (Chapter 9).

3. Necrotizing inflammation: *Clostridium perfringens* and other organisms that secrete very strong toxins cause such rapid and severe tissue damage **that cell death is the main feature**. Because so few inflammatory cells are involved, these lesions resemble infarcts, with disruption or loss of basophilic nuclear staining and preservation of cellular outlines. At times, viruses also cause necrotizing inflammation when cell damage is widespread and severe.

4. Cytopathic-cytoproliferative inflammation: These reactions are usually produced by **viruses**, and are characterized by damage to individual cells, **with little or no inflammatory response**. Some viruses while replicating within cells make viral aggregates that are seen as **inclusion bodies** (e.g., Negri bodies in rabies) or induce cells to fuse and form polykaryons (multinucleate cells, e.g., with herpesvirus). Focal cell damage may cause epithelial cells to form blisters (e.g., chickenpox virus in humans). Viruses can also cause epithelial cells to proliferate and take unusual forms (e.g., warts in animals induced by papillomaviruses). Finally, viruses can cause dysplastic changes and cancers in epithelial cells and lymphocytes (see 'dysplasia').

5. Chronic inflammation: The final common pathway of many infections is chronic inflammation, which may lead either to complete healing or to extensive scarring (fibrosis).

Index

Bold numbers indicate main discussion

A

Abrachia, 542
Abrachiocephalia, 542
Abrasion, 501
Abscess, 156
    sterile, 157
Acanthosis nigricans, 50
Acquired immunodeficiency
syndrome (AIDS), 464
Acrania, 542
Activation-induced cell death, 441
Acute,
    cellular swelling, 28
    chronic inflammation, 167
    phase proteins, 172
    radiation syndrome, 511
    serum sickness, 426
Adactylia, 542
Adaptation(s), **19**, 20
    cellular, 19
    definition, 19
    pathological, 267
    physiological, 267
Addition products, 294
Adenocarcinoma, 279, 373, 378, **380**, 383
    of cow uterus, 381
Adenoma, 279, **379**
    adenomatous polyps, 380
    follicular, 387
    hepatocellular, 391
    intrahepatic bile-duct, 392
    liver cell, 391
    of adrenal cortex, 386
    of sebaceous glands of dogs, 385
    papillary, 380
    polypoid, 380
Adenosine diphosphate (ADP), 230, **233**, **237**, 238
Adenoviruses, 314
Adherence proteins, 556
Adhesion(s), 130
    defects in, 146

molecular mechanisms of, 130
molecules, 130
    on cancer cells, **338**, 340
    of leukocytes, 112, **146**
    of platelets, 231, **232**
Adhesive glycoproteins and
integrins, 212
    fibronectin, 212
    integrins, 213, **214**
    laminin, 213
Adiposity, 47
Adrenal medullary tumours, 386
Adreno-cortical adenoma, 386
Adreno-cortical carcinoma, 386
Aetiology, 2, **4**
Agammaglobulinaemias, 458
Age, as intrinsic cause, 5
Agenesia, 542
Agenesis, 542
Agnathia, 542
Albinism, 50
Alkali disease, 494
Allergens, 417
Allergy, eosinophilia, 149
Alpha-foetoprotein, 350
Amelia, 542
Amyelia, 542
Amyloid, 97
    amyloid associated (AA), 98
    amyloid light chain (AL), 98
    beta-pleated sheet structure, 98
    chemical nature, 98
    physical nature, 97
    staining, 103
Amyloidogenic potential, 100
Amyloidosis, 96
    aetiology, 99
    classification, 99
    harmful effects, 102
    in humans, 100
    macroscopic appearance, 102
    microscopic appearance, 103
    occurrence, 99

563